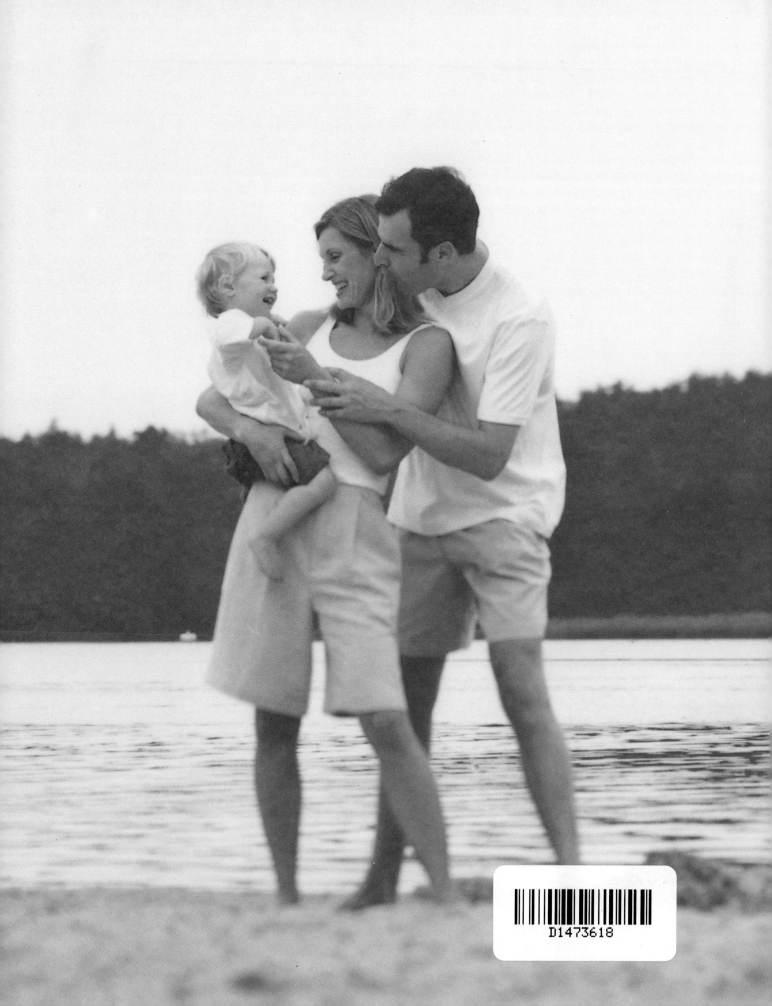

D1473618

THE HAMLYN ENCYCLOPEDIA OF
FAMILY
HEALTH

DR MICHAEL APPLE B.A., M.B., Ch.B., M.R.C.G.P.

HAMLYN

Publishing Director: Laura Bamford
Executive Editor: Jane McIntosh
Editor: Catharine Davey
Project Manager: Jo Lethaby
Contributing Editor: Rowena Gaunt
Copy Editors: Arlene Sobel
           Diana Vowles
Proofreader: Anne Crane
Directory: Jill Cropper
Index: Michele Clarke
Creative Director: Keith Martin
Design Manager: Bryan Dunn
Designer: Les Needham
Illustrators: Philip Wilson
           Debbie Maizels
           Jackie Harland
           Roddy Murray
           Steve Rawlings
           Birgit Eggers
Picture Researcher: Liz Fowler
Production: Karina Han

First published in Great Britain in 1999 by Hamlyn
an imprint of Octopus Publishing Group Limited
2–4 Heron Quays London E14 4JP

Copyright © 1999 Octopus Publishing Group Limited

ISBN 0 600 59254 5

All rights reserved. No part of this publication may be
reproduced, stored in a retrieval system, or transmitted
in any form or by any means, electronic, mechanical,
photocopying, recording or otherwise, without the
permission of the copyright holders.

A CIP catalogue record of this book is available from
the British Library

Printed in China

Note

This book is not intended as an alternative to personal
medical advice. The reader should consult a physician in all
matters relating to health and particularly in respect of any
symptoms which may require diagnosis or medical attention.
While the advice and information are believed to be accurate
and true at the time of going to press, neither the authors nor
the publisher can accept any legal responsibility or liability for
any errors or omissions that may be made.

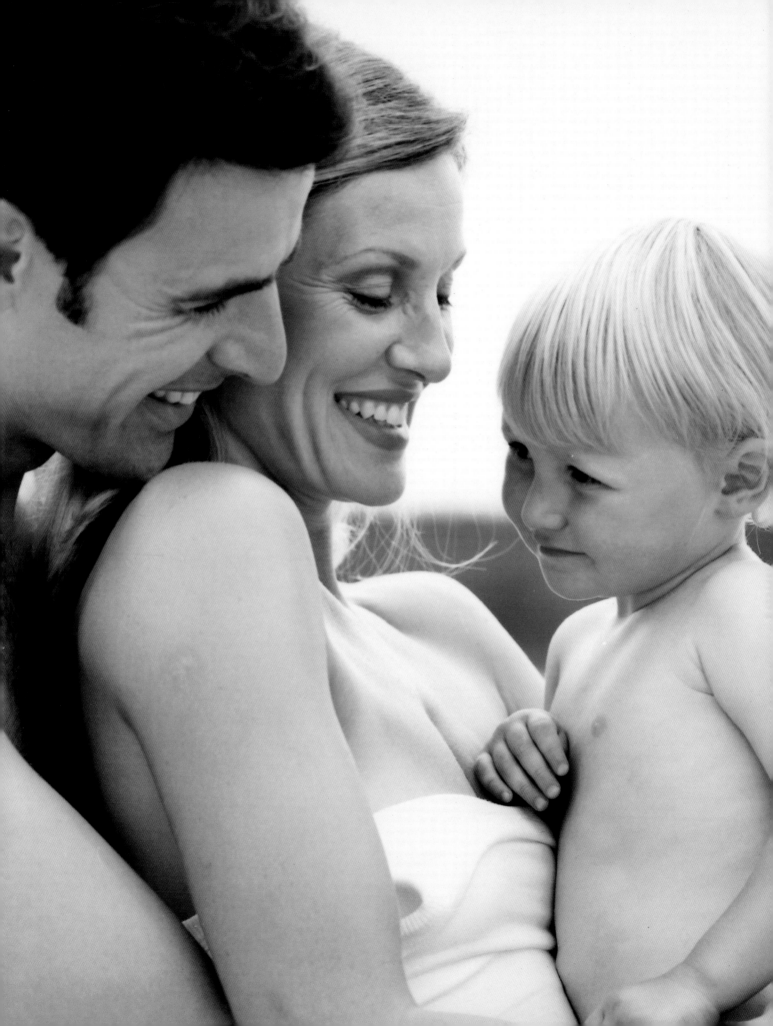

CONTENTS

INTRODUCTION

MODERN MEDICINE is developing at an amazing rate, with new ideas, techniques and treatments appearing almost daily. It is hard enough for the professionals to keep up to date, let alone the lay public. What is more, today's breakthrough may easily be tomorrow's discredited theory.

However, now more than ever people want to become informed about and involved in the management of their health. They want to know the latest information about their illnesses, the options for treatment and the side effects of medication. They want to know how to lead a healthy life, what they should do about screening and what the long-term implications are of any illnesses they do develop.

Most health professionals welcome this trend. A person who is well informed about their illness handles the anxiety of illness more successfully and is better placed to share in decisions on treatment.

This is because the practice of medicine is not an exact science. The early symptoms of illness are usually quite non-specific and do not always allow for an immediate diagnosis. Diagnoses may be in doubt or remain provisional for some time. Even once an illness is diagnosed, its course may vary greatly from one individual to another. Treatments do not always work and may have unexpected side effects. And the extent of a person's recovery may vary enormously, and their attitude to illness will affect how they recover. These are just some of the reasons why most health professionals favour an increased knowledge of illness among their patients as a way of sharing all of these uncertainties.

In this book you will find accounts as up-to-date as possible of a wide range of illnesses, investigations and treatments. There is a great emphasis on preventive care and in adjusting lifestyles to preserve health from birth to advanced old age. There are sections on first aid and safety consciousness at home and at work. Scattered throughout the book are special features on major life events such as birth, and important health hazards such as pollution. Everywhere you will find illustrations and photographs which will illuminate the text.

The book is written from the viewpoint of conventional Western medicine, but complementary therapies are welcomed in its pages. There is advice about complementary remedies throughout, especially about when they may or may not be appropriate.

While this book is intended to be detailed and informative, it is not a substitute for professional medical care. If in doubt always consult a doctor, although we hope that thanks to this book you will become well informed about family illness and take positive steps towards a healthier lifestyle.

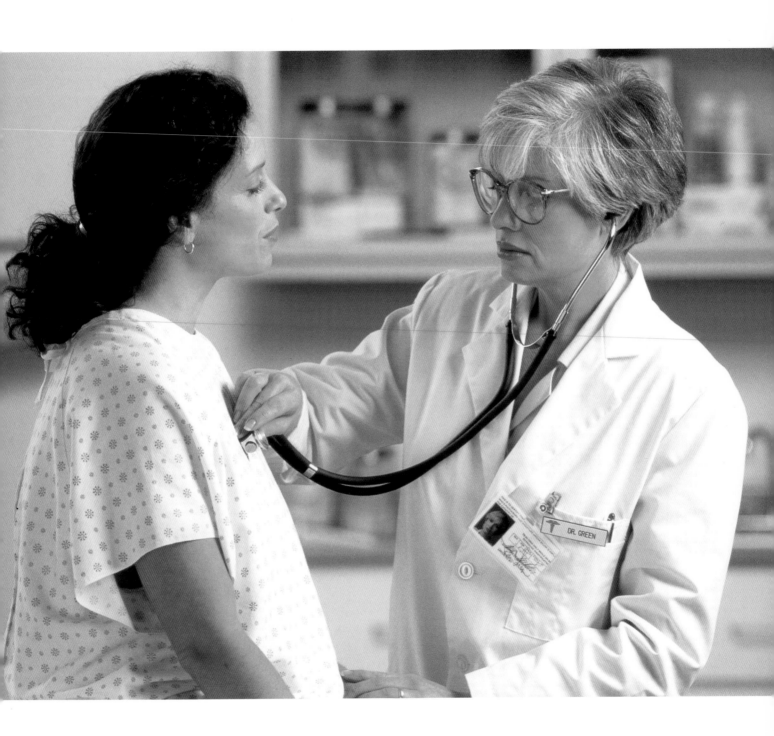

HOW TO USE THIS BOOK

THE BOOK IS DIVIDED into a number of sections. Several deal with the prevention of ill-health in one form or another. There is a major section dealing with many common illnesses, including special features on important topics relating to health (identified in the Contents page and elsewhere by the ☞ symbol), and information about suitable complementary therapies. Other sections cover the process of diagnosis, types of treatment, caring for the sick and first aid. You will also find information about most of the health hazards that a family may face and guidance about what to do or what health professionals may do when illness occurs.

PREVENTION

This section reviews healthy living at all ages, from infancy to advanced old age. It covers important health measures such as immunization, screening procedures appropriate to different ages and gender, and physical safety, such as accident prevention. This is where to find information about having cervical smear tests, blood pressure checks and prostate checks among many other topics.

SYMPTOMS

Look up in the main index the particular illnesses you are interested in. Use the symptoms index for when you are not-sure what a symptom means or you wish to know the possible causes.

AILMENTS

Here you will find information about some two hundred illnesses and common health problems. The ailments are organized within systems of the body, for example the circulatory system, and infectious illnesses. This is how doctors categorize disease. If you cannot find an illness under the system you expect, check in the index of symptoms or in the main index at the back of the book.

Each system begins with an introduction, which explains how that system works and therefore gives an insight into how illnesses begin and are investigated. There is also a special section about childhood ailments.

Each ailment is organized as follows:

A definition of the ailment:

Causes: Examines the typical causes of an illness.

Symptoms: The type experienced and the signs discovered on examination plus tests used in diagnosis.

Treatment: Both conventional and complementary methods are given. Complementary treatments can be easily identified by their coloured icon (see table opposite).

Questions: These commonly asked questions about an ailment will appear when further information is required.

Within some ailments, there will also be cross-references in bold face to other ailments covered elsewhere in the book. At certain points in this section there are also feature articles reviewing an area of medical interest that cuts across conventional classifications, for example blood donation and food hygiene. These features include health information, prevention and treatment.

DIAGNOSTIC

Arriving at a diagnosis is a fundamental aim of medicine, with a wide array of techniques available. Within this section you will find explanations of commonly used tests, including some of the latest available such as MRI scans. Here, too, is a description of how doctors examine patients for signs of illness and how they take a comprehensive medical history.

TYPES OF TREATMENT

Treatment is covered at many points in the book, relevant to specific illnesses. In this section are explanations of general techniques such as chemotherapy and drug treatment, plus information about how they work and side effects.

CARING FOR THE SICK

In this section you will find detailed advice about coping with sick children and the elderly and also what to expect when going into hospital.

FIRST AID

This section covers the emergency treatment of many health problems at home and at work. There is practical advice on treatment and tips on prevent-

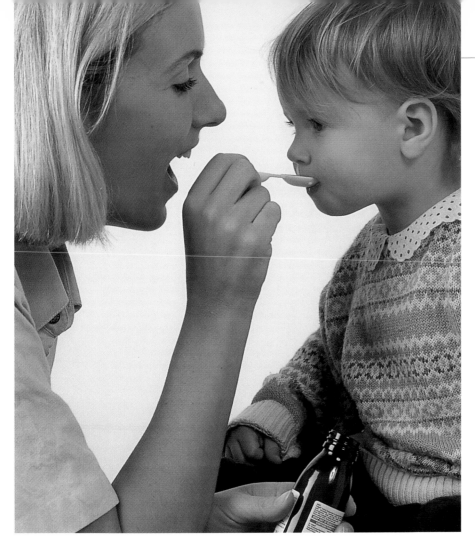

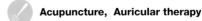 Acupuncture, Auricular therapy

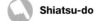 Shiatsu-do

Chinese herbalism

Ayurveda

Chakra balancing

Osteopathy, Cranial osteopathy

Chiropractic

Massage

Reflexology

Aromatherapy

Homeopathy

Nutritional therapy

Western herbalism

Naturopathy

Bach flower remedies

Alexander technique

Hypnotherapy

Yoga

Tai chi/chi kung

Autogenic training

Healing

Cymatics

Biodynamics, Hellerwork, Rolfing

Arts therapies

Play therapy

ing accidents. Included are instructions on how to perform resuscitation and mouth-to-mouth respiration and how to deal with choking. However these are techniques which need to be properly learned at a first aid class.

DRUG GLOSSARY

This covers the most common generic drugs and drugs groups, giving details of how they are used in treating specific ailments and conditions.

COMPLEMENTARY MEDICINE GLOSSARY

Here you will find an authoritative review of the therapies available together with explanations of how they are thought to work and where their use is most appropriate. This is in addition to the many references to complementary therapies elsewhere in the book.

DIRECTORY OF ORGANIZATIONS

This section provides a list of useful organizations. International counterparts are also given where possible.

NOTE

This book is not intended as an alternative to personal, professional medical advice. The reader should always consult a physician in all matters relating to health and particularly in respect of any symptoms which may require diagnosis or medical attention. While the advice and information are believed to be accurate and true at the time of going to press, neither the authors nor the publisher can accept any legal responsibility or liability for any errors or omissions that may be made.

PREVENTION

THE PREVENTION OF ILL HEALTH can be a worthy but boring topic, with its constant repetition of things that we think we already know. The important measures are those that have been known for years. It is rare that breakthroughs in prevention hit the headlines.

Risk

Prevention is really about risk and how best to manage it. This is always a balance. Things that prevent ill health come at some cost – time, personal inconvenience, a challenge to established behaviour or diet. If prevention gave an immediate benefit, surely we would all make changes. But a benefit such as not having a heart attack in 30 years feels like no benefit at all, since we do not feel under an immediate threat. This is why people so often seek advice on prevention only after a colleague has had lung cancer or a heart attack, which brings home the risk of certain behaviours.

Statistics alone can often fail to convey the real level of risk. For example, it has long been known that 25–50% of smokers will die from a smoking-related illness – a threat to stimulate panic on the streets, you might think, but not so. On the other hand, the tiny and still controversial risk of catching BSE from cattle has rocked the agricultural industry.

Public health

While everyone has to take decisions about risk in their own lives, there are certain decisions that governments take for the benefit of the population. Childhood vaccination is deemed so important and well proven that pressure is applied by all health professionals to have children vaccinated, making it difficult although not impossible for parents to refuse. The risk to the population of a reappearance of diphtheria or whooping cough is judged too high to let individuals choose to opt out easily and there is even less choice about testing milk for TB or having fire exits from buildings.

Thinking prevention

The major threats to health in the developed world are cancers and heart and circulatory disease. Measures that have really big effects on these require dietary and behavioural changes, the benefits of which will not be seen for decades.

Fortunately, there are many strategies for safeguarding health which produce quicker results. For example, accident prevention, control of blood pressure and immunization (see page 278) are all areas where immediate protection from risk is possible, while increased exercise improves someone's fitness within a few weeks.

Screening

Screening programmes, such as that for cervical cancer (see page 150), cost a great deal of money. This can be expressed as the cost per life saved, taking into account the costs of early treatment and whether this improves survival. There are also, for individuals, the emotional costs produced by the wait for results, or by misleading results and uncertainty as to the accuracy of the screening procedure.

Governments are cautious about introducing new procedures until there is evidence of benefit. For example, a programme to screen for bowel cancer (see page 180) is currently under trial, while much controversy surrounds screening for prostate and ovarian cancer using blood tests.

Screening will probably become more widespread over the next few years, but this should not allow the fundamental preventive strategies mentioned earlier and those which follow to be forgotten.

Right: A doctor vaccinating a child against smallpox in an 1820 painting by Desbordes.

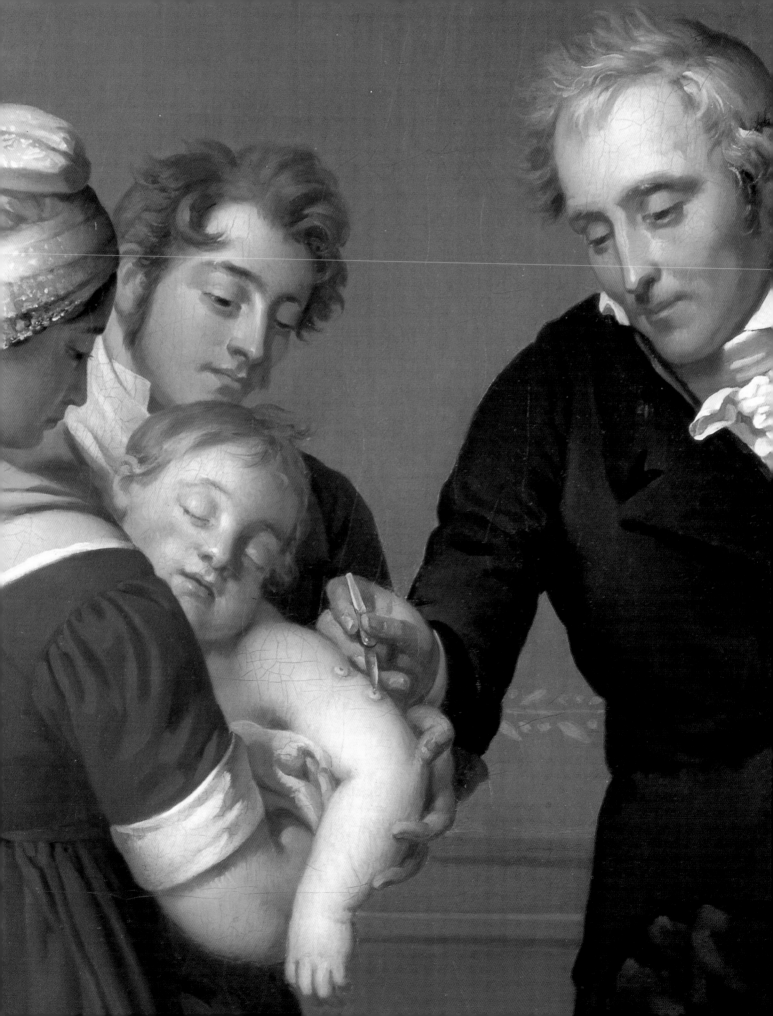

BABIES

Human babies are unique in how helpless they are and how reliant they are on others for feeding, warmth, cleaning and protection. Some argue that this very vulnerability has shaped human development and supported the family system. All parents feel the burden of responsibility that babies put on them.

Physical development

Ninety-eight per cent of newborn babies are physically normal; the two per cent of physical problems are often of a relatively minor or correctable nature such as birthmarks, minor heart murmurs or undescended testicles. Similarly, most babies grow adequately; only the few who do not grow need monitoring or investigation.

Prevention of problems All babies should be physically checked over after birth (a neonatal check), again a few days after birth, again at between six and eight weeks and every few months thereafter. The purpose is to pick up abnormalities as soon as possible, so as to decide which ones require treatment. Neonatal checks are also a baseline for judging later development. For example, a doctor cannot decide if a baby has an abnormally large head without knowing the previous head circumference. Therefore do take full advantage of baby health checks, question the doctor or health professional about any worries and draw their attention to anything that concerns you. After all, you are the person in closest contact with your baby and are therefore more likely to notice possible physical or mental problems.

Minor infections

A newborn baby is a happy hunting ground for all the germs of the world which invade at the instant of birth. This is not all bad; without exposure to infectious challenge the baby will not build his own immunity. It starts with small skin blemishes a day or so after birth and may include infection of the umbilical cord and sticky eyes. It will not be long before the baby has a first cold, especially where eager older children push their faces into the baby's. Soon the baby will have a cough. Most babies can be expected to get mild gastroenteritis, with diarrhoea and vomiting (see page 296).

Prevention If you are bottle feeding, keep all the equipment sterile with a sterilizing solution. Give feeds promptly before they have a chance to go off, and chill or dispose of what is left.

You should keep your baby clean but that does not mean keeping him sterile. Baby soap and water are perfectly adequate for skin hygiene, although spots may require an antiseptic cream. It makes sense for someone with a streaming cold not to breathe over babies. As a parent wash your hands frequently and wear a face mask if you have to care for your baby while you yourself are ill.

If your baby has a fever, be especially careful not to overwrap her. You should bring her temperature down with paracetamol syrup, if necessary undressing your baby and cooling her with a fan. It is natural to want medical advice when a baby is unwell until you gain confidence in dealing with your baby's inevitable minor illnesses. Learn your baby's reactions to minor infection so you can judge when she seems more than usually unwell and therefore when you need medical help (see When to call a doctor – some important symptoms, opposite).

Feeding

It is increasingly suspected that feeding patterns in infancy may lead to later physical problems such as obesity and heart disease, not to mention faddy eating. An average baby should gain about 200 g/ 7 oz a week up to three months and about 150 g/5 oz a week thereafter, approximately doubling birth weight by about six months and trebling it by one year.

Prevention of problems Breastfeed for as long as possible; the mother's milk contains antibodies to infections she has come across and to which she has immunity. These antibodies give breast-fed babies protection, too, quite apart from giving them a perfectly balanced diet. Introducing cow's milk too soon, i.e. before four months, may predispose a baby to allergies and food intolerances.

Have your baby weighed regularly to ensure adequate weight gain, but do not get too fixated on precise weights since the above are only general guidelines. In the developed world overfeeding is likely to be more of a problem than underfeeding. Be prepared for your health visitor to discuss this if your baby appears to be gaining too much weight.

Many authorities recommend giving vitamin supplements to all babies, breast- or bottle-fed; these are A, B, D and C.

Introduce different textures and flavours of solid food from about four months. This early experience of variety and 'lumpiness' reduces the likelihood of faddy eating and food refusal later (see page 312).

Major infections

Infectious disease is by far the most dangerous threat to babies worldwide. Serious infections include measles, mumps, polio, tetanus, whooping cough, diphtheria and many localized threats such as malaria.

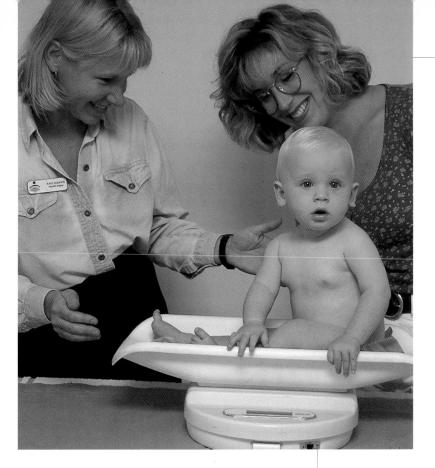

Above: Routine checks are opportunities to judge standards of care and the baby's development and happiness; carers can share pride, worries and frustrations.

WHEN TO CALL A DOCTOR – SOME IMPORTANT SYMPTOMS

♦ Fever lasting more than 24 hours that does not respond to paracetamol
♦ Unusual drowsiness
♦ The sudden appearance of a purple rash
♦ Diarrhoea and/or vomiting lasting more than a few hours, especially if there is no sign of urination
♦ Rapid breathing, inability to feed
♦ Unusual coldness and floppiness
♦ Blue lips or tongue

Prevention Most developed countries offer immunization against the above-mentioned common childhood diseases and often others with smaller but still serious risk such as haemophilus B, which is a cause of meningitis. So successful has immunization been in reducing the risk of infections that paradoxically there are now valid and understandable worries about the risks of immunization itself (see page 278).

Before embarking upon foreign travel, consider whether you may be needlessly exposing your baby to hazards.

Physical comfort

Babies need warmth, since they cannot maintain their own temperature efficiently. On the other hand they must not be overheated, as this can lead to convulsions and may be a factor in cot death. Newborn babies should be kept in a temperature of about 18°C/65°F and be well wrapped up when going outside.

Do not smoke when a baby is in the room. It is well established that children brought up in a smoking environment suffer more coughs, colds and chest infections and are at higher risk of cot death.

Put your baby to sleep on his back; this simple precaution greatly reduces the risk of cot death. (See page 313 for more information on cot death.)

Emotional comfort

Despite a vast amount of literature on the subject it is impossible to be sure how important early emotional experiences are on a baby's later emotional stability. We have to rely on our intuition to give the baby an emotionally healthy environment. It seems sensible to provide a stable family unit where the baby becomes used to being handled by just a few individuals. Handling, even at this stage, should be consistent. For example, if a baby is sometimes comforted when crying and other times neglected it seems likely that the baby's behaviour will become irritable and that he will learn that his environment is always inconsistent. This may have later consequences for discipline, eating and general behaviour.

In truth we just do not know at this stage. We can only guess and do what seems to be the right thing.

Keeping your sanity

A demanding, difficult baby is tremendously stressful; parents may experience resentment, tiredness and depression. It is a short step from these emotions to inflicting physical harm, by shaking, neglecting or worse forms of non-accidental injury. Rather than reach this extreme, talk to friends and health professionals about your feelings, which you will find are common.

TODDLERS

This covers children from about 15 months to about 3 years. The main characteristics of this age are relentless curiosity, combined with an almost complete lack of appreciation of danger. All the things said about babies remain important but there are additional worries as a result of the toddler's mobility.

Immunization

As toddlers increasingly mix in groups as they get older the risks from transmission of infection grow. The great majority of these will be simple colds and minor skin infections; the infectious diseases that are great childhood killers elsewhere – tetanus, gastroenteritis and malaria – are extremely rare in the developed world.

You should continue the immunization process begun in infancy.

Physical safety

External physical dangers are by far the greatest threat to your toddler's wellbeing and you must be constantly aware of them. Some common areas to think about are in the home, in the garden, at play and in the car.

But before you get down to worrying about detail, there is something fundamental about hazards that toddlers have to learn. Until they experience risk they will not know what risk is; until they experience heat they will not know why fire is a hazard; until they fall they will not know what a bump is, or a scratch. These things can and should be taught so that toddlers come to appreciate just why their parents are forever shouting 'careful' or 'put that down'.

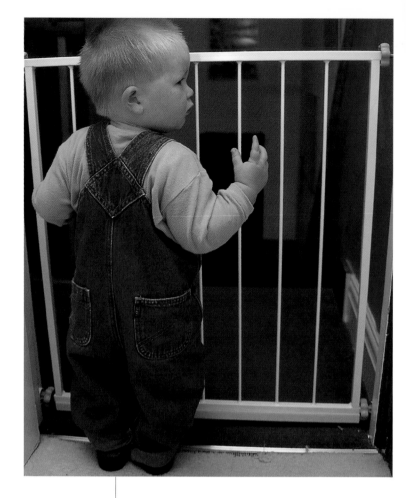

Above: Parents need to allow their children a considered path between gentle risk-taking and unreasonable hazards.

Let your toddler touch a radiator to learn what heat is and feel a pen top to know what sharp is. Bumps and scratches will come for free; your child will get them but after the tears, try to turn it into a learning experience. This is how to give toddlers a proper sense of their environment so that they can start to make judgements for themselves about their personal safety, a lesson they will have to learn for when they are older.

Prevention of accidents

In the home So many things we take for granted can be hazardous for toddlers, looked at from their perspective. Make sure they cannot pull heavy objects on to themselves, for example a plant stand, or a TV resting precariously on a work surface. Toddlers will tug any electrical flex; secure it or hide it and ensure the electrical socket is guarded so they cannot poke objects inside.

Glass, pointed objects and fires are special risks. Keep such risks out of reach or completely guarded. Remember that small objects such as beads, while a source of endless innocent amusement, can also be shoved up the nearest orifice or inhaled. Keep these for play only under close supervision, or else for a later age when the toddler is better at manipulating objects.

Modern kitchens are less of a hazard than once was the case, with electrical hobs and neat units. Even so, there is plenty of danger for the child who clambers on to a work surface, grabs a pan of hot water or finds where the household cleansers are kept. Make your kitchen safe from waist-height down by having toddler-proof locks on cupboards and by keeping sharp and hot things well above your toddler's reach.

Keep medicines where your toddler cannot see or grasp them – including ones prescribed for them – preferably in a locked cupboard. One commonly overlooked drug is the contraceptive Pill, left lying where you won't forget to take it. Keep that out of reach, too.

Stair guards are essential until children are three or four years old. It is not that toddlers are unaware of height. They are, but their sense of curiosity will lead to clumsy and risky attempts to clamber down stairs.

In the garden The pleasures of playing outside are enhanced by a few simple measures. Cover ponds and pools unless you can watch your child constantly – this

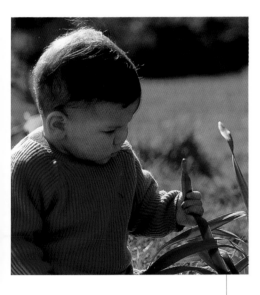

Above: Touching, sniffing and tasting – a toddler's attitude to enjoying gardening.

does mean *constantly*. Do not leave a toddler alone by water even for a few seconds; a child can drown in just inches of water. Teach your child to swim.

Many plants have poisonous berries, thorns or leaves; know what is growing in your garden and what is likely to be hazardous. Keep garden tools and garden chemicals under lock.

At play Toys are generally now designed with safety in mind and are made from non-toxic materials, with no sharp edges and no small parts that can fall off and be swallowed. This is all very worthy but there is another aspect of play that does call for the manipulation of small objects, cutting paper, gluing things or tying them together. Only you can judge when your toddler is ready to learn these skills. The key, of course, is careful supervision while the toddler learns. Do not leave your toddler alone with potentially hazardous objects.

Many toddlers will go to playgrounds or have bikes and swings of their own. No matter how brilliant your toddler is, she will not be safe to play alone in such environments; she will not appreciate that a swing that is such fun swung forward will hit her if she stands behind it as it swings back. In these and in so many other ways, the toddler has to be eased into the world of risk.

In the car Just as no adult should be in a car without a safety restraint, nor should any child. There are many well-designed child seats available. Your toddler should not be allowed to roll down windows to stick out his arms or, almost as bad, to throw things out. For some reason people think that it is all right for children to ride in the boot of an estate car and without restraint, although it is one of the most vulnerable parts of a car. If your family needs that amount of space, consider instead a 'people carrier'.

Emotional problems

The remarks about babies apply as much to toddlers, except that toddlers can give feedback. This may be in the form of tantrums, violence, disturbed sleep or sheer awkwardness. Try to provide consistent handling and consistent messages, whether about eating, playing or discipline. This is a goal, not an essential; no parents will ever be completely consistent, any more than adults are in other situations of life. But an upbringing with broad ground rules and broad limits on behaviour is likely to be emotionally healthier than one without bounds, where a toddler is unaware of what is expected of him and so cannot make sense of the response from his carers.

Physical health

The system of pre-school medical assessments continues. Major congenital problems should have been picked up by now, although some do slip through the net and a few new problems can arise. Hearing loss is probably the most common, whether through congenital deafness or acquired through glue ear (see page 214). If you think your toddler has a hearing problem or is slow in speaking, trust your judgement and seek professional advice. See a doctor for an undescended testicle or a twist in the spine that may have been missed on previous checks.

Other less specific things that might concern you are difficulty in walking, unusual clumsiness, wild, uncontrollable behaviour or lack of emotional response. There will often be perfectly innocent reasons for these and they may just be a phase in your toddler's development. It is the skill of child development specialists to decide whether such behaviour is indeed just a phase or calls for further help. (See also page 300.)

CHILDREN

The age from about three to the teenage years scans a period of enormous mental development and increasing physical independence. Accidents are still the major cause of injury, so accident prevention is a top priority. A balance has to be struck between developing independence and coping with the risks of life.

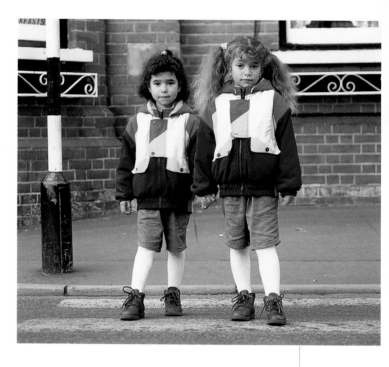

Above: Adults can make the path to independence for children as safe as possible.

Physical safety and accident prevention

Now that the hazards of life as a toddler are a thing of the past, there are other equally worrying causes for concern, although the need for constant parental supervision should be gradually lessening. (See also page 88.)

Road safety Children must be introduced to the realities of roads and traffic. This means learning to:

♦ *Cross a road only at crossings and in a safe fashion*
♦ *Not dash into a road in pursuit of anything*
♦ *Take care not to walk close to the edge of a pavement*

In the author's opinion no child under the age of ten is safe to cross a road alone.

Cycling is enjoyed by most children; there are many organized courses that deal with cycling safety, handling bikes and wearing visible clothing and helmets.

Road safety includes being safe within a car, wearing seatbelts and not opening a car door without a parent's permission and guidance.

Water and sun Teach your child to swim but remember the hazards of swimming unsupervised – swimming pools should have a lifeguard or a responsible adult who keeps an eye on swimmers. Again, do not let children play unsupervised in gardens with pools or ponds.

Remember sun protection: sunscreens and protective clothing. Do not let children burn in the sun. (See also page 236.)

Healthy eating

Evidence suggests that healthy eating habits in childhood will provide benefits into adult life. Introduce your children to a varied and healthy diet: fruit and vegetables every day, fibre in wholemeal bread, low-fat foods and lean meat, if they eat meat. Encourage them to eat fruit for snacks instead of sweets, crisps or biscuits. Steer them towards water, fruit juices and diet drinks rather than heavily sweetened drinks. Support the children's school in its efforts to provide healthy eating options on its menu, or give your child a healthy packed lunch.

Even though you may fail initially – after all, you are up against tremendous advertising and peer pressures – console yourself with the thought that you are giving your children a variety of experience, some of which will rub off.

Healthy eating in childhood will reduce the chances of later obesity, heart disease from high cholesterol, tooth decay, bowel problems such as diverticulitis and possibly even cancers through improving antioxidant and vitamin E intakes from vegetables and fruit. Obesity in children, as much as in adults, is an increasingly worrying health hazard (see page 100), which bodes poorly for the future health of the nation.

Admittedly, telling your children to eat their greens so they won't get diverticulitis will go down no better than telling them to start saving for their pension scheme. It is probably best not to reason with them; just provide healthy food while they remain under your control.

Exercise

Sport and physical exertion should be a natural part of childhood. Some children have an innate ability and will shine in some area, which is a source of great self-esteem. All children should learn the pleasures of sheer physical exertion, again in

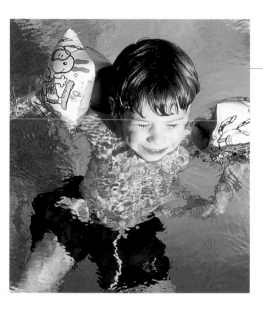

Left: There are some skills all children should acquire for their future security.

the hope that healthy habits will be carried into adult life.

Take your children for walks, let them try all sorts of sports, give them adventure holidays. They will have great fun. At the same time you will be reassured, knowing you are helping them to have healthy bones – which will provide protection against future osteoporosis – and hearts, and to enjoy the more indefinable benefits from playing sport: the winning, the losing and the supporting.

At the same time, do make sure they wear the correct gear, are supervised by properly qualified adults and do not train beyond their reasonable abilities.

Emotional hazards

Your child will soon be faced by the emotional stresses of real life; there may be a younger child who gets more attention or the parents may have relationship problems. At school he has to cope with 'in groups' and 'out groups', with rejection, shifting friendships, bullying and aggression. Incidents trivial to an adult may be devastating for a child. Although you cannot prevent such happenings you can give your child the opportunity to talk

Left: There are some skills all children should acquire for their future security.

about things which are worrying him. Where emotional distress appears excessive you might need professional help through the school. Warning signs would be reappearance of bed-wetting, nightmares, regression of behaviour, unusually disturbed and aggressive behaviour, depression or withdrawal.

Sexual and physical abuse

Neither of these is new; what is new is the openness with which they are now discussed and a readiness much greater than before to take a child's complaints of abuse seriously. Children at greatest risk are those with parents who were themselves abused or who are splitting up, and those with step-parents or who live in institutions, such as children's homes.

Carers should be aware of the possibility of abuse in children whose behaviour changes dramatically, who become withdrawn, run away from home, show ambivalence and wariness about certain adults (or children) in their lives, have unexplained bruises of varying ages, have unusual burns – especially cigarette burns – show precocious sexual behaviour or, of course, make allegations of abuse.

This is a very difficult area in which unwarranted allegations may have devastating consequences. Child protection procedures have become much less heavy-handed in recent years, so if your concerns remain, do discuss them with the school, social services or child-care agencies.

Part of this awareness is to teach children how to protect their personal safety. Teach them to avoid parks and deserted

places if alone and after dark, not to accept lifts from strangers, to be prepared to run away or shout if they feel in danger, and to know they can talk to a trusted adult about things that are troubling them. There are no easy answers as to how to strike a balance between teaching reasonable streetwise behaviour and making childhood lose its innocence.

Abuse of drugs, cigarettes and alcohol

These substances may be dangerous in themselves, lead to criminal behaviour or carry future health hazards. Children who indulge in these usually start by following parental example or peer pressure. The responsibility on parents is to limit such behaviour by not smoking in the presence of children, nor drinking to excess.

Suspect drug abuse if your child's behaviour and school performance alters, if she plays truant, appears emotionally unstable, has sores around the mouth and nose (from glue sniffing) or if she mixes with children known to have these problems. A child who starts to steal money may be doing so to pay for such activities.

It is a parent's responsibility to know where their children are, what they are doing and who they are doing it with. You should be prepared to ask your child about her usage of drugs and so on and to speak to other parents, the school or the specialized police units.

In some cases, drug and alcohol abuse may be part of a greater behavioural or personality problem. The child may be generally uncontrollable, indulging in bullying, aggression or petty crime. In such a case you need help from a child psychiatrist to see if anything can be done to channel your child's abilities in a more positive direction.

Rarely, children well below the age of ten can be mentally ill, with depression and psychosis. This has to be considered if their behaviour becomes bizarre.

ADOLESCENTS

The years from puberty to late teenage are widely accepted as being filled with emotional and physical turmoil. Despite the problems, on the whole this is a healthy period of life, the main serious risks still being from accidents.

Physical health

Any significant health problems are likely to have become apparent well before adolescence. It is still worth being vigilant for previously missed undescended testicles; a scoliosis (twist in the spine) may become more prominent (see page 294). In both sexes, failure to enter puberty by 16–17 calls for specialist assessment, looking for one of the unusual hormonal causes of delayed puberty. Growth should take off just before puberty and again, failure to grow requires hormone studies.

Some girls, conscious of their breast development, adopt a hunched, round-shouldered stance. Try suggesting a bra that has good support and encourage your daughter to maintain an upright posture.

Diet

Teenagers grow rapidly and need large quantities of food to keep going. They will shovel in anything at hand, especially fast or junk food. Even so parents should still try to keep the faint flame of healthy eating alive during these guzzling years, offering fruit and vegetables and discouraging empty, salt-filled snacks. Poor dietary habits now may lead to later obesity, heart trouble and high blood pressure.

A significant number of adolescents – mainly girls but occasionally boys – become anorexic. The pressure seems to be from a culture where thin is good and

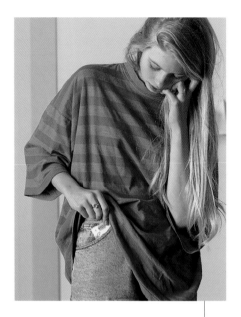

Above: Using a condom greatly reduces the risk of HIV infection.

where anorexic role models abound. Your adolescent may have an eating problem if she loses weight steadily, will not eat at family mealtimes and considers herself overweight despite clearly being normal or thin. Bulimia is compulsive overeating, often followed by self-induced vomiting. Depression and self-mutilation frequently accompany eating disorders. Fortunately most adolescents recover spontaneously but those few who become severely malnourished require psychiatric help.

Sex

Few children now reach adolescence unaware of at least the basic facts of sex and reproduction. While thinking they know it all, however, adolescents are ignorant of the true nature and risks of sexual relationships. It is inevitable that they will experiment. As a responsible parent you should ensure that the risks of pregnancy and sexually transmitted diseases are minimized.

Adolescents should be aware of the legal framework regarding sex with underage children and the consequences.

You should not condone underage sexual activity. However, once your teenagers are of age legally (16 in the United Kingdom) there is little you can do about it if they choose to have sex.

Your adolescent son should know about condoms and how to use them, and should regard using them as the norm and not a sign of weakness. Teenagers should also know that condoms prevent the transmission of venereal diseases and are reasonably good at preventing pregnancy.

Girls who take the contraceptive Pill should ensure their sexual partners also use condoms for the above hygiene reasons, and especially if they do not know a partner's sexual history. Once a girl starts having regular sexual intercourse, she should have a smear test; her risk of cervical cancer, although low, increases the earlier she has sex and the more sexual partners she has (see page 150).

HIV/AIDS and sexually transmitted disease

The risk of HIV/AIDS is low for people having normal heterosexual intercourse in the Western world. High-risk behaviour is having anal intercourse with homosexual men or intercourse with intravenous drug users. HIV can be transmitted by heterosexual intercourse but at present this is a significant risk mainly in parts of Africa and Asia, although it is expected to become important worldwide over the next few decades. Using a condom greatly reduces the risk of transmission and should be used in addition to other more reliable methods of contraception such as the Pill, unless one is entirely certain of a partner's HIV status.

Adolescents should be aware of the symptoms of sexually transmitted diseases such as heavy vaginal discharge, discharge from the penis, painful spots around the genitalia or persistent sores. They should know that they can get confidential help at a sexual diseases clinic. (See also pages 124, 164 and 286.)

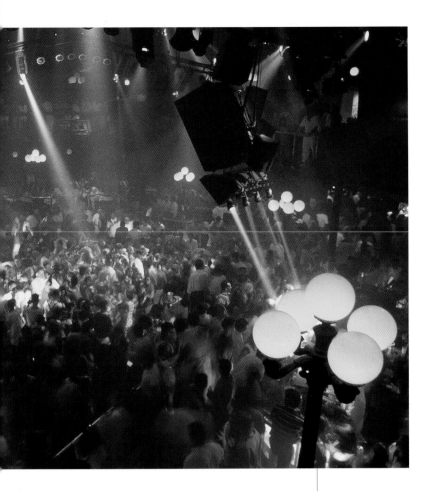

Emotions

The emotional roller-coaster of adolescence leads to apparently irrational attachments and just as irrational abandonment of previously cherished friends. It can be difficult for adult onlookers to detach themselves from these events, which are part of a necessary learning curve. Many adolescents fall foul of emotions too large for them to handle alone and will welcome, albeit reluctantly, a sympathetic non-judgemental ear.

A significant number of teenage girls take an overdose on impulse at a period of emotional turmoil. These teenagers should have a psychiatric assessment as a small number will be in genuine despair and may contemplate suicide. Although the numbers are relatively small, suicide is the most common cause of death in these years after accidents. The same goes for any teenage boy who appears deeply depressed and apathetic. Depression and schizophrenia are not rare in adolescents and are treatable. It takes tact to persuade

Above: Adolescence features group activities in the guise of individualism.

teenagers that they need help. There are self-referral agencies to which they can go in confidence and without stigma.

Aggression and road accidents

Many teenage boys, and increasingly teenage girls, show aggressive gang behaviour which can be unprovoked and vicious. This competitive nature extends to sports and driving, especially in the first years after learning to drive. Road traffic accidents are the major cause of death in the teenage/early adult age group. In this age group half of all deaths in girls are from road traffic accidents, as are two-thirds of deaths in boys.

Stringent driving tests are one way of dealing with risk-taking on the roads.

Other methods are driving with probationary (new driver) plates, taking advanced driving tests soon after passing the basic test and driving a safer, less powerful car. Unfortunately, all these measures count little for the adolescent who is tempted for personal reasons or by peer pressure to show bravado, as the constant stream of statistics of teenagers killed and injured in car crashes proves.

Drink and drugs

Experimentation and peer pressure extend to alcohol and drugs. Alcohol in particular plays a significant role in aggressive behaviour and in accidents – especially road traffic accidents. Drug-taking appears to have become accepted behaviour by many young people in the teenage social scene, mainly using the so-called soft recreational drugs such as ecstasy and cannabis. Responsible parents cannot condone such addictive behaviour, even though the risks of recreational drugs may be less than the risks of the acceptable drugs in our society – alcohol and tobacco. The whole topic is blurred by moral and pseudo-scientific consideration, but the recurrent reports of drug-related deaths should be enough to dissuade anyone from taking these additional risks in what is already a dangerous age for accidents.

Smoking

Smoking is one of the most dangerous activities anyone can voluntarily indulge in. Recent government action in the United Kingdom and in the United States may at last herald a move from the *laissez-faire* attitude to this. It is difficult to get across to teenagers just how dangerous smoking is, because the consequences are a lifetime away. This puts all the greater responsibility on parents and governments to reduce the pressures on teenagers to take up smoking and to make it easier for them to quit.

WOMEN: CHILDBEARING YEARS

As a woman you will enjoy a greater life expectancy than men, even allowing for the common female cancers of breast, ovary and womb. You can enhance this in-built advantage and, by maintaining your physical health, also ensure that you are in peak shape for pregnancy.

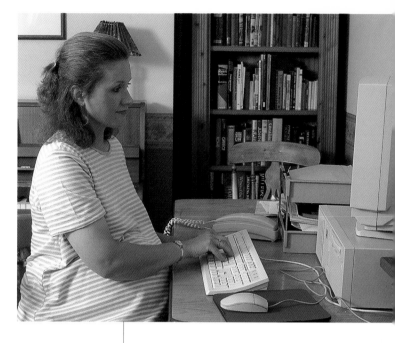

Above: Women today often have to juggle a number of conflicting responsibilities.

Physical wellbeing

During these years women, by virtue of being female and subject to oestrogen, are protected against the heart and circulatory problems to which men are more liable. This protection will ebb away at the menopause; therefore the earlier years are the ones in which to tackle risk factors for later heart disease. Keep to a healthy diet, avoiding hard fats and eating polyunsaturated and low-fat foods. Dietary fibre in fruit and vegetables will avoid constipation, reducing a risk of diverticulitis or cancer of the bowel. These same foods provide vitamin E and other antioxidants, believed to protect against circulatory problems and cancers.

Diet As well as healthy eating, try to keep your weight under control. You should not be more than ten per cent over a healthy body mass index or you may later develop the problems of obesity (see page 100): early osteoarthritis, tiredness, hiatus hernia or high blood pressure. Furthermore, if you are overweight at the beginning of pregnancy, you will find it very much harder to lose weight after the birth of your baby.

Exercise Keep active and try to build exercise into your weekly routine, be it a walk at lunchtime or going to the gym. As well as the sense of wellbeing this provides, you will maintain healthy bones, protecting you against osteoporosis from your 60s onwards.

Sun Bear in mind the guidelines about sun exposure and resist the temptation to use sunbeds for a year-round tan. This is high-risk behaviour for skin cancer 20 years down the line. (See also page 236).

Smoking If you give up smoking now, there is plenty of time for your body to recover from the smoke, tars and nicotine that poison your lungs and affect your blood vessels. Lung cancer is the form of cancer most rapidly increasing in frequency in women. Within one year of giving up your risks are greatly reduced, while by five years they are little more than those of a non-smoker (although the risk is always greater than in someone who has never smoked).

If you smoke during pregnancy, you may cause your baby to miscarry or to be born pre-term. Smoking affects the growth of your baby, reducing birthweight by about ten per cent, in itself a major health risk. Remember, too, that the children of smokers suffer more upper respiratory infections.

Accidents and road safety

The greatest risk to your health from childhood right through to the age of about 40 is from accidents, of which road traffic accidents are overwhelmingly the greatest risk. Between one-third and one-half of all deaths of women in this period are due to road accidents, quite apart from the many thousands left permanently injured. You owe it to yourself and others to drive as carefully as possible, not to drink and drive and not to indulge in 'road rage'. Other causes of serious accidents are sports, recreation such as climbing and, much less in women than in men, industrial accidents.

Whether for sport, recreation or at work, take pride in knowing the right equipment, the right procedures and what to do if something goes wrong. Remember, too, the risks at home and with do-it-yourself projects. (See also pages 88 and 358.)

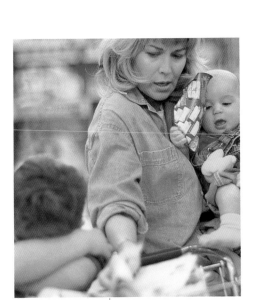

*Above: The responsibility
for parenting is still
mainly a woman's role.*

Cervical smears

Sexually active women should have a cervical smear every three years. Twenty per cent of the 1800 deaths from cervical cancer a year occur in women below the age of 45. These may be preventable by regular screening and detection. More often, a smear at this age reveals inflammatory changes that may lead to cancer of the cervix. These changes, called dyskaryosis, are treatable by laser or by cauterizing (burning) the cervix. Women at greater risk are those who have sexual intercourse from their early teens with multiple partners. (For other female cancers, see pages 148, 151 and 152.)

Breast checks

Check your breasts every few weeks for lumps: nine out of ten are innocent and breast cancer below the age of thirty is extremely rare. There is no scientific evidence to support having mammograms in this age group unless there is a strong family history of breast cancer, in which case you should seek specialist advice.

Sexual health

The advent of HIV/AIDS has made it respectable for women to take the initiative in sexual safety. You should know the sexual background of your partners. If one is bisexual or an intravenous drug user, or comes from a country where AIDS is prevalent, you should take seriously the risk of acquiring HIV through normal intercourse. You should insist that your partner uses a condom, and you should avoid risky behaviour such as oral or anal intercourse. Even if your partner does not appear to fall into a high-risk group, you should still insist on a condom until you are sure of his safe status. Take seriously any symptoms of possible sexually transmitted disease (see page 164), for example genital spots, discharges, cystitis or pelvic pain. Early treatment will help avoid later problems of subfertility.

Anxiety, tension and depression

Many women have to juggle social, work and family commitments, any of which could demand all their time and which at any one time could be mutually exclusive. Discuss the issues with your partner and friends. It is difficult to choose between career progression and economic necessity, or seeing your children grow up, and this has to be a personal choice.

One of the few areas in which women are at greater risk than men is in attempting suicide. Tens of thousands of women a year attempt this; many are below the age of thirty. However far fewer women than men actually commit suicide. There are many anonymous and supportive counselling services available to those who are contemplating a suicide attempt. Depression is a treatable condition and one that you need not put up with alone (see page 72).

Preventive planning for pregnancy

Rubella vaccination In the United Kingdom all babies are immunized against rubella at the age of around 12 months. The vaccine fails to take or to last in a few individuals, so some women are therefore at risk of rubella during pregnancy (see page 280). This illness affects the baby's heart, ears and brain. Have a blood test to see if you are immune a year before you plan pregnancy; this allows plenty of time for revaccination and for repeat blood tests (see page 324).

Folic acid and other vitamins By taking just 0.4 mg folic acid a day, you greatly reduce the chances of having a baby with spina bifida. You should start taking folic acid before you conceive and continue it until 12 weeks after becoming pregnant.

There are not such compelling reasons to take other vitamins, as long as your diet is healthy and includes fruit and vegetables. However, if you have heavy periods and plan to breastfeed – both of which lead to loss of iron – it makes sense to take iron to avoid anaemia at the beginning of pregnancy. Do not worry too much about this – blood tests during pregnancy will show whether you need iron supplements later.

Alcohol Currently, in the United Kingdom, the recommended maximum weekly alcohol intake for women is 21 units – a unit is a glass of wine, 300 ml/ ½ pint of beer or a measure of spirits. There is controversy about whether drinking is harmful to the foetus during pregnancy; babies born to heavy drinkers have a distorted facial appearance. Most doctors think that moderate drinking is OK; some women feel happier to avoid alcohol altogether during pregnancy, and especially during the first three months.

WOMEN:
THE MENOPAUSE
AND AFTER

These years, when day-to-day family responsibilities generally lessen and financial pressures ease, should be fulfilling and healthy. It should be a time to reap the rewards from previous healthy living and to take steps to ensure an active mind and body for the years up to retirement. A number of female cancers become more common from this age, early detection of which improves the outlook.

The menopause

Women enter the menopause on average at around 50 years of age, although the range can be from the late 30s to mid-50s. The event is heralded by increasingly irregular and infrequent periods until they cease altogether. Flushes may appear a year or so before periods cease. If there is any doubt a blood test will confirm it.

With the menopause women lose the protection of their female hormones, which hitherto protected them against heart disease. They also lose bone density rapidly for several years afterwards.

HRT (hormone replacement therapy)

Other than lifestyle changes, the most beneficial preventive strategy at this age is HRT. It reduces flushes, improves skin texture, reduces vaginal dryness and helps mood swings. It protects against heart disease while being taken. HRT maintains bone density and so protects against osteoporosis. These are advantages which many women find helpful.

The most important disadvantages are the return of periods, (although newer forms of HRT avoid this), weight gain and a risk of thrombosis. This risk is greatest in the first year on HRT. After eight years or so, HRT increases the risk of breast cancer. Statistical studies favour remaining on HRT indefinitely but even staying on it for just two to five years, as many women do, is a considerable benefit. Women coming off HRT suffer the usual menopausal symptoms for a few weeks, possibly longer, and should continue with a healthy diet and regular exercise.

Osteoporosis

Prevention of osteoporosis involves regularly taking active, weight-bearing exercise – either walking or something more strenuous. Ensure your diet is rich in calcium and vitamin D by eating dairy products or taking calcium and vitamin D supplements. These measures will maintain your bone density (see page 248). Smoking increases the rate of calcium loss and hastens the onset of osteoporosis.

Certain women run a greater risk of osteoporosis and should have their bone density measured. These include women who have been on steroids, for example for asthma, women who are immobile, have a poor diet, smoke, have a family

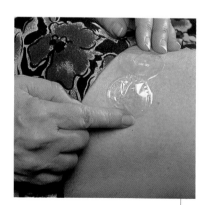

Above: HRT is available in many forms. Here a patch is worn on the skin.

history of osteoporosis and who have an early menopause (before the age of 45). Bone density helps decide whether it is worthwhile taking medication to reverse osteoporosis, for example etidronate or alendronate, and for how long.

Breast cancer

This is the peak time for this disease (see page 148), in recognition of which there is, in the United Kingdom, a breast-screening service using mammography. Currently this invites women from 50 years of age for screening every 3 years. Screening cannot be 100% accurate so continue to check your breasts regularly yourself, reporting any lumps or changes in the nipple, and any bleeding or discharge from the nipple. Even in this age group, most breast lumps prove benign.

Cancers of the cervix, womb and ovary

You should continue to have regular cervical smears every three to five years up to the age of sixty-five. About 70% of the 1800 deaths a year from cervical cancer occur in women over the age of 55. Cancer of the womb is more common from this age; post-menopausal vaginal bleeding or lower abdominal pains should be checked out. A smear test also allows an internal examination, which may pick up an abnormality in the womb or ovary before you notice any symptoms, greatly improving the prospects of cure for these cancers (see pages 150, 151 and 152).

Blood pressure, cholesterol and heart disease

Because of the requirements of contraception or because of pregnancy, most women will have had their blood pressure checked during their reproductive years and high blood pressure should have been dealt with. As blood pressure tends to increase as you get older, have yours checked every couple of years.

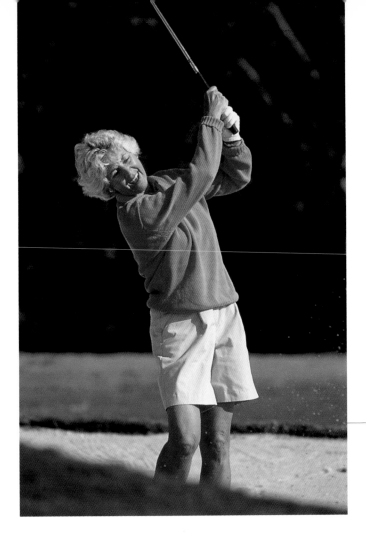

Left: Middle age often coincides with having more time for the pastimes important for your physical and mental health, as well as providing social benefits.

If you have a family history of high cholesterol, you should have had a cholesterol blood test well before now. Otherwise ask for this to be done as a baseline. There are guidelines on handling raised cholesterol which take into account family history and coexisting risk factors, so talk to your doctor about the result.

From the menopause onwards women are at a similar risk of heart disease as men. You should take seriously any chest pains, unusual breathlessness and tiredness, each of which could be due to heart trouble. Heart disease in women tends to progress more rapidly than in men, so you should expect such symptoms to be taken seriously and be properly investigated.

Diabetes

About two per cent of the population are affected (see page 98), and probably five per cent of those over sixty-five – especially the overweight. The screening for diabetes is simple: a sample of urine is tested for sugar. If in doubt your doctor may send you to have blood tests. Have a urine test every couple of years.

Alcohol and smoking

Excessive alcohol affects your liver and pancreas. Smoking will affect your heart, which is no longer protected by female hormones, vastly increasing your risk of heart disease, especially if you have other risk factors such as bad family history, high cholesterol or high blood pressure.

Glaucoma

This condition of raised pressure within the eyes affects about 0.5–1% of this age group and can lead to blindness (see page 200). Have your eyes tested for glaucoma by your optician every few years; more often if a close relative suffers from it.

Diet

It is tempting at this age to let everything go, on the basis of 'what difference can it make now?'. This is a pity; you should be looking forward to another two or three decades of life, so why risk it? It is still important to eat healthily, with a low-fat high-fibre diet. More than ever you should eat high fibre as protection against bowel cancer and diverticular disease. A low-carbohydrate and low-sugar diet will also reduce your chances of diabetes.

Mental health

The menopause often coincides with children leaving home or careers peaking; it may throw into focus marital and relationship problems hitherto ignored. Certain health problems are almost inevitable, for example arthritis, dry skin and loss of stamina. It is hardly surprising that many women find that their self-confidence takes a knock at this stage and they may get depressed on further contemplation of their life. HRT helps mood swings and can ease this transition.

Otherwise talk about your worries before they get out of hand and you fall into a deeper state of depression or anxiety. You might share worries with friends, seek a counselling service or discuss how you feel with your doctor. The sympathetic listening ear is the only medication most women require, but a few become significantly depressed. You may be one of these if you are waking in the very early morning, take no pleasure in life, keep crying, think only black thoughts or lose your appetite. Help is available with one of the effective modern antidepressants, so discuss it with your doctor.

General body awareness

Be alert to changes in your body which could signal early disease. Important symptoms are weight loss, breathlessness, persistent cough, coughing blood or bleeding from the bowels, bladder or vagina. Recurrent abdominal pains, new lumps and old skin lumps that change colour or bleed should also be checked.

YOUNG AND MIDDLE-AGED MEN

This covers men from their mid-20s to the age of 65. It is a large age group with very different health risks at either end. If you have always enjoyed a healthy diet and take regular exercise you are unlikely to meet any serious health hazards until you reach your 50s.

Accidents

Until the age of about 40, accidents on the road, at work or from sport pose the greatest risk of death or serious injury for both men and women. Up to the age of 25 road traffic accidents account for nearly two-thirds of all deaths in men. This is partly through inexperience; partly through male aggressive behaviour and irresponsibility; partly it is the statistical consequence of the numbers of men driving and pursuing hazardous recreations or jobs. Prevent yourself from becoming one of these statistics by driving carefully. Think of it not just for yourself but to protect others from the consequences of you having a serious accident: the loss of a wage earner, the loss of a husband or son.

In a male environment safety procedures may be skimped on as being wimpish or even unnecessary; if your factory or workplace has a safety policy adhere to it, and if it does not, perhaps it should have. The same goes for sports such as climbing or parachuting. The professionals in these sports take safety seriously because they see the things that go wrong more often than the amateur does. Follow their advice and guidance.

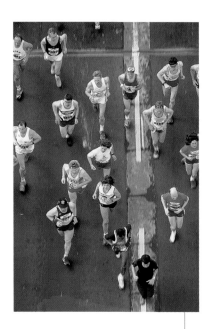

Above: Many sports welcome participants across all ages.

Alcohol

Excess drinking plays a part in many road traffic accidents. It contributes to industrial and sports accidents and reduces efficiency at work. This is over and above the actual medical consequences of alcohol excess (see page 95). Currently in the United Kingdom the recommended maximum intake for men is 28 units a week, where a unit is 300 ml/½ pint of beer, a glass of wine or a measure of spirits.

Smoking

Lung cancer is the single most common cancer affecting men (see page 68). The good news is that men have taken on board the message about smoking less; consequently the rates of lung cancer in men are slowly falling. It still remains a fact that 25–50% of men who smoke will die as a consequence of cigarette smoking, of which lung cancer is just one disease, along with heart disease, chronic lung disease and many other conditions.

Heart disease

Men are 20 times more likely than women to develop heart and circulatory problems by their early 50s, a period of time during which women are protected by female hormones. Little wonder then that there is so much emphasis on men trying to improve their lifestyles to reduce this natural risk. Reducing smoking is the biggest single step you can take. Other important measures are to reduce cholesterol and to have high blood pressure treated.

Cholesterol

If you have followed a healthy diet there is a good chance that your cholesterol levels are reasonably low anyway. You should have a cholesterol check in your mid-40s – and sooner if there is a history of early (pre-60s) heart disease in your close family, i.e. parents or siblings. Thereafter, it is a good idea to have cholesterol rechecked every three to five years. Modestly raised cholesterol can be treated by adjustments to diet; very high levels may need medication. Such a decision has to take account of your overall risk, including smoking and high blood pressure.

Blood pressure

All men should have a blood pressure check at some time in their 20s, and again in their 30s. By the 40s blood pressure should be checked every three to five years. It may be possible to deal with mildly raised blood pressure by adjustments such as losing weight and decreasing the amount of salt in your diet.

Testicular cancer

Although not common (about 1250 cases a year in the United Kingdom), testicular cancer is the most frequent cancer affecting men in their 20s and early 30s (see page 122). It is nearly always curable if caught early. Men should check their testicles regularly for lumps and take notice of persistent pains, seeing a doctor for either.

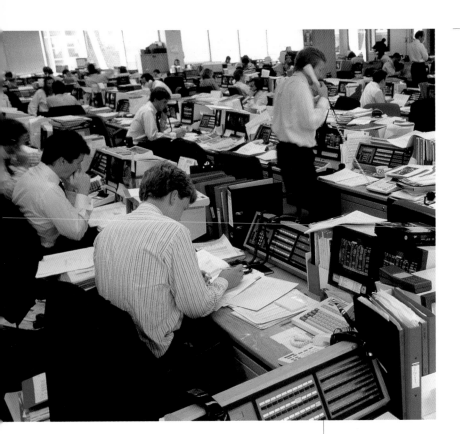

Above: The more stressful your work, the more important it is to find some relaxation.

Prostate cancer

Below the age of 45 prostate cancer is rare and even in men in their 50s it is uncommon, but by their 60s many men will be affected by benign or cancerous prostate problems (see page 120). It is not possible to prevent cancer of the prostate, but it may be possible to screen for it, although this is still a controversial area. Several specialists recommend that men from the age of 50 have an annual rectal examination of their prostate gland, plus a blood test called PSA (Prostate Specific Antigen). At the time of writing it is by no means agreed what is the best course of action on finding an abnormality, so speak to your doctor about the latest opinions.

Suicide and depression

Remarkably, suicide is the second most common cause of death, after accidents, in young men. Although many fewer men than women attempt suicide, those that do seem to have a more serious intent. Men may feel despair caused by work pressures, unemployment or relationship problems. Some men develop a pure depressive illness for no obvious external reason or have another psychiatric condition triggering depression, such as schizophrenia. There are many agencies to help those in despair – in Britain the Samaritans are the best known. Other sources of help are counselling services, your doctor and psychiatric teams. However, the first step is to acknowledge that you have a psychological problem that you cannot deal with on your own and for which you need support and help. This is not an admission of weakness, but sensible self-knowledge and self-assessment.

Glaucoma

This is a condition causing raised pressure within the eyes and possibly blindness (see pages 200 and 202). If you have a family history of this, go to your optician for screening before the age of 40. Others should be screened for this common condition regularly after the age of 60.

Diabetes

By the age of 60, 2–5% of the population – both men and women – will have diabetes (see page 98). It is worth having a simple urine check for sugar every three years from the age of sixty. By avoiding being overweight you greatly reduce the chances of developing diabetes, quite apart from the other health benefits.

Overweight

Middle-aged spread need not be the inevitability it can appear to be. Try not to let your weight edge more than ten per cent above your healthy Body Mass Index (see page 100). Otherwise you run the risks of obesity in your later years – arthritis, heart disease, high blood pressure, diabetes and digestive problems. It is better not to gain the weight in the first place than to have to lose it in later life when mobility and exercise tolerance may already be affected.

Exercise

Try to carry the habit of exercise through from childhood right into old age. Although the theme will be the same the melody will vary. Vigorous contact sports and squash in your 20–30s will naturally give way to gentler, although not necessarily less competitive, exertion later. Tennis, badminton, dancing, swimming, walking and jogging can all carry on into late middle age and beyond, as long as you wear the right clothing and footwear and take notice of unusual chest and joint pains and breathlessness.

Being aware of your body

The warning symptoms for men in these years are weight loss, persistent cough, especially coughing blood, bleeding from the bowel or bladder, difficulty passing urine, chest pains on exertion and unusual breathlessness.

RETIREMENT

The age of retirement from full-time work is no longer the sudden definite event at a predetermined age that it once was. Where many men used to work until 65 and women until 60, it is increasingly common to reduce working hours from the 50s onwards while many people plan to retire at no later than 60, if not before. Whatever the age of your retirement, you will be faced with similar transitional problems.

Maintaining a routine

Those adults who go out to work have to fit leisure time around it: the time they get up, leave the house and return home are largely determined by the demands of work. Irksome as this may be, it does give a structure to the day, which is all too easily lost after retirement. Unless you have activities planned, those free hours are no longer a great opportunity but simply become filled with boredom and worse, as you brood over the loss of status and loss of self-respect. Ideally, increase the time devoted to an interest that you may have taken up well before you retire. It may be bridge, model-making, walking or bingo – it does not matter as long as it gives a pattern to your week and events for you to look forward to.

Keeping active

You would be surprised at how much activity even an apparently sedentary job involves: walking to get there, walking around an office or up and down stairs. Therefore it is as important as ever after retirement to take exercise. Many sports are suitable for older people; particularly

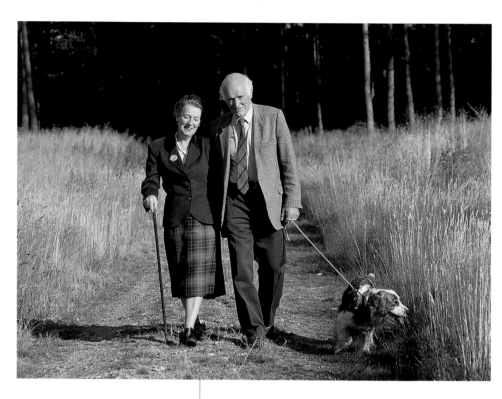

Above: With careful planning, this scene need not be an unrealistically idyllic goal.

ideal ones are swimming, walking, bowls, golf and badminton. But if you feel capable there is every reason to continue tennis, riding, running, climbing and so on. Regular daily exercise keeps your heart and muscles in shape and adds to the structure of your day.

There is nothing like idleness to breed idleness. Have you noticed that it is people who always seem to be on the go who do not run out of energy, whereas those who will not even make an effort somehow become tired in front of your eyes?

Diet

Working people need about 2500 calories a day, even in sedentary jobs. After retirement your need for food should decrease unless you happen to do particularly vigorous exercise. Yet you will be finding it

easier than ever to snack and graze in a way that you may not have done since you were a teenager. Again, it helps to have a routine of regular meals at specific times to avoid overeating all day long. If you need a snack, try to keep to fruit. In this way you will avoid obesity and its effects on your heart, lungs, joints and blood pressure. You will also have the fibre to keep your bowels open naturally without having to turn to laxatives.

Empty calories are as bad for you at this age as at any other. Avoid sugar and fatty foods; in this way you will reduce your risks of diabetes.

Osteoporosis

Both men and women are at risk of this. Keeping active, not smoking and taking calcium are important preventive measures. Women can consider starting HRT or continuing on it, although there is a small risk of breast cancer (see page 22). Men or women with established osteoporosis can take therapy such as alendronate or etidronate to reverse this (see page 248).

Blood pressure

Have this checked every couple of years. Accept treatment if recommended as well as the regular checks every few months that are part of monitoring treatment. The main benefit is in reducing the risk of a stroke or heart disease. Some 40% of the population in this age group have high blood pressure so there is really nothing unusual about this.

Cholesterol

It is not necessary to be obsessive about cholesterol as minor changes at this age will have little effect on health. Very high levels should still be dealt with, but it is not worth worrying about modestly raised cholesterol unless you have heart disease, in which case it is beneficial to get it under control. On the other hand everyone should follow a prudent low-fat diet of fibres, fruit, lean meat and low salt.

Smoking and alcohol

It is still not too late to give up smoking, although the benefits will be relatively small. However, you should drop it in earnest if you develop heart or circulatory problems which nicotine makes worse.

Drinking 3–4 units a day of alcohol appears to offer continuing protection against heart disease (but see also pages 21 and 24). This is probably the first time in your life when you can combine a health message with pleasure, without worrying whether you have to get a column of figures to add up after lunch!

Accidents

Although still an important threat to your wellbeing you probably need take no more precautions than any other prudent adult in order to avoid, for example, household, car or pedestrian accidents.

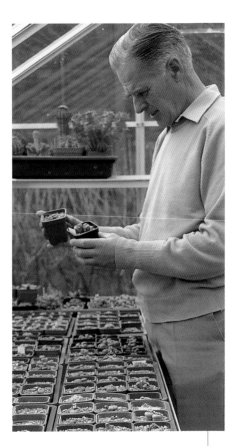

Above: Once the novelty of leisure time wears off, pursuing enjoyable hobbies will provide a structure to your day.

General health screening

Every couple of years it is a good idea to have a basic physical check-up. This should include tests for raised blood pressure, abnormal functioning of the heart and lungs and the presence of diabetes or glaucoma. Now is also the time to have minor but annoying health problems sorted out, for example a hernia, a mole which keeps snagging, a painful hip or prostate symptoms. The reason is starkly simple: you may not be fit enough for surgery if you delay too long.

An aspirin a day

There is good evidence that an aspirin a day helps prevent strokes and heart trouble. Between 75 and 150 mg a day seems effective – ask your doctor about the latest recommended dosage.

Mental health

If you enter retirement without any forward planning you may suffer depression through the sudden loss of status, structure to your days and companionship. This holds true for women as well as men. It is all too common to find that retirement is less financially comfortable than expected so money worries limit your horizons, which makes for a bitter end to a working lifetime.

It is usually a mistake to move home immediately on retirement, leaving behind the memories and networks of previous times. If you do intend to move try to plan it well before retirement, preferably building up a circle of friends in the area where you plan to go. Think very carefully about how you will manage physically – not just now but when your mobility worsens later, as it inevitably will. That short walk to the shops which seems so easy now may be a nightmare if you have angina.

Older people who get depressed get very depressed indeed. If you see this in yourself or your partner get help or try to persuade them to do so. Warning signs are poor sleep, morbid thoughts, loss of appetite and constant anxiety. Take particularly seriously any hint of suicidal intent – when an older person says this they mean it. People especially vulnerable are those who are living alone, recently bereaved, in poor social circumstances, drinkers and those with other serious health problems.

General health awareness

Without being obsessional about your health you should take seriously any new and persistent symptoms. The most important ones include weight loss, loss of appetite, passing blood in urine, bowel or the vagina, coughing blood, skin changes in moles, ulcers, chest pain, bone pains, difficulty passing urine, profound tiredness or lumps in the breast or elsewhere.

ADVANCED OLD AGE

After the age of 75 you must expect to have a number of health problems, with heart disease and arthritic disorders high on the list. Some general preventive measures can help you preserve your mobility, mental alertness and safety.

Accident prevention

The older you get the more you must anticipate accidents, as eyesight fails and agility diminishes. In women 60% of accidental deaths are after falls, especially following a fractured hip; the figure for men is 40%.

In the home Make your home safe. Have good lighting in the most hazardous areas – stairs, front and back steps and kitchen. Look at the risks of tripping: have carpets properly fitted, run electrical flexes by walls and not across a room, secure rugs so as not to catch your foot. Make spaces easy to navigate, placing tables and chairs so you do not keep bumping into them.

It may no longer be wise to cook on gas or to have a gas heater; electrical cooking and heating reduces the risk of fire. Food and cooking utensils should be within easy reach so step-ladders are not needed. Cigarette smoking is a common cause of accidental fires. Never smoke in bed.

In the bathroom, have grab handles to assist getting in and out of a bath, or else a shower seat, with safety handles within the shower. Run a bath in a safe way, letting cold water in first, then adding hot, so reducing the risk of scalding.

Wear well-fitting footwear – get rid of those old loose slippers, while for outdoors wear shoes with non-slip heels,

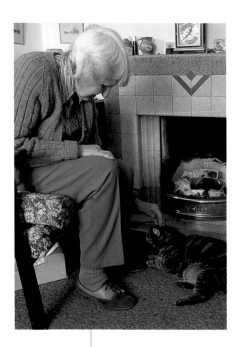

Above: However reduced your horizons, find room for warmth, entertainment and companionship.

which remain non-slip in wet conditions.

Many elderly people feel dizzy when they stand up as a result of changes in blood pressure. Get up slowly, holding something for support for a few moments until you feel ready to walk.

Outside When you go out be sure you know what you want to do. Write a checklist of what you need to buy and the places you have to visit – this way you should not find yourself confused and uncertain of where to go next. In bad weather consider whether your journey is really essential; this is especially so in winter when the risk of a fall on ice or snow is very high.

On the road Most insurance companies insist on a medical check if you continue to drive past the age of 75: your doctor will pay special attention to your eyesight,

alertness and mobility. If a time comes when you fail to meet the required standard, accept that driving is no longer in your best interests.

Road safety also includes safety as a pedestrian, which is why it is important for you still to have regular eye checks, to wear your glasses and to wear a hearing aid, if appropriate. Cross the road only at a designated crossing.

The figures reinforce the importance of these measures. In the over-75 age group, 20% of accidental deaths in men and 10% of those in women are the result of road traffic accidents, the bulk of them as pedestrians.

Activity

Reading the above you may think you should pass these years cocooned in cotton wool; this is not intended. It is important to take as much exercise as you feel capable of. Exercise keeps joints mobile – even those affected by osteoarthritis – and keeps up muscle tone. Gentle exercise will reduce the chances of osteoporosis. There is a psychological benefit from keeping everything moving as well as a social benefit from meeting people and from them expecting to meet you. If you fail to appear for a regular walk, this might trigger legitimate concern for your safety, a morbid but realistic thought.

Even if your exercise consists of simply walking to a corner shop, you should keep it up. Increasingly there are exercise classes and activities for the elderly: swimming or perhaps gentle aerobics and stretching exercises. You will know what level of activity is comfortable for you. Many people in their 80s and 90s can still walk briskly, do the gardening and visit places. Others are confined to their home, but they can still do some exercise – stretching the neck, swinging the arms, bending, lifting their legs. These keep joints mobile and can be done even if you have osteoarthritis.

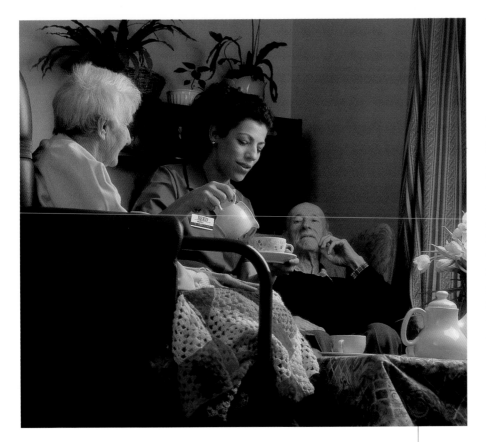

Above: There is often a good network of social support, which allows safe independence well into advanced years.

Diet

The older you get, the less you need to eat as your body's metabolism slows down. The principles of a healthy diet remain: avoid empty calories in bread and cakes, eat fruit, vegetables and fibre, eat dairy products for calcium. The days of worrying about cholesterol are behind you unless you have serious heart disease.

Physical comfort

Because you cannot get out so easily, make sure your home is always stocked with drinks and easily prepared convenience foods.

Warmth The elderly cannot control temperature as well as they once did; being less active affects temperature too. Have efficient heating and use it if you feel cold.

Walking aids However much you may resist it, there comes a point for walking sticks or a walking frame. It is far better to use these than, in mistaken pride, to go it alone and fracture your hip.

Mental agility

Keep your mind as active as possible, since evidence confirms that this delays the onset of memory and confusional problems. Read a daily newspaper and watch the news; this orientates you for time and place. Read books, magazines, racing tips – the subject does not matter as long as something is making you think, plan, remember and anticipate. Your mental stimulation may come from meeting friends and family, from going to bingo, from a day class, theatre trips or the cinema – the more the better.

Do not worry unduly about developing Alzheimer's disease. Even by their 80s about 80% of people do not have any serious memory problems, certainly none that interfere with their daily activities.

Medication

Almost inevitably an elderly person will be on medication for blood pressure, heart disease, diabetes, glaucoma, arthritis or chest problems. It is all too easy for doctors to prescribe one medication after another, any of which may cause you inconvenient side effects. The common ones to look out for are drowsiness, dizziness, constipation, urinary problems and indigestion. If you think your medication may be to blame discuss it with your doctor. Do not discontinue medication without discussion – especially for high blood pressure, the control of which is highly effective in reducing your risk of a stroke.

Depression

Depression is common because of all the losses of old age – loss of partner, family, independence and health. Maintaining as active a life as possible is the preferable way of dealing with this. However, persistent depression is dangerous because of a high risk of suicide and should be taken as seriously as depression in a younger person. Depression in the elderly is less likely to present with crying and morbid thoughts, but more likely in the form of self-neglect, appetite and weight loss and anxiety.

Alertness to symptoms

It is a mistake to think that symptoms should be ignored simply because of your age, while recognizing that there are many symptoms of age that doctors can do little for, such as dizziness, arthritis, poor vision and tiredness. You should still report to your doctor any symptoms that are new or that worry you – in particular, weight loss, persistent pains, bleeding from the bowel, bladder or vagina and palpitations.

INDEX OF SYMPTOMS

⚠ Back to Top

Shipment Details:

Shipping Method: Standard Ground (3 to 8 business days)

Shipping Preference: Ship everything together.
This option saves you money, but it will take longer to receive your order.

Gift Wrap: None

Health and Physical Assessment
Violet Barkauskas, C Darling-Fisher, L. C. Baumann, K. Stoltenberg-Allen, Kathryn Stoltenberg-Allen, Linda Ciofu Baumann
Format: Hardcover
Availability: In Stock. Ships within 24 hours.

Harvard Medical School Family Health Guide
Harvard Medical School, Anthony L. Komaroff (Editor)
Format: Hardcover
Availability: In Stock. Ships within 2-3 days

Our Price: $16.00
You Pay: $16.00

Our Price: $32.00
You Pay: $32.00

Product Subtotal: $59.25
Free Shipping & Handling: $0.00

Shipment Total: $59.25

Terms of Use, Copyright, and Privacy Policy
© 1997-2003 Barnesandnoble.com II

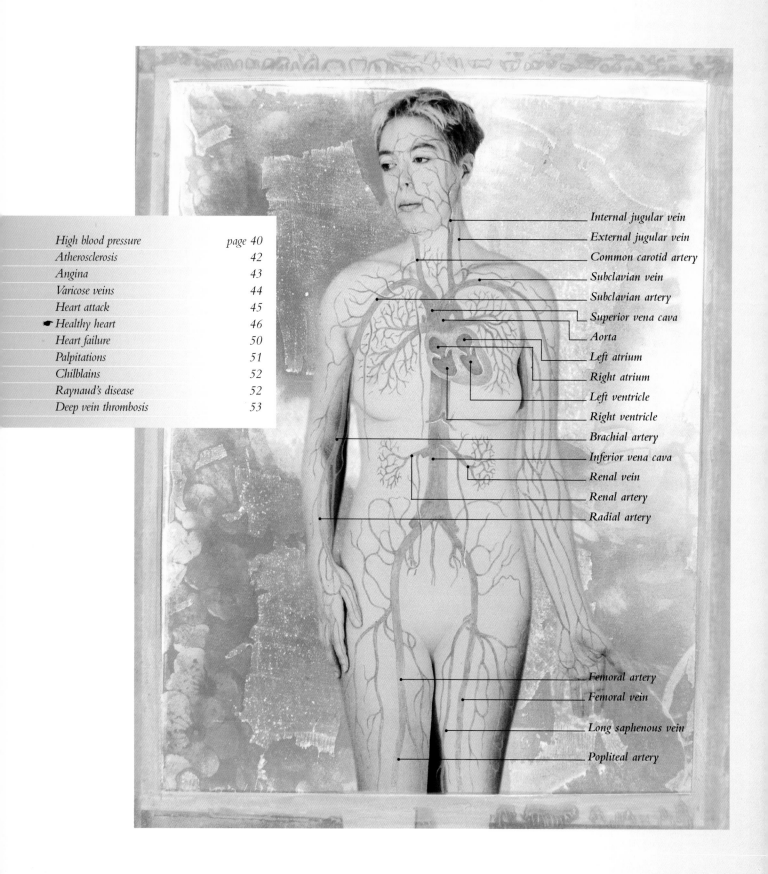

Internal jugular vein

External jugular vein

Common carotid artery

Subclavian vein

Subclavian artery

Superior vena cava

Aorta

Left atrium

Right atrium

Left ventricle

Right ventricle

Brachial artery

Inferior vena cava

Renal vein

Renal artery

Radial artery

Femoral artery

Femoral vein

Long saphenous vein

Popliteal artery

It could be said that the circulatory system, also known as the cardiovascular system, is all a matter of plumbing — but what plumbing! It consists of a pump, the heart, which keeps going for upward of 70 years and which anticipates the body's demands for output, and a system of pipework which is self-sealing and which continues to operate efficiently despite all degrees of cold, heat and posture.

CIRCULATORY SYSTEM

WE NEED A CIRCULATORY system in order to carry essential nutrients to every cell of the body: oxygen to keep energy production going; glucose, which is the basic fuel of the body; and all the chemicals and hormones essential to the regulation of our metabolism. In addition blood carries away waste products from the cells – carbon dioxide to be exhaled by the lungs, and other substances to be handled by the kidneys or by the liver.

The human heart is a four-chambered pump, which maintains a steady blood pressure and flow of blood. It has two sides: the left and the right. Each side has a chamber where blood arrives – the atrium and a powerful ventricle that pumps the blood. The circulation begins with the arrival in the left atrium of blood fresh from the lungs. This blood is carrying maximum amounts of oxygen and is therefore bright red – typical of arterial blood. With each beat of the left ventricle about 70 ml of blood is squeezed into the circulation. It enters the aorta, the great main artery 2.5 cm/1 in in diameter, from which blood flows into ever smaller arteries which eventually become microscopic in size.

The blood now enters the capillary system of blood vessels. These microscopic channels are so narrow that blood can flow through them only one cell at a time, finally reaching the furthermost cells of the body in the fingers and toes. It is at this stage in the system that oxygen is swapped for carbon dioxide and fuel is exchanged for waste products.

This ends the arterial side of the circulation. The blood now begins its homeward journey. Having lost its oxygen, its colour changes to the dark red typical of venous blood, such as we see after a minor cut. The blood returns via the system of veins, channel joining channel until eventually it flows through the great vena cava back to the heart.

Blood enters the right atrium. From here it passes into the right ventricle, from where it is pumped into the lungs. In the lungs carbon dioxide is given up, to be breathed out, and oxygen is picked up. The blood is once again fresh and red, fit to be sent around the body.

How the system is regulated

This whole system of heart, lungs, arteries and veins is regulated by complex controls. There are nerves that open and close blood vessels and that make the heart beat faster or stronger. There are chemicals that have the same effect. The best known is adrenaline, a surge of which sets our pulses racing and our hearts thumping when we are exposed to stress. There are many other subtle mechanisms which fine tune the efficiency of the circulation, including pressure detectors in the neck and within the heart itself.

Clearly there are many possible ways in which the circulatory system can go wrong. This section discusses some of the most common problems that arise.

Left: The heart pumps oxygen rich blood through arteries and capillaries; stale blood returns via the veins.

HIGH BLOOD PRESSURE

The condition of abnormally raised pressure within the arterial system, also called hypertension. It is one of the most common chronic health problems there is.

CAUSES

Overall ten to twenty per cent of the Western adult population has high blood pressure, depending on what definition is used. Most cases remain unexplained; it is not known why one person develops it and another does not. There is a suspicion that something in the Western way of life predisposes to high blood pressure, be it **stress**, diet, being overweight or high alcohol intake. High blood pressure also runs in families.

About five per cent of people with high blood pressure do have a specific identifiable cause – most often kidney disease, because blood pressure is partly controlled by a hormone system involving the kidneys called the renin/angiotensin system. Other rare hormonal causes include hyper- aldosteronism and a disease of the adrenal glands called Cushing's syndrome. Both of these produce changes in blood chemistry detectable in blood tests. In other uncommon disorders, for example phaeochromocytoma, there is a sudden release of hormones which increase blood pressure. These would be considered in a young person who has unusually high blood pressure.

High blood pressure may also be the result of high blood calcium. This, in turn, is caused by other disease and so needs to be investigated. Finally, certain anatomical abnormalities cause high blood pressure, for example coarctation of the aorta, which is a congenital narrowing of that great artery and which is suspected if there are weak pulses in the legs.

SYMPTOMS

Contrary to popular view, high blood pressure rarely causes any symptoms. Although some say they feel headachy or unwell with high blood pressure, objective studies do not bear this out, except in cases of extremely high pressure where there might be a very severe headache plus blurred vision.

How blood pressure is measured

Blood pressure is measured with a sphygmomanometer – a cuff, which is wrapped around the upper arm, connected to either a column of mercury or an electronic gauge.

There is an artery just below the surface at the bend of the elbow and the cuff is inflated to the point at which it closes the artery beneath it. The doctor then places a stethoscope over the artery and listens to its sound reappear. This is the point of systolic blood pressure and is the maximum pressure. It corresponds to the pressure as the heart gives a beat. Then the cuff is relaxed; as blood flows again there are characteristic changes in the sounds until a point is reached called diastolic blood pressure. This is taken to be the lower level of pressure and corresponds to blood pressure in between beats, that is, while the heart is momentarily at rest. Both figures are important and are given equal priority. Ideally, one should have a systolic no higher than 140 mmHg (millimetres of mercury) and a diastolic no more than 90 mmHg; the exact figures aimed at depend on age and associated risk factors.

The doctor will probably take blood tests, to check for kidney trouble or any of the rarer causes of high blood pressure mentioned earlier. Blood tests also help decide which drugs to use, for example someone with a biochemical tendency to **gout** should not be put on a diuretic (commonly known as a water tablet) since this can raise the uric acid responsible for gout. Cholesterol is checked and an electrocardiogram (ECG) and possibly a chest X-ray taken. These show whether the high blood pressure is putting a strain on the heart.

It is usual to check the pressure several times over a few weeks before deciding whether it is truly raised. This is because a single high reading can be a 'one-off' event.

TREATMENT

Why are doctors so keen to treat high blood pressure? Many trials have now shown that the higher the blood pressure the greater the risk of a **stroke**. This is understandable; put any liquid system under pressure and leaks are bound to occur. So it is with the arterial system. If an artery leaks it can cause paralysis and affects sight and thinking. In addition, sustained high blood pressure puts strain on the heart which, in time, can lead to **heart failure**. Lastly, really high blood pressure can damage the kidneys (see KIDNEY FAILURE).

Even a modest reduction in blood pressure lessens these risks, especially the risk of having a stroke. This holds across all ages; even hypertension in the elderly is worth treating to greatly reduce the risk of a stroke.

Self-help measures

Modern medicine has a wide range of drugs available, but before reaching for drugs there are some simple and extremely worthwhile self-help measures you can take. The most important one is to reduce an excessive intake of salt. Next, maintain an ideal weight: your doctor will tell you what to aim for. Relaxation through meditation, yoga or whatever

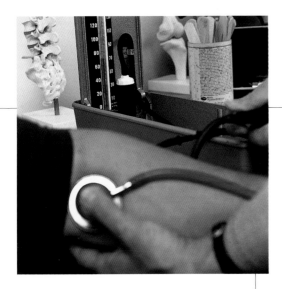

Above: Measuring blood pressure using a mercury-filled sphygmomanometer. Testing blood pressure is one of the most useful health checks.

else suits you has also has been shown to lower blood pressure. These simple measures can make all the difference to blood pressure which is just above borderline.

Assessing risk

There are some other factors to be considered in the treatment of high blood pressure, all of which increase the risk from even mild hypertension. These include smoking, a family history of heart trouble, raised cholesterol and diabetes. Having any of these risk factors makes it more important to treat even mild high blood pressure.

Drugs

If drug treatment is needed, the choice is large. Two classes of drugs stand out as first choice. Thiazide diuretics act on the kidney and, in low doses, are a tried and tested remedy for high blood pressure. Commonly used ones are bendrofluazide and hydrochlorothiazide. Then there are beta-blockers such as atenolol or propranolol. These drugs work on the heart and kidney and have more side effects than diuretics, such as causing cold hands, tiredness and breathlessness. They are very effective drugs and would be a first or second choice.

Newer agents

Angiotensin-converting enzyme (ACE) inhibitors are a fairly new class of drugs, increasingly used in treating younger people. They work on a subtle hormonal aspect of the kidney and also have a strengthening effect on the heart. Their main side effect is that they cause coughing. Common names are lisinopril and captopril. Another widely used class of drugs are calcium-channel blockers, which affect cell metabolism. Drug names include nifedipine and amlodipine.

Many of these drugs can be used in combination; in fact some 40% of people with high blood pressure need to be on two or more drugs to gain control. It often takes time to find drugs that suit the individual and control the hypertension. Thereafter reviews are needed three or four times a year, with occasional checks on blood chemistry and an ECG.

See also PROBLEMS IN PREGNANCY.

See also PROBLEMS IN PREGNANCY.

QUESTIONS

Is treatment forever?
Usually, high blood pressure will require lifelong treatment. However, some people's blood pressure does return to normal, typically on retirement, reducing stress levels or losing weight. In recognition of this fact, doctors might try reducing the patient's medication every few years.

Can nervousness increase blood pressure?
Certainly; doctors call this the 'white coat' effect. Measuring blood pressure continuously over 24 hours shows clearly that blood pressure varies remarkably at different times and in different situations and especially when with a doctor. Twenty-four hour monitoring of blood pressure will probably become more common as the cost of the recording equipment falls.

Complementary treatment

If you are on medication, you should maintain it. **Chakra balancing** – deep relaxation can bring blood pressure down as much as 20/20, a drop which can be sustained over several weeks. **Hypnotherapy** – used when the condition is first diagnosed, this can help reduce blood pressure and maintain the reduction. **Aromatherapy** can help by reducing stress and improving circulation. Try adding six drops of one of the following oils to your daily bath: lavender, neroli, clary sage, marjoram or ylang ylang. **Nutritional therapy** – eat wholefoods, plenty of fruit and vegetables and oily fish like herring. Strictly ration fatty, salty and sugary foods. **Ayurveda** would recommend specific yoga exercises, *panchakarma* detoxification, *marma* therapy, shiro dhara oil massage and steam baths. Oral treatments are also available. *Other therapies to try: tai chi/chi kung; autogenic training; auricular therapy; shiatsu do; yoga; cymatics; Western herbalism.*

ATHEROSCLEROSIS

The accumulation of a fatty material within blood vessels which underlies much heart and arterial disease.

CAUSES

In childhood the linings of the major arteries are smooth and clean. By late adulthood many people have atherosclerosis of the walls of their blood vessels – from atheroma, a mixture of fat and the breakdown products from blood clots. Cholesterol is one major cause of atheroma, deposits gradually building up on the lining of the arteries in the same way that water pipes become furred up with calcium salts. The abnormal layer of cholesterol affects the walls of the artery so that blood is likely to clot on it, something that should not normally happen. Over many years the original patch of cholesterol becomes overlaid and entwined with fibres of old blood cells. Eventually there is a significant obstruction to the flow of blood; symptoms begin to show. The arteries most liable to atheroma are those around the heart, the legs and the brain.

SYMPTOMS

Symptoms only appear when the blood flow is obstructed. If the arteries to the heart are affected, the earliest symptoms are **angina** – pain in the chest on exertion. Often the very first symptom may be an actual **heart attack**, with chest pain and breathlessness. Frequently, there is simply a general reduction in the efficiency of the heart, causing breathlessness and an inability to exert oneself. Some patients will go on to develop **heart failure**.

If the obstruction is in the arteries to the legs, the resulting symptom is pains in the legs, which begin on exertion and go after a few minutes' rest – termed intermittent claudication. Typically the pain is felt in the calf; the leg may feel constantly cold. In severe cases the toes may even start to decay from a form of gangrene. This is called peripheral vascular disease.

Atherosclerosis of the blood vessels in the brain leads to **stroke** or to a slow decline of mental function.

TREATMENT

Cigarette smoking makes atherosclerosis worse by increasing the tendency of the blood to clot, so it is essential to stop smoking. Similarly, **high blood pressure** and **diabetes** make it worse and should be dealt with.

Established obstruction can often be remedied by replacing or bypassing the diseased artery. For the heart this is coronary

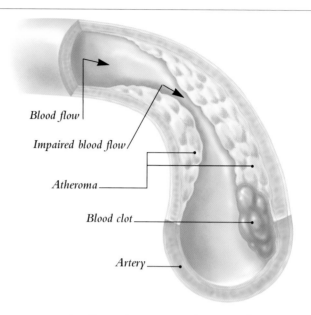

Blood flow

Impaired blood flow

Atheroma

Blood clot

Artery

Above: A cross-section of an artery affected by atherosclerosis, potentially causing pain, death of surrounding tissue and stroke.

artery bypass grafting (see ANGINA). The arteries to the legs can also often be either replaced or bypassed using artificial tubing. In most cases, however, obstruction to blood flow in the legs can be significantly bypassed simply through regular exercise over time. This encourages small new blood vessels to find a way round the diseased area. Only if this does not occur is surgery called for.

At present there are no proven treatments to improve blood flow to the brain (except surgery on the carotid arteries in the neck if narrowed by atheroma.) There is some prospect of drugs for improving brain circulation in the near future.

Raised cholesterol is widely recognized as underlying these problems. Ideally, diets should be adjusted to reduce cholesterol, otherwise a number of drugs can do this effectively.

 Complementary treatment

Autogenic training improves circulation via the relaxation response, allowing greater blood flow and reducing auto-aggression. The warmth from exercise is helpful, slightly raising skin temperature. Diet – a **nutritional therapist** will advise on good and bad dietary fats. Eat fresh wholefoods containing plenty of dietary fibre, B vitamins, and antioxidants – vitamins A, C and E, and selenium. **Ayurveda** would focus on cleansing, detoxification and diet. *Other therapies to try: tai chi/chi kung; cymatics; hypnotherapy.*

ANGINA

Chest pain due to poor flow in the heart's own blood supply, the coronary arteries.

CAUSES

The heart is a highly specialized muscle which, like any other muscle, relies on a steady supply of oxygen-rich blood to function efficiently. Anything that interferes with the blood supply will starve the heart of oxygen and cause angina.

The heart is supplied via four major arteries which are especially prone to blockage with atheroma, a mixture of cholesterol and blood (see ATHEROSCLEROSIS). Blockage builds up gradually over many years until eventually the restriction of blood flow is critical and angina starts.

Occasionally, other conditions cause angina in an otherwise healthy heart, for example severe **anaemia** or disorders of the valves controlling blood flow within the heart.

SYMPTOMS

The cardinal symptom is pain over the heart on exertion; this means pain over the central and left side of the chest. Angina pain also typically radiates away from the heart, so people with angina feel the pain rising up their chest towards the jaw and often down their left arm as well. There can be odd variants on this such as pain in one hand on exertion.

The other typical feature of angina is that it is relieved by a short rest. Unlike the pain of a **heart attack**, which it can closely resemble, angina pains last only as long as you exercise and disappear within a couple of minutes' rest.

TREATMENT

All people with angina need checking out for **high blood pressure**, raised cholesterol and anaemia. Smokers should quit as smoking makes atherosclerosis worse and the overweight should lose weight to reduce strain on the heart.

The simplest treatment is with a class of drugs called nitrates, which are related to tri-nitro-toluene – also known as TNT. These work by opening up the arteries to the heart just enough to bring extra blood flow and relief. They can be taken as single tablets, allowed to dissolve under the tongue, or a spray at the time of need. If angina is more frequent, they are given in longer-acting tablet forms, such as iso-sorbide mononitrate. Fairly recently, nitrates have become available as patches worn on the skin which release nitrates slowly over 24 hours. Other drugs used to treat angina are beta-blockers and calcium-channel blockers (see HIGH BLOOD PRESSURE).

Angina can be further investigated using a stress test, an ECG taken during exercise. This helps confirm the diagnosis and indicates the severity of the condition. If appropriate, the next step is coronary artery angiography: a catheter is guided to the heart from the femoral artery in the groin. A dye is then injected to show how blood flows around the heart. If this reveals serious blockage in the vessels coronary artery bypass grafting (CABG) may be required to replace the obstructed portion of artery with a vein graft. Other options are to dilate the narrowed section of artery via angioplasty (see page 49) or to insert a small tube called a stent. The decision to employ surgical, as opposed to medical, treatment depends on the individual's age and overall state of health and on how many and how severely coronary arteries are narrowed.

QUESTIONS

How safe is coronary artery bypass grafting?
Roughly 95–98% of operations are successful in relieving angina and in improving the quality of life. The main risk is having a stroke during surgery, which happens in about 1% of cases.

Why is low-dose aspirin useful in angina?
This remarkable drug reduces the blood's tendency to clot. Thus it decreases the chances of worsening arterial blockage in the coronary arteries, and is recommended for individuals with angina.

Does angina lead on to a heart attack?
Although a warning of heart circulatory problems, angina is a fairly safe condition to have. Only two to four per cent of cases a year progress to a heart attack. For many people angina can be managed by modest adjustments to lifestyle and simple medication.

Complementary treatment
Acupuncture – a typical point is Pericardium 4, on the arm, plus points on the chest and upper back. **Homeopathy** – possible remedies, depending on circumstances, include cactus, spigelia and naja. **Chakra balancing** can help prevent attacks by reducing blood pressure. Diet is important for prevention; a **nutritional therapist** will be able to advise. **Hellerwork** improves circulation and reduces tension around the heart. *Other therapies to try: Chinese herbalism; shiatsu do; autogenic training; biodynamics.*

VARICOSE VEINS

Unsightly and uncomfortable dilation of veins in the legs.

CAUSES

Varicose veins are one of the prices that human beings pay for standing upright. Being a low-pressure system for returning stale blood to the heart, veins are not sturdy structures and do not cope well with the higher pressure of a column of blood when upright. Their walls stretch and distort and eventually form the familiar worm-like varicosities. This is why people who spend a lot of time on their feet are at risk of these.

Anything that interferes with the return of blood through the veins will also increase pressure and predispose to varicose veins. The most common reason is pregnancy, since the enlarged womb obstructs blood flow from the legs back into the abdomen. For similar reasons, a large growth within the abdomen may show itself as varicose veins. They may also follow years after a **deep vein thrombosis**. However, many people have simply inherited the tendency from their parents.

Varicose veins lead to stagnation of blood flow. There is a tiny but significant leakage of blood from the veins, eventually leading to a brownish discoloration of the lower limb.

SYMPTOMS

There are soft, blue, dilated blood vessels in the legs, usually around the ankles, calf and in the groin. They may ache. As time passes they become more prominent and irregular in shape and are there all the time and not only while the individual is standing. Most people have only cosmetic problems but some develop swelling, scaling and irritation with discoloration of the leg and eventually extensive, chronic ulceration around the ankle.

Phlebitis is a blood clot within the varicose vein, which then looks red, feels painful and is hard. Although uncomfortable, it is not a dangerous condition, as opposed to deep vein thrombosis.

TREATMENT

The varicose veins of pregnancy can be expected to go after delivery. Losing weight reduces pressure within the abdomen and this, too, will relieve mild varicose veins.

Wearing a support stocking helps the return of blood and is a sensible alternative to surgery, but many people do eventually need surgery, either because of the aching or through unhappiness with the appearance of their legs.

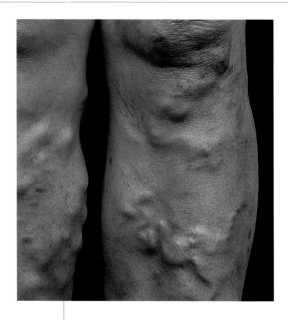

Above: Typical dilated and distorted varicose veins below the knee – one of the most common sites for this condition. Surgical treatment is the only cure for such severe and established varicose veins.

There are two types of surgery. One is to strip out the whole varicose vein from the groin to the ankle. This is rather brutal surgery; moreover this vein may be useful one day for coronary artery bypass grafting (see ANGINA). The other method is to tie off the deeper veins which feed the surface veins. This calls for a series of cuts down the leg to reveal the feeder veins, which are then tied with surgical thread.

Whatever the surgery, varicose veins tend to recur unless lifestyle changes are made to avoid standing or to lose weight.

See also ULCERS.

Complementary treatment

Homeopathy – the treatment depends on circumstances, for example if the varicose veins worsen with warmth and swinging the legs, pulsatilla might be appropriate. **Aromatherapy** can strengthen the circulatory system and improve the tone of the veins. Try adding six drops of one of the following oils to your bath: cypress, geranium or lemon. Inverted **yoga** positions can reduce swelling. **Ayurveda** would recommend *panchakarma* detoxification and *marma* therapy.

HEART ATTACK

◆

Sudden severe chest pain due to blockage of blood flow to the heart. Medically called myocardial infarction (MI).

CAUSES

◆

Most heart attacks are the result of a blood clot suddenly forming in coronary arteries diseased with **atherosclerosis**, thus blocking blood flow to part of the heart. The heart reacts to the drop in blood supply, as any other muscle does, with pain and loss of function. This means that the heart fails to beat efficiently, leading to sudden **heart failure**. It may go into chaotic rhythms or stop altogether.

Sometimes heart attacks happen in the absence of atherosclerosis, and the cause is unclear. The heart might suddenly go into an abnormal pattern of beating for some reason. Sometimes there is disease of the heart muscle itself, a cardiomyopathy, which carries an increased risk of heart attack. Other causes are electrical shocks or a blow to the chest.

SYMPTOMS

◆

The first symptom is severe pain over the breast bone or the left side of the chest. The pain feels like it is deep inside the chest as if something is squeezing or crushing internally. Unlike **angina**, the pain persists for many minutes or hours. There is sweating from the pain and the sufferer looks grey.

Severe heart attacks cause heart failure, with breathlessness; the victim may turn blue from poor blood flow, fall unconscious or collapse. It can happen that the first symptom is when the individual cries out with a sudden chest pain and collapses immediately. Even in this apparently hopeless situation victims should still have cardiopulmonary resuscitation (see page 354) as there is a chance of recovery.

Not all heart attacks are painful. In the elderly especially a heart attack may be suspected because of rapidly appearing heart failure or sudden vague tiredness or **stroke**.

Besides the clinical picture, the diagnosis depends on finding characteristic changes in the ECG or on detecting enzymes released by the damaged heart into the blood stream.

TREATMENT

◆

In recent years there have been some great advances in the treatment of heart attacks, thanks to drugs popularly called 'clot-busters'. These dissolve the abnormal blood clot within the coronary arteries. They should be given by drip immediately, although it is still worth giving them within 24 hours of the heart attack. Drug names are streptokinase and urokinase.

Even before this treatment, a heart attack victim should swallow an aspirin because this humble drug actually reduces the stickiness of the blood and so reduces the size of the blood clot in the arteries. Together, these measures have led to a remarkable 30% drop in the immediate death rate.

Long-term treatment

A low daily dose of aspirin (75–150 mg) reduces the chances of a further blood clot and should be taken lifelong. Drugs called ACE inhibitors and beta-blockers strengthen the heart and help prevent abnormal heart rhythms. Cholesterol should be reduced to low levels by diet or drugs if necessary and, of course, you must stop smoking. Some people, after investigation, may need coronary artery bypass grafting (see ANGINA).

QUESTIONS

Can shock bring on a heart attack?
Sudden emotional shocks set the heart racing and may start an abnormal heart rhythm. This does increase the risk of a heart attack in those people whose coronary arteries are already diseased with atherosclerosis.

How dangerous is a heart attack?
Despite recent medical advances it is always dangerous. About 30% of all heart attacks lead to death within 24 hours. Another 10% of victims die within the next month from complications. Thereafter there is a 5–10% lifelong annual risk of death.

How important is it to reduce cholesterol?
Latest research shows that reducing cholesterol cuts the risk of further heart trouble by up to 40%. This can be achieved by rigorous dieting or, increasingly, by taking cholesterol-lowering drugs.

Complementary treatment
This is a medical emergency and no complementary therapy can help in the immediate short term. Many therapies, however, are excellent in the rehabilitation stage. **Yoga** and **tai chi/chi kung** are gentle forms of exercise that can be very beneficial during recovery. Diet is very important; a registered **naturopath** or **nutritional therapist** will be able to make suggestions tailored to you, your condition and your constitution. *Other therapies to try: see STRESS.*

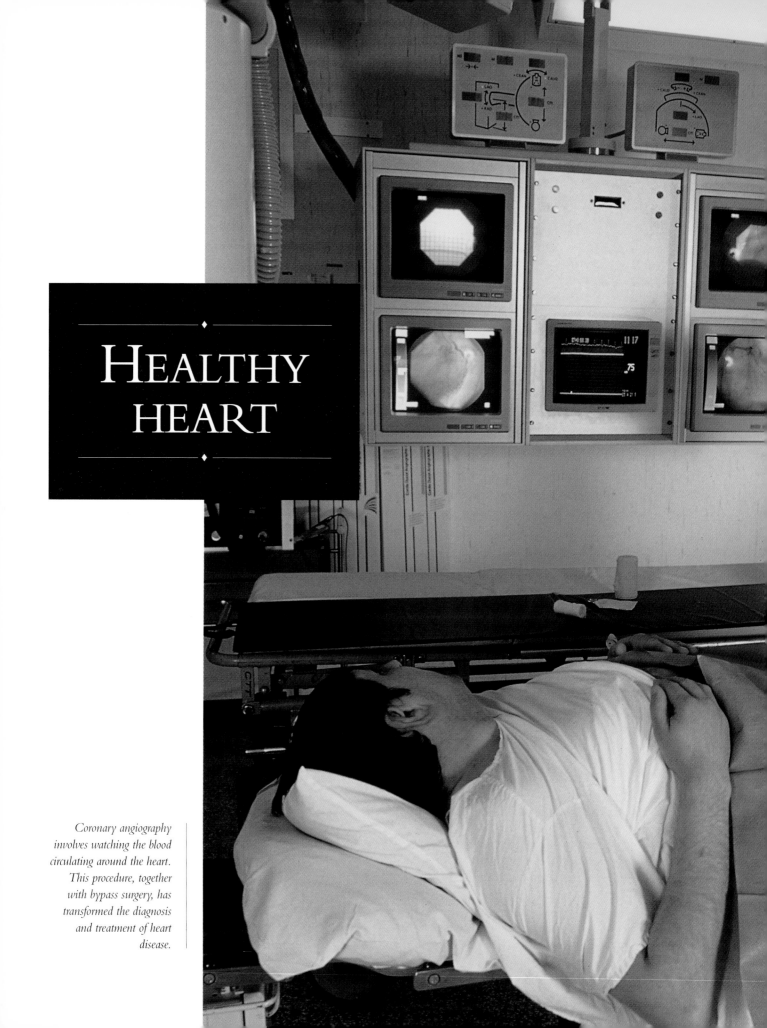

HEALTHY HEART

Coronary angiography involves watching the blood circulating around the heart. This procedure, together with bypass surgery, has transformed the diagnosis and treatment of heart disease.

Risk factors for heart disease can be divided into those you may have some control over and those you do not (see below right). The two sets interlink. For example, if you have a family history of heart disease, it is even more advisable to do something about those things you can control. Moreover, risks do not just add up as in $2 + 2 + 2 = 6$; rather they multiply as in $2 \times 2 \times 2 = 8$. Depressing? Not necessarily. It means that reducing smoking or cholesterol intake has an even greater benefit than you might think.

Your heart must last a lifetime

Smoking and poor nutrition during pregnancy increase the chances of having a low birthweight baby. It would appear that such children have an increased risk of heart disease as adults. Although the link is as yet controversial and unexplained, it is sensible not to smoke during pregnancy and to eat properly.

Childhood Evidence suggests that obese and overfed children grow into overweight adults who are more at risk of heart disease. Set a pattern of healthy eating habits from an early age and also encourage your children to get plenty of exercise and play sports.

Adult life Continue the habits of eating healthily and taking exercise. Check your cholesterol and blood pressure from time to time to make sure that levels are as they should be. Do not smoke.

Old age Now is the time to pay more attention to your blood pressure and to concern yourself less about cholesterol. An active life promotes good health. **Diabetes** is an important risk factor for heart trouble and if it is present it should be carefully controlled.

Early recognition of heart trouble

You do not want your first symptom of heart trouble to be a **heart attack**. Rather, you should take note of the early warning symptoms.

High cholesterol may cause changes in the eye area in some people. You may notice a white ring around the iris (coloured part) of the eye – the medical name for this is an arcus senilis. This is normal in people over the age of 60, but if you are younger than that it is advisable to have a cholesterol check. Another warning sign which needs to be checked by a doctor

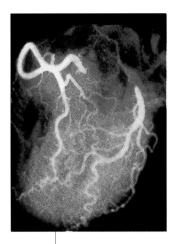

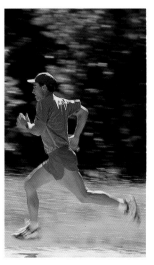

Above: Coronary angiograph showing blood flow through the heart's own arteries. Right: Regular exercise can provide pleasure as well as promoting health.

RISK FACTORS FOR HEART DISEASE

These can be divided into those you may have some control over and those you do not:

No control
- *Being male*
- *Adverse family history*
- *Age (risk increases with age)*
- *Congenital heart disease*
- *Infections such as rheumatic fever or diphtheria*

Some control
- *High cholesterol*
- *High blood pressure*
- *Smoking*
- *Obesity*
- *Lack of exercise*

MISCELLANEOUS FACTORS LINKED WITH HEART DISEASE

◆

These are factors where research suggests a link to heart disease, but the weight to be attached to them is debatable:

Protective factors

♦ *Alcohol – drinking 2–3 units a day (a couple of glasses of wine)*
♦ *Hard water, high in calcium salts*
♦ *Warm climate*
♦ *Higher socio-economic class*
♦ *Vegetarian and vegan diets – people following these diets probably benefit from an improvement in their harmful/beneficial blood–fat ratio*
♦ *Fruit and vegetables – these appear protective thanks to vitamin E and other antioxidants*
♦ *Other trace minerals may be relevant, for example selenium – an area of vigorous current research*
♦ *Taking HRT after the menopause*

Harmful factors

♦ *Stress – people who make their own stress and are hard-driven appear at greater risk*
♦ *The cold – unaccustomed exertion in cold weather is risky, for example shovelling snow*
♦ *Salt intake is probably significant. Do not add salt to food*

is yellow plaques on the skin beneath the lower eyelids – the medical term is xanthelasma.

Chest pain on exertion This is **angina**, the classic warning of heart trouble. It means that the coronary arteries cannot deliver an adequate blood supply to the heart muscle when under exertion. Not all chest discomfort is from angina by any means, but it is the most important possibility to exclude.

Breathlessness A heart with a poor blood supply is inefficient at pumping blood, and breathlessness may be a consequence. Again, there are many more innocent reasons possible, so do get a medical opinion.

Modern investigations

Modern technology allows the clinical impression of heart disease to be objectively proven. The basic tests are harmless and straightforward: first, an exercise ECG, an electrical recording of the heart while running or walking briskly on a treadmill. This shows whether there is a blood flow problem even in people whose resting ECG is normal, and detects about 75% of such cases. If there is still doubt, you might have a radioactive scan of the heart. If that is normal, it is highly unlikely that you have significant heart disease.

Another important investigation is an echocardiogram, to show the valves of the heart beating and to give an idea of how efficiently the heart is working.

A number of people can be diagnosed only by coronary artery angiography (see page 316), where a dye is injected into the circulation around the heart to check for narrowing of the coronary arteries. This carries a one-in-thousand risk of death, so it is used only in order to plan surgery or, rarely, to exclude heart disease in someone getting pains suggestive of heart disease but where all other investigations are normal.

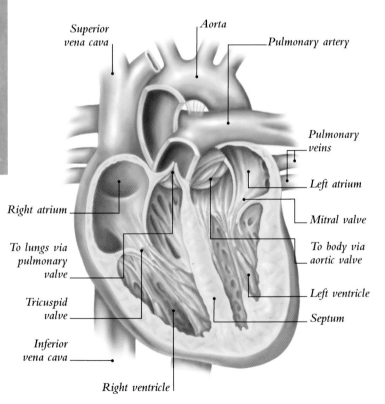

Above: So much in the heart could go wrong, yet it usually remains impressively reliable for many decades.

Angioplasty This means opening up coronary arteries narrowed by **atherosclerosis**. It is an important alternative to coronary artery surgery. A thin tube is guided to the heart from the large femoral artery in the groin. Once it reaches its destination, instruments are inserted through the tube to clear the blockage.

Coronary artery surgery This involves replacing diseased arteries with a vein graft from the leg or from the chest. It is highly effective and can be repeated if the grafts block up, which happens in five to ten per cent of people each year.

Heart transplantation This amazing technology has, in 30 years, moved from experiment to routine. It is reserved for people who have no other hope of survival and who are otherwise healthy. There is now the very real prospect of an artificial heart that can be inserted more easily than those currently available, or even of using hearts taken from specially bred pigs. Such developments would transform the prospects for people with **heart failure** which is treatable by no other means.

Treatment of a heart attack

If you experience a sudden constant central chest pain and breathlessness, assume you have a heart attack until proven otherwise. Early treatment greatly improves the outlook, so ring for an ambulance. Take an aspirin immediately, as this reduces the size of the clot forming in the heart.

Once in hospital, you will be given an injection of a clot-busting drug such as streptokinase, unless you are one of the small number who should not have it, for example if you have had recent surgery or a history of abnormal bleeding, especially from the gastrointestinal tract.

For at least six months after recovery you should take a beta-blocking drug such as atenolol to prevent abnormal heart rhythms. You will probably have to take an ACE inhibitor such as ramipril to reduce the chances of heart failure. These modern measures have lowered the risk of death from a heart attack by some 40%.

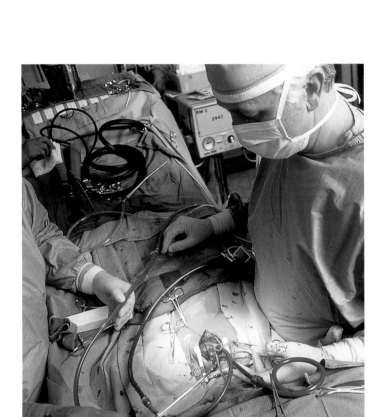

Above: A child has received a new heart. The surgeon inspects his handiwork before removing the pipes that have kept circulation going.

Effective therapy

Never has there been such a wide range of treatment for heart trouble and it should be possible to find something that suits you. Medical treatment is the preferred option, pending exact diagnosis of the state of blood flow in the heart. It may be as simple as taking an aspirin every day. This reduces the tendency of the blood to clot and thereby lessens the risks of a heart attack. It has side effects, especially bleeding from the stomach, so cannot be recommended to everyone, but for those who either have angina or have had a heart attack it is a lifelong option.

HEART FAILURE

An inefficiency of the pumping action of the heart because of some underlying disease or problem.

CAUSES

The heart is made of tough, durable, specialized muscle which beats with impressive reliability for a lifetime. It follows that most cases of heart failure result from a **heart attack** or **atherosclerosis** of the blood supply to the heart. These both diminish the amount of blood flowing through the heart and so reduce how well the muscle can pump, as well as leaving areas of damaged muscle which pump less efficiently.

Other common causes are **high blood pressure** and irregularities of heart rhythm outside the steady 60–90 beats per minute of the normal heart. This rhythm allows for efficient flow of blood around the body. This efficiency is reduced if the heart beats very fast (above about 120 bpm), very slowly (below about 40 bpm), or irregularly (see PALPITATIONS). There are many other uncommon causes of heart failure.

Heart failure affects about one per cent of those over the age of 65. It used to carry a grim outlook but this has changed in recent years thanks to the latest medication.

SYMPTOMS

The earliest symptoms of gradual heart failure are tiredness, breathlessness and swelling of the ankles. These result from the sluggish flow of blood, which is relatively poorly supplied with oxygen. The body responds to the failing heart by retaining salt and water, and a back-pressure effect results in swelling of the legs. Eventually fluid also builds up in the lungs, leading to increased breathlessness especially when lying flat, which is why people with heart failure find they need to sleep propped upright with pillows and wake breathless during the night if they roll off the pillows. Certain basic investigations should be done, for example chest X-ray, blood count and ECG.

Acute heart failure

This usually follows a heart attack; there is sudden breathlessness and coughing of frothy phlegm. The victim often turns blue because of poorly oxygenated blood.

Heart failure can often be diagnosed simply on examination. The doctor hears characteristic sounds of fluid on the lungs and notices neck veins distended with blood returning from the head that the heart cannot pump away fast enough.

There are also signs of fluid on a chest X-ray and of heart strain on an ECG. The most reliable way to detect heart failure is with an echocardiogram of the heart; this also detects otherwise unsuspected disease of the valves of the heart.

TREATMENT

For immediate treatment diuretic drugs by mouth or, in urgent cases, by injection force fluid out of the lungs and cause a high output of urine. This reduces the volume of blood to be pumped and also blood pressure, relieving strain on the heart. They are life-saving measures.

For long-term treatment many people with heart failure need continuous low dosages of diuretics such as frusemide or bumetanide. A class of drugs called ACE inhibitors has emerged as being highly effective in improving heart function; they are increasingly used in all age groups.

Several other less common causes are eminently treatable, for example severe **anaemia**, thyrotoxicosis (see THYROID PROBLEMS) or problems in the valves of the heart. Diseased coronary arteries can be treated by CABG (see ANGINA).

QUESTIONS

Can heart failure be cured?
It cannot really be cured but it can be controlled. Common measures to control it are to treat high blood pressure, to lose weight and to reduce salt intake.

What is the role of a heart transplant?
This is reserved for otherwise healthy people, including those who have suffered heart attacks in the past for whom all other measures have failed. It is a marvellous treatment with a steadily rising success rate, despite the need to stay on powerful anti-rejection medication (see page 331).

Complementary treatment

Do not abandon conventional approaches. **Western herbalism** – treatments for water retention might be useful. **Chinese herbalism** remedies can strengthen the heart and circulatory system. Diet – a registered **naturopath** or **nutritional therapist** will be able to advise on how you can switch to a balanced diet, low in saturated fats. **Healing** can be effective in promoting circulatory function. **Yoga** and **tai chi/chi kung** are gentle forms of exercise with much to offer.

PALPITATIONS

An unusual heart rhythm, often entirely harmless.

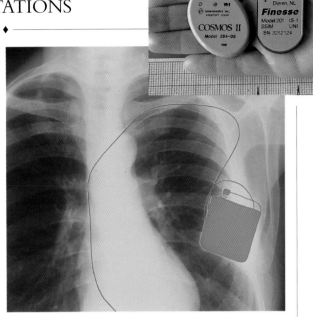

Top: *Electronic pacemakers.*
Above: *X-ray showing a pacemaker implanted below the skin near the armpit; the wire carries electrical signals to the heart.*

CAUSES

The heart beats regularly thanks to a remarkable electrical system that sends the signal to beat along nerves that form electrical pathways from a 'pacemaker centre' to the rest of the heart. This system ensures that the muscle of the heart beats in an orderly and efficient way; problems with it, however, are extremely common. Everyone at some time experiences harmless, innocent variations of rate and rhythm.

There are innumerable causes of unusual heart rhythms, including **stress**, caffeine, alcohol and inhalers for **asthma**. The diagnosis is often difficult to confirm. Modern devices can record all heartbeats for 24 hours, which can then be computer analysed in search of abnormalities.

Rapid rhythms

A heart rate above 100 per minute causes palpitations and is abnormal. Likely causes are atrial fibrillation, where the rate is rapid and irregular, or thyrotoxicosis (see THYROID PROBLEMS). It is very common to have bursts of rapid heartbeats between perfectly normal rates. This may occur in fit young people with no underlying heart abnormality but may also be a feature of underlying heart disease such as **atherosclerosis**.

Slow rhythms

If the heart misses a beat, as it often does, the catch-up beat is unusually hard and will be felt as a thump in the chest. Another common cause is heart block. In this condition there is interference with the electrical flow, so that the heart beats at its own natural rhythm which can be as low as 20 beats per minute. Slow rates can be due to a severely underactive thyroid gland (see THYROID PROBLEMS).

SYMPTOMS

Palpitations are common so take note only if a nuisance or if you notice breathlessness, chest pain or tiredness, which suggest they are putting a strain on the heart and need checking.

TREATMENT

Many cases prove wholly free from disease and need no treatment other than reassuring the patient the heart is basically healthy. Such cases are helped by reducing heart stimulants such as coffee, alcohol, smoking or certain medication.

Rapid rhythms

Several drugs can control these rhythms; the best known is digoxin – most commonly used to treat atrial fibrillation, a rapid and chaotic beating of the heart. Other drugs include amiodarone and verapamil. Beta-blockers are widely used to slow the heart and they also have a mild antianxiety effect. The treatment for really fast rates unresponsive to drugs is to shock the heart back into a normal rhythm. This has to be done because otherwise the heart becomes exhausted.

Slow rhythms

Heart block is treated with a pacemaker. This fires a regular electrical signal so that the heart beats steadily (see page 330).

Complementary treatment

Chakra balancing – the therapist can help by working over the whole heart. **Nutritional therapy** – deficiencies may be to blame, especially deficiency of B vitamins or magnesium. **Healing** can bring an irregular heartbeat into balance. **Hypnotherapy** calms and lowers heartbeat, and stabilizes palpitations. **Ayurvedic** yoga and oil massages would be recommended, possibly with *panchakarma* detoxification as well. *Other therapies to try: tai chi/chi kung; acupuncture; autogenic training; cymatics; auricular therapy; homeopathy.*

CHILBLAINS

Areas of skin that have been damaged by the cold.

CAUSES

Chilblains are a mild form of frostbite. The final stage in the circulation of blood around the body is via the capillaries, minute channels that reach into the furthermost parts of the body – generally the fingertips, toes and skin. In cold conditions some of those capillaries can be damaged, which in turn reduces blood flow to that small patch of skin. The result is that a few skin cells die, the skin surface breaks and a small ulcer forms. Anyone can be affected by chilblains if their skin becomes chilled enough.

SYMPTOMS

The most commonly affected sites are fingers, toes and the nose. The initial cold injury is painless and often overlooked unless you happen to notice a small patch of white flesh.

There then follows intense irritation due to the release of breakdown products from the cells that have died. After a day or two a small ulcer appears as a red spot.

TREATMENT

Protection against the cold is the basic precaution – wearing gloves, thick socks and face protectors. If you notice a white chilled area of skin warm it gently by rubbing. Established ulcers should have a smear of antiseptic cream. Drugs are available that increase blood flow to the skin, for example calcium antagonists such as nifedipine, but are used only in the most severe cases.

Complementary treatment
Aromatherapy – make up three drops of lemon oil in 10 ml of carrier oil. Massaged daily over the toes, this should aid prevention of chilblains. *Other therapies to try: Western herbalism.*

RAYNAUD'S DISEASE

Fingers and toes that go cold and numb unusually readily.

CAUSES

This is a problem with the tiny blood vessels in the fingers and toes. In people with Raynaud's disease these blood vessels are oversensitive to cold; they narrow in response to very minor changes in temperature and are slow to relax again on rewarming. The disorder is more common in women and often other family members are affected.

Occasionally there is some other underlying condition that attacks the blood vessels, such as **systemic lupus erythematosus**, but this would give other symptoms as well. In such cases the condition is called Raynaud's phenomenon. It can also result from using vibrating machinery for long periods of time, and from taking beta-blockers for **high blood pressure**.

SYMPTOMS

When the fingers or toes get even slightly chilled they go first white, because of constriction of the tiniest arteries in the digits, and then blue, because of the resulting poor and stagnant blood flow. They feel numb; as they warm up they gradually

regain normal colour, and often ache until fully recovered. In severe cases the skin becomes fragile, possibly breaking down into small **ulcers**. The whole cycle can last minutes or hours.

TREATMENT

Use common sense; dress warmly and avoid exposure to the cold. Avoid smoking, too, since nicotine causes blood vessels to constrict. Those with severe disease can obtain electrically heated gloves and specially insulated footwear.

There are safety regulations about the use of vibrating equipment in factories. If beta-blockers are the cause, there are many alternatives. Drugs called calcium-channel blockers can help by opening up the blood vessels, but are used only for extreme cases. You may need blood tests to check on the rare illnesses that can underlie severe cases.

Complementary treatment
Nutritional therapy – try supplements of fatty acids. **Ayurveda** would use detoxification, oil massage and steam baths with oral circulatory stimulants. *Other therapies to try: cymatics; tai chi/chi kung; chakra balancing; autogenic training; Western and Chinese herbalism.*

DEEP VEIN THROMBOSIS

◆

The result of blood clotting, usually in the veins of the legs.

CAUSES
◆

Blood flow through the veins is a more leisurely affair than the urgent rush of blood through arteries. This increases the risk of blood clotting – a risk that is increased by anything that further reduces blood flow such as bed rest, especially after a **stroke** or **heart attack**, immobility as on long flights and, most commonly, immobility during operations. There are also tiny risks from taking oestrogen in the contraceptive Pill and hormone replacement therapy (HRT).

The veins in the legs, deep within the calves and thighs, are the ones most at risk of thrombosis. A further risk is that a small clot in the calf later extends up the leg and even into the major veins within the abdomen. The greatest worry from a deep vein thrombosis is that a portion of the blood clot may fly off and lodge in the lungs, causing a **pulmonary embolism**.

SYMPTOMS
◆

There may be no symptoms at all but often the affected limb suddenly swells up and feels painful. It is usually the calf that swells but it can be the whole leg. The calf looks red and is extremely tender to pressure. Without tests it is frequently impossible to tell whether the cause of a red swollen calf is infection or thrombosis. One test is an ultrasound scan of the veins in the leg, which is good at detecting large clots. The other test is a venogram. This involves injecting a dye into a vein in the foot in order to reveal on X-ray the whole system of veins in the limb. This can detect much smaller clots.

TREATMENT
◆

The aim is to prevent further clot formation, which is done by taking warfarin, a drug that reduces the 'clottability' of the blood. A course of eight to twelve weeks is usual. If there is a major blood clot extending into the abdomen, surgery may be a possibility to remove it, but this is a dangerous procedure. Small clots are left alone; the body gradually dissolves them.

Deep vein thrombosis is such a hazard of surgery that great effort has gone into finding ways of preventing it. One method is to inject heparin at and around the time of surgery. This drug reduces the clottability of the blood but not so much that it increases bleeding during surgery. Another technique is for the patient to wear compression stockings during the operation; these increase the rate of blood flow and so reduce the

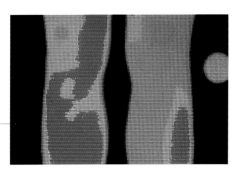

Right: Thermography (heat measurement) revealing thrombosis in the right calf.

chances of stagnation. Finally, all patients are encouraged to become mobile as soon as possible after surgery, in order to reduce the risk of thrombosis. A woman who has had a thrombosis must not take the ordinary contraceptive Pill.

QUESTIONS

How does phlebitis differ from deep vein thrombosis?
Phlebitis is a blood clot within a surface vein, causing a tender, firm, inflamed area. This is not dangerous and responds to anti-inflammatory drugs such as ibuprofen.

How big a risk is deep vein thrombosis?
It is extremely common after a stroke or heart attack, abdominal surgery or hip replacement. The associated pulmonary embolus is one of the major complications after these types of surgery.

Can deep vein thrombosis recur?
Having one increases the chances of having another, so always inform a surgeon if you have had a thrombosis. You should also avoid anything which increases the risk such as the contraceptive Pill and prolonged bed rest. On long journeys you should try to walk around regularly or move your legs about.

    Complementary treatment
If you suspect a deep vein thrombosis, you should seek a conventional medical opinion immediately. **Yoga** and **tai chi/chi kung** are gentle forms of exercise which can be beneficial after recovery. Diet is important in preventing recurrence. A **naturopath** or **nutritional therapist** could help you switch to a balanced diet, containing plenty of wholefoods. Eat plenty of fish, not just white fish, and take fish oil supplements. Also supplement your vitamin E intake, and take garlic supplements.

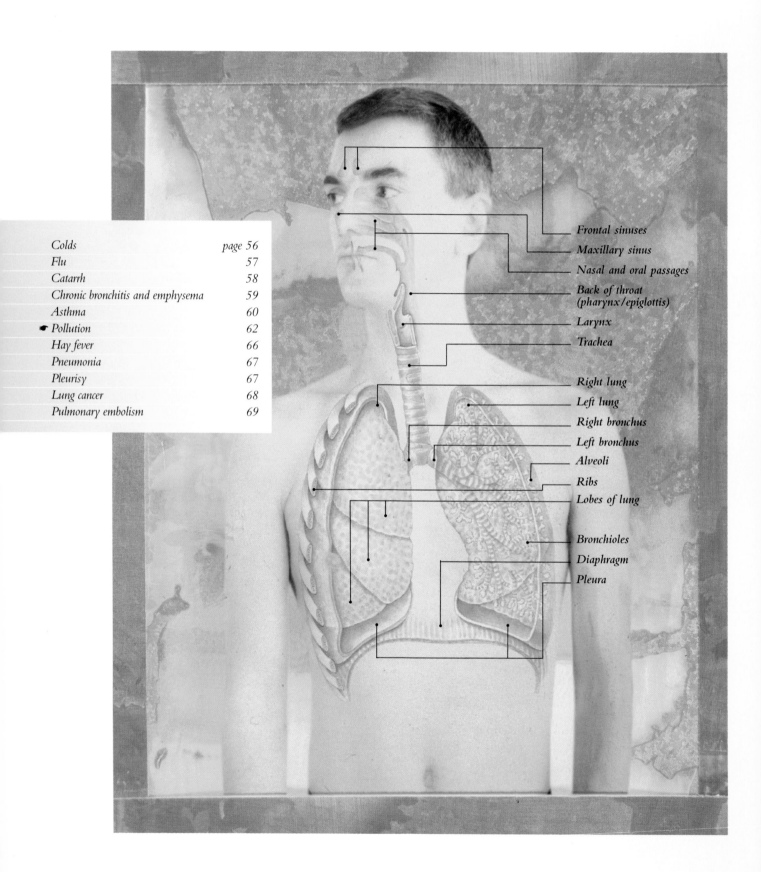

Frontal sinuses

Maxillary sinus

Nasal and oral passages

Back of throat
(pharynx/epiglottis)

Larynx

Trachea

Right lung

Left lung

Right bronchus

Left bronchus

Alveoli

Ribs

Lobes of lung

Bronchioles

Diaphragm

Pleura

*Like any engine, the body needs oxygen to burn fuel.
It also needs a means of disposing of carbon dioxide, which is a
byproduct of the process of generating energy. The respiratory
system performs both of these roles efficiently.*

RESPIRATORY SYSTEM

THE FUNCTION OF THE respiratory system is to bring fresh air into as close a contact as possible with blood within the lungs. This is achieved at air sacs, called alveoli, which form the bulk of the sponge-like lungs. In the alveoli air is separated from blood by the thickness of just two cells. This allows oxygen to permeate into the blood, where it is snatched up by the haemoglobin molecules. At the same time carbon dioxide also diffuses across the membrane from the blood stream into the air sacs. When you breathe out, carbon dioxide is released into the atmosphere; when you breathe in, oxygen-rich air rushes into the lungs.

The pathway to the alveoli is via tubes of ever-narrowing diameter – the bronchi and bronchioles. The great airway is the trachea; this splits into left and right main bronchi, which further subdivide in a branching pattern down into the lungs. The smaller airways, the bronchioles, have a muscle layer which can constrict or dilate them and so adjust the amount of air passing through the lungs.

An adult's lungs have some 300 million alveoli with a total surface area of 60–80 m²/645–860 sq ft. The lungs are designed to filter out dust particles from the inhaled air by trapping them in a layer of mucus; specialized cells then sweep the dust up and out of the lungs. By the time air reaches the alveoli it has become warmed or cooled to body temperature and made just moist enough to optimize gas exchange.

The breathing process

The actual process of breathing is mainly the result of the diaphragm descending, as well as the muscles between the ribs lifting them. The net result is to expand the volume of the chest – and the lungs expand into that volume. Expiration follows through relaxation of the diaphragm and the muscles between the ribs, plus the elastic recoil of the lungs.

Breathing is mainly an unconscious activity that is controlled by the brain, but you can take control of your own breathing to some degree. The depth and rate of breathing responds to the acidity of the blood, which, in turn, is a reflection of how much carbon dioxide it contains. This is detected by specialized cells within the brain and major arteries, which also detect oxygen concentration. You can force yourself to breathe slower or faster but you cannot will yourself to stop breathing, nor can you breathe rapidly for more than a few minutes without causing chemical changes in the acidity of the blood, which trigger the brain to take back control.

The human respiratory system is a very flexible one. Whereas at rest the lungs will be shifting 5–8 litres of air a minute they can increase this 20–30 fold to up to about 200 litres a minute.

Breathing disorders can arise in many different ways – some are caused by environmental problems – and they are extremely common.

*Left: Within the myriad air sacs
of the lungs, blood exchanges waste
carbon dioxide for fresh oxygen.*

COLDS

A viral infection of the nose and upper airways.

CAUSES

There are over 120 different viruses that may cause colds. The first time you meet such a virus it is likely to cause a cold because you have no natural immunity. This is why children get so many colds and adults, who have acquired some immunity, get far fewer. Even so, three or four a year is common. People in offices or areas with poor ventilation are more at risk because of their exposure to others with colds.

SYMPTOMS

The first symptoms are a sore throat, a vague feeling of tiredness and aching muscles. You may have a fever, even though you feel cold and shivery. This lasts for two or three days, then the nose begins to run. You start sneezing and coughing and feel pretty miserable for two to three days. Most colds take seven to ten days from start to finish, although it is normal to continue to cough for a week or two afterward.

In children, complications often occur, especially **ear infection** with pain and perhaps a discharging ear, or a chest infection with coughing and wheezing. Adults can get these secondary infections, but far less often than children. More common in adults are inflamed sinuses, giving pain over the front of the face and a feeling of pressure above or below the eyes on bending forward.

TREATMENT

In the early stages stay warm, take plenty of fluids (to relieve pain in the throat) and paracetamol to reduce temperature and aching. Adults can take aspirin if they prefer, but children under 12 should not have aspirin as it can cause Reye's syndrome, with convulsions and liver damage. Although Reye's syndrome is rare, it is usually fatal. Paracetamol (Calpol) is safe for children, or an alternative called ibuprofen.

Antibiotics are of no value at this stage. They usually make no difference to the illness and there is the chance of side effects, such as rashes, **diarrhoea** and **thrush** in the mouth or vagina. Only if you develop a complication such as a painful ear or a mild bronchitis might an antibiotic be advisable. Even then antibiotics hasten recovery only by a couple of days and so should not be seen as a miracle cure.

Other helpful measures are taking aromatic sweets, which help unblock congested passages, and avoiding smoky or

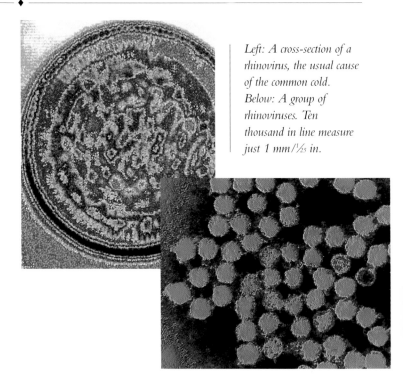

Left: A cross-section of a rhinovirus, the usual cause of the common cold. Below: A group of rhinoviruses. Ten thousand in line measure just 1 mm/$\frac{1}{25}$ in.

fume-filled atmospheres, which set off sneezing or coughing.

There are many cold cures available at the chemist. These contain a combination of a painkiller, such as paracetamol, and caffeine which gives a 'lift' to your spirits. Some contain a drug which narrows the blood vessels in the nose and thus relieves the runny nose for a few hours (this is also how nasal sprays for colds work). There may be an antihistamine, which also relieves the stuffiness and helps you sleep. These remedies are helpful, but should only be used for a few days and only if they do not interact with any regular medication you are taking (your pharmacist will advise if in doubt).

The common cold is usually easily recognizable and does not need medical attention unless you or your child seem to be suffering more than you might expect.

Complementary Treatment

Aromatherapy – see FLU. **Nutritional therapy** – at the first symptoms take a level teaspoon of pure vitamin C dissolved in water or juice. Repeat every two hours until symptoms subside, then tail off slowly, reducing the dosage and increasing the time interval between doses. If any bowel discomfort occurs, reduce the dosage. Continue to take vitamin C and a cod liver oil capsule daily as a preventive measure. *Other therapies to try: most have something to offer.*

FLU

A viral illness causing sweats, aches and high fever.

CAUSES

Flu, or influenza to be precise, is an infectious illness caused by a number of viruses. Every two or three years a new strain of flu virus emerges from the Far East, works its way across Asia and eventually arrives in Europe. There are always large numbers of otherwise healthy people who catch the illness simply by chance, especially those working or living in institutions, old age homes or offices, where the virus can spread easily. Vulnerable people, for example the elderly and people with chronic illnesses such as heart disease, **chronic bronchitis** and **diabetes**, do not catch the virus more easily but are much more prone to develop serious consequences from the infection such as **pneumonia**.

Unfortunately, resistance to any one strain of the flu virus is only short-lived; in addition, the virus changes from year to year which is why flu is an annual problem. About once every decade the virus becomes particularly aggressive for some reason and causes a serious epidemic.

SYMPTOMS

Flu typically begins abruptly with high **fever**, intense shivering and aching in all and any of the muscles. Backache is a common feature, as are headaches. There is usually a sore throat and often a cough develops after a couple of days. Unlike the common cold, there is no sneezing or running nose. However, in the early stages it can be impossible to decide whether someone is going down with flu or whether they are in the early stages of a common cold. Occasionally people can deteriorate rapidly with a serious chest infection and confusion. For most people, however, the illness lasts for five to seven days and gradually goes. Post-flu tiredness is common and can last for several weeks after the original infection.

TREATMENT

Because flu is a viral illness there is no specific treatment that will cure the infection. Instead doctors concentrate on treating any complications that arise. These are most commonly chest infections, which would be treated with antibiotics. Otherwise the patient should stay warm and drink lots of fluids. Fever should be treated with aspirin (but not for children under 12 years old – see COLDS) or paracetamol. This also relieves the muscular aches and pains. In some cases hospital treatment may be needed, for example if the patient is becoming dehydrated or has a serious chest complication.

Flu vaccination is a good idea if you fall into one of the higher risk groups such as diabetics. The single vaccination is given in late autumn, in time to allow a build-up of immunity before the peak flu season, which is late December/January in the northern hemisphere. There is a trend to offer vaccination to everyone over 65 because flu hits the elderly hardest and carries a risk of death in severe cases. Flu vaccination should also be considered by people working in institutions for the elderly and sick, where flu may spread very rapidly.

QUESTIONS

Why do I get flu several times a year?
You are probably getting a flu-like illness, with fever, aches and pains. Any viral illness causes these symptoms in the early stages. Many people call the common cold flu, which drives doctors to distraction. People are surprised at how much more severe true flu is than what they have been calling flu.

Is flu vaccination harmful?
There is no serious risk associated with this vaccine. As it is made from egg protein anyone allergic to eggs must not have it. Also, as with any vaccine, it should not be given if you are already ill with another infection.

Is any other treatment helpful?
A drug called amantadine, originally used for Parkinson's disease, reduces the severity of flu. It is an under-used treatment. Vaccination against the bacterium pneumococcus gives long-term resistance to infection from this germ, which causes many of the complications of flu.

Complementary Treatment

Western herbalism – ginger and cinnamon tea will provide warmth; infusions of elderflower, yarrow and peppermint will help regulate temperature. The following **aromatherapy** oils are helpful: eucalyptus, cajeput, tea tree, sage, thyme. Use them as chest rubs (three drops to 10 ml carrier oil), inhalations (two to four drops in a bowl of hot water or on a handkerchief) or in the bath (six drops). **Nutritional therapy** – see COLDS. *Other therapies to try: most have something to offer.*

CATARRH

◆

Sticky mucus that builds up in the nose or throat.

CAUSES

Mucus is a natural product of the body and protects against infection by trapping germs. In the nose, throat and airways of the lungs there is an elegant system which produces a thin layer of mucus on those linings. The mucus is cleared from the lungs and sinuses by specialized cells with minute hairs which beat it away. When infection occurs, the lining responds by increasing its production of mucus; in addition it sends in large numbers of white cells to attack invading germs. This turns the normally clear mucus into mucus that is stained yellow or green by the debris of invaders and defenders and this is the discoloured mucus that people call catarrh when they cough it up, blow it out or feel it dripping down the back of their throat.

Some people complain that the flow of mucus is constant or is excessive, although what one person finds excessive is normal to another.

SYMPTOMS

Catarrh usually begins after a cold or cough. Those affected have to keep clearing their throat or blowing their nose and are aware of thick secretions at the back of the throat. They may lose their sense of smell and have bad breath and a nasal twang to their voice. There is often a dull ache in the front of the face over the sinuses. People with chronic catarrh lead their lives within reach of handkerchiefs and boxes of tissues.

TREATMENT

Mucus is a natural defence mechanism of the body and it is by no means necessary to have treatment for temporary increases in the flow of mucus where the body is simply doing its job. If the mucus is very heavy, persistent and yellow or green it is reasonable to have an antibiotic. The exact choice of antibiotic depends on where the catarrh is coming from. Decongestant sweets clear sinuses through their aromatic oils. Most cases of catarrh will settle naturally in time over a few weeks.

For chronic cases the path is less straightforward. The doctors will search for chronic infection in the sinuses or lungs by taking X-rays and culturing the mucus to see if a specific antibiotic is required. A child with persistent mucus from one nostril may have pushed a toy or bead up his nose;

this is usually easily discovered on inspection and is a very satisfying diagnosis all round.

Catarrh is more common in smokers and those working in dusty atmospheres. Excessive alcohol and constant emotional stress also contribute to chronic catarrh by affecting the lining that secretes the mucus. However, this leaves many people in whom no obvious cause can be found. Steroid nasal sprays can help by reducing swelling of the lining of the nose, as do antihistamines as given for hay fever. As a last resort an ENT (ear, nose and throat) specialist might cut out the mucus-secreting lining of the nose.

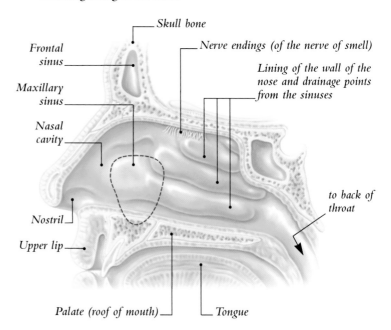

Above: Catarrh comes from the lining of the nose and the sinuses, which drain into the nose. The quantity increases in response to infections and allergies.

Complementary Treatment

  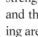

In **auricular therapy** mucus is held to be a by-product of a weak digestion, so the treatment aims to strengthen the function of both the digestive system and the lungs. In **aromatherapy** treatment the following are excellent as inhalations (two to four drops in a bowl of hot water or on a handkerchief): cajeput, eucalyptus or ravensara. **Nutritional therapy** – avoid dairy produce for a week. **Ayurveda** offers nasal inhalations, alongside dietary advice.

CHRONIC BRONCHITIS AND EMPHYSEMA

Two closely related lung diseases, both associated with coughing, wheezing and breathlessness.

CAUSES

Underlying both of these common conditions is chronic irritation of the lungs. This irritation is most often from cigarette smoke and its associated tars; other sources are air pollution, dust from industrial processes and coal mining. These irritating pollutants stimulate the lining of the small airways of the lungs to produce large quantities of mucus. Mucus is the sticky material that traps dust particles; specialized cells then normally sweep the mucus away from the narrowest parts of the lungs to the larger airways and ultimately the gullet, where the mucus can be swallowed or spat out.

Over time – meaning decades – the irritated lungs produce ever greater quantities of mucus, leading to a persistent cough. In addition, the airways narrow, leading to wheezing and breathlessness. In emphysema the further complication is that the tiny sacs at the ends of the lungs decay into large cavities. These are inefficient for gas exchange and add to the feeling of breathlessness.

SYMPTOMS

The earliest features of bronchitis are persistent cough and the constant bringing up of mucus. The cough gradually lasts longer until the individual is coughing all year round. **Colds** keep going to the chest, causing increased amounts of mucus and worsening breathlessness. People with emphysema have similar symptoms with, additionally, an over-inflated chest, giving a barrel-chested appearance. However, there is much overlap between bronchitis and emphysema and the exact diagnosis may not be clear without tests of lung efficiency. Eventually sufferers of both diseases can become constantly breathless even when walking a few steps and are effectively housebound. Severe cases also put a strain on the heart.

TREATMENT

At the earliest signs, it is essential to stop smoking and avoid irritating dusts. Although this will not repair the damage done, it reduces the chances of further deterioration. Medical treatment is with a gas inhaler, of which there are many types. These contain drugs called bronchodilators, which relax the muscles that otherwise tend to squeeze the already narrow airways even narrower. Those affected need to use these

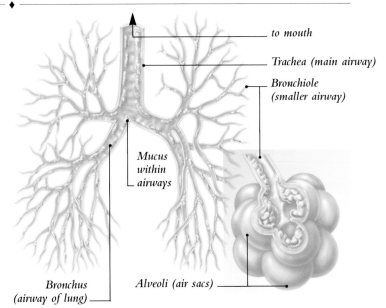

Labels: to mouth; Trachea (main airway); Bronchiole (smaller airway); Mucus within airways; Bronchus (airway of lung); Alveoli (air sacs)

Above: In chronic bronchitis the airways of the lungs over-produce mucus. In emphysema, the alveoli break down into large cavities, where air stagnates.

inhalers several times a day, often in combination. Examples of drugs used are terbutaline and salbutamol. Steroids given via inhalers are very helpful in reducing inflammation within the airways; the most commonly used is beclomethasone.

As well as being used in an inhaler, all these drugs can be given via a nebulizer, which produces a cloud of gas easily breathed in from a face mask. During flare-ups it may be necessary to take high doses of steroids by mouth.

Infections have to be treated aggressively with antibiotics because each infection can damage more of the lung. Many patients need to have oxygen available at home or in portable cylinders for when they go out. Very recently there has been interest in performing operations to remove the part of the lung damaged by emphysema, allowing the other parts to expand and so work more efficiently.

Complementary Treatment

A Chinese herbalism remedy would be *Quing Qi Hua Tan Wan* (clean air and transform phlegm). **Acupuncture** points for the lungs include Bladder 13 on the upper back and Lung 5 on the arm. **Nutritional therapy** – ensure your diet is rich in vitamin C and other nutrients. **Ayurveda** offers dietary advice and yoga breathing exercises. *Other therapies to try: auricular therapy; Alexander Technique.*

ASTHMA

Wheezing and breathlessness caused by reversible narrowing of the airways in the lungs.

CAUSES

For oxygen to enter the blood stream and carbon dioxide to leave it, blood has to come into close contact with inhaled air. Within the lungs this takes place in innumerable tiny sacs reached by ever narrower tubes. Here inhaled air passes over blood vessels and the exchange of gases takes place – the stale carbon dioxide passes out of the blood stream and oxygen passes in. The walls of these tubes contain muscle, which, if it contracts, squeezes the tube narrow and conversely lets it widen as it relaxes. In asthma, this muscle is abnormally sensitive and so the walls can be squeezed narrow unusually easily, thereby obstructing the free flow of air. Often, these small airways are also oversensitive to irritants in general, so asthmatics frequently also suffer from **hay fever** and **eczema**.

The easiest way to gauge this obstruction to airflow is called PEFR (peak expiratory flow rate). This is measured by blowing hard into a meter that shows how much air you can shift in litres per minute. This measure is useful in deciding the diagnosis and in monitoring treatment.

Just why certain individuals are affected by asthma is not known. However, about ten to fifteen per cent of children get asthma and a high percentage of adults, too. These numbers are increasing as a result, it is believed, of worsening air pollution as well as commonly found irritants such as cigarette smoke and the house dust mite. It may also be that mild asthma is being recognized more readily by doctors.

SYMPTOMS

During an asthmatic attack, people become increasingly wheezy and feel breathless; their rate of breathing rises and they literally have to force their lungs hard to get air in and out, which can be quite exhausting. An asthma attack is a dramatic event but fortunately is relatively uncommon as a first sign of asthma.

A common early symptom of asthma is a persistent cough with a little wheezing, especially during the night – frequently the first symptom in children. They may feel fine until they exert themselves, which brings on the wheezing. These symptoms are made worse by anything that irritates the lungs; this includes dust, fumes, emotional excitement, changes of temperature, furry pets and pollen. Certain drugs can also bring on attacks in susceptible people, for example beta-blockers (for high blood pressure) and anti-inflammatory drugs.

In babies with asthma simple **colds** will always 'go to their chest' and any cough is complicated by accompanying wheeziness. If the baby also has eczema it is highly likely that the child will develop true asthma as she gets older.

There is often a period of uncertainty before the diagnosis is definite. The key to making the diagnosis is to show that the obstruction to airflow – the wheezing – can be reversed quickly by treatment. This is where the peak flow test is useful. During even mild asthma there will be a measurable reduction in peak flow. For example, an adult woman who should have a peak flow of around 550 litres per minute may achieve only 350 but after a couple of puffs of an inhaler the peak flow rises back to normal. Thus both the doctors and the individual can keep a record of how effective treatment is. It is frequently a question of trying various antiasthmatic treatments to see how the individual responds.

TREATMENT

The modern treatment of asthma has three strands. These are removing irritants, reducing the sensitivity of the lungs and treating acute problems.

Removing irritants
All asthmatics should stop smoking. It is more difficult to control household dust but measures can include fitting special bags to vacuum cleaners to filter dust and wiping surfaces frequently so dust does not build up. Many people worry about the house dust mite, an insect found in enormous quantities in the cleanest home. Asthma is made worse by sensitivity to their droppings. It is impossible to eliminate these mites but regular cleaning helps and very sensitive individuals can cover pillows with polythene before placing them in pillowcases. Think carefully before you buy a furry pet as people with asthma may develop sensitivities to animals, especially cats, and it is hard to remove a much loved pet.

Prevention
Preventive treatments consist mainly of inhaled steroid drugs, which have revolutionized the treatment of asthma in the last 20 years. They deliver very small quantities of steroids straight into the lungs, where they reduce the sensitivity of the lining of the lungs. Understandably, people worry about the side effects of steroids, such as weight gain, **diabetes** and poor growth. These are possible only where large quantities are taken by mouth over many months. Inhaled steroids are very

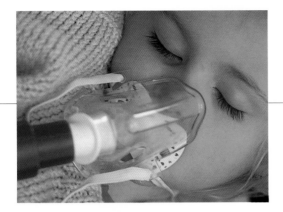

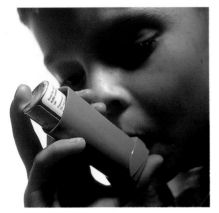

Above and left: Asthma treatment works best as a gas. Older children can handle self-triggered inhalers; young children need a mask.

safe and have not been shown to carry any significant risk. Drugs include beclomethasone and budesonide. There are many devices to deliver these drugs – all rely on producing a fine spray of gas to be breathed deep inside the lungs.

Cromoglycate is an alternative non-steroid preventive drug, very effective in some people. Again, it works by reducing the irritability of the linings of the lungs.

Acute treatment

Drugs called bronchodilators are used to treat acute attacks. They have a direct action on the muscles in the walls of the airways, forcing them to relax, thereby allowing the airway to open up and so ease the flow of air. Drug names include salbutamol and terbutaline. These drugs are given by inhaler, injection, nebulized fine spray or tablet.

In severe attacks it is normal to add a steroid by mouth; this delivers a very high dose with the aim of reducing inflammation rapidly. Typically this would be given for five to ten days. Even young children can benefit from a short course of steroids during a severe attack.

In-hospital treatment might include oxygen and broncho-dilating drugs given directly into the blood stream via a drip.

The most difficult group to treat is very young children, because their immature lungs do not respond to the standard treatments in the same way as the lungs of older children and adults. Even so, nebulized bronchodilators can help from about nine months of age. Syrups are also available.

Measuring the effectiveness of treatment

Treatment should allow the individual to follow a normal life, which includes exercise and sport. This may not be achieved in the most severe cases, but it is the goal for the great majority and if their treatment does not achieve this then it needs reviewing. Regular PEFR measurement helps show how good treatment is and also warns of any deterioration.

People with severe asthma may have to adjust their lives by giving up jobs involving dust or fumes and giving away pets.

QUESTIONS

Is allergy testing useful?

Generally it is not, because most asthmatics will prove to be sensitive to predictable things such as the house dust mite or pollen. It can be useful if asthma occurs in certain settings or is of recent severe onset, which suggests something very specific is responsible. Allergy testing might help establish whether or not to keep a pet.

Do people grow out of asthma?

A large percentage of mildly wheezy children grow out of it by late childhood. People who still have asthma by late childhood or who develop it as adults are likely to have it lifelong.

Complementary Treatment

Do not abandon conventional approaches. **Chinese and Western herbalism** both offer herbs to reduce the oversensitivity of the airways – experienced practitioners will advise. **Homeopathy** can be extremely effective, but it is impossible to generalize about treatment, which depends on many variables. The **Alexander Technique** is particularly effective in dealing with breathing difficulties and chest problems. It encourages a release of undue muscle tension in the neck and chest, which can lead to a gradual increase in chest capacity. Diet – consult a **nutritional therapist** or a **naturopath** for advice. **Chiropractic** manipulation in the upper back can help loosen the chest area and aid breathing. **Ayurveda** offers *panchakarma* detoxification, yoga breathing exercises, dietary advice and *marma* therapy. **Hellerwork** improves breathing dramatically, and eases tension caused by difficulty in breathing. *Other therapies to try: chakra balancing; acupuncture; healing; autogenic training; hypnotherapy; tai chi/chi kung.*

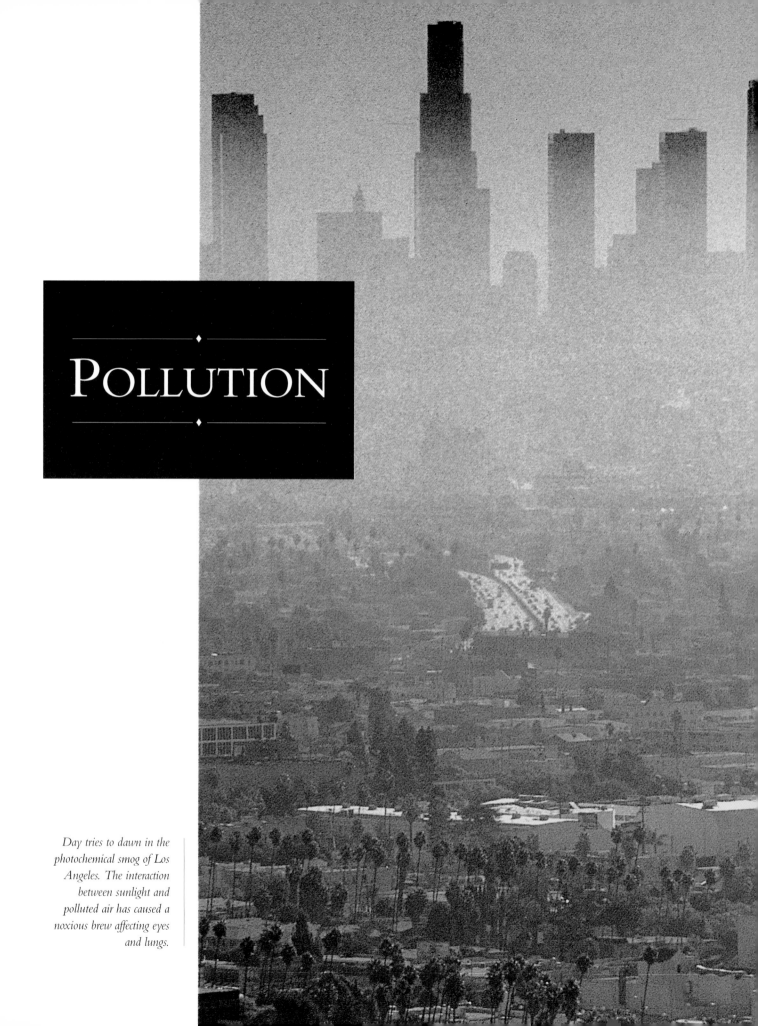

POLLUTION

Day tries to dawn in the photochemical smog of Los Angeles. The interaction between sunlight and polluted air has caused a noxious brew affecting eyes and lungs.

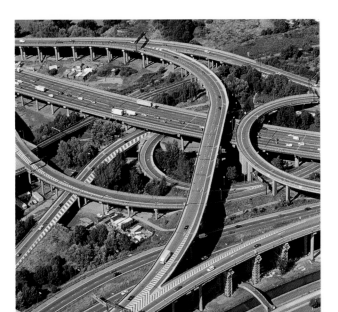

Above: Fumes from vehicles (shown here at a busy interchange in the United Kingdom) are potentially controllable causes of air pollution.

WHILE OUR HIGHLY INDUSTRIALIZED, technological society has many benefits in terms of advanced medical care, economic growth and improved living standards, the Earth is paying a price that is already impacting upon our lives and will do so even more in the future. The 200 years of the Industrial Revolution have introduced waste products of an unprecedented nature and scale that threaten the stability of the whole Earth's environment.

It was probably the photographs taken of the Earth from space that first made us realize that ours is really quite a small planet, limited in its capacity to absorb pollution. The composition of the whole atmosphere is endangered by destruction of the ozone layer, global warming and acid rain.

Ozone depletion

Ozone is a molecule of three oxygen atoms, formed by ultraviolet radiation splitting oxygen molecules in the upper atmosphere. The 'ozone layer' refers to a concentration of ozone in the stratosphere about 15–50 km/9–31 miles above the surface of the Earth. This is a beneficial shield protecting life from the damaging effect of ultraviolet radiation emitted by the sun. In contrast, the ozone formed in the lower atmosphere by sunlight reacting with pollution such as that from car exhausts, industry and the burning of fossil fuels is harmful to animal and plant life.

It is believed that the ozone layer formed some 400 million years ago as plants emitted oxygen, a byproduct of photosynthesis, the conversion of carbon dioxide and water into organic chemicals. By reducing the intensity of ultraviolet radiation, the ozone layer allowed life to venture out safely on to dry land from the protective waters.

The ozone layer has always been affected by natural environmental influences such as volcanic eruptions and solar flares. Now there is evidence that it is being reduced by human activity, mainly by the use of chemicals called CFCs (chlorofluorocarbons) in refrigeration, solvents and aerosols.

What happens? Increased ultraviolet light multiplies the risk of **skin cancer**, **cataracts** and possibly genetic damage. It may damage micro-organisms, affecting fish populations and food production. However, much of this is still theory.

What can be done? In 1992 more than 70 countries signed the Montreal Protocol, an agreement that CFCs would be phased out. However, because they remain in the atmosphere for decades, it will be many years before regeneration of the ozone layer is possible; a reduction in the speed of its decline is the most that can be achieved in the short term.

Global warming

The temperature of the world has always fluctuated and has been a major factor in driving evolution. The Earth's temperature depends largely on the insulating properties of the atmosphere and the balance between heat gained from the sun and heat lost by radiation from the earth. This balance is threatened by gases given off by industry, especially carbon dioxide, largely from burning coal and wood and from car exhausts; methane, from agriculture and rubbish tips; nitrous oxide, from burning coal and oil, and from nitrogen fertilizers; and CFCs.

What will happen? These gases trap more heat in the atmosphere leading, in theory, to global warming. The concentrations of these gases have risen as a consequence of the 100-fold increases in global energy use in the last 200 years. As the world emerged from the last ice age, global temperatures rose by about 5°C/9°F over several thousand years. Now, computer models used by the Intergovernmental Panel on Climate Change predict a rise in temperature of 1.5–4.5°C/2.7–8.1°F by the end of the 21st century – an astoundingly rapid rise. This rate of change is 2–5 times faster than that to which ecosystems are able to adapt.

It is believed that the result of global warming will be much more unstable weather, with more droughts, cyclones and floods, bringing increased susceptibility to disease and to heat-related deaths. Tropical diseases such as **malaria** may spread to previously temperate zones. Some low-lying islands may be lost altogether as polar icecaps melt and the sea levels rise.

What can be done? The way ahead is not at all clear. Experts do not agree whether global warming is a true phenomenon or just a temporary blip in climate. There is not yet any worldwide agreement on the threat, let alone coordinated action to counter it. Many developing countries continue to rely on coal and wood burning, while in the developed world people remain wedded to their cars. Scientists fear that pollutant gases will actually increase as a consequence of escalating industrialization.

Acid rain

This phrase is not an invention of the modern Green movement but was first used in the 1850s in Manchester. Acid rain is mostly from sulphur dioxide dissolved in water, forming sulphuric or sulphurous acid. Some is from nitrogen oxides, from vehicle exhausts. These gases are given off in vast quantities by industrial processes that burn wood or coal; the worldwide output into the atmosphere has increased from 7 million tons per annum in 1860 to over 150 million tons by the late 1980s.

What does it do? By increasing the acidity of rivers and lakes, acid rain kills fish, damages forests and so indirectly affects human wellbeing. Drinking slightly acidified water appears not to have any direct effect on human health.

What can be done? Stringent environmental industrial controls in the developed world are reducing the output of sulphur dioxide gases. These are still major pollutants in the developing world, especially China and India.

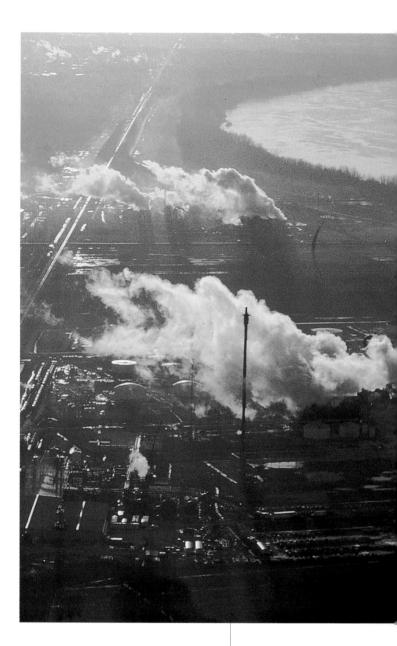

Above: Fumes drift from chemical plants in the United States. The developed countries have the technology to reduce such emissions, if they have the will.

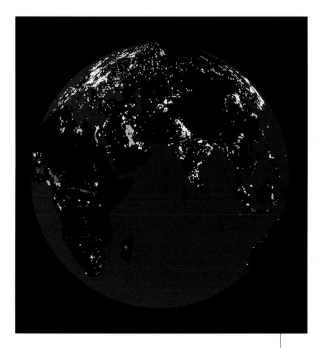

Above: Europe (upper left), Africa (lower left) and Asia (right) at night. City lights glow white, forest fires red, burning gas yellow.

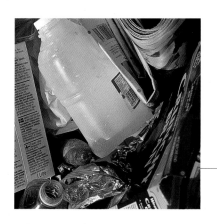

Left: Another day's trash: plastics, metal, chemicals, paper. Life is unimaginable without them, but becoming unbearable with such refuse.

Pollution – localized issues

Our economy depends on thousands of industrial processes using thousands of chemicals, many of which are toxic if they escape into the air, food and water.

Air Our air is contaminated by gases, dusts and tiny particles called particulates. It appears not so much that one single component causes damage but rather the cocktail of pollutants if further degraded by ultraviolet light. This can cause photochemical smog, as in Los Angeles.

The effect on health of the output of a single factory or power station is hard to measure except in the case of unusual accidents, for example the release of toxic fumes at Bhopal in India, which killed 2500 in 1984. However, general atmospheric pollution is responsible for a great increase in **asthma**,

chest conditions and eye irritation. Carbon monoxide is emitted by vehicles, cookers and heating devices, an excess causing headaches, drowsiness and even coma and death.

Lead pollution was much greater in previous centuries than now; output has more than halved in the last 25 years thanks to control of lead in petrol, paints, toys and plumbing. The effect of lead in the air is controversial but it does appear to reduce IQ in children. If eaten, lead causes **anaemia**, abdominal pains and nausea.

Dust is a serious atmospheric pollutant, linked with asthma and chronic chest diseases such as **bronchitis**. There is increasing concern about dust from diesel fumes.

Water Negligent disposal of waste – chemical residues, pesticides and metals such as lead, copper and mercury – almost inevitably ends in pollution of rivers, lakes or seas, thereby reducing fish stocks and aquatic life in general. Specific examples of toxic effects on humans are harder to come by. The worst documented example was in Japan in the 1950s, where discharge of mercury wastes into Minamata Bay was linked to hundreds of deaths and deformities.

Otherwise, evidence is more circumstantial, for example inhabitants of polluted areas of the former USSR have worse infant mortality, lower life expectancy and greater incidence of cancers, although other socio-economic factors do complicate the picture.

Food From contamination of water it is a short step to contamination of food, again with heavy metals such as lead, mercury and other organic compounds. It is hard to show examples of definite general harm except where a single contaminated food is involved. However, much current concern revolves around organophosphate pesticides, which may contaminate via air or skin, causing nausea, muscle weakness, difficulty in breathing and **depression**.

The future

Many lessons have been learnt about the safe disposal of chemicals and control of industrial gases and dust, although the controls set in place are not totally effective. The biggest questions remain unanswered regarding the future of the ozone layer and global warming, the effects of which may transform climatic conditions in ways that still cannot be accurately predicted.

HAY FEVER

*For many a seasonal annoyance, for some a year-round nuisance.
Also known as allergic rhinitis.*

CAUSES

Flowers, trees and grasses release pollen or spores in vast numbers. Each has its own protein fingerprint, which causes an allergic reaction in the nose, throat and lungs. They are called allergens – something that provokes allergy. Furry animals are another source of allergens, whether hairs or fragments of skin (dander). In hot weather, car fumes and pollution may combine to cause a chemical effect that irritates the eyes and noses of those who do not normally suffer from hay fever. Different people are sensitive to different allergens: some have a general hypersensitivity to all allergens and have symptoms all year round – termed perennial rhinitis.

SYMPTOMS

The most common symptoms are itchy eyes and sneezing. The red eyes stream with tears; the nose runs. There is often a constant tickle in the throat. In severe cases the lungs are affected; there is a persistent cough or wheezing, like **asthma**.

There are all degrees of severity from mild nuisance to fighting a battle each summer against breathlessness and discomfort. Fortunately, there is a tendency to grow out of hay fever during adult life. After years of hay fever one nostril may feel constantly blocked. This may be due to a polyp, which is a harmless fleshy growth that can be surgically removed.

TREATMENT

A selection of modern remedies is available for hay fever. Antihistamines are, for most people, the mainstay of treatment. They reduce the severity of the allergic response and a single tablet helps all the symptoms. Modern antihistamines such as astemizole or loratidine are taken just once or twice a day and rarely cause the drowsiness which the older types do. They are available in liquid form suitable for children.

Antiallergy eye drops contain substances that block the allergic response, for example cromoglycate. Extremely safe, they have to be applied several times a day for full effect.

Nasal sprays contain either low doses of steroids, for example beclomethasone, or the same antiallergy substances used in eye drops. They are safe for long-term use because the steroids are absorbed within the nose itself and only negligible amounts are absorbed into the body as a whole. Nevertheless,

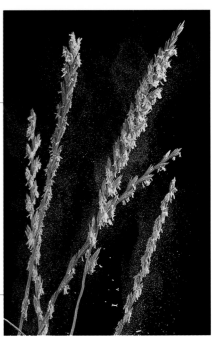

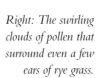

Right: The swirling clouds of pollen that surround even a few ears of rye grass.

do not be tempted to exceed the recommended dose.

The whole range of drugs used in asthma may also be used in severe hay fever, for example steroid sprays and substances to dilate the airways such as salbutamol and cromoglycate.

General measures and surgery

To reduce the impact of hay fever avoid bright sunlight; drive with car windows closed and try to keep windows at home shut in the heat of the day. Avoid animals you know you react against. While inconvenient, these measures are unavoidable if symptoms are not fully controlled by other methods.

Surgery is a possibility for those who are not helped by standard remedies. The lining of the nose is removed, relieving the persistent stuffiness and discharge.

Desensitization and allergy testing

In practice allergy testing is rarely useful (see ASTHMA).

Desensitization is done by giving stronger and stronger injections of whatever the individual is allergic to. There is a risk of provoking a serious allergic response, sudden collapse or even death, however, so it is no longer recommended, except in specialized clinics with full resuscitation facilities.

Complementary Treatment

Bach flower remedies – Rescue Remedy and crab apple diluted in water to bathe sore eyes. **Shiatsu-do** can help reduce sensitivity to allergens. Diet – allergy to food and to pollen may be linked; consult a **nutritional therapist** or a **naturopath** for advice. **Hypnotherapy** can be used in conjunction with a desensitizing programme. *Other therapies to try: Chinese and Western herbalism; tai chi/chi kung; chakra balancing; healing; homeopathy.*

PNEUMONIA

A chest infection involving the whole of one lobe of a lung.

CAUSES

Pneumonia can be caused by any of the bacteria or viruses that cause milder chest infections. These infections usually cause mild inflammation of both lungs. Pneumonia occurs when the infection is concentrated in one lobe of the lung, which carries a higher risk of complications. Pneumonia is common in the elderly, in patients following operations and in people who are run down for other reasons.

SYMPTOMS

At first the symptoms of pneumonia are non-specific – a **fever**, feeling cold and a cough. These symptoms then rapidly worsen with high fever, shivering, a harsh cough and aching over the affected part of the chest. Phlegm may contain blood streaks. In the elderly, pneumonia is often less dramatic. On examination the doctor hears characteristic noises over one section of the lung. Occasionally, a number of germs cause pneumonia in younger people but they do not manifest the classic symptoms; instead there is just a vague feeling of ill health, sweating and a mild cough. These germs include mycoplasma and legionella.

TREATMENT

Most cases respond to high doses of an antibiotic, rest and recuperation. Hospital admission might be needed in severe cases, especially if the individual cannot take antibiotics by mouth and needs a drip. Chest X-rays taken afterwards check for complete recovery of the lung and see if there is any underlying lung problem that allowed pneumonia to set in.

Pneumonia has some possible complications. Often fluid accumulates at the base of one lung, called a pleural effusion, and can take several weeks to go. An abscess may form in the lung, although modern antibiotics have made this a rare event.

   Complementary Treatment
There is no substitute for antibiotics. **Chakra balancing** reduces pain and loosens sputum. **Naturopathy** – large dosages of vitamin C can shorten recovery time. The **Alexander Technique** can help after recovery.

PLEURISY

A knife-like chest pain, worse when breathing deeply.

CAUSES

The pleura are thin layers of tissue forming a kind of insulating layer between the lungs and the chest wall. Pleurisy means inflammation of the pleura. The most common cause is infection of the lung, which spreads to the adjacent pleura; this often happens with **pneumonia** but can accompany even a minor chest infection. Sometimes the pleura become inflamed without other lung disease.

SYMPTOMS

Pleurisy gives rise to a sharp pain in the chest, which feels like a knife sticking into the side. The pain is worse on breathing in as this stretches the pleura. There may be a cough and **fever**, too, if there is a lung infection. On listening to the lungs through a stethoscope, the doctor may be able to hear a characteristic creaking sound over the area of pleurisy as the patient breathes in, which is called a rub.

Pleurisy itself is not dangerous but pleurisy associated with pain in the calf or with coughing blood could mean **pulmonary embolism**, which is dangerous.

TREATMENT

All cases benefit from painkillers; the best type is an anti-inflammatory such as ibuprofen. As well as letting you feel more comfortable, painkillers allow you to breathe deeply, which is important in getting over a chest infection. If there are signs of infection, then you will need an antibiotic. Pleurisy settles over a few days.

   Complementary Treatment
Chakra balancing reduces pain, relaxes the whole body, including the thorax, and loosens sputum. The **Alexander Technique** can help after recovery. Diet is important for prevention – a **nutritional therapist** will be able to advise you on this.

LUNG CANCER

A common tumour that grows within the airways of the lungs.

CAUSES

The evidence is overwhelming that the main cause of lung cancer is cigarette smoking. Cigarette smoke contains hundreds of different components and tars, so just which component is actually to blame is unclear. None the less, reputable research has shown beyond all reasonable doubt that the more cigarettes people smoke and the longer they smoke, the higher their chances are of getting lung cancer. The chances become even higher if the individual is also exposed to other irritant atmospheres such as coal mining or to asbestos. It appears that constant exposure to these substances irritates the lining of the main breathing tubes (bronchi), eventually turning cells malignant.

About 15% of cases of lung cancer occur in non-smokers, a percentage of which can be attributed to passive exposure to cigarette smoke.

SYMPTOMS

Most cases begin in an undramatic way as a persistent cough or with dull aching over part of the chest. Other suspicious features are coughing up blood and recurrent chest infections that are slow to improve. As the disease progresses there may be other features of cancer, for example weight loss, a vague feeling of ill health or loss of appetite. Lung cancer commonly spreads elsewhere in the body and so can produce symptoms in bone (with pain), within the brain (epileptic fits, confusion) and the liver (jaundice). When faced with such symptoms in smokers doctors will think immediately of lung cancer and order a chest X-ray.

If the X-ray shows a tumour, the diagnosis has to be checked by obtaining a sample of it. This is commonly done by a technique called a bronchoscopy (see page 323) where a flexible fibreoptic tube is guided to the tumour so that a sample can be taken for analysis.

TREATMENT

Unfortunately, lung cancer can rarely be cured. However, it is possible to give worthwhile relief by cutting out the affected part of the lung. Also, radiotherapy (see page 338) will shrink the tumour for a while, so relieving cough or breathlessness. Radiotherapy is also used in treating the spread from the tumour, for example secondary cancer in the brain or in bone.

There have been many attempts at developing chemotherapy (see page 339) for lung cancer but so far without finding a cure. At present chemotherapy may halt progress of the disease by about a year at the cost of side effects such as nausea and hair loss.

Why wait to get lung cancer? Stopping smoking results in a steady reduction in risk; even two years after quitting smoking the risks of getting lung cancer are much lower and carry on falling for many years thereafter.

QUESTIONS

Why don't all smokers get lung cancer?
Not all mountaineers fall, but if you're not a mountaineer you can't fall off a mountain . . . Smokers often comfort themselves by arguing that many smokers do not get lung cancer. About 25% of all smokers will die from a disease caused by smoking, be it heart disease, chronic bronchitis or lung cancer.

Is there any way of screening for lung cancer?
Not as yet. Trials have shown that while regular X-ray screening will detect early cancers it does not improve survival. It is important to report to your doctor any of the early symptoms mentioned previously.

Are low-tar cigarettes safer?
They are. Part of the fall in the numbers of cases of lung cancer in men in recent years is thought to be due to a switch to these types of cigarettes, athough there is always the danger that smokers who switch to low-tar cigarettes will compensate by inhaling more deeply. Low tar is safer, but it is not safe.

Complementary Treatment
Complementary therapies cannot cure cancer, and they should be used only alongside conventional approaches; in this way they can offer much support. **Chakra balancing** is a deep relaxation technique, which will help with symptom control and energy balance. **Hypnotherapy** can help you visualize your tumour being attacked by drugs. **Aromatherapy**, especially combined with gentle **massage**, is excellent for reducing the stress and tension of coping with cancer. **Reflexology** can encourage a positive attitude during treatment. *Other therapies to try: see* STRESS.

PULMONARY EMBOLISM

The dangerous condition of a blood clot lodging in the lungs.

CAUSES

Pulmonary embolism is a risk after major surgery and in individuals who are bed-bound with illnesses such as a **heart attack**, **stroke** or **pneumonia**. It is an important cause of post-operative illness and much research has gone into trying to reduce the risks after surgery.

The problem begins when blood clots within the veins in the calves and thighs. This is the condition of a **deep vein thrombosis**. Fortunately, most of the clots remain within the leg. However, there is a risk that a portion of the blood clot, called an embolus, might become detached and be carried off in the bloodstream to the lungs. The clot then becomes stuck in the blood vessels, causing the symptoms below.

For unknown reasons the risk of pulmonary embolism is higher with certain general illness, especially cancer. This is probably due to some effect that makes blood clot abnormally easily. There is also a very small increased risk of pulmonary embolism in women taking oestrogen in the contraceptive Pill or hormone replacement therapy (HRT). The risk depends on the type of Pill; those containing hormones called gestodene or desogestrel pose a higher risk. Recent research suggests the period of highest risk from HRT is in the first year of treatment.

SYMPTOMS

There may be the symptoms of a deep vein thrombosis, for example a painful swollen calf, but often there is no warning and the legs appear normal. A small embolus may cause **pleurisy** or slight breathlessness. Doctors think of a pulmonary embolus if these symptoms occur after a high-risk procedure such as hip replacement or in someone who has just had a heart attack or been bed-bound for some reason.

A large pulmonary embolus blocks off a major portion of one lung, with resulting sudden severe breathlessness, faintness, chest pain and often coughing of blood.

An embolus can also be detected by the absence of sounds over part of the lung and changes on the ECG (an electrical recording of the heart). Ordinary chest X-rays are not especially helpful in making the diagnosis. It is better to have a lung scan. Here a radioactive injection is given, which should spread evenly through the lungs (see page 320). Failure to spread suggests a large embolus.

If the embolus is big enough it will completely block blood flow through the lungs, resulting in sudden death.

TREATMENT

Treatment aims to reduce the risk of abnormal blood clotting after surgery and to prevent a deep vein thrombosis. One way to reduce the chances of thrombosis is for the patient to wear compression stockings during surgery. Drugs, for example heparin, are given to make the blood less likely to clot. If there has been a small embolus, therapy is started with heparin by injection or warfarin by mouth.

Treatment of a large clot can be successful if immediate skilled chest surgery is available to remove the blood clot from the blood vessels of the lungs. This is only possible in a few centres, which emphasizes how important it is to reduce the risks in the first place.

QUESTIONS

How can I reduce my risks of pulmonary embolism?
If you need surgery, see what steps the hospital takes to reduce risk. This might include wearing compression stockings and being given heparin during surgery. Start walking as soon as possible after surgery, a heart attack or stroke. Stop smoking and stop the contraceptive Pill before major surgery.

What risk of pulmonary embolus does the contraceptive Pill carry?
About double the natural risk – less than a one in one hundred thousand chance per annum. This is still less than the health risks from pregnancy.

Can a pulmonary embolism recur?
There is an increased risk in anyone who has had one before. Frequent emboli may result from unusual auto-immune disorders, a source of blood clots within the heart or a hidden cancer.

Complementary Treatment
This is a medical emergency and needs urgent treatment in hospital. Postoperatively, a number of complementary therapies can help the body to heal, for example **chakra balancing**. **Yoga** and **tai chi/chi kung** are gentle forms of exercise which could help after recovery. Diet – to prevent recurrence, a **nutritional therapist** would probably recommend you switch to a diet rich in fish oils and take supplements of vitamin E and garlic.

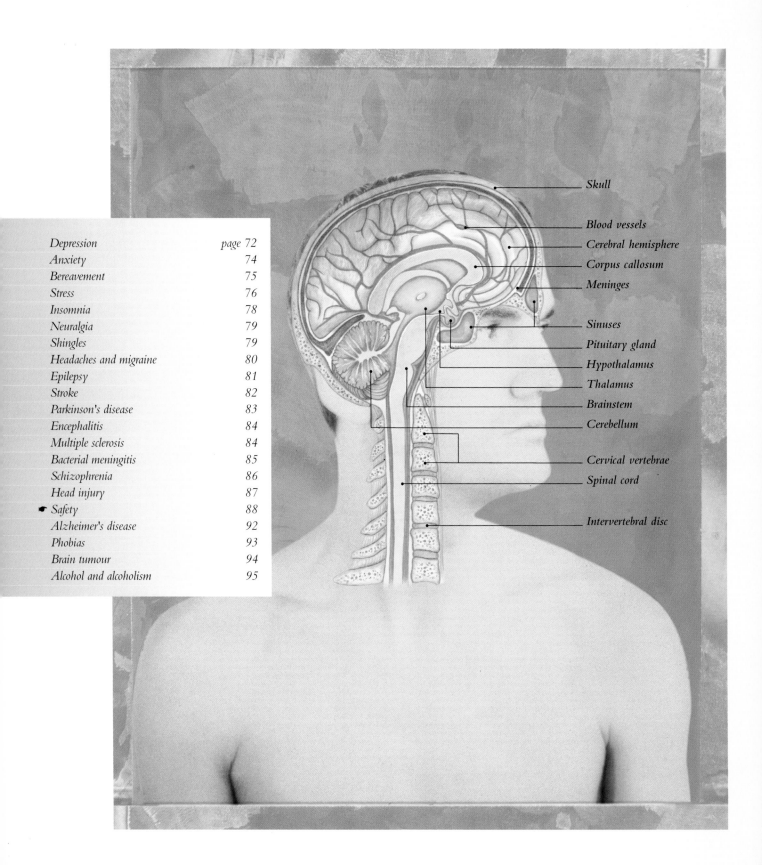

Skull

Blood vessels

Cerebral hemisphere

Corpus callosum

Meninges

Sinuses

Pituitary gland

Hypothalamus

Thalamus

Brainstem

Cerebellum

Cervical vertebrae

Spinal cord

Intervertebral disc

*Next time you use your personal computer, spare a thought
for the amazing components within your skull. Always
'on-line', it needs no plug and runs on sugar.*

MIND, BRAIN AND NERVOUS SYSTEM

THE BRAIN HAS TWO halves (hemispheres) and is a structure of some hundred thousand million nerve cells, supported by billions of additional cells. Each nerve cell, or neurone, has a thin extension called an axon, along which electrical signals pass. Axons of nerve cells within the brain can be just a fraction of a millimetre long, whereas the nerve cells in the spinal cord that control the muscles of the legs have axons 1 metre/3¼ ft long. Each axon makes contact with up to thousands of other neurones at junctions called synapses. The electrical signal cannot jump this synapse; instead the signal is normally carried by chemicals called neurotransmitters to the next cell, setting off an electrical signal for further transmission.

Somewhere within this dance of electrochemical interconnections are the fountains of memory, thought, foresight, emotion, imagination, speech and activity. Although our vocal cords make sound it is the brain that gives speech meaning; although muscles score a goal, control is within the head; and the most agile fingers are only channels through which the brain expresses itself. It is possible to locate quite precisely the parts of the brain that control these activities. However, the location within the brain of personality, consciousness and all the things we call 'higher human functions' is still a mystery.

Much is known about the anatomy and chemistry of the brain; there are many specialized areas responsible for definite activities such as speech or controlling temperature and breathing. Surrounding these areas there are millions of less specialized cells that seem to relate to the function in a diffused way. For this reason it is possible to have destruction of large parts of the brain resulting in little apparent effect on function; conversely there are some areas so critical that damage to just a few square millimetres causes paralysis, arrests breathing or destroys speech.

Messages and signals

Messages get into the brain through the sense organs. The well-known ones are, of course, vision, touch, hearing, smell and taste. However, there are many other less obvious senses, too: detectors in the aorta tell how much oxygen is in the blood, the cells in the brain stem monitor carbon dioxide concentrations in the blood and messages from the inner ear to the cerebellum enable it to maintain balance.

Signals leave the brain via nerves that end in muscles or glands; hence we speak and move, and also body temperature, appetite and thirst are regulated. These pathways leave via the spinal cord and via special nerves called the cranial nerves to the structures around the face.

Hard at work

The brain works flat out and demands a staggering percentage of the body's total energy. Twenty per cent of the heart's output goes to the brain. Even brief interruptions in blood flow lead to confusion or unconsciousness, as does lack of sugar, the fuel of the brain.

Brain diseases are most commonly the result of problems with blood flow (clots or bleeds), tumours or brain cell degeneration. Head injuries are a major cause of disability in all communities.

*Left: The brain's electrical networks
control and interpret movement, the senses,
speech, thought and imagination.*

DEPRESSION

◆

A feeling of sadness that can range from occasional low spirits to constant and overpowering despair.

CAUSES

Depression is commonly a natural response of the individual to life, with its disappointments, relationship problems and stresses, for example serious illness, **bereavement**, divorce or money worries. Psychiatrists call this type reactive depression and, in general, both the reason and the degree of depression are understandable to an onlooker sharing the same culture.

Biochemical reasons

Depression beyond understandable limits is thought to have a largely biochemical cause. Within the brain nerves communicate by means of biochemical messengers called neurotransmitters. There are hundreds of types, several of which are thought to be linked with moderate and severe depression – these include noradrenaline, dopamine and serotonin.

Depression considered mainly biochemical in origin is called endogenous or psychotic depression. There is no hard cut off between endogenous and reactive types of depression; rather they merge into each other and overlap, although extremes of each type are clearly of a different order of magnitude.

Other causes

Depression is sometimes the expression of some underlying problem – commonly alcoholism (see ALCOHOL AND ALCOHOLISM). The elderly, especially if suffering from early dementia, become depressed probably in reaction to awareness of their deteriorating health and memory. Depression after childbirth affects up to 20% of women and can fast become very severe. Depression in young people can occur because of early **schizophrenia**, where the individual is struggling to cope with disordered thought. Rarely, depression can result from brain disease, although there are usually additional features more specific to brain disease, such as paralysis or **epilepsy**.

Depression runs in families, as do other serious psychological illnesses such as schizophrenia. The close relatives of severe depressives are therefore two or three times more likely to become severely depressed than the general population.

SYMPTOMS

◆

Depressed individuals get no enjoyment out of life; they feel sad and may tell others how sad they feel. They dwell on the things that go wrong to the exclusion of the things going right.

As depression deepens they cry more easily and are increasingly preoccupied by thoughts of death, decay or bad events. They suffer sleep disturbance and often wake in the early hours of the morning, worrying (see INSOMNIA). This is the usual pattern of reactive depression of one degree or other.

If symptoms go beyond this point, the depression is more endogenous in nature. Often great agitation accompanies the depression while other sufferers become withdrawn and apathetic. Eventually, they think of suicide or even attempt it. In the most depressed state, the individual may end up mute and unresponsive, shut away in a world where they feel themselves rotting from within and where suicide is not awful but a logical release. Clearly such profound psychotic depression goes way beyond our normal experience of depression, and is not something out of which one can 'pull oneself together'.

Physical symptoms and investigations

Beyond the recognizable look of sadness, severely depressed people neglect themselves and lose their appetite. Often they suffer from constipation and complain of generalized pains for which no physical cause can be found. Except in the most obvious cases, doctors will do a physical examination and basic blood tests. The conditions most often confused with depression are an underactive thyroid gland (see THYROID PROBLEMS) and, much less commonly, brain disease such as a **brain tumour** or dementia. An underlying cause may be discovered, such as alcohol abuse, which needs specific handling.

TREATMENT

◆

It is common human experience that sharing problems is comforting. Psychological treatment of depression is based on this, although the actual theories may vary. The best known, psychoanalysis, holds that many psychological problems are the result of unconscious conflicts between repressed desires, conflicts influenced in turn by childhood experiences. Psychoanalysis aims to uncover and come to terms with conflicts, and can take years of therapy.

Classic psychoanalysis is too time-consuming for most people and so is less available than counselling, of which there are many varieties with differing theoretical frameworks. Counselling lets people talk about what underlies their depression (or many other emotions), while the counsellor gently tries to guide their thoughts towards a positive outcome. Counselling does not have to be given by a professional to be effective and there are undoubtedly people who are naturally 'good listeners', who help others simply by psychologi-

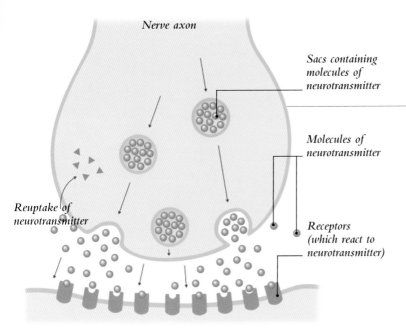

Nerve axon

Sacs containing
molecules of
neurotransmitter

Molecules of
neurotransmitter

Reuptake of
neurotransmitter

Receptors
(which react to
neurotransmitter)

*Above: A synapse – where nerves
meet, chemical transmitters relay
electrical activity from nerve to nerve.*

cal support, although it is difficult to prove this scientifically.

Psychological approaches are most useful in mild to moderate depression, which appears to be a reaction to sad life events but where the individual can still cope with life.

Drug therapy

Serious depression that is long lasting or profound needs treatment in addition to psychological support. It is a dangerous condition since five to ten per cent of sufferers will attempt suicide. (This is why everyone treating them has to be constantly judging the risks and deciding if they should be referred to a psychiatric unit – for enforced treatment if necessary.) Drug treatment reduces depression and this suicide risk rapidly. It also brings the individual to a point at which he can look more rationally at his problems and so get more out of psychological support. Drug treatment is continued for six to twelve months on average.

It is controversial whether antidepressants are of any benefit for people with mild depression but psychiatrists are gradually coming to believe that they are useful in people whose depression, although mild to an outsider, is significantly affecting their quality of life.

Tricyclic antidepressants are the drugs most widely used. They work by altering the levels of neurotransmitters in the brain, taking two to three weeks to do so. Drug names include imipramine, amitriptyline and dothiepin.

Each drug varies a little in its type of action and side effects, but they all share the common side effects of drowsiness, dry mouth, blurred vision and, in overdose, dangerous heart rhythm irregularities. The danger of overdose is critical, because of the constant risk that a depressed person may attempt suicide. Nevertheless, tricyclic drugs remain extremely useful and effective in treating serious depression.

SSRIs (selective serotonin reuptake inhibitors) are increasingly popular. The name refers to levels of a neurotransmitter in the brain – in this case serotonin. These drugs have fewer side effects and, crucially, are much safer in overdose than tricyclics and are therefore the drugs of choice for anyone posing a serious suicide risk. As they do not generally cause drowsiness they are especially useful in treating people who are still working or having to cope with family responsibilities. Drug names include fluoxetine and paroxetine.

Other treatments

There are many other drugs for selected cases. In particular, lithium is useful for people who swing between depression and excitement – bipolar affective disorder (manic depressive psychosis). Electroconvulsive therapy (ECT) is a controversial option for the most severe and resistant cases of depression where there is a major suicide risk. For some reason, passing a high voltage across the brain cures depression, so ECT may be the only therapy left for someone in the deepest depression.

Complementary Treatment

Western herbalism – St John's wort can be helpful. **Bach flower remedies** – try mustard if the depression comes for no apparent reason, gentian if you know the cause, gorse for a sense of hopelessness, sweet chestnut for utter despair, willow for bitterness and self-pity. **Art, dance movement, drama or music therapists** can help you become aware of the underlying unconscious causes of depression by enabling you to express feelings through the arts. Greater understanding of emotions can lead to improved self-esteem and motivation. **Shiatsu-do** calms the nervous system and has positive benefits on the emotions. Useful **aromatherapy** oils include neroli, rose, jasmine and bergamot. Use as inhalations (two to four drops in a bowl of hot water, or on a handkerchief) or in the bath (six drops). **Nutritional therapy** – try supplementing B vitamins. *Other therapies to try: healing; cymatics; yoga; hypnotherapy; tai chi/chi kung; acupuncture; auricular therapy; Alexander Technique; homeopathy; Ayurveda; chakra balancing; autogenic training; biodynamics.*

ANXIETY

A feeling of generalized worry and apprehension out of proportion to the objective stresses in someone's life.

CAUSES

Humanity is distinguished by its capacity for thought. With thought comes imagination, with imagination comes apprehension and with apprehension comes anxiety. It is normal for human beings to try to look ahead and to plan for that which has yet to happen, or to try to work out how to deal with an immediate problem. Until the problem is resolved there will be a feeling of tension mingled with worry – the 'what if' or 'suppose that' feeling. This we recognize as anxiety; a mild degree is a part of normal existence and may be helpful as a stimulus to action.

Abnormal anxiety – anxiety that dominates thought – happens to ordinary people who find themselves in constantly stressful environments. It also happens to those who develop **depression** or who are faced with such an array of stressful events that they see no way out of the situation. Severe anxiety is a debilitating, destructive emotion and is in no way simply an inability to cope. Illnesses which can mimic anxiety are thyrotoxicosis (see THYROID PROBLEMS) and depression.

SYMPTOMS

Mild anxiety leads to preoccupation with the problem at hand; there may be disturbed sleep and an inability to relax but on the whole the individual still copes with life. As anxiety gets more severe, however, it starts to interfere with normal activity. The mind cannot be turned to rational thought and it becomes ever more difficult to cope with day-to-day responsibilities, which become neglected. There may be irritability and a short temper. The person might turn to drink or drugs to relieve the anxiety.

In even more severe cases there is a constant tremor of the hands, crying and a complete inability to think normally.

TREATMENT

The mild anxieties of life generally resolve with time and thought. Support from outsiders is helpful in guiding the individual to a solution of her immediate problems. More severe anxiety, by blocking productive thought, feeds on itself. Here tranquillizers are helpful if only to allow the individual to start thinking productively about her problems. Useful drugs are the benzodiazepines (diazepam, lorazepam). These give

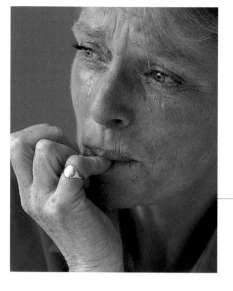

Left: Mild anxiety is common in everyday life. Severe anxiety is harmful, interfering with normal activity and leading to physical and psychological problems.

immediate relief but there is a risk of addiction if taken regularly for more than a few weeks – not in the sense of craving more, but from the withdrawal effects of increased anxiety and tremors, among others.

Beta-blockers, which in much higher dosage are used to treat high blood pressure, are good for reducing tremor and relieving the vague sense of being on edge. These are not addictive and can be taken as needed. Stronger again, there are major sedatives such as chlorpromazine and antidepressants such as amitriptyline.

Many doctors recommend trying relaxation techniques, learning how to structure your day and avoiding drugs or alcohol for relief. Changes that can be made to your life or work should, of course, be followed up, especially since excessive stress on employees is coming to be seen as something that employers have a legal responsibility to control.

Complementary Treatment

Bach flower remedies – the remedy depends on the cause, for example red chestnut for anxiety about loved ones. **Acupuncture** – see STRESS. **Arts therapies** help you become aware of the unconscious causes of anxiety by enabling you to express your feelings through dance, art, music or drama. Gaining insight with the therapist's help can enable you to feel emotionally stronger. **Aromatherapy** – see DEPRESSION. **Nutritional therapy** – try supplementing B vitamins, magnesium and calcium. **Hypnotherapy** changes unwanted patterns of behaviour produced by anxiety. *Other therapies to try: most have something to offer.*

BEREAVEMENT

◆

The loss of a close relative or friend, which has an emotional impact and can lead to months or even years of mourning.

CAUSES
◆

Bereavement usually means loss through death but the same reaction can follow divorce or the disappearance of a friend or relative, i.e. the permanent loss of someone who was central in the lives of others. It does not matter whether the person was deeply loved or not; simply to lose someone whom you were used to living with can be enough to provoke problems.

It is really only in the 20th century and in the developed world that bereavement has become a relatively unusual event. This is because the illnesses that used to cause high child mortality and poor life expectancy have been greatly reduced. Whereas even 75 years ago most people would have come across early deaths almost routinely, now death occurs mainly among the elderly. This means that the first bereavement experienced at close hand could be the death of a parent when the son or daughter is themself well into middle age.

Ironically, we are surrounded by images of death in newspapers and films and on television but these are absolutely no preparation for the reality of the death of someone close to us.

SYMPTOMS
◆

There are three well-recognized phases to bereavement. Initially, there is often disbelief, especially if the death is unexpected. Although the person may have been ill and expected to die, the actual event comes as a psychological blow which we seek to reject. This phase lasts a day or two.

Frequently, there then follows a reaction of anger mingled with bewilderment. Questions tumble out. Why this person? Why now? Why in this way? The circumstances are picked over. Were they on the right treatment? Could this have been prevented? If they had taken a different route would they have avoided an accident? This phase can last many weeks and may never be entirely resolved.

Most bereaved people eventually reach the third stage of acceptance and reconciliation; things get back into context: the elderly do die, accidents do happen, tragedies do occur.

TREATMENT
◆

Bereavement rarely needs medical treatment except, possibly, the short-term help provided by sedatives or sleeping tablets. Even medication such as this is probably best avoided for

what, after all, is a fundamental human experience.

Someone experiencing profound sadness that lasts for longer than a few weeks may be slipping into a depressive illness, especially if there are other symptoms of **depression** such as disturbed sleep, self-neglect and morbid thoughts. In this case an antidepressant is often helpful.

Prolonged grieving can suggest unresolved emotions towards the person who has died. One of the most common emotions is guilt for something that had not been sorted out by the time of death – 'unfinished business' as it were. These feelings, which are actually very common, are best handled by specialized counselling.

QUESTIONS

What assists mourning and acceptance?
The process of mourning should include recalling as much as possible of the relationship, difficult memories as well as happy ones. This way each emotion can be dealt with and not left to engender guilt or resentment.

How can friends and relatives help?
Their immediate support is essential, especially in handling the administrative matters. They can help guide mourners through the process of remembering, putting an emphasis on the best memories. After the funeral they should keep in touch regularly because that is when grief can grow.

Should children be told about a death?
They will find out eventually so why conceal things? Young children, below eight years old or so, will not take it in, unless by relating the emotions to those they felt on, for example, the death of a pet. Older children follow the same pattern of mourning as adults but will need more help to express their emotions.

Complementary Treatment
Bach flower remedies – star of Bethlehem for the shock and grief of sudden loss, sweet chestnut for utter dejection, pine to relieve feelings of guilt, willow if there is inclination to bitterness. **Acupuncture** – see STRESS. **Aromatherapy** – see DEPRESSION. **Autogenic training** is a self-administered psychotherapy that can help. *Other therapies to try: yoga; hypnotherapy; tai chi/chi kung; biodynamics; healing; shiatsu-do; auricular therapy; homeopathy; massage; chakra balancing.*

STRESS

A form of pressure that leads to the associated psychological feelings of tension and anxiety.

CAUSES

It might be said that life is all about stress: the stress of dealing with family; the stresses of personal growth and development; stresses of study, of job finding and job keeping. In the modern developed world the most primeval sources of stress are in general taken care of, that is, the stresses of finding food, shelter and security. Far from this fact relieving stress, we find other things to get stressed about. It might not be immediately clear what is stressful about having to wear up-to-date fashions, but millions of people find it so. Nor is it clear why, having a superabundance of food in the local supermarket, the act of going there to shop should provoke stress; but it does, and so on.

These might seem frivolous examples but they do make a serious point. What is benign to one person is stressful to another and this is what makes dealing with stress so difficult. People who are struggling to make ends meet will probably show little sympathy towards someone obsessed with keeping up with the latest fashion. But everyone lives within a particular environment and the stresses are no less real for being bizarre to another person in another environment.

That said, the stresses imposed by life in a modern complex society are heavy and demanding. Increasingly, it is being recognized that unreasonable stress leads to poor performance, which is ultimately counterproductive to society in general and to employers in particular.

SYMPTOMS

Stress produces **anxiety**. This is a feeling of general worry plus poor concentration and a range of possible physical symptoms from headaches, tremors and sweating to abdominal pains and **indigestion**. As stress increases, anxiety becomes more prominent with a constant fear of doing something wrong and worrying about your performance. Family life suffers; the individual becomes irritable and snappy; he loses interest in sex and may turn to drink. As stress builds up further, individual tasks are neglected because of the need to turn attention to some more pressing problem. This poor performance ultimately leads to even more stress in a self-perpetuating vicious cycle.

It is fairly easy to see how things can then deteriorate into a state of **depression**. The type of depression most likely is

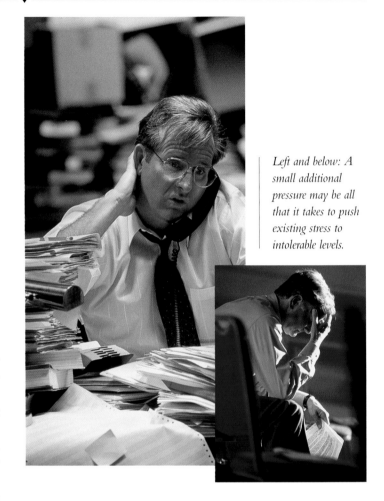

Left and below: A small additional pressure may be all that it takes to push existing stress to intolerable levels.

called agitated depression: the individual is on edge, appears hyperactive and talks freely – unlike classic depression where thought and activity slow down. However, outsiders will notice that the activity is empty and that it achieves little. Tasks that are quickly begun are just as quickly abandoned unfinished, causing yet more stress. Finally there may be a complete breakdown of the ability to cope; all the stresses build into one apparently insoluble threat; the individual collapses in tears and bewilderment. This is what is commonly called a nervous breakdown.

Evidence suggests that stress lasting over months or years increases the risks of developing a peptic ulcer and may increase the risk of heart disease. The condition called 'burn out' may result from years of stress; it is characterized by lack of enthusiasm, neglect of responsibilities, delaying even important tasks, chronic irritability and a feeling of worthlessness in one's job or life generally.

TREATMENT

◆

A degree of stress is not in itself unreasonable and is indeed a necessary stimulus to high performance. We all recognize the benefits of having a deadline, while juggling priorities is simply a fact of life for many. There may be times when these stresses build up and seem for a while overwhelming, even though each itself is not excessive. This is where counselling is helpful, together with time management and setting priorities.

The aim is rarely to transform your life, which would be unrealistic. Rather the counsellor guides you towards agreeing your own agenda for dealing with demands, sorting out what is essential and what can be delayed. Time management helps by organizing your week, devoting time in a preplanned manner instead of reacting to the latest demand. Where excessive stress is leading to anxiety, treatment may include further counselling or sedatives. In extreme cases the individual needs complete rest in a tranquil environment before being gradually encouraged to resume responsibilities.

Constant stress is not healthy. People should try to arrange their schedules so that they have protected time not subject to demands and interruptions, perhaps developing hobbies or pastimes. Talking problems over is always worthwhile and helps put stresses into perspective. In the end, people may be faced with choices about their lifestyle or jobs and may simply have to opt for alternatives if they cannot negotiate changes or cope with what is expected of them.

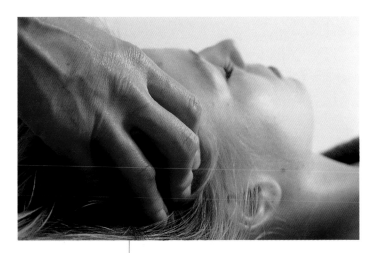

Above: Aromatherapy head massage is one of several complementary therapies that can help you defuse stress without resorting to conventional tranquillizing medication.

QUESTIONS

Surely some people just cannot cope with stress?

People do vary in how well they handle stress and so there is self-selection in the lifestyles that people choose. For example, you do not become a test pilot if you cannot deal with multiple demands. However, for any individual there will be a point at which stress becomes unreasonable.

What can be done if severe stress is unavoidable?

People do cope under extraordinary stresses but the question is for how long. If there really are no changes possible to a person's lifestyle, he or she will eventually develop an anxiety state. Whether this progression takes a matter of weeks or years will depend on the individual.

What about using drugs to cope?

Most societies have found certain drugs to alleviate stress: alcohol, tobacco and coca, for example. Although they are helpful in the short term, excessive use simply adds to stress, quite apart from providing their own health hazards.

Complementary Treatment

Bach flower remedies – Rescue Remedy is a stand-by for stressful situations; otherwise the remedy depends on the cause. For example, vervain suits people who get stressed by injustice. **Acupuncture** is good at calming and strengthening the spirit. Typical points include Heart 7, whose name is *Shenmen*, gate of the spirit, and Pericardium 6. **Chakra balancing** can help suppress the body's biochemical responses to stress, thus boosting the immune system. **Arts therapies** – therapists can help you to become aware of the underlying, unconscious factors contributing to stress by helping you to express your feelings through the arts media. Increased understanding allows you to make informed decisions about your life. **Reflexology** – your practitioner will concentrate on areas that correspond to the zones in the head. **Ayurveda** would recommend meditation, breathing mediation and yoga, along with *panchakarma* detoxification. **Osteopathy** can help if stress causes pain in the musculo-skeletal tissues, particularly the neck and shoulders, but also the lower back. *Other therapies to try: most have something to offer.*

INSOMNIA

Strictly speaking, insomnia means complete loss of sleep, but is usually taken to mean sleep disturbances varying from poor quality of sleep to an inability to sleep.

CAUSES

Insomnia is defined in relation to one's normal pattern of sleep. As people grow older their need for sleep decreases. Whereas babies naturally sleep for upward of 16 hours a day, adults need on average 7–8 hours and the elderly just 5–6 hours. It is when the pattern of sleep deviates from what is usual for the individual that there may be a problem.

By far and away the most common cause is worry, including worry about getting to sleep itself, so that a run of bad nights can be self-perpetuating. Although worry leads to difficulty in getting to sleep there is a reasonable night's sleep once asleep.

Depression, by contrast, is not associated with difficulty in getting to sleep. Instead the sufferer wakes and worries in the early hours of the morning.

Environmental disturbances might include noisy neighbours or hot nights. Eating or drinking to excess disturbs sleep through discomfort or the need to pass urine during the night. Many people find that stimulants, especially tea and coffee, keep them awake. In older people illness often leads to insomnia – the pain from **osteoarthritis**, a chronic cough or the need to pass urine associated with prostate trouble.

SYMPTOMS

There may be constant tiredness and daytime drowsiness. Losing some sleep on a regular basis will lead to poor concentration, tension and irritability. A complete lack of sleep even for just one night results in a serious fall in performance at skilled tasks or tasks involving judgement.

TREATMENT

Short periods of insomnia are self-limiting: eventually the need for sleep catches up on you and you return to your normal pattern. Firstly, do something about whatever is disturbing sleep, be it noise, excess alcohol or pain. Then adjust eating or drinking patterns to avoid stimulants and reduce the amount of fluid you drink for a few hours before going to bed.

It often helps to make a ritual for going to bed: preparing the bed, having a warm bath and a small warm drink. This sets up the mind for sleep psychologically. Avoid daytime snoozes since this time will be lost from night-time sleep.

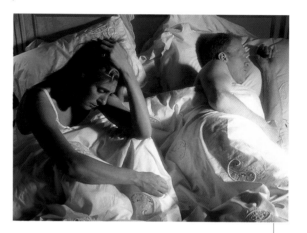

Above: When sleep escapes you, nothing seems longer than the night hours.

Once you are awake, the usual advice to get up and do something useful until you feel drowsy is rarely practical. It is better to make a warm drink, read and go back to bed. If you regularly wake, delay going to bed until you feel drowsy even if that is in the early hours of the morning.

It is difficult to treat the effects of **stress** and **anxiety**; a short course of sleeping tablets (see below) may be unavoidable.

Drug treatment

So-called hypnotic drugs are useful in the short-term treatment of serious insomnia. Modern sleeping tablets are very safe unless taken with alcohol. People can get used to them within a couple of weeks of regular use, so they should be kept for occasional use only. The drugs most commonly used are short-acting benzodiazepines, such as temazepam. Even so, these may have a hangover effect the next day. Some newer drugs such as zopiclone are claimed to avoid this. Depression should be treated specifically.

Complementary Treatment

 Bach flower remedies – the remedy depends on the cause, for example agrimony for sleeplessness caused by hidden worries behind a cheerful facade.
 Acupuncture – see STRESS. **Massage** fosters calm, especially if given by your partner last thing at night.
 Aromatherapy – try adding six drops of lavender or chamomile oil to your bath, or sprinkle them on to your pillow. **Nutritional therapy** – cut out coffee; try taking supplements of B vitamins and magnesium.
Other therapies to try: most have something to offer.

NEURALGIA

Pain in a nerve of a recurrent and persistent nature.

CAUSES

Any irritation of a nerve through pressure or inflammation will cause neuralgia, although often no definite disease is found. This is particularly so with nerve pains around the face and upper body. Even though they appear severe and upsetting exhaustive investigation may reveal nothing, leaving the diagnosis as 'neuralgia'.

States of **anxiety** and **depression** are associated with neuralgia. It is not clear whether they lead to pain through muscular tension, such as clenching of teeth, or through lowering the tolerance threshold for the minor pains everyone experiences.

SYMPTOMS

The most common symptoms are pain around the face, shooting from the jaw to the ear, or pain across the lower chest. Neuralgia together with altered sensation in the fingers and muscle weakness suggests causes such as **multiple sclerosis** or other nerve damage.

TREATMENT

It can be curative simply to know that investigations are negative. In the case of facial pain, adjustments to the dental bite can help by relieving stress on the joints in the jaw. A painkilling injection into the tempero-mandibular joint, between the upper and lower jaws, will relieve this common source of facial neuralgia. Always mention facial pain or headaches to your dentist. He or she might be able to offer some other useful suggestions to ease the pain of neuralgia.

Where no definite cause is apparent, treatment with a low dose of an antidepressant or an antiepileptic drug is often effective although it takes several weeks to work. If pain is specific to one nerve, for example pain below one rib, it is worth trying a nerve block, which is done by injecting an anaesthetic into the nerve.

Complementary Treatment

Acupuncture achieves excellent results. **Chiropractic** helps if neuralgia is triggered by nerves in the neck. *Other therapies to try: healing; tai chi/chi kung; shiatsudo; hypnotherapy; Ayurveda; chakra balancing.*

SHINGLES

A painful skin rash caused by the herpes zoster virus.

CAUSES

On first contact with the herpes zoster virus you get **chickenpox**. Afterwards the virus does not completely disappear from the body. It lives on in a dormant state within collections of nerve cells called ganglia, which are found along the spinal cord. For reasons not well understood, the virus can become active again decades later, this time causing shingles.

You cannot catch shingles from shingles – but you may catch chickenpox from shingles if you have not had it before. The virus is spread by skin-to-skin contact.

SYMPTOMS

At first there is an uncomfortable sensation over an area of skin. This may be facial pain, pain across the ribs or down one limb, and appears to be **neuralgia**. After seven to ten days a blistery rash appears over the site of pain. In cases of chest or abdominal pain the rash spreads around one half of the trunk only, which is unique to shingles. The rash takes about three weeks to fade. Afterwards pain is common where the rash was, which in some cases can last months or years.

TREATMENT

During the puzzling neuralgia stage the treatment is with painkillers. Once the typical rash appears, treatment is with an antiviral drug such as acyclovir or famciclovir. These reduce the severity of the illness and the chances of persistent pain afterwards. Shingles on the upper part of the face needs more specialized treatment to avoid ulceration of the eye.

Complementary Treatment

Nutritional therapy – supplement vitamins C, B_{12} and E. **Homeopathy** – if you have been exposed to shingles, try taking variolinum as a preventive measure. *Other therapies to try: Western herbalism; acupuncture; chakra balancing; healing; hypnotherapy.*

HEADACHES AND MIGRAINE

◆

Extremely common conditions that affect everyone occasionally and some people more often than others.

CAUSES

◆

The causes of most headaches are uncertain, although many are clearly the result of muscular tension arising from the muscles of the neck and spreading across the scalp. Migraine is caused by abnormal dilation (widening) of blood vessels within the skull and around the brain. This can be provoked by tension, certain foods, the menstrual cycle, overtiredness, eye strain, overuse of painkillers and excitement.

Many people fear more serious causes of headaches or migraine but in practice sinister causes are rare. The box (right) shows features that would suggest a more serious cause. It is a myth that high blood pressure causes headaches, unless it is exceptionally high. Headaches and migraines affect all ages and are surprisingly common in children, when the child often also gets stomach ache.

SYMPTOMS

◆

Headaches are described as a pressure on the top of the head, a band drawn across the skull, or a constant throbbing pain.

Classic migraine follows a pattern: at first there is a foreboding of something happening within the head, often with nausea; there may be a shimmering in the field of vision, called a fortification spectrum, and, more dramatically, some people go blind in one eye, develop slurred speech or get an odd sensation in one limb. There then follows a severe headache, affecting one side of the skull ('migraine' means half of the skull), more nausea and vomiting.

Headaches and migraines can last hours or a few days.

TREATMENT

◆

Most headaches and migraines respond to simple painkillers such as aspirin or paracetamol. Often these are combined with an antisickness drug such as prochlorperazine. It is important to take these early in the attack because once the nausea sets in painkillers are poorly absorbed from the stomach. There is a temptation to take stronger and stronger painkillers but these can actually make headaches worse.

A drug called sumatriptan is very effective at cutting short severe migraine. People having frequent attacks may find it worth taking preventive treatment; the most widely used are beta-blockers, which also have a mild calming effect, or pizo-

tifen. Both of these have to be taken every day for full benefit.

It is worth keeping a diary to see if headaches or migraines link up with certain foods, days of the week and so on. Foods commonly provoking migraines are cheese, chocolate, red wine, oranges, bananas and nuts. Certain drugs can cause migraines, especially the contraceptive Pill and calcium-channel blockers (for high blood pressure), and may have to be stopped. A constant vague headache may be caused by **depression** and may respond to a low dose of a sedative or an antidepressant. It is difficult to control **stress** underlying headaches but relaxation techniques may help.

Investigations are rarely necessary unless the headaches or migraines include the features in the box below.

SYMPTOMS THAT MAY POINT TO SERIOUS CAUSES OF HEADACHE

◆

- ◆ *Sudden onset over seconds or minutes (bleeding around the brain)*
- ◆ *A fever, neck stiffness and aversion to bright lights (meningitis or encephalitis)*
- ◆ *Loss of use or clumsiness in a limb (brain tumour or blood clot on the brain)*
- ◆ *Following a head injury (blood clot on the brain)*
- ◆ *Worse in the mornings and with nausea or change of personality; the new onset of epileptic fits (brain tumour)*
- ◆ *Migraine for the first time or worsening after beginning the contraceptive Pill (sensitivity to the hormones)*

Along with these, doctors would look for irregular pupils, disturbed thought or behaviour, weakness in limbs and raised pressure within the skull as seen by examining the back of the eyes.

Complementary Treatment

The **Alexander Technique** encourages the release of muscle tension in the neck. **Chiropractic** and **osteopathy** – loss of joint movement and flexibility in the neck with associated muscle spasm contribute to headache and migraine. These manipulative therapies can help, although they work on different principles. Diet – a **naturopath** or **nutritional therapist** could offer dietary advice which would help reduce the severity and frequency of headaches. *Other therapies to try: most have something to offer.*

EPILEPSY

◆

An electrical disturbance within the brain, leading to bizarre behaviour or sensations.

CAUSES

◆

Like a computer, the brain relies on an orderly flow of electrical current to work efficiently. Epilepsy is the result of a major electrical storm within the brain. Any scarring or area of damage is a likely focus for the disorder. This may accompany **cerebral palsy** or follow a **head injury**, a **stroke**, brain surgery, drugs or excess alcohol (see ALCOHOL AND ALCOHOLISM).

High **fever**, especially in children, is an extremely common cause of fits, fortunately with no long-term consequences. Other causes are heat stroke, **brain tumour** and disorders of body chemistry such as **diabetes** and lack of oxygen. After all these have been excluded there are about 75% of epileptics where no cause can be found despite extensive investigation.

SYMPTOMS

◆

The classic epileptic fit begins with a sense of something about to happen, called an aura. Auras may consist of an odd sensation, an emotion or a smell. They come from electrical activity in the part of the brain where the fit is beginning. Then there is a phase of generalized muscle activity, first stiffening up, followed after a few seconds by regular jerking of limbs, often with frothing at the mouth and incontinence of urine. This is the time when epileptics may come to harm through falls. After a few minutes most fits end, followed by a period of drowsiness that can last several hours. There are many variations on this classic fit. The fit may consist of unusual behaviour or a momentary lapse of consciousness.

A reliable eyewitness account is a good way to make the diagnosis; otherwise an EEG may show characteristic electrical wave forms from the brain. Most cases nowadays would be investigated with a brain scan (see pages 318 and 319).

TREATMENT

◆

Treatment is not always essential for single or very infrequent fits, as in a feverish child. Treatment aims to stabilize the electrical activity of the brain and so reduce, if not stop, further fits. Drugs in general use include phenytoin, valproate, vigabatrin, carbamazepine and several others. Each suits different people. The correct dosage is found by experience and by monitoring blood levels of the drug. Any precipitating causes such as alcoholism or high fever need to be dealt with.

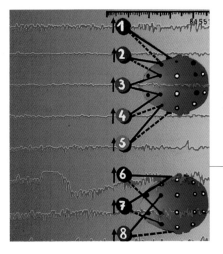

Left: An EEG, *which shows disordered electrical activity throughout the brain during an epileptic fit.*

If someone is having an epileptic fit, the only action to take is to put him into a safe position on his front so that he will not choke. After the fit has ended he should be allowed to recover from the ensuing drowsiness. Only if a fit is prolonged might active treatment be necessary – injection of a sedative such as diazepam.

It is possible to perform brain surgery for certain highly localized types of epilepsy, with the aim of cutting off the part of the brain where the abnormal electrical impulses begin.

Providing an epileptic remains fit free for a number of years, he can lead a completely normal life, including driving a car, although some occupations are forbidden such as driving public service vehicles or flying a plane. Deciding whether medication can be stopped is difficult, depending on the consequences if fits recurred. It is helpful to show first that brain activity is normal with an EEG, then the dosage of drugs is slowly reduced. Withdrawing medication is often done for children. Adults may be reluctant to stop medication despite years of being fit free because of implications for their job or driving licence if fits restarted.

✿ Complementary Treatment

There is no substitute for orthodox treatment; however, any of the relaxational therapies will be useful on a day-to-day basis. **Bach flower remedies** – try taking Rescue Remedy immediately after a fit. **Nutritional therapy** can offer some long-term help; recommendations might include supplementing vitamin B_6 and magnesium, zinc and selenium. Through **healing** the frequency and severity of attacks can be reduced, as this therapy has a calming effect on the whole being. *Other therapies to try: see* STRESS.

STROKE

A brain injury occurring as the result of some kind of interference with blood flow within the brain.

CAUSES

The brain relies on a constant flow of oxygen-rich blood via the great carotid arteries in the sides of the neck and the vertebral arteries up the back of the neck. Disruption, even for seconds, leads to giddiness and blackouts; loss of blood flow for more than a couple of minutes leads to death of nerve cells and a resulting stroke. Nerve cells cannot regrow so any loss is permanent but recovery is possible by other cells taking over the functions of the dead cells.

Some strokes follow leakage of blood from one of the arteries in the brain; most result from blockage of arteries with a blood clot. Least common are strokes due to **brain tumour** or brain injury. The risks of a stroke are increased by anything that increases the risks of diseased blood vessels. This includes, most importantly, **high blood pressure**, raised cholesterol and smoking. Strokes become much more common with age, due to a general deterioration in the otherwise remarkable reliability of the circulation in the brain. They are a major cause of disability in old age and a common reason for death in the elderly.

SYMPTOMS

The symptoms can range from momentary to permanent. The most obvious symptoms are paralysis of muscles, for example sudden loss of use of an arm or a leg or both, drooping of half the face, slurred speech and difficulty in swallowing. There are more subtle changes in the senses, for example blindness for part of the field of vision, inability to feel part of the body, loss of balance and giddiness.

There is loss in the so-called higher brain functions: an inability to read or articulate correct words, loss of emotional control and confusion – in fact a complete change of personality. The most serious strokes cause sudden unconsciousness then death; others lead to chronic ill health with immobility, incontinence and the increased risk of chest infections.

TREATMENT

After a stroke, the treatment is to provide skilled nursing care while time does its healing. About 25% of stroke victims will recover rapidly and completely. A brain scan (see pages 318 and 319) will localize the site of damage and confirm the type of stroke: bleeding, obstruction or unexpected disease. It is important to control blood pressure and to stop smoking.

Aspirin, in a dose of 75–150 mg a day, reduces the tendency of the blood to clot and so lessens the risks of a future stroke by up to 30%. Investigations may reveal that a blood clot has come from deposits of cholesterol in the carotid arteries; surgery can reopen these vessels (carotid endarterectomy).

Rehabilitation ideally involves a team of physiotherapists, speech and occupational therapists as well as relatives, all pushing the individual to make the best use of her remaining abilities. It can be a long, demanding business because of the changes in personality produced by strokes. Many practical problems need addressing such as learning to transfer in and out of chairs or beds, help with swallowing and with feeding.

QUESTIONS

What is a TIA?
A transient ischaemic attack, or so-called mini-stroke. By definition a TIA has all the features of a stroke but complete recovery occurs within 24 hours. They are caused by small blood clots and should lead to as full an investigation as a complete stroke. Aspirin is very effective treatment for a TIA.

How long can recovery take after a stroke?
Most recovery occurs within three days but worthwhile improvement happens for at least 12 and possibly 24 months. During this period the brain 'reprogrammes' itself to overcome the damaged area of permanently lost nerve cells.

Is it worth treating blood pressure in the elderly?
Yes, even in the very old. However, doctors do not look for such tight control as they do in younger people.

Complementary Treatment

Stroke requires prompt hospital treatment. Complementary therapies have a role in prevention and rehabilitation. **Nutritional therapy** – a high intake of oily fish and vitamin E, with a wholefood diet, helps prevent small clots in the brain, which cause strokes. **Western herbalism** – ginkgo promotes cerebral circulation. **Acupuncture** is excellent in conjunction with physiotherapy, as is **chiropractic**. **Ayurveda** – regular treatment helps restore muscular strength. *Other therapies to try: shiatsu-do; reflexology; tai chi/chi kung.*

PARKINSON'S DISEASE

A degeneration of the brain marked by shaking of limbs and a generalized stiffness of movement.

CAUSES

In individuals with Parkinson's disease, for reasons not understood, there is an abnormally rapid loss of certain specialized cells within the brain. These cells produce a chemical called dopamine, which is involved in the fine control of muscle activity. Dopamine is one of a number of neurotransmitters, chemicals through which one nerve cell communicates with another.

Parkinson's disease is mainly a disease of ageing, affecting about two per cent of over-80 year olds, but it is not unknown in younger age groups. A few cases are caused by drugs that have reversible Parkinsonian side effects, for example sedatives such as chlorpromazine. There are a number of other rare neurological diseases that mimic Parkinson's disease but are differentiated on investigation. In this case the condition is called Parkinsonism.

SYMPTOMS

The early symptoms are easily mistaken for the effects of ageing: lack of mobility, dizziness, slow speech and a mild tremor of the hands. The diagnosis becomes more obvious once the more typical symptoms appear, for example a tremor of the hands at rest in a pattern where the thumb keeps rubbing the index and middle fingers – a so-called pill-rolling movement. There is a general rigidity of the limbs. For example, walking is with a stiff gait with the arms held rigidly at the sides and the whole body bent over. As the condition worsens patients have an immobile, expressionless face. They have difficulty in starting to walk, making a few shuffling paces before getting into their stride. In addition, there is frequently **depression** and **constipation**.

Interestingly, handwriting becomes small and cramped and the diagnosis has been suspected on this evidence alone.

TREATMENT

The drugs available work by boosting the levels of dopamine in the brain. Probably the best known is L-Dopa, given alone or in combination with other drugs, such as carbidopa, which improve the brain uptake of L-Dopa. Side effects such as nausea, low blood pressure and confusion are common. Unfortunately, most patients develop resistance to these drugs after a few years. There are a few alternative drugs, such as selegiline, which can relieve symptoms and so put off the need to go on to L-Dopa.

Physiotherapists and occupational therapists can be of use, helping people with Parkinson's to make their home environment as safe and convenient as possible.

Surgery can be performed on the brain, cutting certain nerve pathways in order to relieve disturbances of movement. This is less commonly done since L-Dopa has been available. There is the possibility of implanting brain cells taken from a foetus to replace the dopamine-producing cells in the brain. This is still an experimental and controversial treatment with unpredictable results but may lead to an eventual cure of this relatively common and distressing condition.

QUESTIONS

Is there anything other than drug treatment?
Physical aids are important, e.g. something as simple as slip-on shoes that don't need lacing up. Enthusiastic physiotherapy encourages people to make the best use of their remaining mobility.

Does it affect the mind?
Parkinsonism does not cause dementia; it can be difficult to accept this when faced with a severely disabled individual, but the mind does remain intact. Having a normal mind in a diseased body is one reason why people with Parkinson's frequently get depressed.

What is the long-term outlook?
Many people have mild symptoms with little progression even over several years. A few people deteriorate rapidly. For the majority there is a gradual decline over ten to twenty years; life expectancy is little affected.

Complementary Treatment

WARNING: Vitamin B$_6$ should only be administered by a doctor to Parkinson's patients. **Biodynamics** can help in the early stages of the disease. Regular exercise via **tai chi/chi kung** can help delay the progress of the disease in its earliest stages, as can the **Alexander Technique**. Diet – **nutritional therapy** can be helpful. Ask your therapist about a low-protein diet. Various vitamin and mineral supplements could help, for example vitamins B$_1$, C and E – but note the warning above with regard to vitamin B$_6$.

ENCEPHALITIS

Inflammation of the brain leading to confusion and drowsiness.

CAUSES

Any infection that irritates the brain can result in encephalitis. The most common cause is a non-specific viral infection although it can accompany **mumps** and **chickenpox**. Probably the headache so common with these viral illnesses is a mild form. Certain biochemical disorders can cause encephalitis, for example alcoholic poisoning. Infection with the herpes virus is one potentially treatable cause. There is a rare and incurable form caused by **measles**, one reason for offering vaccination against this disease. There are several tropical insect-borne diseases which cause encephalitis.

SYMPTOMS

It begins as a typical viral illness with widespread muscular aches and headache. After a day or two the sufferer becomes drowsy, the headache worsens and the sufferer may lapse into a coma. There may be epileptic fits and paralysis of certain facial muscles. The coma can become profound. The diagnosis is confirmed by detecting viruses on a lumbar puncture, showing brain inflammation on a brain scan and, occasionally, taking a biopsy of the brain to detect the herpes virus.

TREATMENT

Most cases of encephalitis can be treated only with nursing care and steroids to reduce inflammation within the brain. A brain scan may show some treatable cause such as a brain abscess. If caused by herpes, the treatment is with high doses of antiviral drugs. Although most victims do recover, encephalitis is always a serious condition with a risk of death or of permanent neurological damage.

Complementary Treatment
Complementary therapies are not an appropriate response to encephalitis. During recovery any of the relaxational techniques could help – see STRESS.

MULTIPLE SCLEROSIS

Degeneration of the central nervous system leading to widespread weakness and changes in sensation; commonly called MS.

CAUSES

The cause of MS remains unproven, but wide international variations in frequency suggest an environmental cause, possibly a virus. It is the most common serious neurological condition in young adults. It is caused by degeneration of the cells that surround the nerve cells like insulation.

SYMPTOMS

In a first attack there is blurred vision or loss of vision, numbness in various parts of the body, weakness of a limb or difficulty controlling urination. The symptoms appear rapidly and disappear within weeks. It may be years before any further problems develop. A pattern eventually emerges of recurrent neurological symptoms affecting different parts of the body at different times. An MRI scan (see page 319) will reveal abnormal nerve structures scattered throughout the brain. The disease does not affect thought processes or intelligence.

TREATMENT

For a first attack nature is usually left to take its course. Occasionally steroid tablets are used to control symptoms and help acute flare-ups. Interferon-B reduces the frequency and severity of flare-ups slightly and at very great expense, therefore currently it is not widely recommended.

In first attacks the future pattern of the disease is unpredictable. It is likely to progress, but many people with MS find that their disability is manageable and only a minority deteriorate to the point of needing intensive nursing.

Complementary Treatment
Complementary approaches cannot cure MS. **Chakra balancing** relaxes spasms and eases aching muscles and pain from bladder infections. **Chiropractic** is useful as part of an overall treatment regime, helping the individual keep as mobile as possible, using manipulation and soft tissue massage of the spine and other joints. **Ayurveda** can help in the early stages. Oil **massage** is given, along with *marma* puncture. *Other therapies to try: biodynamics; tai chi/chi kung; naturopathy.*

BACTERIAL MENINGITIS

An infection of the brain with potentially very serious effects.

CAUSES

The brain is surrounded by delicate layers of specialized tissue called the meninges; meningitis means infection of this tissue. Most cases arise from viral infections that reach the brain via the blood stream. Fewer cases are caused by bacterial infection but these are always more serious. Meningitis is actually rather difficult to catch but the risks are higher in institutions where many people are close together. This is why outbreaks often spread through schools and colleges. Meningitis can follow any penetrating injury of the skull such as may occur in a road accident. The peak time for meningitis is winter.

SYMPTOMS

The illness begins as an unremarkable infection with **fever**, mild headache, muscle aching and possibly a cold. Over a few hours or a couple of days the severity of the illness becomes rapidly worse. The headache becomes intense, bright lights hurt the eyes and there is pain on attempting to bend the neck. Eventually, features of **encephalitis** occur, such as drowsiness, irritability, epileptic fits and possibly coma. These symptoms are caused by irritation of the meninges over the brain, which is made worse by anything that stretches them such as bending the neck.

If the cause is bacterial, for example meningococcal meningitis, then there may be a widespread purple rash in the skin which consists of tiny bruises. This rash appears over just a few minutes and is a sign that the infection has spread into the blood stream (septicaemia) and is destroying the blood's ability to clot.

In babies the disease is often much less dramatic and therefore more difficult to recognize. The baby may be simply irritable, drowsy, possibly vomiting and possibly with a bulging fontanelle – caused by pressure within the skull.

TREATMENT

If bacterial meningitis is even suspected, the first essential is to give an injection of penicillin. The diagnosis is confirmed by lumbar puncture – this means withdrawing fluid from around the spinal cord and analysing it for the bacteria responsible. If the cause is bacterial, the patient is maintained on high doses of the appropriate antibiotic. If the cause is viral, the illness will settle with just nursing care. The terrible

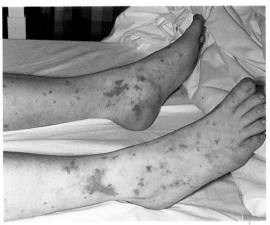

Above: The sinister scattered purple rash of meningococcal meningitis, which signals septicaemia. Get medical help immediately.

effects of septicaemia lead to bleeding not only in the skin but in internal organs. These individuals are desperately ill, requiring intensive care, blood transfusion, artificial respiration and control of epileptic fits.

In bacterial meningitis, people who have been in close contact should have antibiotics to reduce the risks of contracting it. Ninety-nine per cent of people who contract **viral meningitis** make a full recovery; unfortunately, bacterial meningitis is more dangerous with about a ten per cent risk of death. After-effects such as **epilepsy** and partial paralysis are common.

A vaccination against haemophilus B is now offered routinely in childhood. This one bacterium causes about 50% of all cases of bacterial meningitis. Even though this vaccination has been routinely used for only a few years, the number of cases caused by haemophilus B has plummeted.

See also VIRAL MENINGITIS.

Complementary Treatment

Complementary therapies are not appropriate in response to the medical emergency of meningitis. However, many therapies will be able to offer help during the recovery stages. Any of the relaxational therapies mentioned under STRESS will help with the tensions of illness. There are many therapies that can help boost the immune system, for example **Western** and **Chinese herbalism**, **homeopathy** and **acupuncture**. The gentle arts of **tai chi/chi kung** and **yoga** can help restore the battered system.

SCHIZOPHRENIA

A disturbance of thought often marked by delusions, hallucinations, self-neglect and paranoia.

CAUSES

Schizophrenia is considered a disorder of brain chemistry. Probably there is disease in the system of neurotransmitters – chemicals through which one nerve communicates with another. Of these, the dopamine system is under suspicion.

It has a strong hereditary tendency, with a chance of one in seven to ten of the offspring of a schizophrenic parent developing it – a much greater-than-average risk. There are similarly increased risks if a sibling has the condition.

Although most psychiatrists accept that environment and upbringing also play a role in schizophrenia, it has been difficult to prove scientifically and many such theories have largely been abandoned for lack of evidence.

SYMPTOMS

In its mildest form the individual simply seems a little eccentric: a loner, poor at socializing, reticent and wary of eye contact. This is the schizoid personality and may progress no further; such individuals often find solitary occupations and lead a quiet, withdrawn life.

If the condition worsens schizophrenics start to experience bizarre events, voices commenting on their behaviour and hallucinations. Thinking becomes disordered: certain ideas become absolute certainties resistant to any reasoning. For example, a schizophrenic may be convinced that radio waves are being emitted by a light switch and influencing his mind

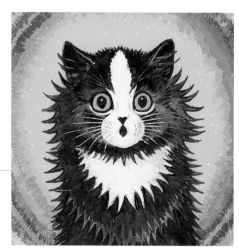

Right: A drawing by Louis Wain, a well-known schizophrenic who drew cats. The drawings became more bizarre whenever he relapsed.

and that his own thoughts are being broadcast to the world at large. These are termed delusions, unshakeable beliefs based on no objective evidence. There is a strong feeling of being under the control of others, be it voices from the television or a central heating unit or just vague, menacing 'others'.

This paranoia is a common feature of schizophrenia, as is **depression** and extreme **anxiety**. These symptoms increase the chances of schizophrenics becoming aggressive towards their supposed persecutors or harming themselves, and suicide is a risk. As the disease deteriorates there is disintegration of the personality and increasing self-neglect.

TREATMENT

Drug therapy has revolutionized treatment since chlorpromazine was first discovered 40 years ago. Various drugs control symptoms in individuals who would otherwise languish in psychiatric institutions or drift on to the streets. These drugs are given by mouth or regular injection to ensure reliability of dosage. Schizophrenics cannot cope with normal stresses of life; calm, orderly and careful handling is important in their management, which can be at home or in hostels.

Up to 40% of schizophrenics have just one episode of schizophrenia and return to normal life eventually. Pointers to eventual full recovery are if the condition came on rapidly and was accompanied by minimal hallucinations or delusions, and the patient had a previous reliable personality within a stable family. About 10% of schizophrenics remain seriously disturbed despite treatment. The rest will experience relapses from time to time. Severely paranoid schizophrenics may pose a major risk to the safety of others and may remain so dangerous that they have to stay in special secure psychiatric prisons.

Families need much support in caring for schizophrenics, whose bizarre, unpredictable behaviour strains family loyalty.

Complementary Treatment

WARNING: Visualization, hypnotherapy and deep relaxation techniques, including chakra balancing, are extremely dangerous for schizophrenics and should never be used *except* by people trained in psychiatry. They bring about altered states of consciousness and schizophrenics have reported seeing lights and disturbing visions during treatment. Complementary approaches cannot cure schizophrenia. **Yoga** and **tai chi/chi kung** are calming forms of exercise which might benefit schizophrenics. **Reflexology**, **massage** and **aromatherapy** are generally supportive.

HEAD INJURY

Any blow to the skull is serious, potentially risking brain damage.

CAUSES

The brain is a soft structure with a filigree of delicate blood vessels entering and leaving it. It is protected from hard blows and shaking by the strength of the skull all around it.

Head injuries may have a direct impact on the brain by fracturing the skull and damaging the brain beneath, or a less obvious effect by shaking the brain. Any injury causes the brain to swell within the rigid skull, which compresses the base of the brain against the skull. The base of the brain controls certain vital functions, in particular breathing and regulation of the heart, so it is pressure on this structure which often causes more problems than the head injury alone.

Common reasons for head injuries are falls, road traffic accidents and deliberate blows to the skull, especially boxing.

SYMPTOMS

A severe head injury has effects similar to those of a **stroke**, the exact effect depending on which part of the brain is damaged. There may be paralysis, loss of speech and variable consciousness, if not coma. Less severe effects, such as those caused by shaking, lead to confusion and loss of memory. Injuries that cause bleeding or swelling around the brain may not result in any immediate symptoms until the blood clot or swelling has become large enough to put pressure on the underlying brain. The effects of this pressure can be confusion, double vision, nausea and vomiting, progressive drowsiness, coma or simply a rapid change in personality. If not treated this situation may lead to death through further pressure on the brain's vital centres.

Brain scans (see pages 318 and 319) have greatly increased the accuracy of diagnosis of head injuries and especially in detecting blood clots (subdural haemorrhage, extradural haemorrhage) – previously confirmed only by exploratory surgery in which a tap hole was driven through the skull.

TREATMENT

A serious head injury requires immediate stabilization of breathing and circulation, both of which are controlled by the brain, while removing debris and dealing with the other injuries that so often accompany a severe head injury. Once stable, patients may have to be maintained on a respirator until they regain consciousness. Where the injury appears milder and there is no obvious damage, it is still important to be vigilant over the next 24–48 hours for any symptoms that might reveal that damage is taking place and is causing increased pressure within the brain.

Rehabilitation follows similar lines to those given to stroke victims, pushing individuals to use their remaining faculties. Head injuries are particularly common in the young but fortunately, younger brains have a better chances of recovery than older brains; even so, rehabilitiation may take years.

WARNING

Even though someone may appear perfectly well immediately after the injury, there are features to be vigilant for afterwards which may indicate underlying brain damage:

Short-term symptoms *(i.e. appearing within hours or days)*
◆ *Unusual drowsiness*
◆ *Severe persistent headache*
◆ *Double vision*
◆ *Difficulty in using a limb, walking unsteadily or slurred speech*
◆ *Vomiting for no apparent reason*
◆ *An epileptic fit*

Longer-term changes *(i.e. appearing over a few weeks)*
◆ *Alteration in personality*
◆ *Unusual drowsiness*
◆ *Progressive paralysis of a limb*

Mild confusion and drowsiness are common signs of simple concussion, which should improve over 24–48 hours.

Complementary Treatment
Chakra balancing can help relaxation during rehabilitation, as can the **Alexander Technique**. **Chiropractic** treatment or **osteopathy** can help patients with head injuries, as often they will have also suffered from neck and back injuries. Treatment aims to restore spinal joint function and mobility, as part of an overall treatment regime. Any of the treatments listed under STRESS can help relieve tension during rehabilitation.

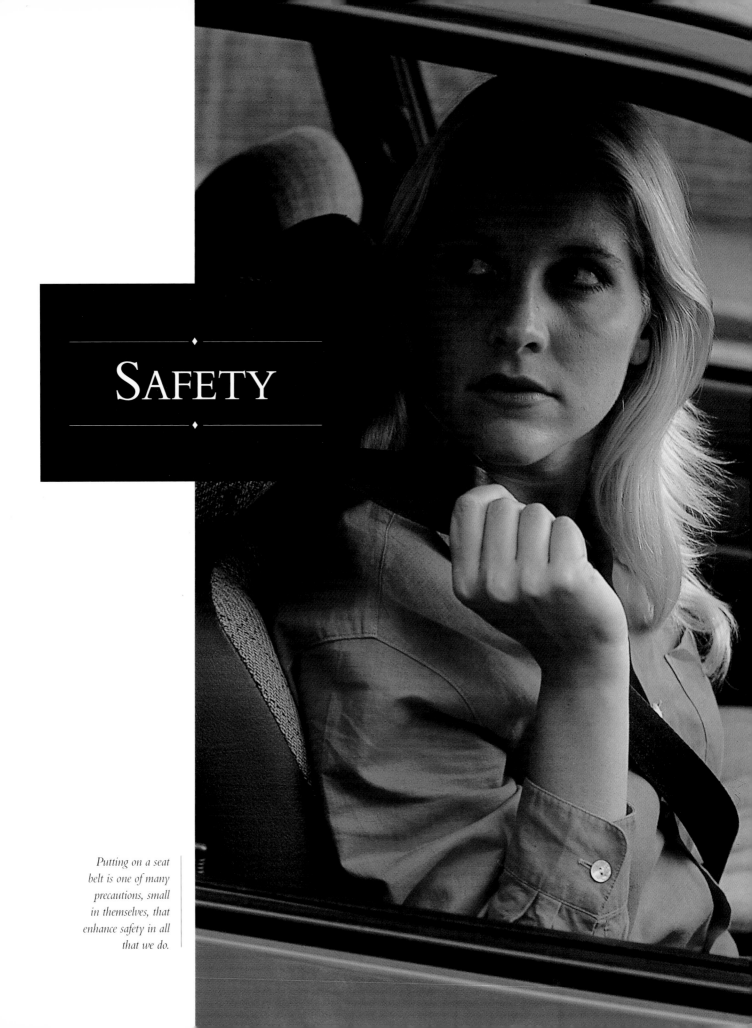

SAFETY

Putting on a seat belt is one of many precautions, small in themselves, that enhance safety in all that we do.

I N DEVELOPED COUNTRIES, as medical advances have reduced the threat of fatal birth injury, malnutrition and many infections, so health promotion and accident prevention have been given greater resources. Physical danger has always taken its toll on human society; archaeological remains often show old injuries, fractures and other signs of violent injury or death. There are great differences in safety and accident rates between different countries. This discussion is based on experience in the United Kingdom.

An overview

While accidents account for approximately two per cent of all deaths, between the ages of one and thirty-five they are the single greatest cause of death. Above thirty-five they are steadily overtaken by age-related illnesses such as heart disease, cancer and stroke.

While most accidents occur at home, since this is where we spend the greatest part of our time, the majority of accidental deaths occur on the road. Domestic accidents, particularly

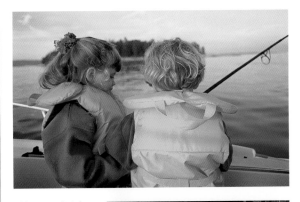

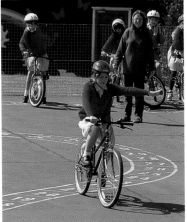

Above and right: Life involves balancing adventure and risk against sensible although possibly boring precautions.

falls, can be fatal, however, as can workplace and sporting injuries. The consumption of alcohol plays a part in at least 30% of all accidents.

What are accidents?

In this context an accident can be defined as an unforeseeable event leading to injury. In practice, and with the benefit of hindsight, many accidents are predictable although not necessarily preventable. It is an important goal of public health to try to reduce the incidence of accidents, while realizing that some accidents are, by their very nature, unavoidable. The risk and nature of accidents vary greatly at different ages.

The lure of the familiar The more often we perform a familiar task the more likely we are to take risks, for example when going up a ladder to clean windows or remembering not to tread on a loose floorboard. It is better to do something about a hazard now than to be saying in hospital, 'I always knew I ought to do something about those slippery stairs.'

Safety and children

The aim is to encourage exploration in a safe environment. The onus is on carers to anticipate hazards, especially those that adults take for granted, such as being careful with pointed objects. Checklists can be tedious – just about anything can be a hazard if misused – and common sense should guide you.

The home Secure objects which children might pull on to themselves; fit guards to the top and bottom of stairs; remove trailing electrical flexes, sharp objects and poisonous substances such as bleach, medicines and garden chemicals. Fit socket guards; lock doors leading to hazardous areas such as the garage. Do not leave children unattended near fires, hot pans or other hot objects.

Always test the temperature of baths, food and drinks meant for children. Keep only safe domestic pets and avoid leaving children alone in a room with a dog, no matter how well behaved it normally is.

Secure the area around garden ponds or swimming pools and never allow young children to go near them without close adult supervision.

Transport Fit safety seats and use them; always strap children in the car and do not let them hang out of an open window. Children love bikes but make sure they get into the habit of wearing safety helmets and reflective clothing. Teach road safety from the earliest age, while remembering that no child under the age of ten is safe alone on roads.

Other Satisfy yourself about the safety of playgrounds and the degree of supervision on trips and special outings.

Unless you are going to cocoon your child in an unrealistic world, accidents in childhood are unavoidable. You can, however, make sure that any accidents that do occur are as minor as possible.

Safety from the age of 13 to 35
The aim is to enjoy life without endangering someone else's. Adolescence is a period of flexing all the muscles and trying everything. So, not surprisingly, this is the period where accidental deaths peak, mainly through road traffic accidents.

Road safety Nearly half of all male deaths in this age group are through road traffic accidents. The means to reduce risk are simple: wearing seat belts whether you are a driver or a passenger, driving at a safe speed, not drinking and driving. Pedestrian safety is equally important; many accidents occur to inebriated pedestrians.

Sports and workplace safety Although far less important numerically, workplace accidents and sporting injuries account for significant numbers of deaths and disabilities

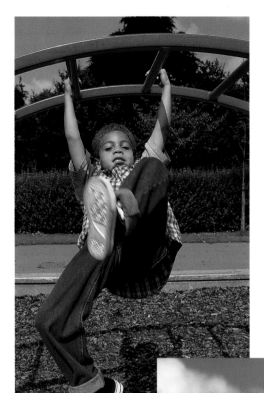

Above: Soft ground covering in a playground will protect against injury while allowing uninhibited play. Right: Safety measures can be made attractive and even desirable.

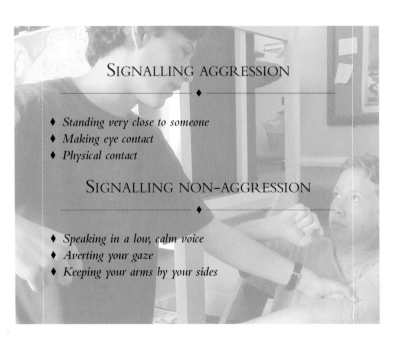

SIGNALLING AGGRESSION

* *Standing very close to someone*
* *Making eye contact*
* *Physical contact*

SIGNALLING NON-AGGRESSION

* *Speaking in a low, calm voice*
* *Averting your gaze*
* *Keeping your arms by your sides*

each year. Young people may feel they jeopardize a macho image if they use safety equipment, but office and factory personnel and sports instructors should keep emphasizing the safe way of doing things.

Aggression Violent assaults make a small but important contribution to injuries in teenage years and early adulthood. Most societies find youth aggression a difficult problem, with no simple answers. It is tied in with socio-economic disadvantage, unemployment, alcohol and drugs, but, at root, young

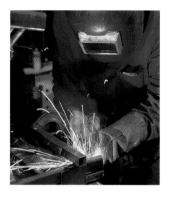

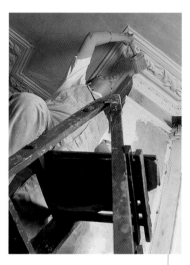

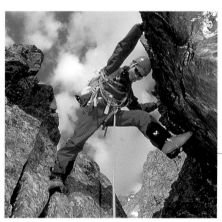

Above left: In certain occupations, safety cannot be left to individual choice. Above: In other activities the responsibility is ours.

Left: Many hazardous sports recommend safety standards that you would be foolish to ignore.

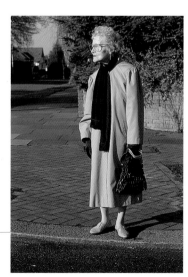

Right: Accidents to elderly pedestrians are a common cause of injury and death.

people are aggressive and large groups are aggressive towards each other. Those wishing to avoid confrontation must keep away from troublespots and learn to recognize anger in themselves so they can alter their body language and walk away from hostile situations.

Safety from the age of 36 to 64

The aim for this age group should be to benefit from wisdom and experience! Road traffic accidents are still the major hazard, less so workplace, home and sports injuries. Alcohol still continues to play an important role.

Safety beyond the age of 65

The aim at this age is to maintain independence despite deteriorating senses and balance. Accidents become increasingly prevalent the older you get, although as a percentage of death and disability they appear less important. Falls alone account for 60% of all deaths due to accidents in women above the age of 75, and 40% in men. Road traffic accidents account for 10–20% of deaths through accidents, most of which relate to elderly pedestrians rather than elderly drivers.

General Make sure your glasses and hearing aid, if worn, are as efficient as possible because you will be relying on your eyes and ears for your safety.

The home Look at the potential hazards in the home. The simplest things are the most important to fix. Secure loose rugs, fit handrails on stairs and tidy up trailing flexes. Do not lift things beyond your capability. Try not to have open flames or candles, which could start a fire. Have bright lighting, especially in dangerous areas like the stairs.

Many elderly people feel giddy on standing up or turning their head; allow for this by taking your time moving around. Consider getting a personal alarm, especially if you have fallen before, and let neighbours have a key for an emergency.

Outside Wear well-fitting shoes with non-slip heels. Think twice about going out in the ice or snow – just a minor fall can fracture your wrist or thigh. Take advantage of handrails and support from a friend or partner and if the time has come for a walking stick do not let pride stop you from using one.

Crossing the road is a potential hazard for the elderly: you should choose your spot with care at a proper marked crossing and cross with the lights. Do not assume that being elderly suspends the laws of motion, so give traffic time to stop.

ALZHEIMER'S DISEASE

A progressive brain disease with loss of recent memory, confusion and eventually dementia.

CAUSES

Personality, thought, emotion and foresight reside somewhere within the billions of cells of the brain and their complex intertwinings. Alzheimer's disease is the result of the degeneration of these interconnections. Instead of being orderly the connections become tangled; as the tangling increases so personality decreases. Evidence is growing that there is a defect in the acetylcholine system, one of the neurotransmitter chemicals in the brain.

A number of sub-variants of dementia are recognized, for example Lewy body dementia, but, as yet, they can only be differentiated post-mortem. Premature dementia – before the age of 60 – should be investigated for the uncommon but treatable disorders which can cause a similar picture such as a blood clot on the brain or a slow-growing **brain tumour**.

There is a very small hereditary risk factor in people with dementia which begins before the age of 60. However, even among the elderly only a minority are affected; about 80% of the over 80s have no particular problems. Alzheimer's affects two to three per cent of people aged between 65 and 75.

SYMPTOMS

The basic symptom is loss of recent memory; individuals still maintain clear recollections of events that occurred decades earlier. Early symptoms mimic the benign forgetfulness of age, such as mislaid glasses and people not recognized. Soon it becomes clear that there is more of a problem: even offspring go unrecognized, the individual starts wandering from her home and her life drifts into a permanent gloom of confusion. At some point there is **incontinence**, and often aggression shown towards family, as a result of complete confusion as to what carers are trying to do.

TREATMENT

It is important to exclude treatable causes by blood tests, used to detect severe **anaemia**, thyroid disease and syphilis. A brain scan may exclude blood clots or brain tumours (see pages 318 and 319). Otherwise the diagnosis rests on showing loss of short-term memory plus confusion, but all in clear consciousness, i.e. the sufferer is not drowsy or comatose. Drugs should be reviewed in case they are adding to confusion.

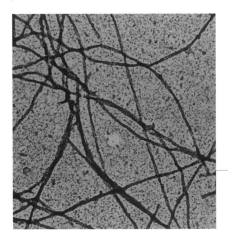

Left: A micrograph of brain tissue, showing the tangle of fibres characteristic of Alzheimer's disease.

As yet, there is no recognized treatment for Alzheimer's disease. Drugs becoming available are claimed to delay the deterioration but these are still unproven.

What can be done?

People with Alzheimer's should be kept stimulated by talking, reading and going out. It is important to keep them aware of time and place by talking about where they live and what they do each day. A regular schedule helps to root people in whatever remains of their appreciation of events. Many people get by, despite being quietly demented, while there is a routine and someone to keep an eye on them. This precarious hold on reality can be broken by moving into unfamiliar surroundings, loss of a companion who looked after them or other illness. Ultimately, people may need constant nursing care to help with all aspects of daily life. Agitation and physically wandering can be major problems, often treatable only by sedation.

People suffering Alzheimer's can live long after the onset of their illness, and usually die of an unrelated illness although chest infections are a common cause of death.

Complementary Treatment

Complementary approaches cannot reverse Alzheimer's disease. A **Western herbalist** might be able to help alleviate symptoms of the disease through the controlled use of ginkgo. **Massage**, especially when combined with **aromatherapy**, can offer support. An experienced **reflexologist** might be able to delay the progression of the disease. **Ayurveda** can offer oral preparations, along with oil baths to the head. Carers must try to ensure detoxification programmes are followed. **Tai chi/chi kung** can be beneficial in the earliest stages of the disease.

PHOBIAS

An abnormal degree of anxiety and fear provoked by one situation or object, leading to excessive steps to avoid that object or situation.

CAUSES

Mild phobias are common but about one in a hundred people has a phobia serious enough to cause them significant **anxiety**. There is no one agreed cause but there are some theories.

Certain things are common subjects of phobias: spiders, heights and by extension a fear of flying, and fear of open or crowded spaces. One theory is that these phobias derive from our prehistoric forebears, for whom poisonous insects were a real hazard; heights carried the risk of falling and open or crowded spaces the risk of being some other animal's lunch.

The psychological theory is that a phobia is a conditioned reflex. Through pure chance something provoked an episode of severe fear and thereafter the thing and the emotion it caused have become firmly entwined. A large friendly dog jumping up and scaring a toddler, for example, can become the source of a lifelong phobia of dogs. This theory has been extremely useful in planning treatment.

Psychoanalytic theories view objects of phobia as symbolic, stirring deeply buried emotions. Thus fear of open spaces is a mourning for loss of the womb and the mother; fear of snakes is a fear of male sexuality. Although thought provoking, such interpretations have not led to successful treatment.

SYMPTOMS

The prime symptom is anxiety at the sight or thought of the feared thing. For arachnophobes the mere thought, let alone sight, of a spider is enough to set them sweating and their heart racing. Severe phobias dominate one's life, turning it into a constant enterprise, for example, to root out spiders and to avoid anywhere that spiders might lurk. Clearly, such phobias become personally destructive.

Mild phobias can often be laughed off by people whose mental health is otherwise good. Severe phobias are socially disabling; the more bizarre they are, for example a fear of electricity leaking out of plugs, the more they might be symptomatic of other problems like alcoholism or **schizophrenia**.

TREATMENT

Mild phobias respond to sympathetic support plus sometimes a mild sedative, as experienced by those who share a slight phobia of flying but overcome it by encouragement and maybe an extra glass of wine.

Severe phobias are very successfully treated using desensitization techniques. With spiders, for example, arachnophobes first visualize one until they can cope with the emotion. They move on to looking at pictures of spiders, then observe real spiders in glass tanks and perhaps eventually handle one.

This slow process uncouples the anxiety from the object by the process of deconditioning and is now the preferred treatment for most phobias. There will be cases resistant to even this, for whom sedatives are the only answer. Any underlying mental illness of course needs treatment, too.

Complementary Treatment

Bach flower remedies – mimulus for known fears, aspen for inexplicable fears, rock rose for absolute terror, cherry plum for a fear of losing control and crab apple for a phobia relating to cleanliness. **Hypnotherapy** is excellent for changing unwanted patterns of behaviour. **Autogenic training** is self-administered psychotherapy which can help. **Ayurveda** might include *panchakarma* detoxification, meditation and *marma* therapy. *Other therapies to try: homeopathy; healing; Alexander Technique.*

Left and below: Flying, spiders and snakes: some of the most common things that stimulate people's phobias.

BRAIN TUMOUR

A growth originating in the brain itself or a growth that has spread from a cancer elsewhere in the body.

CAUSES

Brain tumours can be malignant (cancerous) or benign. The benign ones, called meningiomas, are very slow growing and cause symptoms not through destruction of tissue but by placing pressure on the brain.

Malignant growths within the brain are actually relatively uncommon, despite the enormous numbers of cells that make up the brain and its supporting structures. There are a hundred thousand million nerve cells alone. In theory, any one of these could turn malignant but in fact such primary tumours are unusual. It is far more likely that a brain tumour has spread from a cancer elsewhere, for example the breast or the lung. (Cancers similarly often spread into the bones, lungs and liver, which also have exceptionally good blood supply.)

Brain tumours in children may follow from the abnormal development of the foetus' nervous system.

SYMPTOMS

These depend on where the tumour is growing. There are parts of the brain where tumours can grow large without obvious problems, as in the frontal lobes. Yet even a tiny tumour in the pituitary gland produces symptoms. More destructive tumours lead to the loss of use of various functions, similar to the effects of a **stroke** but happening over weeks rather than instantly. So there may be progressive loss of use of an arm, giddiness, slurred speech or epileptic fits.

Most brain tumours eventually cause headaches. The particular features of these headaches are that they are worse in the morning and awaken you during the night. Often there is nausea and, if more advanced, abrupt vomiting without any warning. These are effects from pressure on the brain.

A particular feature of tumours in the frontal lobes is a change in personality: the individual tends to become moody and irritable. Tumours in the pituitary gland can cause unusual hormone disturbance leading to, for example, acromegaly, which is excessive bone growth.

Examination involves testing tendon reflexes, looking for weakness or unusual briskness. By examining the back of the eye through an ophthalmoscope it may be possible to detect signs of increased pressure within the brain called papilloedema. The diagnosis of brain tumours has been revolutionized by CT and MRI scanning (see pages 318 and 319).

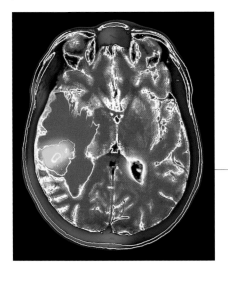

Left: An MRI scan clearly showing a large tumour in the left half of the brain.

TREATMENT

Some brain tumours can be successfully cut out – this is so with meningiomas and can lead to complete recovery. Even malignant tumours can sometimes be removed to give sufferers some relief of symptoms.

Unfortunately, most cannot be dealt with so directly. In this case the main option is radiotherapy (see page 338) to try to shrink the tumour. Steroid drugs also relieve the swelling around the tumour. The decision on treatment depends on the precise type of brain tumour, since some are more sensitive than others to radiotherapy.

Chemotherapy (see page 339) has not proved helpful in most cases, although some tumours do respond.

For all these reasons, the outlook for an adult with a malignant brain tumour is very poor. Although brain tumours are especially aggressive in children, they are often more sensitive to radiotherapy than in adults and are therefore more likely to be curable.

 Complementary Treatment
Complementary therapies will not be able to kill the tumour itself; however, many can help postoperatively. **Chakra balancing** will help with symptom control and energy balance, and also aid relaxation during orthodox treatment. **Hypnotherapy** can encourage a positive attitude. **Aromatherapy**, **massage** and **reflexology** are generally supportive. Any of the therapies listed under STRESS will be able to help ease the tensions associated with this disease.

ALCOHOL AND ALCOHOLISM

Alcoholism means compulsive drinking taking precedence over other activities, with withdrawal effects if alcohol is unavailable.

CAUSES

Alcohol is really a brain sedative: the pleasure comes from a mild degree of sedation of the brain, the pain comes from oversedation. A small amount of alcohol just slightly inhibits the brain's higher functions – thought, emotion and social inhibition. The shy become more extrovert, the anxious relax, the tongue-tied find unexpected eloquence.

With more drink the brain becomes more sedated, releasing controls on behaviour on which we can usually rely. We take a sharp comment as an insult; we stop noticing social cues such as the expression that says 'OK, stop there'; but we still imagine we are in control. As drinking continues muscle control becomes poor, with staggering and slurred speech; there is difficulty concentrating, then a slide into unconsciousness.

SYMPTOMS

Alcohol makes the blood vessels dilate, causing a flushed face and heat loss. (This is why it is a bad idea to give people too much alcohol to warm them up – they will experience an initial flush, but followed by a feeling of cold as they lose heat.)

Alcoholism is basically a dependence on alcohol. This means craving a drink, even in the morning, drinking a lot each day, drinking so much the drinker loses track of time. Drink or drunkenness begins to interfere with work and with the drinker's relationships.

Chronic alcohol abuse is associated with poor nutrition, because the energy derived from alcohol reduces appetite, leaving the drinker short of protein and vitamins. This can give rise to a permanently abnormal gait and tingling in the fingers. There is an increased risk of heart disease in drinkers, through a direct effect of alcohol on the muscle of the heart. In time the brain deteriorates, too, with a loss of memory and possibly even epileptic fits.

Heavy drinkers are at risk of **pancreatitis**, a painful inflammation of the pancreas. This gives rise to recurrent abdominal pain and **diabetes**. Cirrhosis of the liver is another long-term risk: the liver becomes hard and inefficient, with jaundice, easy bruising and potentially life-threatening bleeding from enlarged veins in the gullet (see LIVER PROBLEMS).

In addition to causing harm to the drinker, alcohol in excess is involved in much crime and violence and is still a major contributor to road traffic accidents.

TREATMENT

Acceptance by the drinker that they have a drink problem is a major step in the treatment of alcohol abuse. When people are given evidence as to how their health is being affected as well as guidance on sensible levels of alcohol, many people manage to pull back from alcoholism. Those people with a serious drink problem often need skilled support to reinforce their own will power. Sometimes drugs are given to aid rapid withdrawal of alcohol. This is called detoxification, but must be given under medical supervision.

STEPS TO COPING WITH A DRINK PROBLEM

- *Accept that there is a problem*
- *Recognize the effects on health, work and family*
- *Adopt safe limits*
- *Use medication short term to aid withdrawal*

There are many support groups that offer drinkers help: Alcoholics Anonymous is the best known.

Safe alcohol intake
The current British recommendations of maximum alcohol intake for men are 28 units a week and for women 21 units a week (see below).

The consumption of alcohol is measured in units:
- *A glass of wine = 1 unit*
- *A measure of spirits = 1 unit*
- *A pint of beer = 2 units*

Complementary Treatment

Massage promotes feelings of self-esteem and fosters a positive body image. **Auricular therapy** can help reduce harm during periods of alcohol abuse, ease the detoxification process when you come off, and help maintain abstinence. **Hypnotherapy** is excellent at changing unwanted patterns of behaviour and reducing cravings. Diet – seek help from a **nutritional therapist** or **naturopath**: you may well be malnourished because alcohol provides empty calories. *Other therapies to try: healing; acupuncture; Hellerwork; Ayurveda; chakra balancing.*

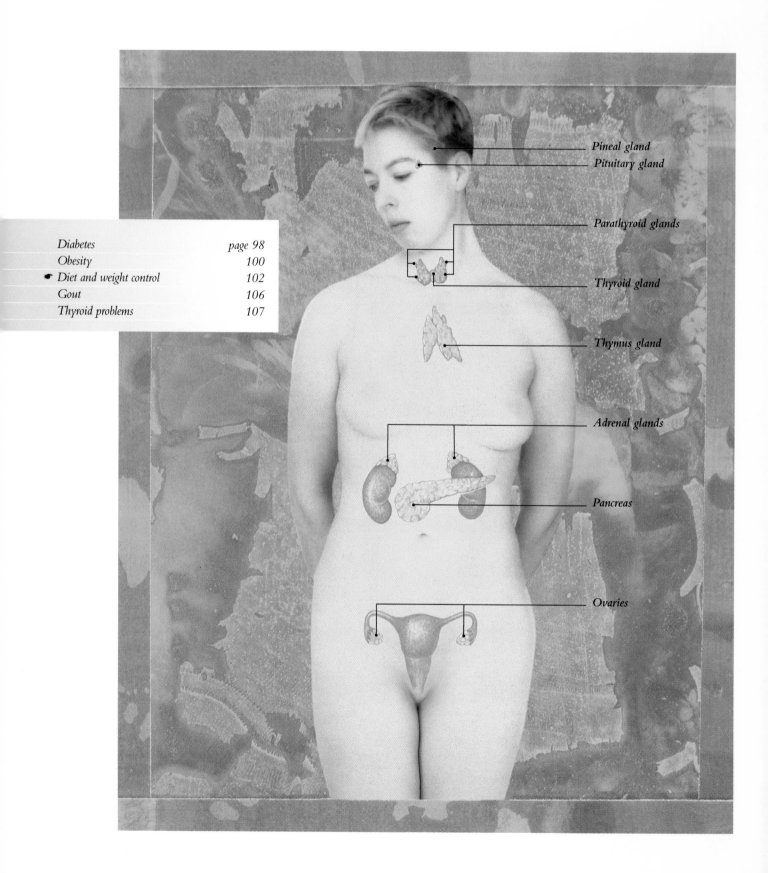

Pineal gland

Pituitary gland

Parathyroid glands

Thyroid gland

Thymus gland

Adrenal glands

Pancreas

Ovaries

*All living organisms need to exert control over their more distant components —
the most well-known control system is the nervous system with its pathways of
muscle-controlling nerves. The endocrine system is less obvious and relies on glands.*

ENDOCRINE SYSTEM AND METABOLISM

T HE GLANDS OF THE endocrine system are specialized tissues, which release biochemically active
substances called hormones. Hormones move
around the body in the body fluids. The cells on
which hormones act detect them by means of receptors on
their surface, which latch on to the hormone molecule and
trigger a desired effect within the cell. Most hormones, such
as adrenaline, are small molecules; some, like insulin, are
much larger and more complex molecules.

Insulin and thyroid hormones are well known; less recognized but vitally important are calcitonin and parathormone,
involved in the calcium balance needed for muscle activity
and bone density. These are produced in the parathyroid
glands which are in the neck. The ovaries and womb produce
progesterone and oestrogen, which control the menstrual
cycle and pregnancy. The adrenal glands secrete adrenaline,
noradrenaline and cortisol, which enhance the body's reaction
to stress. Yet more hormones stimulate growth, sperm formation and blood pressure. There is a whole array of hormones
that help control the intestinal tract and they play a crucial
role in regulating metabolism.

Metabolism refers to all the biochemical processes within
the body by which it survives and grows. It includes especially
the digestion of food, and how it is used to create proteins and
the innumerable other biochemical ingredients of life.
Metabolic disorders include **gout**, which involves abnormal
handling of protein, and **obesity**, due to excess food intake.

Many hormones are regulated by elegant feedback loops,
involving the hypothalamus and pituitary gland. This pea-
sized gland located beneath the brain is the origin of some
hormones, called releasing factors, that regulate the concentration of other hormones. The hypothalamic/pituitary unit

*Left: Hormones from glands affect digestion,
energy use, emotion and menstruation, among
many other aspects of metabolism.*

monitors the blood levels of these other hormones and
increases or decreases their production accordingly by sending releasing factors to stimulate the endocrine glands. This
is why disease of the pituitary gland can have widespread
effects on health. Examples are growth deficiency, gigantism
(acromegaly), **subfertility** and collapse of blood pressure.

How the system can go wrong
Endocrine disorders are often the result of an auto-immune
condition. In such illnesses the body turns against its own
tissues and destroys them with antibodies, which can be
detected in blood samples. Examples of auto-immune hormone disorders are thyroid disease and adrenal insufficiency.
Growths (usually benign) in endocrine glands are a common
cause of excess secretion of hormones. The critical hypothala-
mus/pituitary complex is most often affected by benign
tumours or by deterioration of blood flow to the gland.

Detecting and treating disorders
Fortunately many deficient hormones can be replaced or, if
the problem is an excess of hormone, the output of the gland
responsible can be biochemically blocked. For this reason
many hormone disorders can be successfully treated.

Hormone disorders are detected by measuring concentrations of hormones in the blood. The interpretation of these
tests is complex because hormone levels are affected by the
time of day, stress, medication and even how long it takes to
analyse the blood sample. Additional investigation of hormone disorders may call for brain scans to detect disease of
the hypothalamus or pituitary gland, or scans of the neck or
abdomen to detect disease of important glands such as the
pancreas, the thyroid and the adrenal glands.

This section concentrates on four conditions that are linked
with hormones. Many other parts of this book deal with other
hormonal problems, such as menstruation, **pregnancy
problems**, subfertility and **osteoporosis**.

DIABETES

An abnormality in the body's handling of sugar.

CAUSES

Sugar, in the form of glucose, is the basic fuel of the body, obtained from carbohydrates (bread and starch) or made within the body by a complex biochemical pathway. It circulates within the blood stream to all body cells; close biochemical control ensures the quantity of sugar in the blood matches the body's needs. Too little blood sugar leads to light-headedness and tiredness; too much blood sugar is diabetes.

A constant high sugar intake in the diet takes its toll on this control system, which eventually can no longer control the blood sugar accurately. Blood sugar then remains persistently high and the individual becomes diabetic – known as Type II, maturity-onset or non-insulin dependent diabetes.

Insulin

Without insulin little sugar would be absorbed by most cells (the brain is an exception since it absorbs sugar regardless of insulin levels). Insulin is the hormone switch that tells cells to let sugar in. It is produced by the pancreas gland and released into the blood stream in response to the body's needs for energy. Any disease of the pancreas causing a deficiency of insulin will lead to high levels of blood glucose. This insulin deficiency is the other major cause of diabetes, called Type I, or insulin-dependent diabetes.

Just why the pancreas fails to produce insulin is not well understood. Certain illnesses, such as **pancreatitis**, cause damage to the pancreas, but this is not the case for most diabetes; yet something causes the insulin cells to switch off. This switching off can be a dramatic event in young people in whom diabetes can develop over a few weeks.

SYMPTOMS

Diabetes causes both immediate and long-term problems. The immediate problems are the direct chemical consequences of high blood sugar while the long-term problems are the result of damage to cells after years of exposure to high blood sugar.

Short-term effects

Excess urine output/increased thirst: High sugar levels present the kidneys with too much sugar to be properly reabsorbed, so sugar leaks out with the urine. Large amounts of fluid leave with the sugar, thus one of the early symptoms of diabetes is passing a lot of urine. Because of the fluid loss,

the diabetic feels thirsty and drinks much more than usual. In extreme cases the individual cannot keep pace with the fluid loss and becomes seriously dehydrated, with confusion and weakness, ultimately lapsing into a coma. Before insulin was discovered, this was how many young diabetics died.

Tiredness: Despite a superabundance of sugar in the blood stream, without adequate insulin the body cannot transport it into the cells where it is needed as fuel.

Weight loss: Unable to use sugar, the body turns to making its energy from fat and even protein from muscle, hence the weight loss. This presentation is especially dramatic in diabetics whose pancreas has failed – the younger diabetics. They become rapidly ill with weight loss and dehydration.

Infections: Bacteria feed on sugar. Diabetics have masses of the stuff in their urine and blood. This makes them walking banquets for bacteria, leading to **thrush** (a fungal infection of the groins, armpits and vagina), boils and abscesses.

Long-term effects

Over years the high blood sugar levels damage blood vessels all around the body permanently. Within the retina blood vessels leak and overgrow and may lead to **blindness** – diabetes is the most common cause of acquired blindness. Small blood vessels in the legs become diseased, thus diabetics are prone to leg **ulcers** and poor blood flow to the legs. Disease of the kidneys reduces their efficiency and can lead to **kidney failure**. Disease of the circulation of the heart and brain explains why diabetics are at greater risk of heart disease and **stroke**. It is therefore very important to detect and to treat diabetes.

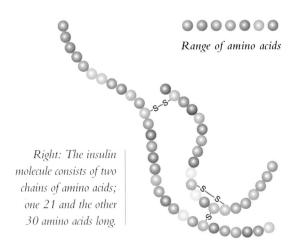

Range of amino acids

Right: The insulin molecule consists of two chains of amino acids; one 21 and the other 30 amino acids long.

Detection

The urine can be checked for sugar using a biochemical testing strip. If sugar is present then a blood test is taken to see whether blood sugar really is high. If there is still doubt then a glucose tolerance test might be required: you drink a very sweet drink and have half-hourly measurements of blood sugar for the next two hours.

TREATMENT

♦

The aim of treatment is to keep blood sugar levels as close to normal as possible. This is done by reducing sugar intake with a balanced diet and by using drugs or insulin.

Diet

A diet with balanced amounts of fat, protein and sugar is important for diabetics. The sugar should be in a natural, unrefined form, as in fruit and vegetables. Diabetics should aim to lose excess weight. Most people with maturity-onset diabetes find that diet alone will give good control.

Drugs

These are used where diet is insufficient but they are not a substitute for a diet. The sulphonylurea drugs stimulate the pancreas to release more insulin and are best for those who are not overweight and who therefore have some reserve of insulin. Drug names include gliclazide and glibenclamide.

Biguanide drugs help sugar to be absorbed by cells as well as reducing the absorption of carbohydrates from the intestinal system. A kind of insulin substitute, they are used in diabetics who are overweight. The best known is metformin.

Insulin

There is no substitute for insulin for severe diabetics and especially for young people with acute diabetes. Modern devices allow diabetics a high degree of control of their insulin dosage – for example discreet syringes, which look like pens, are used to give a boost of insulin when needed, on top of a regular dose once or twice a day. Almost anyone can learn to self-inject with these user-friendly devices. Because insulin is a protein it is not possible to take it by mouth – the body would just digest it. Research is aiming to overcome this.

Quality of control

The aim is to keep blood sugar levels within a fairly narrow normal band; it is checked by taking finger-prick samples of blood for analysis in glucose meters. Testing urine for sugar is a more rough-and-ready check but adequate for non insulin-dependent diabetics.

Diabetics need regular medical checks so complications can be detected and treated early. They should check their feet for ulcers and have chiropody to avoid injuries ulcerating. Annual eye checks will reveal disease in the retina or **cataracts**, which are more treatable at an early stage. Kidney function is monitored by testing urine for protein. Since they have a high risk of heart and circulation trouble, diabetics should avoid other risk factors, including **high blood pressure** and smoking.

QUESTIONS

Who needs insulin?
Most young diabetics with disease of sudden severe onset require insulin. Otherwise, it is considered when diet and drugs have failed to gain control and the individual is running into complications.

What are the hazards from drugs or insulin?
An excessive dosage will send blood sugar below normal, called hypoglycaemia. This starts with light-headedness; severe hypoglycaemia causes confusion, sweating and then unconsciousness, including a risk of epileptic fits. Diabetics, especially those on insulin, and their companions should learn to recognize the early signs of hypoglycaemia. Treatment is to take a sweet drink or an injection of glucagon, a hormone which raises blood sugar rapidly.

Complementary Treatment

Diabetes becomes a medical emergency if it is not properly controlled, so do not abandon conventional treatment. **Autogenic training** allows mind and body to rebalance themselves; hormone levels may rise and fall according to the system's needs. Severe insulin-controlled diabetes will probably not respond but, in combination with dietary control, good results can be achieved for late-onset diabetes. Diet – changing to a wholefood, even vegan, diet, can help all diabetics. Nutritional deficiencies can be implicated in adult-onset diabetes, for example zinc, chromium, magnesium and B vitamins. Consult a **nutritional therapist** about supplementation. Increased vitamin E may be needed. **Ayurveda** can help if diabetes is linked to diet, when a number of preparations are available; **yoga** and *marma* puncture also help. **Tai chi/chi kung** is a gentle form of exercise which may benefit diabetics.

OBESITY

◆

Carrying a great excess of weight in relation to your build and height.

CAUSES

◆

In the developed world the days are gone when eating was purely and simply for survival. The 1500–3000 calories that most people need are there in plenty.

Eating has become a focus for many other things: a social affair, a business event, even a fashion statement. Food is marketed in appealing and convenient ways. It is cheap, abundant and desirable, ready to eat at the flick of a switch. Little wonder that babies are overfed, becoming children who graze all day, then adults who eat instant convenience foods containing sugar and large quantities of fat and salt.

It is important not to overfeed babies as there is evidence that fat children grow into fat adults, and obesity is an increasingly serious problem in childhood. The fat child will experience ridicule quite apart from future health problems.

A slow route to obesity

The obese are rarely relentless gluttons who have guzzled themselves into fatness. It takes just a small but regular excess intake of food over many years to accumulate into obesity.

Whatever calories are not needed each day the body turns into fat and puts by, for a 'rainy day': a bit on the hips, a bit on the belly until eventually there is more than a bit everywhere and the rainy day never comes.

Physical causes or inherited from parents?

There is some truth that obesity is all to do with glands or genes, or parents or **depression**. Underactivity, however, is a more likely cause. People who do not walk or exercise but eat as much as an athlete are heading straight for trouble. Comfort eating is universal. Never has it been so easy, nor the comfort so dangerous, with salt-, sugar- and fat-enriched cakes and biscuits rather than fruit or vegetables.

There are a few gland problems that lead to overweight. The most probable is an underactive thyroid gland, but this is less common than many believe (see THYROID PROBLEMS).

There is some evidence that obesity is partly inherited. Doctors do not yet know how significant the 'obesity gene' is. It may explain obesity in some individuals who are apparently resistant to normal dietary control, but it is inconceivable that the gene has spread in a generation or two to cause the widespread obesity that is now seen across the developed world. (See also page 102.)

SYMPTOMS

◆

After being weighed and measured, you can be compared to a table of 'normal' height and weight. But what if everyone is already overweight? If you weigh an 'average' weight the table will tell you that you are average even though, objectively, you are overweight. A more meaningful statistic overcomes this problem with averages; it is called the body mass index (BMI) (see below).

The formula for BMI is:

$$BMI = \frac{Weight\ (in\ kilograms)}{Height\ (in\ metres)\ squared}$$

For example, for a woman weighing 90 kg/14 st and 1.75 m/5 ft 9 in tall, the calculation is:

$$BMI = \frac{90}{1.75 \times 1.75}$$

which gives a BMI of 29.39. A BMI between 19 and 24 is normal for a woman, and between 20 and 25 for men. A BMI above 30 is obese. Clearly, there are degrees of overweight short of obesity.

General effects

Imagine a large sack of potting compost weighing 25 kg/ 55 lb. This is equivalent to a modest degree of overweight. Mentally place that across your shoulders and stand up. You would experience pressure on your hips while sitting; as you stand your knee joints will groan and your hips twinge. Although you have only stood up, already a thin film of sweat coats your brow. You walk, feeling clunks in your ankles, knees and hips on each step and that is just on the level. You plod up a gentle slope that feels like a mountain; by now your heart is racing, your breathing is short, your shoulders ache, you feel tired. You are experiencing obesity.

Your joints, heart and lungs are under strain and you face early **osteoarthritis** and **high blood pressure**, increasing the risks of **heart disease** and **stroke**. In terms of specific effects, the overweight are prone to skin infections, especially in warm moist areas beneath the breasts and between the upper thighs. **Diabetes** is a likelihood. The sheer enjoyment of life is reduced because of awkwardness and self-consciousness.

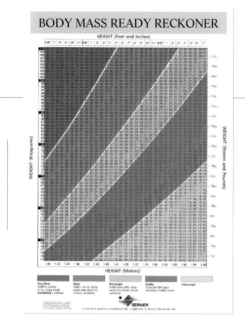

BODY MASS READY RECKONER

Right: Very high and very low BMIs are abnormal, as shown on this chart.

TREATMENT

♦

Overweight people have to take the mental step of accepting that the control of the problem is in their own hands. It is unproductive and too easy to blame the food industry, **stress** of work or depression, although these may all play a part.

Targets and diets

Using the BMI, calculate your target range of healthy weights – you may feel more comfortable a little heavier or lighter within that band. Then calculate how long it will take to reach that weight on the basis of losing 0.5–1 kg/1–2 lb a week. This may seem a surprisingly long time, but it has taken you a lifetime to reach your current weight. By losing weight slowly you lose true excess fat. Crash diets appear successful but it is mainly fluid that is lost, which reaccumulates rapidly.

All diets share one property: eating less, although the details vary. The aim is to eat 1000–1200 calories a day. This must include all snacks and nibbles, which are so easily 'overlooked'. Most people lose weight steadily on such a regime. Some people are truly more resistant and need an 800–1000 calorie diet; these must be specially designed for the individual to be nutritionally sound, balancing fat, carbohydrate, protein and vitamins. There is a weight-loss diet for everyone, although for some it will be uncomfortably low in calories.

Exercise and other manoeuvres . . .

As well as reducing energy intake, you should increase your energy output. Walking just 1.5 km/1 mile as briskly as possible three times a week is a target that everyone should be able to incorporate into their lifestyle.

Appetite-suppressant drugs are frowned on, because their effects are temporary and they can be addictive. Also, they have worrying stimulant side effects. There is a case, however, for using them under careful supervision when first embarking on a diet.

Surgery for obesity fluctuates in popularity. It is possible to staple the stomach, clamp the jaws or even remove part of the intestine. These drastic measures are resorted to only after careful psychological assessment.

QUESTIONS

How dangerous is overweight?
Modest overweight, i.e. a BMI of 25–30, is not necessarily a significant health risk. True obesity – a BMI above 30 – carries significant hazards for the heart and joints.

How should I choose a diet?
Health diets should include fat, carbohydrate, minerals and vitamins – it is unhealthy to exclude one thing, such as fat, completely. Do check the nutritional content of dietary drinks and foods. You will lose weight on any crash diet in a week, but it is not good for long-term results.

Can I lose weight without following a particular diet?
Aim to eat less and exercise more. Strategies include using smaller plates (which still look satisfyingly full), eat only at meal times, eat slowly. Don't snack; if desperate nibble on fruit or vegetables.

Complementary Treatment

Complementary therapists are likely to recommend gentle exercise, reducing calories and healthy eating, as well as specific treatments. Be wary of any tablets for weight loss, no matter how natural the ingredients appear. No diet should make you feel ill or involve bizarre foods. **Aromatherapy** is excellent for raising self-esteem; try one of the following oils in the bath (six drops) or as inhalations (two to four drops in a bowl of water or on a handkerchief): cypress, fennel, rosemary, lemon, juniper or black pepper. Diet – it is important to get sound advice from a **nutritional therapist** or a **naturopath**. **Hypnotherapy** can identify and release emotional or psychological causes; suggestion is used to change eating and lifestyle habits. **Ayurveda** – some preparations restore metabolism and eliminate toxins. *Other therapies to try: homeopathy; tai chi/chi kung; autogenic training; healing; chakra balancing.*

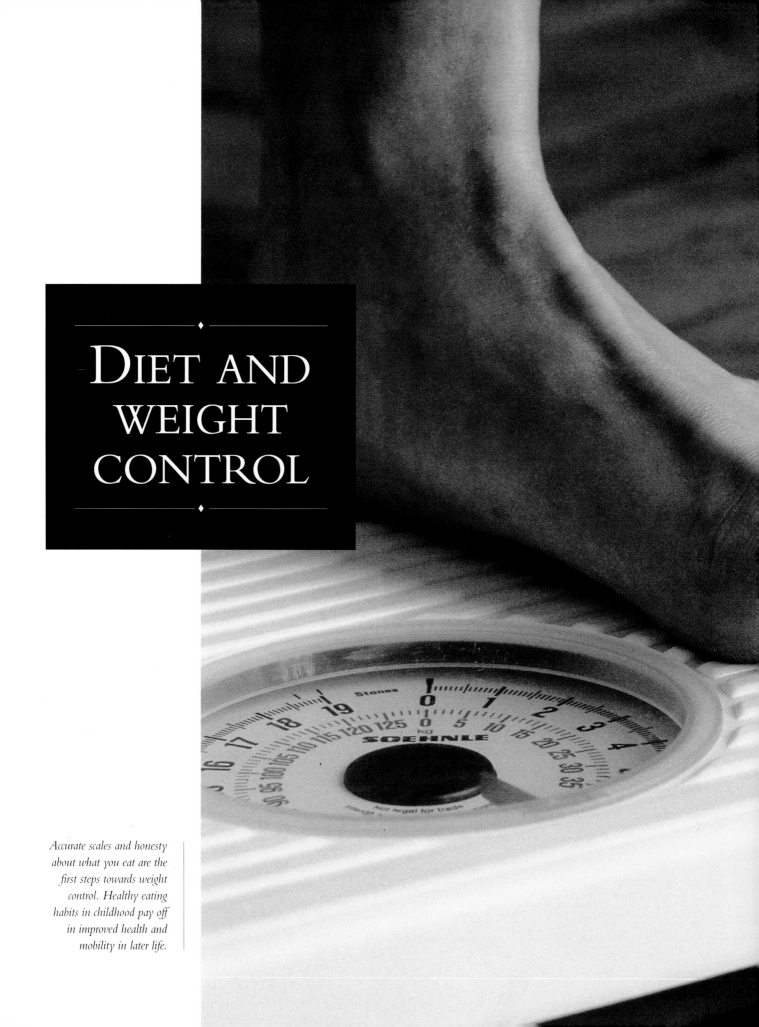

DIET AND WEIGHT CONTROL

Accurate scales and honesty about what you eat are the first steps towards weight control. Healthy eating habits in childhood pay off in improved health and mobility in later life.

OURS IS PROBABLY THE FIRST century in which large numbers of people in some countries have had more food than they need. This welcome change from widespread starvation and malnutrition, still so common in much of the world, has brought its own problems in the form of diseases of affluence. There are health consequences from the sheer fact of being overweight, and from the types of food we eat.

Diseases of affluence

The consequences of overeating include heart disease, **diabetes** and the physical effects of **obesity**. What is the route to this? Why have **heart attacks** moved from being rare to being the most common cause of sudden death?

It appears that the affluent diet leads to high levels of cholesterol, and thus to **atherosclerosis** and heart attacks. Saturated fats (hard fats) are ubiquitous in our Western diet – in cakes, biscuits and chocolate especially – and these are thought to be a major factor in cholesterol levels.

Fat, fibre and physical exertion

In some ways the 20th century has been an enormous experiment with regard to what the human body can get away with. Can we eat more saturated fat and get away with it? The answer appears to be no. We develop high cholesterol, followed by atherosclerosis and then **high blood pressure**, **strokes** and heart disease. The experimental conclusion? 'Nice but nasty.'

Can we safely eat less fibre? We do not go out of our way to eat less fibre – it is just that it seems so boring to eat all those breads and grains. As for brown rice . . . Instead, we have turned to high protein/low fibre food – essentially meats and fewer green vegetables and potatoes. The experimental conclusion? Increased **constipation**, **diverticular diseases**, possibly **irritable bowel syndrome** and probably an increased risk of **bowel cancer**.

As well as changes in diet there have been profound changes in our physical activity: we walk less, move less and exert ourselves less. Lack of activity, by leaving our cardiovascular system unchallenged, compounds the effects of diet, increasing our susceptibility to circulation problems. Increasing obesity is linked to decreasing general fitness.

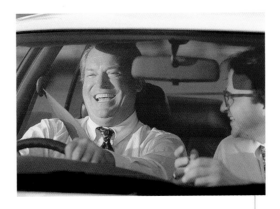

Above: Our increasingly sedentary lifestyles can result in health problems.

Other factors

There are a number of other dietary factors that affect health and weight control.

Salt Salt is an ubiquitous flavour enhancer, particularly in processed food where it is used in everything from custard to cakes. It is clear that high salt levels increase high blood pressure and therefore heart disease. Some evidence suggests that salt may also play a role in **stomach cancer**. The World Health Organization recommends no more than 5 g/¼ oz a day. Avoid crisps, biscuits and instant foods.

Sugar Sugar in all its forms is an answer to a human dream. We cannot get enough of it. In ancient civilizations people risked their lives to get honey, so deeply was sweetness craved. Now that we can get it out of a vending machine our desire knows no bounds. Why is it bad for us? Refined sugar predisposes to obesity and exhausts the pancreas, leading to diabetes. It contains no supplementary health benefits and blunts our appetite for more health-giving foods. This is over and above **tooth decay**, once a rarity but now common.

Vitamins These chemicals play vital roles in the body's metabolism but the body cannot make them for itself. Though they are required in only small quantities, deficiency can cause many illnesses. Vitamin deficiency is uncommon in affluent societies among those who eat a broad and balanced diet. Strict vegetarians may become deficient in Vitamin B_{12} if they eat no animal or dairy products and pregnant women may become deficient in folic acid, otherwise vitamin deficiency is most likely to result from deliberate self-neglect, for example in alcoholics, or diseases such as pernicious anaemia.

Minerals The body requires many simple elements such as iron, zinc, copper, selenium, calcium, sodium and potassium. All play more or less vital roles in metabolism. Excess is more likely than deficiency, most notably in the case of sodium, in salt. In large parts of the world iodine is naturally deficient in food, leading to **thyroid problems** and goitre. It is therefore often added to salt and dairy products. Iron deficiency is very common, especially in women, who lose it in pregnancy and through menstruation, and in children coping with the demands of growth.

Vitamin and mineral supplements There is little need for these in adults who eat a normal healthy diet. They may be advisable for the elderly if they eat little fresh fruit or for rapidly growing children, whose eating habits are also picky.

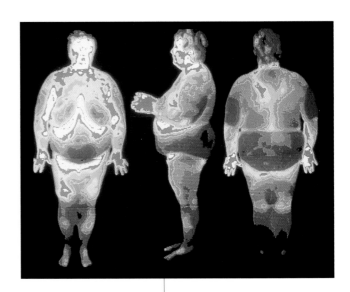

Above: Heat radiation in an obese person; the lighter coloured areas are mainly over the warm fatty parts.

A STRATEGY FOR HEALTHY EATING

◆

♦ *Try to eat something from each food group (see Food Values table on opposite page) every day*

♦ *Eat more carbohydrates in the form of pasta, potatoes, rice, pulses and bread*

♦ *Eat more fibre from fruit, vegetables and wholemeal bread. You need at least 25–30 g/1 oz a day*

♦ *Eat more fruit and vegetables – as well as providing fibre and vitamins these contribute antioxidants, which may be important in preventing cancer of the stomach or lung by scavenging free radicals – naturally occurring biochemicals, which are believed to have a role in causing disease. Green leafy vegetables are particularly good for you. Eat three helpings of vegetables and two of fruit a day. It makes no difference whether these are fresh or frozen; salads and fruit juices can be counted as helpings*

♦ *Select processed foods that are low in salt, sugar and saturated fat*

♦ *Eat less fat – reduce your intake to 77–87 g/3 oz a day. Select sources of non-saturated fat, e.g. fish. Select milk and dairy products low in fat and eat only lean meat*

Children and the elderly equally benefit from healthy eating, but if you plan to make wide-ranging changes to your children's diet take your health visitor's advice first.

Obesity

The physical effects of obesity are those to be expected from carrying more than your recommended body weight: arthritic pains, breathlessness and **gallstones**, which are common in affluent countries but rare elsewhere. **Breast cancer** shows an association with high-energy and high-fat diets.

Being obese means having a body mass index (BMI) of at least 30 – implying at least one-third over ideal weight (see page 100). This index has been steadily creeping up: in 1980 seven per cent of the population of the United Kingdom had a BMI over thirty. By 1995 this figure had more than doubled: 15 per cent of men and 16.5 per cent of women were obese.

Dieting

Most sensible diets restrict fat and empty calories (sugar) while maintaining the necessary amounts of protein, minerals, complex carbohydrates and vitamins. The amount of carbohydrate you need depends on your activity levels. Most people will lose weight if they restrict total calorie intake to about 1100 calories a day. Do this by restricting fat and simple carbohydrates – sweets, biscuits and cake. A healthy daily calorie intake for men and women aged 19–60 is 2550 and 1940 calories respectively, assuming average physical activity and that there is no need to lose weight.

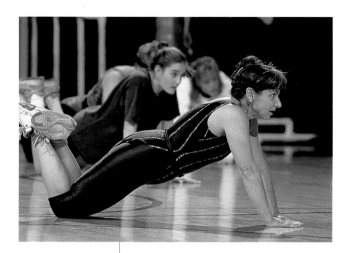

Above: Exercise is complementary to sensible eating for a healthy life style.

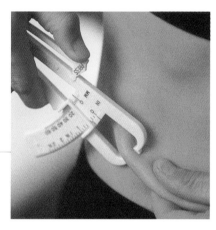

Right: Skin fold thickness reliably indicates total body fat.

LOSING WEIGHT — THE PRINCIPLES

◆

- ◆ *Work out a target weight*
- ◆ *Review your food intake, especially empty calories from alcohol, sweet drinks, snacks, crisps, sweets and chocolate*
- ◆ *Remember you still need some carbohydrate and fat*
- ◆ *Choose a balanced diet – you're more likely to stick to it, preferably for ever*
- ◆ *Diet with a friend*
- ◆ *Aim to lose slowly but certainly (250–500 g/½–1 lb a week), not 'dash and crash'*
- ◆ *Eat slowly, from small plates and only at meal times*
- ◆ *Combine dieting with increased exercise – three half-hour walks a week will do*
- ◆ *Reward yourself for success – but not with food!*

Always take professional advice before beginning strict dieting or greatly increased activity.

FOOD VALUES

◆

This simple table gives some idea of what each type of food provides. Clearly a vegetarian diet can be perfectly healthy, although one lacking dairy products and eggs could lead to vitamin and mineral deficiencies.

Food	Provides
Meat, fish, eggs, pulses, nuts	Protein Carbohydrates Fat Minerals (iron, potassium, copper, selenium, zinc, phosphorus) Vitamins (B_{12}, thiamine, niacin)
Dairy products	Protein Carbohydrates Fat (especially saturated fat) Minerals (calcium, phosphorus, zinc) Vitamins (especially A and B_{12})
Fruit and vegetables	Carbohydrates and fibre Vitamins (folic acid, A, C) Minerals (potassium, magnesium)
Cereals (includes bread, pasta, rice)	Protein Carbohydrates and fibre Minerals (iron, calcium, zinc) Vitamins (B complex and E)

GOUT

A disease of joints due to an excess of uric acid in the blood.

CAUSES

Somewhat unfairly, gout has the image of a self-inflicted disease, the result of overindulgence on heavy wines and red meat. In fact, most cases have little to do with lifestyle.

The condition is due to excess uric acid within the body. Uric acid is produced by the digestion of protein and is usually excreted in urine. If the blood contains too much uric acid, it can crystallize inside the joints, the earlobes and the kidneys.

People who have gout nearly always have an inherited tendency to high blood levels of uric acid. There are certain drugs that can increase uric acid levels, notably thiazide diuretics used to treat **high blood pressure** such as bendroflu-azide. A much less common cause is anything that increases cell turnover, and therefore protein load; this includes certain forms of **leukaemia**.

Those with a tendency to gout may indeed find that overindulgence in rich foods or alcohol brings on an attack, probably by giving a little more protein than the body can handle. The disease is very unusual in women. It is most common in middle-aged men; finding it in a young person should prompt a search for an underlying blood disorder.

SYMPTOMS

The most common initial symptom is sudden and excruciating pain in one joint – most often the big toe, although any joint can be affected including the knees, elbows and shoulders. The pain is a result of crystallization of uric acid within the joint, which becomes swollen, hot and reddened and tender to the slightest movement. Pain lasts for several days.

After repeated attacks the joints become misshapen and stiff. Crystals also precipitate in the ear lobes and the tissues around joints. Crystals may form within the kidneys, affecting kidney efficiency. These complications are unusual nowadays because the disease is recognized early and treatment is straightforward. The diagnosis is confirmed by finding high blood levels of uric acid, or by showing that fluid from an affected joint contains crystals of uric acid.

TREATMENT

Immediate relief is the first priority in the treatment of gout and this is effectively given by an anti-inflammatory drug such as ibuprofen, indomethacin or diclofenac but *not* aspirin.

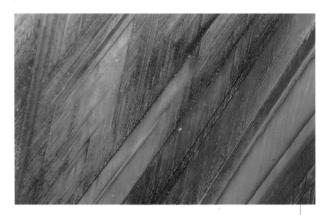

Above: These crystals of uric acid, seen here glowing under polarized light, are the cause of gout.

Failing that, one old remedy for gout is colchicine, although this does tend to cause **diarrhoea** as a side effect.

It is important to review any medication people with gout may be taking in case certain drugs are to blame and, if so, to stop or alter their dosage. A blood count will detect the rare blood disorders that can cause gout. Some adjustments to lifestyle may be sensible, especially reducing alcohol intake and being cautious about rich foods.

Many people with gout have only occasional attacks, which are adequately handled by pain relief alone. However, if attacks are frequent, if there is kidney damage or if the blood uric acid is persistently very high, then long-term treatment usually becomes advisable. Allopurinol is the mainstay. This is a drug that increases the output of uric acid in the urine by making it into a more water-soluble form. Taken just once a day and with few side effects, allopurinol now makes the complications of gout a thing of the past for the great majority of sufferers.

Complementary Treatment

Western herbalism remedies containing celery seed can speed up uric acid excretion, helping to reduce pain and inflammation. Celery seed is particularly useful in cases of recurrent gout. **Chakra balancing** can be used for pain control. **Hypnotherapy** can be used for pain relief, and to change unwanted patterns of behaviour. Possible **Ayurvedic** treatments include *panchakarma* detoxification, oral medications and diet. *Other therapies to try: Chinese herbalism; homeopathy; cymatics; autogenic training.*

THYROID PROBLEMS

Disease of the thyroid gland is a common cause of vague ill health, weight loss or weight gain.

CAUSES

If there is one switch that controls the body's activity it is the thyroid gland. This shield-shaped gland lies in the neck on either side of the windpipe. Thyroid hormone regulates the level of metabolic activity of the cells of the body: too much and they go into overdrive (hyperthyroidism); too little and there is a sluggish underactivity (hypothyroidism).

Thyroid disease is usually a result of an auto-immune condition, where the body treats its own tissues as a foreign invader. It sends in white cells and other immune factors which destroy the thyroid gland. This holds both for over- and underactive glands. Underactive glands can also result from treatment of a previous overactive gland. Iodine is essential to the formation of thyroid hormone and iodine deficiency leads to underactivity of the gland.

SYMPTOMS

Both under- and overactivity of the thyroid begin in a slow way and are often overlooked by family, friends and doctors.

Overactivity

The body's rate of activity is speeded up. People feel on edge and notice a fine tremor of their hands. They sweat, feel hot and seem in a rush. The heart rate is raised well above the normal 60–90 beats per minute and they may feel **palpitations**. Weight loss is common as the body burns energy at a rapid rate; the appetite is good to ravenous. In Graves' disease a staring eye appearance is due to abnormal tissue deposited behind the eyes. Left untreated, hyperthyroidism (thyrotoxicosis) ends in exhaustion and, ultimately, **heart failure**. It is most common in women between 20 and 50.

Underactivity

The picture is in reverse: people feel sluggish and tired and might gain weight despite a normal appetite. Their skin feels cool and rough and their features look coarse and puffy. The heart rate is below 60. There is often **constipation** and **depression**. Hypothyroidism can lead to severe hypothermia (very low body temperature), apathy, self-neglect and heart failure. It is common in middle age and very common in the elderly. Underactivity is rare in children. It is detectable by a blood test which is done routinely in many countries at birth.

TREATMENT

The diagnosis is confirmed by blood tests of the exact level of thyroid hormone. These tests can also monitor treatment.

Overactivity

Two drugs are used to bring the gland under control: carbimazole and propylthiouracil. Both take several weeks to work, during which time a beta-blocker helps relieve the sense of agitation and palpitations. Treatment continues for several months. Many cases settle like this. If the illness recurs the options are to remove part of the gland (a thyroidectomy) or destroy it with a radioactive, but harmless, form of iodine.

Underactivity

Replacement thyroid hormone is given as a daily tablet of thyroxine. It is initially used as a very low dose – as the hypothyroid heart is very sensitive to it – and guided by blood tests as to the right dose. Once stable, the patient remains on thyroxine for life, requiring regular blood tests to check control.

Complementary Treatment

Complementary approaches should not replace conventional treatment. **Autogenic training** allows mind and body to rebalance themselves; hormone levels may rise and fall according to the system's needs. Nutritional deficiencies may be implicated in some thyroid problems, for example zinc, vitamin A, selenium and iron – a **nutritional therapist** will be able to advise on supplementation. *Other therapies to try: cymatics; yoga; tai chi/chi kung; reflexology.*

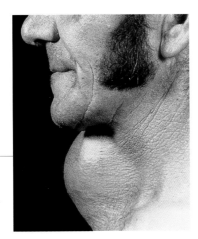

Right: Graves' disease (hyperthyroidism) has here caused an enormous goitre. Underactivity (hypothyroidism) can also cause goitres.

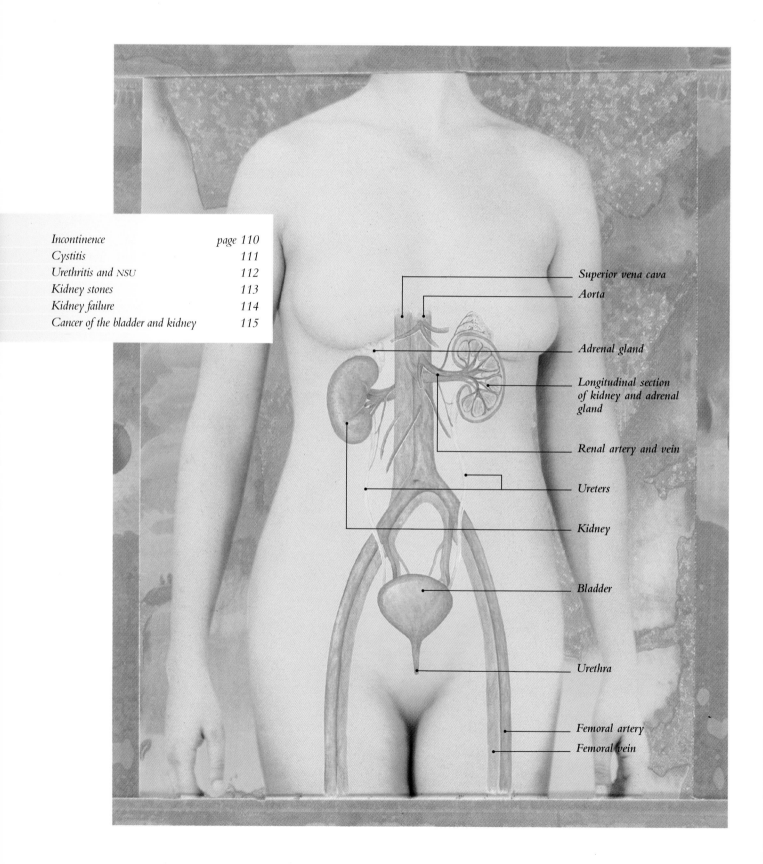

Superior vena cava

Aorta

Adrenal gland

Longitudinal section of kidney and adrenal gland

Renal artery and vein

Ureters

Kidney

Bladder

Urethra

Femoral artery

Femoral vein

The urinary system is one of the body's mechanisms for disposing of waste products, especially urea, a breakdown product from the metabolism of protein. The system comprises the kidneys, ureters, bladder and the urethra by which urine empties from the bladder.

URINARY SYSTEM

THE KIDNEYS ARE INCREDIBLY sophisticated filtration units, which process about 1.3 litres/2¼ pints of blood per minute to make urine at about 1 ml per minute. This urine drains through the ureters – muscular tubes that descend down the back of the abdomen, ending in the bladder. Contractions in their walls help propel the urine and prevent it from stagnating. The kidneys and ureters are under automatic control and they function unobtrusively.

The bladder is a storage vessel capable of holding 1 litre/1¾ pints or more of fluid. The outlet from the bladder is under more conscious control; we can decide when to hold and when to expel urine. Thus far this system is exactly the same in both men and women and is subject to similar disorders with similar symptoms.

Male and female urinary systems

The differences begin from the bladder onward. The urine empties via the urethra, a narrow tube ending just inside the vagina or at the tip of the penis. The female urethra is very short, so bacteria can easily ascend from the perineum. This is why women are far more likely than men to get urinary infections or **cystitis**. In addition, the bladder and urethra are supported by the muscles of the perineum, which are often weakened by childbirth. Women are therefore prone to prolapse leading to urinary problems such as **incontinence**, which is mainly, although not exclusively, a female problem.

The male urethra is much longer, so it is far more difficult for bacteria to ascend. This is why urinary infections in men are unusual and need more investigation than in women. The male urinary system, from the bladder on, joins with the reproductive system to allow sperm to be ejected through the urethra and penis. The male system experiences fewer problems than the female system because changes in supporting muscle structures are less likely and less critical to its efficiency. On the other hand men can expect to get trouble eventually from the prostate gland through which the urethra passes and which obstructs the urethra in about 30% of men by late middle age (see DISORDERS OF THE PROSTATE GLAND).

Potential problems

The urinary system is fundamental for health. In recognition of this there is great overcapacity in the system. It is possible to enjoy normal, and often reasonable, health with only one kidney, even if that remaining kidney is working at half capacity. This fact – that we can survive perfectly well with one kidney – makes kidney donation possible for transplantation.

Primary kidney disease is uncommon. Disease is more often due to infections, **kidney stones**, one of the many drugs that affect kidney function or simply through deterioration in efficiency of the kidneys with age. Other than congenital disease, the other common reasons for acquired kidney trouble are **diabetes**, **high blood pressure** or very low blood pressure after major blood loss or septicaemia.

Left: The kidneys continually filter blood to make urine, which the bladder stores until a convenient moment.

INCONTINENCE

The inability to hold urine, resulting in leakage or wetting.

CAUSES

As the bladder fills, its muscular walls involuntarily contract. This would lead to urination except that a sphincter of muscle around the outlet from the bladder remains closed under voluntary control until the desired time to release urine.

Urge incontinence

The natural tendency of the sphincter is to relax once the bladder is moderately full, as happens in infants. Children and adults gain voluntary control over the sphincter so that they can hold and release urine at will. However, ageing, dementia and disease of the nerves, such as **multiple sclerosis**, can weaken this voluntary control, so that once again the bladder empties automatically when it is only partially full. Urge incontinence can also be as a result of nerve damage caused during bowel and prostate surgery.

Stress incontinence

In stress incontinence anything that increases abdominal pressure, for example sneezing, coughing, laughing or simply standing, causes leakage of urine through the inefficient sphincter. This is a major cause of adult incontinence.

The anatomy of the neck of the bladder is critical to the control of urine. In women childbirth often results in changes to this anatomy and weakens the muscles of the pelvic floor. These factors commonly lead to prolapse (descent) of the womb and stress incontinence.

Incontinence may be made worse by minor infections; this is more common in women, particularly after the menopause.

SYMPTOMS

Urine leaks occur. If leaking follows straining, the likelihood is stress incontinence, that is, weakness of the sphincter. If there is an urge to pass small, frequent amounts of urine there is probably a nerve problem or chronic irritation of the bladder neck. There may be signs of dementia such as memory loss and breakdown of personality. There may be a previous history of **stroke** or abdominal surgery.

It is important to detect infections or **diabetes** by testing the urine. The diagnosis of the type of incontinence is aided by very precise tests of urine flow and bladder pressure, called cystometric studies. These help predict the value of treatment with drugs as opposed to physiotherapy or surgery.

TREATMENT

Assuming any infection has been treated, incontinence in women is helped by hormone replacement therapy (HRT), which restores the health of the sphincter muscle. The several drugs which decrease unwanted bladder muscle contractions, for example flavoxate and oxybutinin, work best for women, less well for men.

For stress incontinence, pelvic floor exercises strengthen the muscles around the bladder that assist continence, and are recommended after childbirth. In cases of severe stress incontinence, surgery can restore the anatomy around the bladder neck (repair of prolapse).

For incontinence with brain disease, the above-mentioned drugs can reduce the frequency of incontinence, as does restricting fluid intake before bed and taking the person to the toilet regularly. In the worst cases it may be best to drain urine with a catheter. Modern catheters are non-irritant and designed to stay in place for several weeks.

Lastly, it is possible to divert urine into the bowel or into a bag on the abdomen, called a urostomy. Such operations are done for incontinence after bowel surgery.

QUESTIONS

How common is incontinence?
Exact figures are not available; by the age of 70 probably at least 10% of women and 2–5% of men experience incontinence. The figure rises rapidly above that age.

Why do so many people simply put up with it?
Incontinence has a bad public image with overtones of self-neglect and dementia. Evidently, this is quite unjustified. Also there is a lack of knowledge about treatments available for both men and women, regardless of age.

Complementary Treatment
Shiatsu-do techniques calm the nervous system and have positive benefits on the emotions; they also boost immunity – all factors in combating incontinence. Some **yoga** positions can help, in conjunction with specific exercises to strengthen the pelvic floor. **Hypnotherapy** – the therapist will use visualization, suggestion and regression to strengthen the bladder and uncover the origin of the incontinence.

CYSTITIS

Discomfort on passing urine, often the result of infection.

CAUSES

This very common condition is often caused by infection around the outlet from the bladder or within the bladder itself. Women suffer far more than men, because it is a shorter journey for germs to spread from the anus across the perineum (the area between the legs) up the short urethra and into the bladder. In women, this journey is only 3–4 cm/ 1¼–1¾ in, while in men it is 15–20 cm/6–8 in.

Often, in women, infection may not be found despite repeated urine tests. Such cystitis is thought to be a chronic inflammation of the bladder neck, making it irritable and giving rise to a burning sensation and a need to pass urine frequently. This inflammation could be caused by a mild infection not detectable on samples. It could be provoked by vaginal douches or wipes, or even bubble baths. Cystitis often follows sexual intercourse through sheer mechanical irritation. If a man has cystitis it points to a urethritis (see URETHRITIS AND NSU).

People who suffer recurrent infections may have an abnormality either within the bladder, such as a bladder stone or a tumour, or further up the system in the ureters. Some people find that certain fruits or acidic foods provoke cystitis.

SYMPTOMS

In women there is an urgent need to pass urine and the urine feels hot and stings. Within minutes the urgent desire returns; this cycle goes on for hours, passing just small amounts each time. There is often a trace of blood in the urine, which may smell fishy and look cloudy because of infection.

Men have similar symptoms, often with an additional aching in the perineum. If a man has a discharge with cystitis, NSU is a possibility. Both men and women may have a dull ache in the lower abdomen over the bladder.

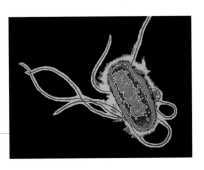

Right: The E. coli bacterium, which commonly causes cystitis and other urinary infections.

Testing urine reveals protein from pus in the urine, and blood from the inflammation of the bladder and urethra. An MSU is a test to grow the causative organism, which is frequently a bowel organism called *E. coli*.

TREATMENT

The body deals with minor episodes of cystitis naturally over a few days. It is helpful to drink extra fluids to keep washing out the bladder. The MSU result will dictate the appropriate antibiotic to be used. Commonly used drugs are trimethoprim and cephalexin. Any blood in the urine has to be treated seriously.

People with recurrent infections will need a cystoscopy, a procedure to look inside the bladder with a light source, or X-rays (see page 316) to outline the ureters.

Post-menopausal women are particularly prone to cystitis, and are helped by hormone replacement therapy (HRT). It is sensible to avoid vaginal deodorants and douches, which remove natural lubricants, to pass urine before and after intercourse and to wash carefully after opening the bowels.

QUESTIONS

How do over-the-counter remedies help?
These contain salts that make the urine more alkaline. This relieves the stinging and also hampers the growth of the infection responsible. A teaspoon of ordinary sodium bicarbonate dissolved in water may be just as effective.

What if no infection is found?
Even so a regular low daily dose of an antibiotic can help. The doctor will consider irritability in the bladder, which requires cystoscopy to prove. Treatment is often a matter of trial of agents including drugs used for urinary incontinence such as oxybutinin.

Complementary Treatment
Chinese and **Western herbalism** – many antiseptic herbs act on the urinary system to reduce irritation and increase urine output. **Nutritional therapy** – drink plenty of water. Cranberry juice and extracts prevent bacteria from adhering to the bladder walls. **Aromatherapy** – tea tree oil improves even chronic cystitis, take sitz baths daily (six drops). **Shiatsu-do** boosts immunity. **Healing** rebalances internal ecology. *Other treatments to try: acupuncture; homeopathy; Ayurveda.*

URETHRITIS AND NSU

Infection of the urethra, with inflammation and possible discharge.

CAUSES

Infection of the urethra, the narrow outlet tube through which urine leaves the bladder, leads to inflammation and often a thin clear discharge. Women may mistake the discharge for their usual vaginal secretions, whereas in men a discharge from the penis is obvious and always abnormal.

NSU means non-specific urethritis. It is considered a sexually transmitted condition but, by definition, no organism can actually be identified as responsible. The most common identifiable infective causes of urethritis are gonorrhoea and chlamydia, which may also cause **pelvic inflammatory disease** and affect a woman's fertility.

As with **cystitis**, women are affected more often than men as it is easier for bacteria to ascend the urethra. In women, urethritis is often due to infection from the perineum or irritation from bubble baths, vaginal deodorants or sexual intercourse. In a particularly troubling type of post-menopausal urethritis the walls of the urethra become thin and dry.

Strictly speaking, the term cystitis means inflammation of the bladder wall but it is often used to include both urethritis, where no definite infection can be found, and a true urinary tract infection with an identifiable bacterium. The terms are thus used interchangeably.

In about one-third of cases of chronic urethritis no cause is found and it is possible that psychological factors play a part.

SYMPTOMS

A burning of the walls of the urethra causes stinging on passing urine plus the urgency to pass small amounts of urine repeatedly. Often in NSU there is also a clear or cloudy discharge. Urine analysis fails to find an infection in the urine itself, which differentiates the condition from urinary infection. Many cases of NSU are asymptomatic and can be detected only by tracing the sexual contacts of people with known NSU.

TREATMENT

The first step is to take swabs from the urethra to try and identify the germ responsible. It is particularly important to detect gonorrhoea, which causes a heavy discharge in men but may cause no early symptoms at all in a female partner, yet lives on within her reproductive system to cause problems of chronic infection later. It is usual to test for other **sexually**

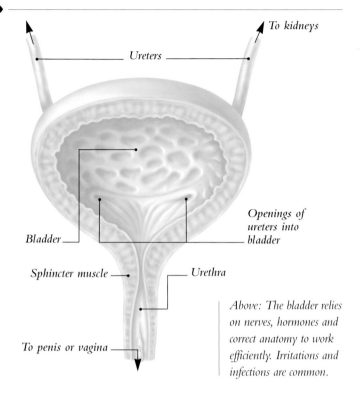

Ureters
To kidneys
Openings of ureters into bladder
Bladder
Sphincter muscle
Urethra
To penis or vagina

Above: The bladder relies on nerves, hormones and correct anatomy to work efficiently. Irritations and infections are common.

transmitted diseases with appropriate blood tests and swabs.

If an organism is identified the appropriate antibiotic is given. Where none is identified – truly non-specific urethritis – it is usual to give a 'best-guess' antibiotic such as oxytetracycline or doxycycline. Again, it is important to trace sexual contacts who may be infected but symptom free themselves.

It is difficult to cure chronic urethritis in women. One method is to dilate the urethra under anaesthetic, a procedure performed during cystoscopy. Post-menopausal urethritis responds well to hormone replacement therapy (HRT) or to oestrogen cream rubbed into the urethra. Careful hygiene is sensible and passing urine before and after intercourse.

   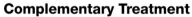

Complementary Treatment

Chinese and **Western herbalism**, **nutritional therapy** and **shiatsu-do** – see CYSTITIS. **Ayurveda** – a therapist will recommend *panchakarma* detoxification and specific oral preparations to prevent recurring attacks. In **reflexology** the heels reflect zones on the urinary system. **Homeopathy** – many remedies are available, depending on specific symptoms. **Aromatherapy** – try sitz baths with tea tree oil (six drops). **Hypnotherapy** – cell command therapy could have a beneficial effect. *Other therapies to try: acupuncture; chakra balancing.*

KIDNEY STONES

Common abnormalities that are a source of pain and infection.

CAUSES

Kidney stones, in common with stalagmites and furred-up water systems, are formed by deposits of salts precipitating out from filtered fluid. Kidney stones are made of calcium salts and can be tiny or fill the whole kidney.

Some people are prone to kidney stones, having a constantly high level of calcium in the blood. Any abnormality in the kidney's anatomy increases the risk. Another reason is low urine output, which is why stones are more common in hot countries and in summer, as a result of dehydration. Bladder stones form for much the same reasons as kidney stones.

SYMPTOMS

Curiously, the larger stones cause fewer symptoms than the small ones, remaining stable within the kidney. There may be a vague ache over the kidney and an increased risk of urinary infections but, because of their size, the large stones cannot migrate. Small stones, however, eventually begin a journey from the kidney down the ureter to the bladder, with excruciating pain each time one moves, called renal colic. The pain is from spasm in the muscular walls of the ureter plus back pressure from obstruction to the flow of urine down that ureter.

The sickening pain (see also GALLSTONES) radiates from over the kidney across the abdomen down to the vagina or tip of the penis. During an attack the individual is sweating, nauseated and in true agony. There is always some blood in the urine. Most stones make this painful journey to the bladder successfully over a few days or weeks, punctuated by several episodes of renal colic. The passage out from the bladder is also uncomfortable but less than that previously experienced.

Classic renal colic is unmistakable. Minor colic is easily misinterpreted as lumbago or non-specific abdominal pain.

TREATMENT

For immediate relief, only the strongest painkillers dull the pain. Pethidine is widely used and diclofenac by injection is as effective and less sedating. Drinking copiously helps flush the stone through. As 90% of stones show on an abdominal X-ray, it is easy to follow their progress.

Long term, an ultrasound scan (see page 317) of the urinary system is a reliable way to detect and monitor stones. Otherwise sufferers have an IVP, an injection of a dye which is

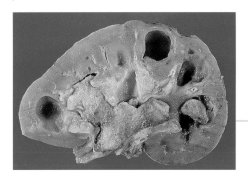

Left: Despite filling the base of the kidney, large stones cause remarkably few symptoms.

concentrated in the kidneys, so outlining the urinary tract. With patience, fluids and ample painkillers the stones pass.

If a stone sticks the preferred treatment is to shatter it using lithotripsy (see page 337) and the smaller fragments pass out without trouble. Thanks to this, surgery is now uncommon. If necessary, it involves opening the kidney to remove a large stone or passing a clever basket-type trap up the ureter to snare and pull out the stone. Stones are analysed to investigate their composition and blood tests are taken, seeking any biochemical disorder that increases the risks of further stones.

QUESTIONS

Do kidney stones recur?
Unfortunately they do. There is a high probability of a second kidney stone within a few years of the first one.

Do stones do any permanent damage?
In theory a stone completely obstructing a ureter could cause permanent damage to that kidney. In practice the stone is surgically removed before this. A large stone within the kidney does interfere with the efficiency of that kidney but only rarely is this significant.

Complementary Treatment

Chinese and **Western herbalism** – anti-inflammatory herbs and herbal diuretics might help. **Shiatsu-do** boosts immunity. **Nutritional therapy** – avoid calcium-rich foods, including dairy produce. Stone formation has been linked with vitamin B_6 and magnesium deficiencies, so consider supplementation. Drink plenty of hot, sweet drinks. **Hypnotherapy** – there are cases of kidney stones shrinking and being passed, possibly in response to hypnotic suggestion. *Other therapies to try: homeopathy; healing; tai chi/chi kung; reflexology.*

KIDNEY FAILURE

Failure of the kidneys to function efficiently for various reasons.

CAUSES

The kidneys filter about 180 litres/40 galls of blood daily, extracting the waste products of metabolism, especially urea – a breakdown product from protein. Besides filtration, the kidneys also regulate blood pressure (via the renin/angiotensin system), blood volume, vitamin D and calcium balance and red blood cell production.

Filtration takes place at a delicate membrane layer, which is the usual site for chronic kidney disease. Damage to this membrane is caused mostly by inflammation of the filtration apparatus or blockage with protein complexes, from an immunological cause. **High blood pressure** damages circulation within the kidneys, while kidney disease itself leads to high blood pressure. The other common cause of kidney failure is **diabetes**, which damages the filtration surface and the blood flow. Less common but still serious causes of kidney failure are infections, large **kidney stones**, obstruction to urine flow, serious falls in blood pressure, certain drugs, tumours and congenital abnormalities of the kidneys.

SYMPTOMS

These are rarely dramatic at the onset; you pass urine that is a little more dilute than usual, blood pressure creeps up. If things deteriorate you feel tired and nauseous as waste products accumulate within the blood. Blood pressure may reach high levels, there is **anaemia** and swelling of limbs. Eventually there is profound tiredness, nausea, itching, bone pain and ultimately confusion or convulsions.

Kidney failure is confirmed by blood tests showing raised levels of the breakdown products urea and creatinine, and specialized measures of the efficiency of the kidneys. Often a kidney biopsy (see page 321) is required to establish the cause. Abrupt kidney failure is usually the result of either low blood pressure, for example after haemorrhage in an accident or major surgery, or acute infection.

TREATMENT

Clearly, blood pressure, obstruction or diabetes must be controlled or eliminated. Special diets control a number of salts poorly handled in kidney failure, such as sodium, potassium, calcium and phosphate. A low-protein diet reduces the load on the kidneys and may slow progression of the disease.

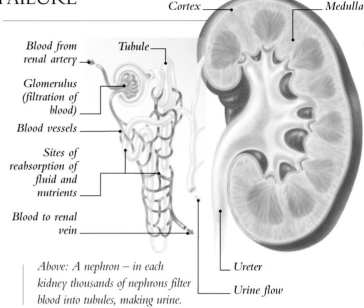

Cortex — Medulla

Blood from renal artery — Tubule

Glomerulus (filtration of blood)

Blood vessels

Sites of reabsorption of fluid and nutrients

Blood to renal vein

Above: A nephron – in each kidney thousands of nephrons filter blood into tubules, making urine.

Ureter

Urine flow

Anaemia used to be untreatable but is now helped by injections of synthetic erythropoietin, which the kidneys normally produce to maintain red blood cell numbers.

Eventually the kidney patient may require kidney dialysis (see page 335) or a kidney transplant (see page 331).

QUESTIONS

How common is kidney failure?
Chronic failure resistant to all but transplant affects about one person in ten thousand per annum. Many more people have a more modest degree of kidney failure requiring dialysis or special diets.

Can it be avoided?
Most cases are unavoidable, the cause being some as yet unknown immune condition. However, good control of blood pressure and diabetes reduces the chances of kidney failure.

Complementary Treatment

Kidney failure is a medical emergency and needs to be treated in hospital. However, many complementary therapies can aid recuperation. Those listed under STRESS could all help ease the tension associated with being ill and in hospital. See DIABETES and GASTRO-INTESTINAL ALLERGY for kidney disease linked to these conditions. Depending on the cause of the disease, traditional Chinese medicine (**acupuncture, herbalism, tai chi/chi kung**) may offer help, as may **Ayurveda**.

CANCER OF THE BLADDER AND KIDNEY

Cancer within the kidney, the ureter or the lining of the bladder.

CAUSES

There is evidence that suggests that half of the bladder cancers in both the United States and the United Kingdom are caused by cigarette smoking. Exposure to certain chemicals called amines, which are concentrated in the bladder and which are found in the rubber and chemical industries, probably account for another ten per cent of bladder cancer cases. In addition, schistosomiasis, a parasitic tropical disease, is an important cause of cancer of the bladder in Africa, South America and Southeast Asia.

Bladder cancer can extend into the urethra, the narrow outlet that leads from the bladder, and the ureters, the tubes that drain urine from the kidneys.

In children cancer of the kidney is usually caused by cells that have been left over from the embryonic development process. (This is also the case with most of the other rare childhood cancers.) Kidney cancer in children is treated much more successfully than it is in adults, in whom kidney cancer develops from normal cells that turn malignant.

In adults there is some weak evidence linking kidney cancer to smoking or chemicals at work. Some cases are due to taking the painkiller phenacetin, now banned in most parts of the world. The majority, however, are of unknown origin.

SYMPTOMS

The prime symptom in both cancers is blood in the urine. Unlike infection, where there is stinging as well as blood, this is normally painless. Even so doctors are cautious if someone with apparent **cystitis** has blood as well. It is a sensible precaution to test urine samples after antibiotic treatment in case microscopic amounts of blood are still present. The same goes for recurrent urinary infections. At some point a specialist must further investigate the urinary tract.

The diagnosis of bladder cancer is made by cystoscopy, looking inside the bladder and sampling any suspicious-looking areas on the walls of the bladder, urethra or ureters.

In cancer of the kidney, pain over the kidney is likely, as well as the general cancer effects of weight loss and loss of appetite. This cancer is an unusual but well-recognized cause of persistent **fever** and sweats. It may be possible to feel an abnormal mass in the abdomen, which is the way in which it is often detected in children. Diagnostic aids are scanning with ultrasound, CT or MRI (see pages 317, 318 and 319).

TREATMENT

Treatment of bladder cancer depends on the stage of the tumour. If the tumour is just on the surface it can be burnt away, with a very high probability of cure. However, you will need to have check cystoscopy for several years to deal with any recurrence of the cancer.

If the tumour is growing deeper into the bladder the options include removing the bladder, radiotherapy (see page 338), chemotherapy given into the bladder or general chemotherapy (see page 339). However, the outlook is much less good.

A kidney affected by cancer nearly always needs removing, after which radiotherapy or chemotherapy may be tried, although results are not good. The tumour may respond to hormones and more recently interferon has proved useful. If the cancer is confined to the kidney there is a 60–70% 5-year survival, which drops if it spreads to the liver, bones or lungs.

QUESTIONS

How common are these tumours?
Growths in the bladder are quite common (nearly five per cent of all cancers) and can usually be treated successfully. Kidney cancer (one to two per cent of all cancers) causes vaguer symptoms so tends to be more advanced by the time of diagnosis.

And in children?
Kidney cancer affects about one in a hundred thousand children up to three years of age, then becomes extremely uncommon until late adult life. In children it is called a nephroblastoma or Wilm's tumour and is much more likely to be curable than in an adult.

How serious is blood in the urine?
It should never be ignored even though the great majority of cases will be due to infection or no detectable serious reason.

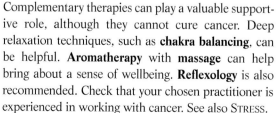

Complementary Treatment

Always have blood in urine checked by a doctor. Complementary therapies can play a valuable supportive role, although they cannot cure cancer. Deep relaxation techniques, such as **chakra balancing**, can be helpful. **Aromatherapy** with **massage** can help bring about a sense of wellbeing. **Reflexology** is also recommended. Check that your chosen practitioner is experienced in working with cancer. See also STRESS.

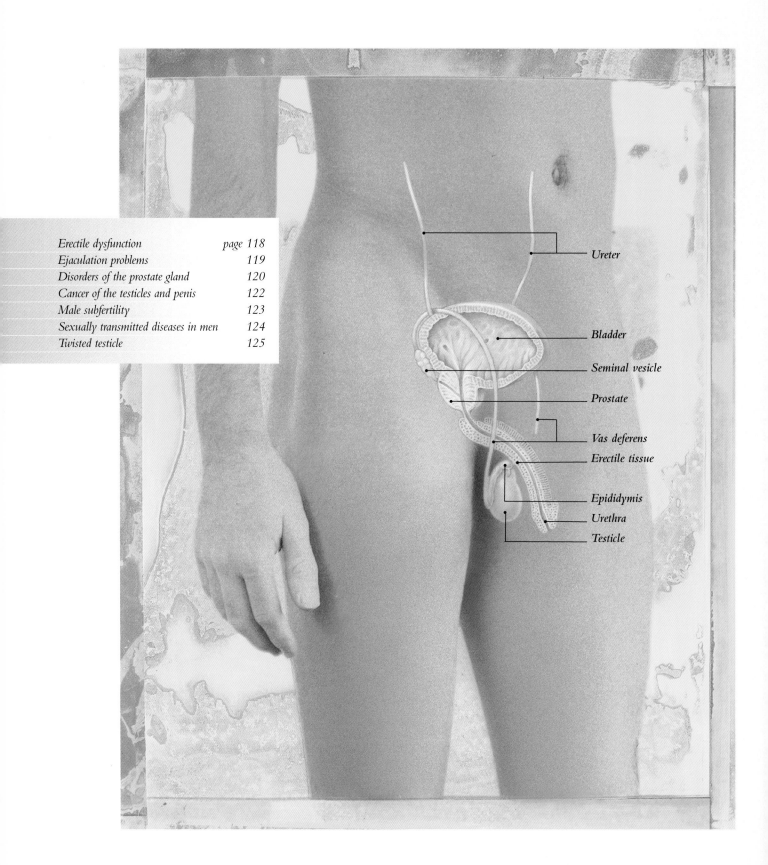

Ureter

Bladder

Seminal vesicle

Prostate

Vas deferens

Erectile tissue

Epididymis

Urethra

Testicle

Although this complex system works reliably in the main, sexual problems affect all men occasionally, while prostate trouble annoys many by late middle age.

MALE REPRODUCTIVE SYSTEM

THE MALE REPRODUCTIVE system shares structures with the urinary system to deal with the tasks of releasing urine and delivering sperm. Urine is stored in the bladder and leaves through the urethra, which runs through the penis. Sperm mature within the testicle and the epididymis – a small structure behind the testicle. They are given nutrition by secretions from the seminal vesicles and the prostate gland, then also leave via the urethra and penis. Sperm and urine do not normally mix thanks to a valve system, which prevents back-flow of urine from the urethra to the seminal vesicles and epididymis. At the time of ejaculation this same system ensures sperm go forward out of the penis and not backward into the bladder.

Most of the male reproductive system is visible, comprising the penis, testicles and scrotum. The prostate gland is hidden in the perineum – that part of the anatomy between the legs – and can only be examined via the rectum or with ultrasound. This visibility is a source of both pride and concern for men, as much male literature testifies. Men worry about size, performance and potency. As far as nature is concerned, however, all that is required is for large quantities of healthy sperm to be delivered into a female reasonably efficiently. Although it is tempting to dismiss all else as vanity, evolutionary theory teaches that there are genetic advantages favouring the potent and aggressive male.

What are sperm?

Sperm are packets of genetic material, each containing 23 chromosomes. Fertilization occurs when the 23 chromosomes from a sperm merge with the 23 chromosomes in the female egg in order to produce the normal human cell of 46 chromosomes. It is the shuffling of these chromosomes and the chance assortment within the fertilizing sperm that underlies and maintains the genetic variations of humanity. Sperm are programmed to swim as fast as possible to deliver that genetic material to the egg (see page 129).

Male hormones

This section concentrates on disorders of the genitalia themselves. However, the overall system of male sexual maturity and fertility relies on complicated hormonal control from the pituitary and hypothalamic glands within the brain, plus hormones from the testicles themselves. These hormonal influences are less noticeable than those of women, because there are not the obvious hormonal cycles of menstruation and pregnancy. They are no less vital for all that but disorders of those factors are not included in these pages because of their rarity and complexity.

An important difference between men and women with regard to the reproductive system is that men's sexual performance is affected by psychological factors and illness, plus a range of depressants of which alcohol is the most common. More controversial is the 'male menopause', a fall in testosterone levels with age, which is yet to be accepted as being an abnormality that requires treatment.

Changing attitudes

Men have been traditionally reluctant to talk about problems of sexuality and the prostate gland, despite the fact that these are exceedingly common. Such attitudes are changing, coinciding with research offering a better understanding of impotence, **subfertility** and **disorders of the prostate gland**.

Left: Several glands and elaborate pipework let the male system work both for sex and passing urine.

ERECTILE DYSFUNCTION

An inability to have or maintain an erection sufficient for satisfactory sexual intercourse – commonly known as impotence.

CAUSES

Erection of the penis occurs when blood flows into large sponge-like chambers along the length of the penis. The blood vessels involved are controlled by the autonomic nervous system, which works largely at an unconscious level but which can be stimulated by conscious will. When those blood vessels dilate blood rushes in and erection occurs; when they contract blood flows out and is not replaced so the penis shrinks. Men with poor blood flow to the lower body or with spinal cord or brain damage are liable to impotence, and research suggests that these factors are the most likely causes in older men.

Psychological factors are also important. **Anxiety** and **depression** in general, and attitudes to sex in particular, frequently cause impotence. Less important, although still significant, are abnormal levels of male hormone – testosterone.

Many drugs affect potency, for example alcohol, which, as Shakespeare said, raises the desire but decreases the ability. Other culprits are drugs for **high blood pressure** such as beta-blockers and diuretics.

Diabetes is very often accompanied by impotence through damage to the nerves and interference with blood flow.

SYMPTOMS

As a general rule, in men who are unable to get an erection at all there is probably a physical cause, whereas men who are impotent but get a nocturnal erection or wake with an erection are more likely to have a psychological cause for their impotence. Other symptoms suggesting a psychological cause are if impotence occurs with certain partners but not with others, or if there is a background of anxiety or depression.

It is important to have a general physical check-up, looking especially for normal blood flow and testing for diabetes.

TREATMENT

Occasionally, blood flow can be improved by microsurgery to dilate the arteries or veins of the penis. Steps are taken to reduce progression of circulatory problems by controlling blood pressure, cholesterol and diabetes, if detected.

Physical treatment with drugs such as alprostadil, induces an erection when injected into the penis. With training, most men can learn how to self-inject into the penis.

Recently available to treat male impotence is a new drug called sildenifil (Viagra), which, if taken an hour before sexual activity, improves erection in most impotent men. The main side effect is headache.

Other devices include rings that fit around the penis, keeping blood within it, and vacuum devices that fit over the penis and draw blood in. Another treatment possibility is to implant mechanical devices that are inflated at will; these are becoming more sophisticated and reliable. Proven lack of male hormone can respond to testosterone.

Treating psychological impotence is a specialized area. It involves exploring attitudes to sex ('dirty', bad experiences), learning to give mutual sexual pleasure short of intercourse with stroking and stimulation, and de-emphasizing penetrative intercourse as the only goal of each sexual encounter.

QUESTIONS

What is self-injection?
An injection into the side of the penis, via a very fine needle, of a drug in a dosage sufficient to give an erection for about an hour. The risks are of a prolonged erection (more than four hours), pain at the injection site and effects on blood pressure.

How important are psychological factors?
These were long thought to account for the great majority of cases of impotence. Research is increasingly showing that in fact physical factors cause well over 50% of cases.

Is impotence an inevitable consequence of ageing?
Only in that blood flow problems and other physical disease are more common with increasing age. Although levels of testosterone do decline with age, this plays a relatively minor part in impotence.

Complementary Treatment

Auricular therapy can increase blood flow to the genitals. **Aromatherapy** stimulant oils include jasmine, ginger and black pepper. Try three drops of one of these in 10 ml of carrier oil, to make and use as a **massage** oil. **Hypnotherapy** – sex therapists sometimes use hypnotic suggestion and regression as part of a treatment plan. Many **Ayurvedic** preparations are available to improve sexual potency. **Homeopathy** – see MALE SUBFERTILITY. *Other therapies to try: tai chi/chi kung; acupuncture; healing; chakra balancing; homeopathy.*

EJACULATION PROBLEMS

Common problems with the expulsion of sperm and seminal fluid at the time of orgasm.

CAUSES

The mechanics of ejaculation are quite well understood. It begins with the release of sperm from the testicles, which mixes with seminal fluid from the prostate gland and seminal vesicles. Reflex contractions of muscles at the base of the penis then pump out the 2–5 ml of a normal ejaculate. An internal valve closes to prevent back-flow of semen into the bladder. These reflexes are under unconscious control by the nervous system. Accompanying this is the intense sexual sensation of an orgasm, which is the response of the brain to sexual stimulation. Orgasm includes additional reflex consequences such as rapid heart rate and breathing as well as a rise in blood pressure.

After orgasm the penis goes limp and there is a feeling of relaxation lasting a half hour or more. There is also a period during which it is not possible to have another full erection or orgasm. This period depends greatly on age, ranging from minutes in a young man to 24 hours or more in the elderly.

The main ejaculation problems are complete failure, usually because of disorder of the nervous system, retrograde ejaculation and premature ejaculation. Retrograde ejaculation is often an inevitable and permanent consequence of surgery on the bladder or prostate gland, which damages the valve mechanism that normally prevents it. Premature ejaculation is so common that it is probably normal, especially in young men.

SYMPTOMS

Failure of ejaculation means little or no semen appears at orgasm. In retrograde ejaculation little appears at orgasm but the urine is clouded with semen that has flowed backwards (retrograde) into the bladder.

In premature ejaculation orgasm occurs rapidly after sexual activity begins, whether during manual stimulation or within a brief time of inserting the penis into the vagina. There are usually feelings of guilt or shame at failing to prolong the sexual act or failing to bring the partner to sexual satisfaction.

TREATMENT

In terms of treatment there is little that can be done about retrograde ejaculation, but it is worth realizing that it is harmless – although it does reduce fertility. Nor can anything be done for failure of ejaculation that follows nerve damage.

Although common, premature ejaculation has become so entangled with sexual mythology, notions of potency and of giving sexual satisfaction to partners that few men will admit to experiencing it. The first step for treatment is therefore to acknowledge the problem.

The treatment is similar to that used for treating impotence (see ERECTILE DYSFUNCTION). The focus is moved away from penetration and orgasm and on to wider sexual gratification, such as gratification by stroking and mutual stimulation. In addition, the man lets his partner know when he feels orgasm is approaching. His partner can then squeeze the base of the man's penis, which very effectively inhibits the reflex. Over time the urgency of the sexual act is modified so that premature ejaculation becomes less likely.

Other treatments for premature ejaculation involve taking relaxants, including alcohol (but see ERECTILE DYSFUNCTION). The latest antidepressants, selective serotonin reuptake inhibitors (SSRIs), appear helpful in retarding ejaculation (see DEPRESSION). However, a quick non-psychological answer for treating premature ejaculation has yet to be established.

QUESTIONS

Is premature ejaculation necessarily abnormal?
Premature ejaculation is only a problem if the couple finds it so. If the man's partner is not bothered by him ejaculating quickly, then there is no need to seek medical help.

Are erection and ejaculation necessarily linked?
They involve different nervous mechanisms, although there is great overlap. This is why it is possible and common to have an orgasm with a limp penis, especially during 'wet dreams'.

Complementary Treatment

Auricular therapy – if the problem is emotional, treatment can be weekly; if physical, it should be more frequent, to increase blood flow to the genitals. **Aromatherapy** and **hypnotherapy** – see ERECTILE DYSFUNCTION. **Healing** helps to dispel negative feelings which can manifest in physical problems. Many **Ayurvedic** preparations are available to delay orgasm. If the cause is emotional and not physical, **chakra balancing** can help by balancing energies. *Other therapies to try: homeopathy; acupuncture.*

DISORDERS OF THE PROSTATE GLAND

Benign and malignant disease of the gland that encircles the urethra, the tube which runs from the bladder to the penis.

CAUSES

The function of the prostate gland is not entirely clear. It does, however, produce secretions that mix with the sperm and help to transport and nourish them.

Benign enlargement

By the age of about 60 most men will have some enlargement of the prostate gland – this can be double the usual size. The reason is thought to do with changing concentrations of oestrogen and testosterone as men get older. Benign (non-cancerous) enlargement appears to be a pure function of age and evidence suggests that every man will get it if he lives long enough. The enlarged gland squeezes the urethra, obstructing urine flow to a greater or lesser degree.

Cancer of the prostate

In the United Kingdom cancer of the prostate accounts for about seven per cent of all cancers. After lung and bowel cancer it is the next most common cause of death from cancer in men. Male sex hormones are part of the cause of prostate cancer but these are by no means entirely to blame since heredity and diet also have a role to play.

Small nests of malignant cells in the prostate gland are extremely widespread in older men, being found in about 80% of men by their 80s. However, only a small percentage of these cells develop into symptomatic prostate cancer.

SYMPTOMS

Both benign and malignant disease of the prostate gland cause similar symptoms so that investigation is needed to differentiate between the two. Both cause pressure on the urethra, constricting it and thereby weakening the flow of urine and causing difficulty in beginning to pass urine, which may just dribble out. There is an irritability to the bladder, with a need to pass urine frequently but, unlike **cystitis**, there is no stinging on passing urine.

The pressure on the urethra causes stagnation of urine in the bladder and a risk of bladder infections. Because of incomplete emptying of urine the bladder enlarges and can reach as high as the belly button. This back pressure can be transmitted to the kidneys, causing aching in the loins.

There is always the risk of urinary retention, which is complete obstruction to outflow, with pain and further distension of the bladder. This is a medical emergency treated by passing a catheter into the bladder in order to drain the urine.

Cancer of the prostate can cause all of the above symptoms. In addition, there may be symptoms from the spread of cancer into bones. For this reason doctors suspect prostate cancer in any older man who presents for the first time with back or hip pain and who also has prostatic symptoms.

Examination of the prostate gland

All cases need examination of the prostate gland, which is done by passing a finger into the rectum to feel the gland. The benign gland is enlarged and smooth whereas a cancerous gland feels hard and has irregular areas. A very helpful blood test for detecting malignancy is Prostate Specific Antigen (PSA). A high reading almost certainly means cancer, a low reading almost certainly means benign enlargement. Borderline results or the response to treatment can be monitored by checking the PSA every few months.

TREATMENT

In the case of benign enlargement of the prostate not all men require treatment, especially if the only symptoms are a need to pass urine a couple of times a night and a poor flow of urine. As long as the bladder is not distended and blood tests show that kidney function is normal, it may be several years before treatment is needed, although a slow deterioration in the gland is inevitable.

Benign enlargement

The first choice in medical treatment is using drugs, such as finasteride, that shrink the prostate gland by blocking the action of testosterone on the gland. Other drugs, called alpha-blockers, relax the smooth muscle of the urethra enough to reduce symptoms to acceptable levels, but do not reduce the size of the gland – indoramin is an example.

If these measures fail or if there is complete blockage, a prostatectomy is necessary. This is an operation to trim away the gland. It is usually performed using slim fibreoptic instruments passed into the urethra. The gland is then dissected away by a heated wire or by a laser (see page 333).

There is great current interest in implanting metal tubes to prevent the prostate from squeezing the urethra closed but these are not yet fully evaluated. Other possibilities involve heating or freezing the gland and, again, these are relatively experimental. Different specialists favour different methods.

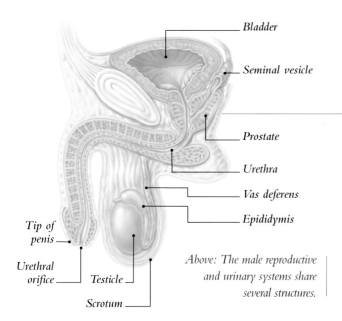

Bladder

Seminal vesicle

Prostate

Urethra

Vas deferens

Epididymis

Tip of penis

Urethral orifice

Testicle

Scrotum

Above: The male reproductive and urinary systems share several structures.

Cancer of the prostate

It is usual to confirm the diagnosis of prostate cancer by taking multiple biopsies through the rectum, although this is being replaced by high-definition ultrasound images of the gland. It is important to know whether the disease has spread elsewhere, so a bone scan is performed.

If there is just a tiny focus of cancer confined to the gland, the current British approach is to keep it under regular review. In the United States more aggressive treatment is usual, which means removal of the whole gland.

There is a choice either to remove the prostate gland, called a radical prostatectomy, or to irradiate it. Both methods appear to give comparable results. The drawback of surgery is the likelihood of **incontinence** of urine and impotence (see ERECTILE DYSFUNCTION), although improved microsurgical techniques are reducing these risks. Radiotherapy can also cause impotence and there may be radiation damage to the bowel, causing pain and **diarrhoea**.

If the disease has spread outside the gland or to bone, then radiotherapy is favoured, together with drugs that reduce testosterone levels. These are cyproterone, taken by mouth, or injectable drugs such as goserelin, which need to be given every three months only. These drugs have thankfully removed the need to perform a castration, which used to be the standard way of reducing testosterone.

Screening for prostate cancer

The discovery of PSA appeared to open the prospect of screening for disease. This is still controversial, however, because not enough is known about the natural history of prostate cancer. As has already been mentioned, up to 80% of men over 80 will have microscopic cancer and may have an abnormal PSA but it is simply not known how many of such deposits may go on to cause problems.

Regardless of the lack of scientific evidence, men over the age of 50 are increasingly asking for screening by way of a yearly rectal examination and PSA. However, if these results are abnormal, the man will then be faced with decisions about which there is not yet medical agreement.

QUESTIONS

Is surgery/radiotherapy essential?
If cancer is a chance finding, current British practice is to monitor it, because there may be no problems for many years. However, treatment of cancer that is causing symptoms improves survival.

What is the outlook?
Surgery for benign enlargement relieves symptoms for a decade or more and can be repeated if necessary. Sixty to eighty per cent of men treated for early cancer are still alive after ten years, an encouraging result considering that these are men already in their 60s and 70s. Unfortunately, once cancer has spread into bone there is about a 20% survival to 5 years.

Why is screening not recommended?
Currently, screening detects many men with cancer that causes no symptoms and where the rate of progression is unknown. This is why screening is controversial.

Complementary Treatment

Cancer: Complementary therapies cannot cure cancer. Herbal and vitamin therapies, however, could be useful for cancer of the prostate, but it is very important to have a conventional medical assessment before embarking on complementary treatment, and to keep conventional practitioners informed of what you are doing. Herbal and vitamin therapies could be provided by a **Western herbalist**, **Chinese herbalist**, **Ayurvedic** practitioner, **naturopath** or **nutritional therapist**. **Reflexology**, **aromatherapy** and **chakra balancing** can all offer support during orthodox treatment for cancer. *Benign enlargement:* Zinc deficiency and/or essential fatty acid deficiency appear to be common factors in the onset of benign enlargement of the prostate. **Nutritional therapists** work to reverse such deficiencies, and might also use herbs, for example clinical trials have shown saw palmetto to be useful. **Homeopathy** can also be of benefit – treatment depends on individual circumstances.

CANCER OF THE TESTICLES AND PENIS

Both of these are unusual, but cancer of the testicles is becoming more common. It is curable, so early detection is important.

CAUSES

In the case of cancer of the testicles, the one agreed cause is undescended testicles. This means that the testicles stayed within the abdomen instead of dropping into the scrotum at or around birth. If untreated, there is about a five per cent risk of later malignancy. Other causes of testicular cancer arise from malignant changes in the cells within the testicles that make sperm, although the trigger for this change is not understood. For unknown reasons testicular cancer is more common in men from higher socio-economic groups and is becoming more common.

In the case of cancer of the penis it is thought that poor hygiene contributes to this uncommon tumour. It is extremely rare in circumcised men. The role of environment and heredity is important in other unclear ways. For example, the tumour is up to 20 times more common in parts of South America and Africa than it is in the United States.

SYMPTOMS

In testicular cancer there is a lump in the testicle that may or may not be painful; this testicle often feels heavier than the other. There might be swelling of the scrotum with inflammatory fluid, called a hydrocele. The tumour can spread to bones or lung; if this happens the first symptoms might be pain or breathlessness. Importantly, ten per cent of tumours cause no symptoms at all but can be detected by self-examination. Most testicular cancers occur in men in their 20s and 30s.

In cancer of the penis there is a persistent sore or ulcer on the penis and often enlarged lymph glands in the groin. The disease is most common in men in their 60s or older.

In both cases the diagnosis has to be confirmed by taking a biopsy, plus scans and chest X-rays to show whether the cancers have spread. This is important in planning treatment and in deciding the prospects for cure.

TREATMENT

Depending on the precise type of the tumour, the treatment for testicular cancer will involve radiotherapy, chemotherapy or both (see pages 338 and 339). Removal of the affected testicle is not always necessary but again it depends on the type of tumour. Treatment is now so good that nearly every man can be cured, although it is important that follow-up for recurrence is continued for many years. Follow-up is aided by the discovery of biochemical substances in blood tests that give early warnings of the recurrence of cancer. These are alpha-fetoprotein and beta-chorionic gonadotrophin, both of which are easily measured.

Many cases of penile cancer can be dealt with by removal of the growth itself, leaving most of the penis intact, depending on the site of the cancer. If it has spread to the glands in the groin these must be removed in a major operation, performed only if the cancer has not spread elsewhere. Chemotherapy or radiotherapy have not proved very effective in the condition. Even so, there is up to a 90% 5-year survival, although falling to much less where there is spread to glands or bones.

QUESTIONS

How important is testicular cancer?
Although it ranks far behind lung or bowel cancers, it is the most common tumour in men in their late teens to early 30s (about 1300 cases per annum in the United Kingdom).

Why is early detection of these cancers important?
The prospects for cure of both these conditions is much higher in the case of early disease.

Can these cancers be prevented?
All young men should check their testicles regularly every few weeks. Feel for lumps or ulcers and have anything remotely suspicious checked. Undescended testicles should be surgically corrected at an early age. Any persistent sore on the penis should be reviewed by a doctor. The role of circumcision in preventing cancer of the penis is controversial.

Complementary Treatment
Complementary therapies cannot cure cancer. However, many of them have a role during treatment. **Chakra balancing** will help with symptom control and energy balance, as well as aiding relaxation during orthodox treatment and offering support during rehabilitation programmes. **Reflexology** can offer support during orthodox treatment. **Aromatherapy**, especially when combined with **massage**, is excellent for reducing stress and tension associated with disease. *Other therapies to try: see STRESS.*

MALE SUBFERTILITY

Subfertility is the failure to conceive despite a year of regular intercourse (once or twice a week). Male causes are a factor for 30–40% of couples having difficulty in conceiving.

CAUSES

First, it is important to distinguish between subfertility in the male as opposed to some problem with sexual technique. There may be impotence (see ERECTILE DYSFUNCTION) or inaccurate ideas about sexual intercourse, so that sperm is being deposited outside the vagina.

Low sperm count

Then it is a matter of whether the man is producing adequate quantities of healthy sperm that can reach their target. Sperm are produced in huge quantities by the testicles, then stored until expelled at orgasm. The life of a sperm is short (90 days) and almost entirely disappointing, bar one brief moment of hope at the time of orgasm. Sperm are little energized cells whose destiny is to race against a hundred million other sperm in order to be the one that fertilizes the egg, thereby passing on genetic material. So what interferes with this?

The testicles need male hormones; any lack of these will affect sperm formation. Many drugs affect the testicles, as do any serious illnesses, especially liver disease, kidney disease and excessive alcohol intake.

A varicocele, a kind of collection of varicose veins behind the testicles, reduces sperm count by increasing the temperature of the epididymis where sperm mature. The sperm themselves may be abnormally formed or lack forward drive. There may be blockages in the pathway from testicle to penis. Antisperm antibodies may be produced by the man against his own sperm or by his partner, which reduce the number of effective sperm despite an otherwise adequate sperm count.

SYMPTOMS

Before focusing on the woman if there is failure to conceive it is essential to look for male causes. Basic investigations are examination of the testicles and penis and a sperm count.

The sperm count should show large quantities of normal sperm. By convention 'normal' is taken to be at least fifty million sperm, of which at least 60% are mobile and most are normally formed. Although it is true that it takes only one sperm to achieve fertilization, the wastage is such that a low sperm count reduces the chances of conception considerably. More sophisticated tests involve measuring sperm antibodies

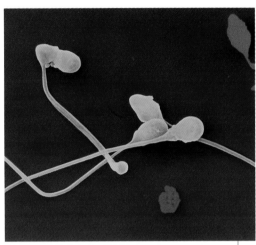

Above: Sperm with abnormal lumps on their heads, which prevent them from successfully penetrating the egg.

and performing a post-coital test – collecting sperm from the vagina after intercourse to establish whether sperm are moving and living within the environment of the vagina.

TREATMENT

Avoiding smoking and alcohol are known to improve the sperm count. The number and quality of sperm improve up to about seven days of abstinence from intercourse, after which they decline. The optimal sperm quality should therefore be timed to coincide with the woman's time of maximum fertility. Treatment is possible in cases of hormone disease such as underactive pituitary gland. Removing a varicocele may improve the sperm count. Attempts to deal with antibodies are not widely successful as yet. The most encouraging work is in artificial insemination (see FEMALE SUBFERTILITY).

Complementary Treatment

Homeopathic remedies include agnus for ineffectual erection, conium for inability to sustain erection and sepia for lack of libido. The effectiveness of these remedies depends on individual circumstances. Diet – low sperm counts may be linked with deficiencies such as vitamin C and zinc; a **nutritional therapist** could advise. **Hypnotherapy** could help if subfertility is linked to subconscious fears about fatherhood. *Other therapies to try: tai chi/chi kung; naturopathy; acupuncture; autogenic training; Ayurveda.*

SEXUALLY TRANSMITTED DISEASES IN MEN

Infections spread by sexual contact, known as STDs. Many are detected through tracing the contacts of those already infected.

CAUSES

These are caused by micro-organisms, most of which prefer living in the genital system and surrounding skin. Some of these are serious, causing gonorrhoea, syphilis and **AIDS**.

Gonorrhoea is caused by gonococcus, a micro-organism unique to humans and spread only by sexual contact. Syphilis is caused by *Treponema pallidum*, which can also pass from mothers to the unborn foetus, leading to congenital syphilis. In recent years the micro-organism chlamydia has come to be recognized as an important cause of **urethritis** and, in women, of subfertility. The herpes simplex virus is a common and persistent infection causing much discomfort. The fungus candida is often carried by men, although rarely giving symptoms as annoying as for women, in whom it causes vaginal **thrush**. Then there are viruses that cause warts around the genitalia and those that cause AIDS and hepatitis B and C. Apart from HIV (the virus responsible for AIDS), the above are most common in the West; there are other STDs common in the tropics.

SYMPTOMS

Usually, there is some combination of itching around the genitalia, pain on passing urine and a discharge from the penis. Depending on the cause there may be a rash or warts on the genitalia or the anus, enlarged glands in the groin and possibly a more widespread rash on the body. These symptoms occur any time from a few days after infection to several weeks later.

Urethritis may settle without treatment. Syphilis causes an initial rash and generalized ill health which disappear, only for more serious symptoms to recur years later, for example **ulcers** on the skin, damaged and weakened bones, difficulty with walking, dementia and damage to the heart.

TREATMENT

Genito-urinary clinics deal with diagnosis, treatment and tracing sexual contacts. This is done in the strictest confidence – even your own doctor will not be informed without your permission. Diagnosis is arrived at by taking swabs from the urethra, anus and mouth to try to grow the organism responsible. Blood tests confirm syphilis, HIV and hepatitis B and C.

Treatment may be simply an antifungal or antiviral cream for thrush or herpes. Gonorrhoea is treated by a single short

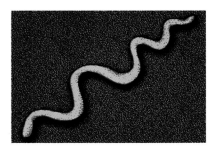

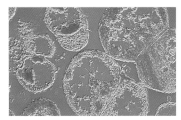

Top left: Spiral-shaped Treponema pallidum *is the micro-organism that causes syphilis.*
Bottom left: Pairs of kidney-shaped gonococci, the bacteria responsible for gonorrhoea.

course of an antibiotic such as amoxycillin or ciprofloxacin. Syphilis requires about 10 days of penicillin injections. Urethritis also responds to antibiotics. There is a very high probability of cure in most cases; even with early syphilis, although the damage done by late syphilis cannot be cured.

Tracing sexual contacts

The importance of this cannot be overstated. Men know when they have a problem but women may not, especially with gonorrhoea and chlamydia, which may silently destroy a woman's fertility. Syphilis and HIV may ruin both partners' lives, and those of future sexual partners. You are encouraged at the clinic to list recent sexual partners. Staff then diplomatically contact them, explain any risks and invite them for investigation. They will not be told who might have infected them.

See also SEXUALLY TRANSMITTED DISEASES IN WOMEN.

Complementary Treatment

There are serious consequences from the inadequate treatment of STDs, so always seek a conventional opinion. Complementary therapies can boost the immune system to help the body resist further attack. **Western herbalism** – echinacea boosts the immune system. In traditional Chinese medicine a combination of **herbs**, **acupuncture** and **tai chi/chi kung** could help. **Ayurveda** would suggest a combination of detoxification, oil massage and yoga. **Aromatherapy** may have some effect on herpes – an experienced practitioner could advise. *Other therapies to try: homeopathy.*

TWISTED TESTICLE

◆

A cause of pain in the groin, with implications for future fertility.

CAUSES
◆

The testicles dangle within the scrotum on the spermatic cord, which is a combination of blood supply, nerves and the vas deferens through which sperm leave the testicles. In theory, this should carry a high risk of the testicle twisting. In fact the testicle is held in place by a surrounding layer of tissue.

It is not known exactly why the testicle sometimes twists but it is thought to follow a vigorous contraction of the muscles that pull up (retract) the testicles. If they contract rapidly enough the testicle twists – called a torsion – cutting off the blood supply, which is a medical emergency. It most often affects boys in their early teens.

SYMPTOMS
◆

There is a sudden severe pain in one testicle, which swells and is extremely tender to even gentle examination. The overlying scrotum becomes reddened, and there may be nausea, vomiting and pain in the lower abdomen. The affected testicle hangs noticeably higher than the other one.

Babies suffering a torsion will cry through pain and draw up their legs. Unless the scrotum is carefully examined it is easy to overlook the diagnosis in a baby.

There are other causes of pain in a testicle: epididymitis gives pain behind the testicle; any injury may cause pain and swelling. Orchitis is inflammation of the testicle and occurs for no obvious reason. These are valid alternative diagnoses to consider in an adult but are unsafe diagnoses in any boy below the age of about 16. This is because it is impossible to tell the difference between these conditions for sure.

In some cases there is little pain, but just a suddenly swollen red scrotum. Within about four hours of torsion there is serious damage to the testicle through blockage of blood flow. Unless torsion is corrected within about 12 hours that testicle will shrink and be permanently less fertile.

It is possible to differentiate these conditions with a radioisotope scan of the testicles but most surgeons prefer to operate to see the situation for themselves.

TREATMENT
◆

It may be possible to manoeuvre the testicle back into position under a local anaesthetic. The more usual treatment is to open up the scrotum, untwist the testicle and stitch it to the

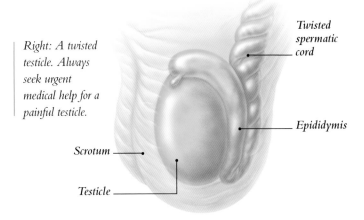

Right: A twisted testicle. Always seek urgent medical help for a painful testicle.

Twisted spermatic cord

Epididymis

Scrotum

Testicle

scrotum to prevent future problems. If one testicle has twisted there is a higher chance of torsion of the other, so it is advisable to stitch both testicles into place.

If the testicle has been irredeemably damaged it may be best to remove it all together.

QUESTIONS

How common is torsion?
Complete torsion is uncommon; minor episodes of pain in the testicle are common and may be the result of twists that correct themselves. Any prolonged discomfort should be taken seriously.

How important is early treatment?
After 12 hours of torsion the testicle will probably be permanently damaged. Therefore pain in a testicle in a young boy should be medically assessed as an emergency.

By how much is fertility affected?
Although a single testicle makes adequate amounts of sperm, losing one will reduce the total sperm count and just tip the odds towards reduced fertility. Of course, it increases the risk of total infertility should an accident happen to the surviving testicle.

Complementary Treatment
Never ignore pain in your testicles. This should always be reported to a conventional practitioner because there are serious long-term consequences from inadequate treatment. Postoperatively, **acupuncture** can be used to control pain. **Chakra balancing** and **healing** can help speed recovery.

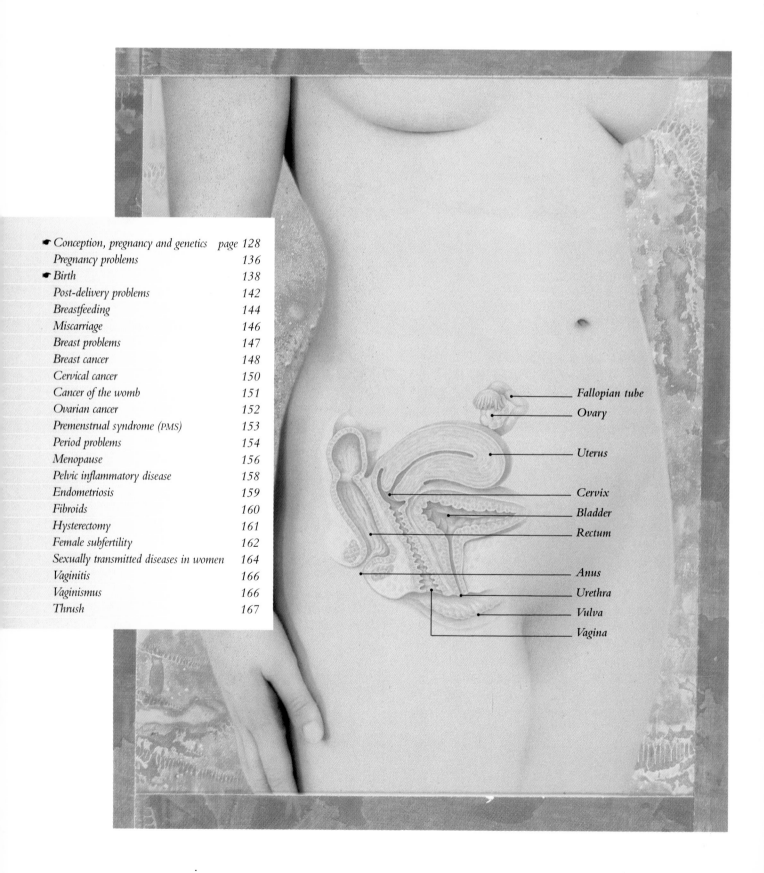

Fallopian tube

Ovary

Uterus

Cervix

Bladder

Rectum

Anus

Urethra

Vulva

Vagina

*Most societies regard with awe the menstrual cycle and pregnancy,
an awe enhanced as scientific research reveals the intricate interplay
of hormones and specialized tissues involved.*

FEMALE REPRODUCTIVE SYSTEM

THE MAIN COMPONENTS of this system are the womb (uterus), Fallopian tubes and ovaries. The ovaries contain all the eggs a woman will ever have. By just six weeks' gestation the baby girl already has all the genetic material that will be used during her reproductive lifetime. At birth the ovaries contain some two million cells that could turn into eggs; this falls to a few hundred thousand by puberty. During a reproductive life of say 35 years, only about 400 eggs are released. The rest degenerate.

The onset of puberty

Puberty begins when something as yet unknown triggers the hypothalamus in the brain to stimulate the ovaries to produce oestrogen, the female hormone. With this stimulation the girl starts to develop secondary sexual characteristics, such as growth of breasts, pubic hair and, eventually, the commencement of menstruation. Puberty may begin anywhere from nine to sixteen years and is probably triggered in part by the amount of body fat.

The reproductive process

In the mature woman the ovaries work under the influence of hormones from the hypothalamus and pituitary glands, undergoing the cyclical changes of menstruation (see PERIOD PROBLEMS). Most months an egg is released from the ovary and caught by frond-like outgrowths at the end of the Fallopian tubes, which guide it into the tube. Over the next few days the egg travels to the womb; when it occurs, fertilization takes place during this journey.

The womb is where the fertilized egg embeds itself; the womb's walls provide a rich blood supply to the developing embryo via the placenta. The bulk of the womb is made up of muscle which expels the baby at term. The outlet of the womb is the cervix, which projects into the vagina.

The vagina is a muscular tube, guarded at the outside by the labia. The vagina distends during intercourse and, of course, during childbirth to allow the baby to exit. The labia have no particular function, although they do distend during sexual arousal. Tucked just before the entrance to the vagina is the clitoris, which is the female equivalent of the penis and like the penis responds to stimulation, leading to orgasm.

The female reproductive system includes the breasts, which are designed to supply milk to the baby but respond to sexual stimulation as well.

Hormonal control

The whole system is under the control of hormones secreted by the hypothalamus and pituitary glands in the base of the brain, with input from several other sources. Such influences include the adrenal glands, the fat layers, the thyroid gland, growth hormone and the ovaries themselves.

Many women's problems are hormone related, through aberrations in the delicate hormone balance from day to day and from cycle to cycle. The breasts, womb and ovaries are all environments with great cell activity and are subject to tremendous hormonal changes, which is why they are common sites for cancer. Quite unlike in men, infections can gain access to the interior of the body via the vagina and Fallopian tubes; thus pelvic and vaginal infections are common and potentially extremely serious.

At the **menopause** hormonal changes cause women to experience widespread effects throughout the body.

*Left: Within the mostly hidden female
system are the structures which produce
eggs and nurture the foetus.*

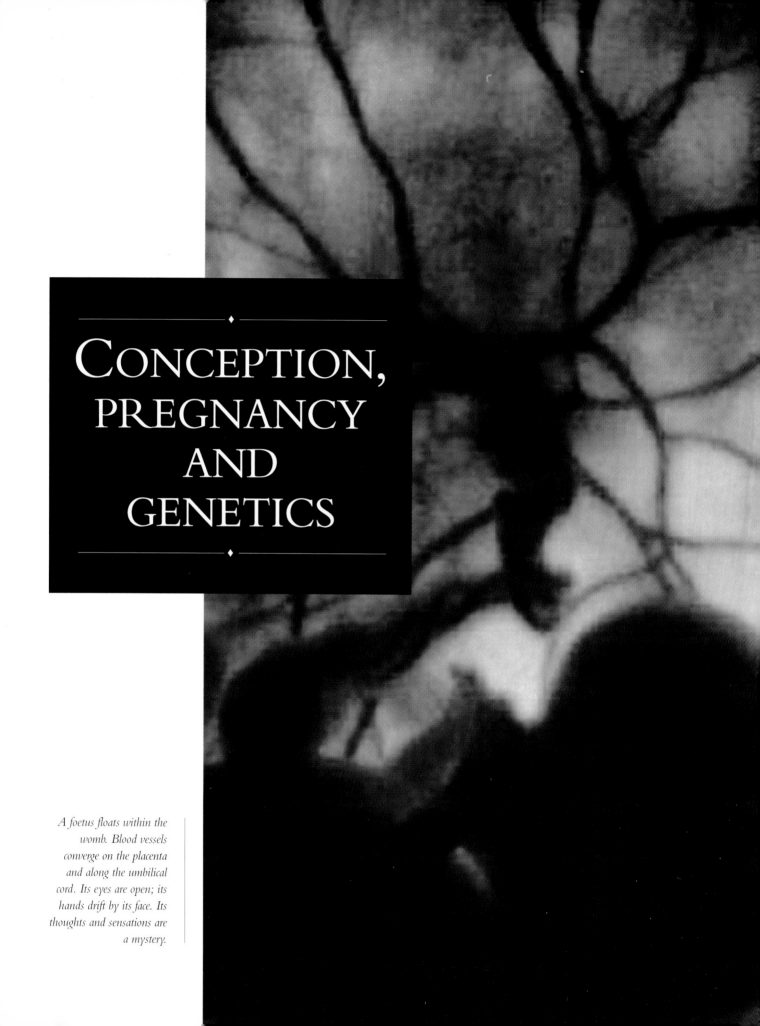

CONCEPTION, PREGNANCY AND GENETICS

A foetus floats within the womb. Blood vessels converge on the placenta and along the umbilical cord. Its eyes are open; its hands drift by its face. Its thoughts and sensations are a mystery.

THE CREATION OF A NEW LIFE begins with the fusion of a sperm and an egg. These two microscopic elements contain between them the blueprint to create over the next 40 weeks that amazing organism called a human being.

At ejaculation, the man deposits 100–500 million sperm into the woman's vagina. The freshly ejaculated sperm must then penetrate the cervical mucus, which is possible only when the vaginal secretions are of a certain acidity and the mucus is of a certain viscosity.

Fertilization

The sperm are capable of living for three days within the genital tract; they swim through the cervix, through the womb and into the Fallopian tube to meet the newly released ripe egg. It is not yet known exactly what drives sperm, but it is thought they are probably responding to a biochemical pull towards the egg.

Of the hundreds of millions of sperm, a mere hundred or so actually reach the egg. One single sperm penetrates the egg by digesting its way through the surface. At that instant of penetration, a biochemical change occurs in the coating of the egg which prevents any other sperm from penetrating it.

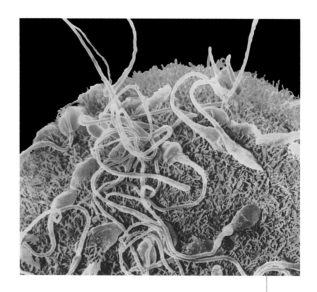

Above: A few successful sperm (green, with tails) on the egg (orange). Of the millions that strove to reach this egg, just one will fertilize it.

Egg and sperm then merge, their genetic contents intermingling. Thirty hours later the egg divides in the firstcritical division into two cells, then into four, then into eight which, within a few weeks, will have formed the billions of cells of the embryo.

Implantation and the placenta

The fertilized egg moves along the Fallopian tube until it reaches the womb after five to seven days. Here it implants into the wall of the womb by sending outgrowths into the womb which mature into the placenta. This remarkable structure combines foetal and maternal tissues to form a large disc where the baby's and the mother's blood capillaries come into intimate contact, but remain separate. The placenta is where oxygen, carbon dioxide and waste materials pass between mother and baby. At the same time the placenta excretes a variety of hormones in order to ensure the continuation of the pregnancy.

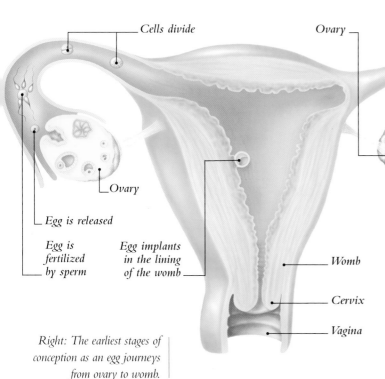

Cells divide — *Ovary*

Ovary

Egg is released

Egg is fertilized by sperm

Egg implants in the lining of the womb

Womb

Cervix

Vagina

Right: The earliest stages of conception as an egg journeys from ovary to womb.

Preconception

You can take certain health measures to secure the best possible start for you and your baby even before you are pregnant.

Diet Ensure a balanced intake of fruit, vegetables and protein. Vegetarians may need to take iron supplements.

Folic acid Taking this natural vitamin greatly reduces the chances of having a baby with **spina bifida** – a child whose backbone fails to fuse, leaving the spinal cord exposed. Folic acid should be taken prior to conception and during the first 12 weeks of pregnancy. The dose is 0.4 mg a day.

Alcohol Excess alcohol can cause brain damage in the baby as well as affecting its appearance. The risk increases with the more alcohol you drink; some authorities recommend avoiding alcohol completely during pregnancy.

Smoking If you smoke during pregnancy, your baby will be smaller and weigh less than if you did not smoke and may remain smaller throughout its life – an avoidable legacy.

Rubella *(German measles)* Routine vaccination programmes in childhood now offer protection from this illness, which causes multiple abnormalities in the baby if contracted in the first four months of pregnancy (see page 280). A simple blood test will show whether you are immune.

Exercise: Continue your usual routine of exercise. The first three months is the time of greatest risk of miscarriage, but there is no evidence to suggest that an active lifestyle contributes to this risk. On the contrary, regular exercise is good for maternal and foetal health.

An outline of pregnancy

The course of a pregnancy is normally considered in three sections called trimesters. Each trimester is approximately three months.

The first trimester

The baby These months are the most critical time in the baby's development. All its vital organs are formed, including the brain. Having begun as a single microscopic cell, by just four weeks the embryo has the rough outline of a human baby, although it is just 4 mm/³/₁₆ in long.

How does this happen? It is a process like origami: the twisting and folding of a flattish layer of cells into a cylinder,

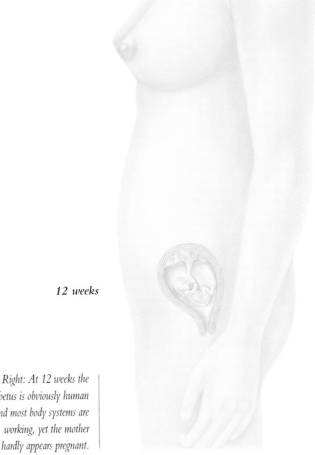

12 weeks

Right: At 12 weeks the foetus is obviously human and most body systems are working, yet the mother hardly appears pregnant.

which further differentiates into the brain, spinal cord and all the internal organs.

At eight weeks' pregnancy the embryo is clearly recognizable as human and is about 2.5 cm/1 in long. Its heart is beating and it can use some muscles. Eyes and ears are present, although primitive. Yet you have only missed one period and may only just suspect that you are pregnant.

By three months' pregnancy the baby will be about 5 cm/ 2 in long, with well-formed limbs and face. It will be kicking, but too faintly to be felt.

The mother So much is going on yet there is little to show for it except for a few natural, although inconvenient, symptoms caused by hormone changes.

Women vary greatly in how much nausea they experience. Nausea is very rarely serious. Tiredness appears to be a real hormonal effect, although compounded by the need to care for other children or to work.

Bladder irritation is a result of yet more hormonal effects on the neck of the bladder; it is often one of the earliest signs of

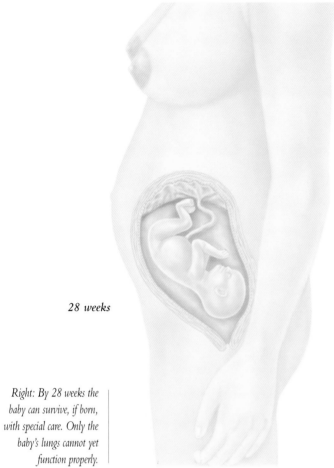

28 weeks

Right: By 28 weeks the baby can survive, if born, with special care. Only the baby's lungs cannot yet function properly.

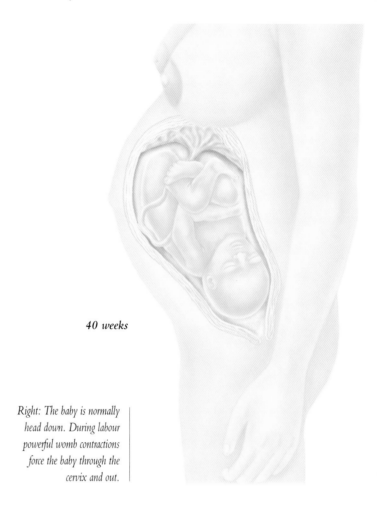

40 weeks

Right: The baby is normally head down. During labour powerful womb contractions force the baby through the cervix and out.

pregnancy. Breast tenderness is from the effect of proges-terone causing glands within the breast to swell in preparation for producing milk.

The second trimester
The baby All the baby's organs are formed and from now on it is a question of continued growth and maturation. Movements can be felt from about 16 weeks. At 16 weeks' pregnancy the baby has definite limbs, fingers and toes, is 18 cm/7 in long and weighs about 100 g/4 oz; it is recogniz-ably male or female. Its kidneys are secreting urine and it swallows amniotic fluid. At 24 weeks' pregnancy the baby is 24–32 cm/9$^{1}/_{2}$–12$^{1}/_{2}$ in long and weighs 750–900 g/1$^{3}/_{4}$–2 lb. It moves regularly and vigorously, has skin and is covered with fine hair. Its eyes are open, but whether it is able to see or not is not known. Most of its organs are reasonably mature, except for the lungs.

A baby born at 24 weeks has a chance of survival within an incubator but will need artificial respiration because the muscles for breathing are too weak to expand the lungs.

The third trimester
The baby Except for its lungs, the baby is virtually mature and can survive if born at any time during this stage. Over the last three months the main changes are growth and the deposition of fat under the skin. Babies born before 36 weeks may need special care. By 40 weeks the average baby is 50 cm/19$^{1}/_{2}$ in long and weighs about 3.4 kg/7$^{1}/_{2}$ lb.

The mother You have the increasing anticipation of a happy outcome to your pregnancy which outweighs the discomforts of this last stage. These include backache, feeling ungainly, **constipation**, **piles** or **varicose veins**. Movements are easily felt and often you are aware of contractions of the womb called Braxton Hicks contractions, especially in the last few weeks. In first pregnancies the baby engages at about 36 weeks, which means that its head sinks low into the pelvis, ready for birth. In later pregnancies the baby usually engages only just before labour starts.

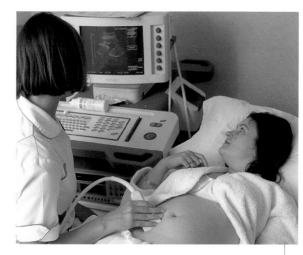

Routine antenatal care

Pregnancy is not an illness, yet there is much that can go wrong: poor growth of the baby, **high blood pressure**, urinary infections, **anaemia**, **diabetes** and many more, quite apart from the hazards of birth itself. Fortunately, serious complications are uncommon but routine antenatal monitoring (see page 324) aims to detect abnormalities as early as possible. In addition to providing time for discussion and reassurance, routine antenatal care includes checks on:

♦ *Heart*
♦ *Blood pressure*
♦ *Urine*
♦ *Weight gain*
♦ *Growth of the womb*

Investigations during pregnancy *Pregnancy tests* are done on a urine sample and are highly sensitive and reliable. They detect the presence of HCG (human chorionic gonadotrophin), a hormone released by the fertilized egg and detectable in blood or urine from six days after fertilization, when the fertilized egg is implanting into the womb.

Blood tests are necessary to detect anaemia, blood group, rhesus factor and whether there are unusual antibodies in the blood stream. Later, blood tests can indicate problems with the growth of the baby by measuring a hormone called oestriol, which is an indication of the health of the placenta.

Ultrasound scans allow precise monitoring of the growth of the baby and can detect abnormalities in the heart, back, kidneys and other organs.

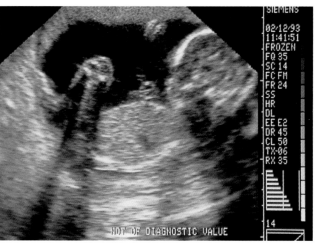

Above: High-definition ultrasound scanning is invaluable for monitoring the health, development and position of the baby. In the lower image the head of a 20-week foetus is visible at the right, knees and feet to the left.

Amniocentesis is sampling of the fluid surrounding the baby, performed in cases of suspected abnormality such as **Down's syndrome**.

Chorionic villus sampling can be done from about ten weeks to detect foetal abnormality. A tube is passed through the cervix to take a fragment of the tissue surrounding the foetus.

IMPORTANT WARNING SIGNS IN PREGNANCY

♦

♦ *Abdominal pain or bleeding may indicate miscarriage, premature labour or problems with the placenta, depending on the stage of the pregnancy*
♦ *Rapid weight gain or headaches and blurred vision may indicate pre-eclampsia if there is also a sudden rise in blood pressure*

See also PREGNANCY PROBLEMS *and* MISCARRIAGE.

Right: Pregnancy is a natural sequence of events for which a woman's body is designed. Modern antenatal care makes pregnancy safe while still fulfilling.

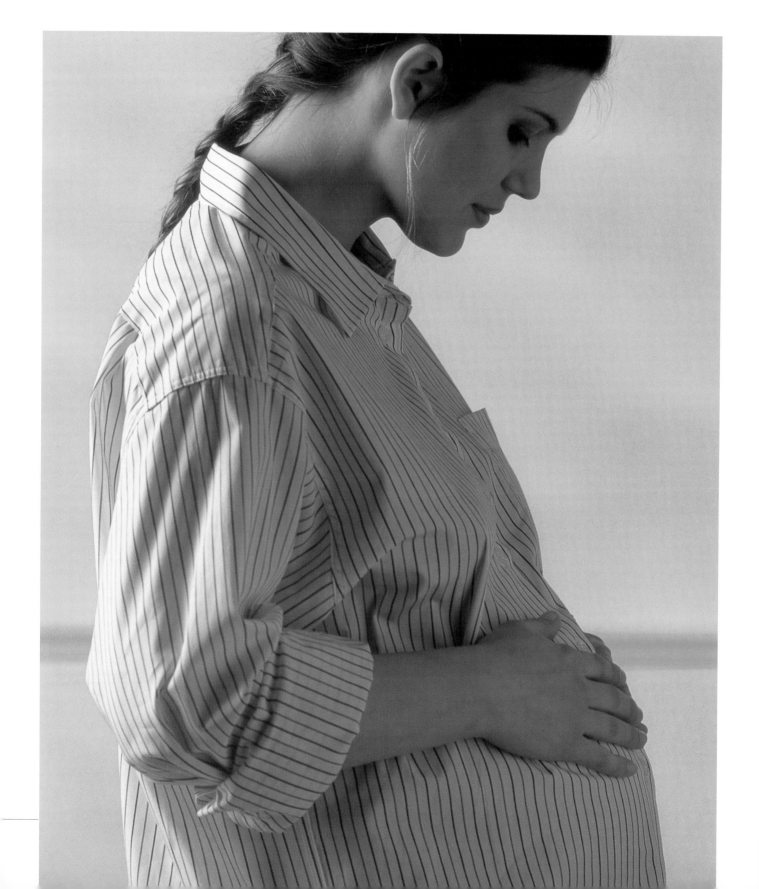

Genetics

There has been an explosion of knowledge about human genetics in the last 20 years. More and more of the genes responsible for human characteristics are being identified and the complete description of DNA is foreseeable. The following is an introduction to this complex and rapidly changing area of knowledge.

DNA (deoxyribonucleic acid) DNA is made of two molecular strands which spiral around each other in what is called a double helix. It is a record of how to make the proteins that are essential for life. All cells contain DNA because this is the blueprint to which they constantly refer in order to make the myriad proteins required by cells.

DNA is formed using just four simple chemical building blocks called nucleotides. Groups of three nucleotides specify (or code for) particular amino acids (see proteins, below). To translate a section of DNA, RNA (ribonucleic acid) is formed from the DNA in a way that copies the nucleotide sequence. That RNA moves elsewhere within the cell where it is in turn read by other forms of RNA carrying the amino acids specified by the original DNA code. The strand of amino acids lengthens into a protein. A gene is a section of DNA that carries the instructions to build one protein. This is the genetic code.

A strand of DNA contains three to four billion nucleotides, more than enough to code for the one hundred and fifty thousand or so proteins used by life.

Proteins These large molecules are built up from combinations of the 20 different human amino acids. As the amino acids are fitted together, the lengthening chain twists and takes a shape. The shape of a protein is often a vital part of its function, for example four haem proteins join to make haemoglobin (see page 268), the shape of which allows it to carry iron and oxygen. Other well-known proteins are those in muscles, connective tissue (collagen), blood clotting factors, antibodies and insulin.

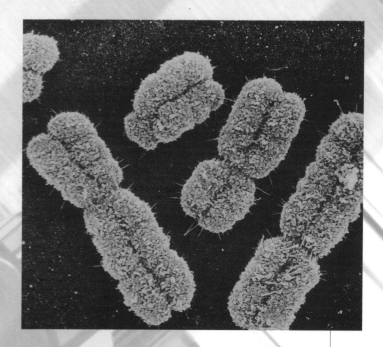

Above: Pairs of chromosomes highly magnified. Each comprises DNA tightly curled in such a way that it can be accessed in order to read the genetic information.

Inheritance

Within most cells the DNA resides in chromosomes, a condensed form of DNA, packaged to make it easier to reproduce itself. Humans have 23 pairs of chromosomes. There is one pair of sex chromosomes, called X- and Y-chromosomes, that determine whether an individual is male or female. A female has two X-chromosomes, while a male has an X- plus a Y-chromosome. The sex chromosomes carry many genes other than those involved in sexual differentiation. These other genes are called 'sex linked' because they are linked with the chromosomes that determine sex. This is why certain genetic conditions are found only in one sex or another. In general, only X-linked recessive genes are of importance in disease, for example haemophilia, which affects males only.

When a cell divides, the double-stranded DNA splits in two,

immediately replicating itself from the pool of nucleotides within the cell. Each daughter strand of DNA is a duplicate of the mother DNA, with all its genes.

Eggs and sperm All the eggs a woman will ever have form within the female embryo just a few weeks after fertilization – some seven million in all. Five million of these will have died even before the baby is born; yet more die during childhood. This leaves about 200,000 eggs when puberty begins, just a few hundred of which will ever develop into fully mature eggs during ovulation.

Sperm, on the other hand, are generated continuously from germ cells that activate at puberty.

Eggs and sperm each contain 23 single chromosomes formed by a complex rearrangement of chromosomes and genes and including a sex chromosome. The female egg always carries just an X-chromosome whereas a sperm may carry an X- or a Y-chromosome. It is therefore the father's sperm that determines the sex of a baby – a girl being XX, a boy being XY.

Once fertilized the egg has 23 pairs of chromosomes – a set from the mother and one from the father. Although many of the genes inherited are similar there are subtle differences that will influence how the child will develop – from the shape of his nose, the colour of eyes and overall size to the child's susceptibility to various diseases.

Dominance Certain genes are dominant, that is, they take precedence over the corresponding gene in the other set – for example, the gene for brown hair is dominant over other hair-colour genes, which are non-dominant, or recessive. This means that if the baby gets the gene for brown hair from one parent it will have brown hair whether the hair-colour gene from the other parent is for brown or fair hair. But it may not get that dominant gene because, in the genetic lottery that precedes the formation of eggs or sperm, the gene may not be passed to the particular egg or sperm involved in fertilization.

The genetic diversity from this system is continually altering the human gene bank and is responsible for much of our individuality. However, genetic inheritance is only one strand in human potential, although an immensely important one; environmental factors may help or hinder the expression of natural capabilities. The transmission of culture through the family and society can be regarded as another form of inheritance and is the more important factor in the slow, often painful, evolution of the human race.

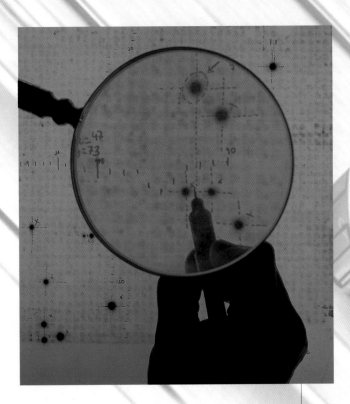

Above: Close examination of DNA sequences on a photographic plate enables scientists to carry out specialized analysis.

A fragment of DNA, enormously enlarged. Its billions of nucleotides encode the information needed for life. The elegant double helix structure was discovered by Watson and Crick in the 1950s.

PREGNANCY PROBLEMS

There are particular problems associated with each of the three trimesters of pregnancy:

FIRST TRIMESTER

Tiredness, possibly overwhelming, affects most women at this time decreasing by about 12 weeks. It may be due to the hormones of early pregnancy and **anaemia** (see below).

Ectopic pregnancy

Causes: This implantation of the fertilized egg outside the womb occurs in one in three hundred conceptions. The risk is higher if a woman has had an ectopic pregnancy before or conceives with a contraceptive coil in place. The ectopic egg can grow for a few weeks before rupturing surrounding tissue.

Symptoms: There is persistent pain in the lower left or right abdomen (central pain is more suggestive of **miscarriage**). The previous period may have been entirely missed or scanty and brief. There may be other symptoms of early pregnancy – nausea and breast tenderness. Internal examination shows the cervix very sensitive to gentle movement. If the ectopic pregnancy ruptures the Fallopian tube there is sudden severe abdominal pain, vaginal haemorrhage and collapse.

Treatment: An ultrasound scan locates the ectopic pregnancy before emergency surgical removal of the fertilized egg and the Fallopian tube on that side. Sometimes the ectopic egg alone can be removed and the Fallopian tube repaired – preserving future fertility, although it is perfectly possible to conceive with just one Fallopian tube.

WARNING SYMPTOMS IN PREGNANCY, WITH POSSIBLE SIGNIFICANCE

- *Any bleeding (miscarriage, placenta praevia, premature labour)*
- *Abdominal pain, especially if one sided (ectopic pregnancy, premature labour)*
- *Severe nausea (multiple pregnancy)*
- *Failing to feel baby's movements (problems with foetal growth)*
- *Fingers or feet that swell rapidly (pre-eclampsia)*
- *Severe headaches, especially if with flashing lights (pre-eclampsia)*
- *Breathlessness at rest (anaemia, heart disease, pulmonary embolus)*
- *A swollen painful leg (deep vein thrombosis)*
- *A feeling that things are not right (most experienced doctors will respect the mother's instinct about this and arrange tests of the baby's health)*

Nausea

Causes: This is assumed to be due to pregnancy hormones. Severe early nausea may indicate twins or multiple pregnancy.

Symptoms: Nausea is greatest each morning, decreasing during the day. Only occasionally is it so bad that the woman vomits continuously and becomes dehydrated – hyperemesis.

Treatment: It is best to have a snack before getting up in the morning. Antinausea medication is not prescribed unless nausea is severe. Hyperemesis needs intravenous rehydration in hospital, with a scan to detect any multiple pregnancy.

Infection/drug damage

Causes: The baby is insulated from most infections. **Rubella** is the main risk but is virtually eliminated by vaccination. A few drugs can damage the developing foetus; others such as some antibiotics are safe but are best avoided unless essential. Alcohol and smoking to excess affect the baby's growth.

Symptoms: Women who smoke have babies about ten per cent (250 g/8 oz) lighter than predicted. Babies born to heavy drinkers have a recognized abnormal facial appearance.

Treatment: There is such a high risk of foetal damage from rubella (30–40%) that non-immune women exposed to it are offered a termination. If a woman has taken a potentially harmful drug she will be offered a detailed ultrasound scan to try to detect any malformation of the foetus.

SECOND TRIMESTER

Foetal abnormality

Causes: Often, this is pure genetic chance. Drugs, infections and parental age account for just a few foetal abnormalities.

Symptoms: The most serious abnormalities end in miscarriage or failure of the baby to grow normally. Ultrasound scans check the appearance of its organs for **spina bifida**, brain, kidney and heart anomalies or **Down's syndrome**.

Treatment: Some abnormalities can be treated in the womb by foetal surgery. Others give early warning that the baby will need special care, sometimes raising difficult ethical issues.

Placenta praevia

Causes: Placenta praevia means that the placenta is implanted low down in the womb (instead of on the side), covering the cervix and obstructing normal delivery.

Symptoms: Occasionally there is bleeding in late pregnancy. If previously undetected, the first symptom is obstruction at the time of birth. One reason for scanning pregnant women is to check for this condition.

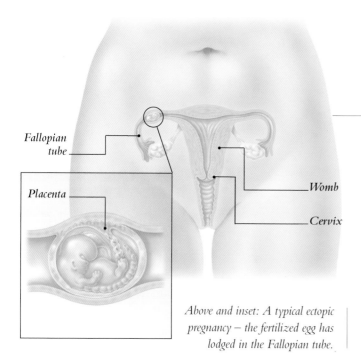

Fallopian tube

Placenta

Womb

Cervix

Above and inset: A typical ectopic pregnancy – the fertilized egg has lodged in the Fallopian tube.

Treatment: Nothing can be done to prevent placenta praevia, but a Caesarean section (see page 141) can be planned in advance and makes safe delivery possible.

THIRD TRIMESTER

Anaemia

Causes: Even in well-nourished women this almost always appears in pregnancy as a result of expansion of blood volume. The risk increases with each pregnancy and in breast-feeding since iron passes into the milk.

Symptoms: There are often none; blood tests show whether it is serious enough to treat.

Treatment: Mild anaemia needs none. Otherwise one or two iron tablets a day are sufficient. It is rare for a woman to be so anaemic by delivery that she needs blood transfusion.

High blood pressure (pre-eclampsia)

Causes: After ectopic pregnancy, this is potentially the most serious complication of pregnancy. The cause is probably an immune reaction against the placenta.

Symptoms: Fingers and feet may swell, appearing and worsening over a few days; there may be severe headaches with flashing lights. Blood pressure is raised, sometimes greatly; there is protein in the urine. This is pre-eclampsia, and may progress to eclampsia with epileptic fits, unconsciousness and a risk of mother and baby dying. Fortunately eclampsia is very rare.

Treatment: Mildly raised blood pressure usually responds to rest as long as there are not the other features above. Severe hypertension is treated with drugs like labetalol. Eclampsia is a medical emergency: the mother has to be deeply sedated and blood pressure controlled by intravenous drugs. The baby must be delivered by Caesarean section immediately.

Premature delivery

Causes: It is not understood why normal labour begins, let alone premature labour. Sometimes the neck of the womb is lax and cannot contain the pregnancy to term.

Symptoms: These are the same as normal labour: a show of mucus, leakage of fluid and blood and rhythmic contractions.

Treatment: The aim is to delay labour until the baby is as old as possible: 32 weeks is desirable, although babies as premature as 24 weeks can survive. A few drugs can delay premature labour which, combined with rest, might gain those vital extra weeks. If the cause is a lax cervix, it is kept closed with a stitch, later removed to allow normal vaginal delivery.

Indigestion, constipation and piles

Causes: The large mass of baby and womb obstructs the gastrointestinal tract. Acid is literally squeezed out of the stomach into the gullet and the bowels are partially obstructed – not helped by taking iron tablets. Piles (see HAEMORRHOIDS) are a direct consequence of the increased abdominal pressure on blood vessels around the anus.

Symptoms: **Heartburn** is common; the bowels may be opened with difficulty, only every few days. Piles are often associated with **varicose veins** at the top of the thighs and in the labia.

Treatment: **Indigestion** lessens once the baby's head engages at about 36 weeks. There are entirely safe antacids available. **Constipation** responds to high fibre or laxatives if necessary. Nothing can be done to reduce piles, which will nearly always disappear after the birth; soothing creams help the itching.

Complementary Treatment

WARNING: In **Western herbalism**, herbs should not usually be taken during pregnancy except under professional guidance. However, ginger tea is a safe and effective remedy for morning sickness.

Always check your chosen practitioner is experienced in pregnancy problems. **Nutritional therapy** – improving your diet and supplementing with folic acid, vitamins B_6 and B_{12} and zinc can help reduce a number of problems, such as nausea and fatigue. **Chiropractic** manipulation can relieve pain in the low and mid-upper back, which is common as a result of enlarging breasts. Specific **yoga** postures can alleviate some symptoms, such as haemorrhoids. **Hypnotherapy** is good at banishing morning sickness. *Other therapies to try: aromatherapy; Chinese herbalism; homeopathy; acupuncture; biodynamics; Bach flower remedies; shiatsu-do; naturopathy; chakra balancing; healing.*

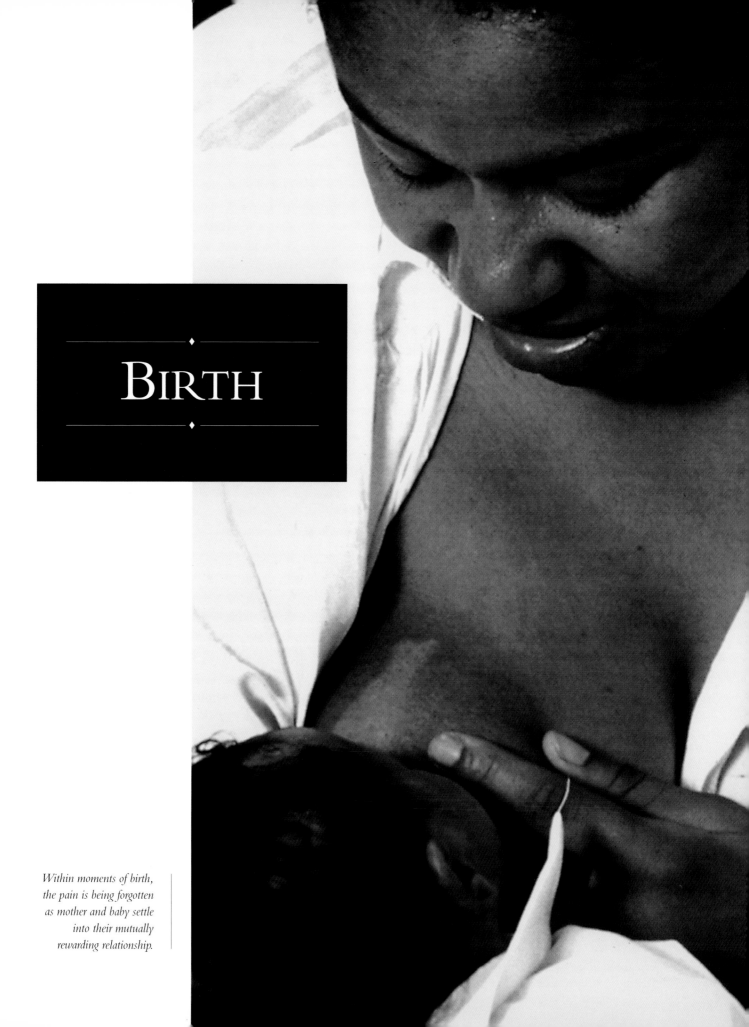

BIRTH

Within moments of birth, the pain is being forgotten as mother and baby settle into their mutually rewarding relationship.

ODERN OBSTETRICS, the care of women in pregnancy, is largely concerned with making birth as rewarding but safe as possible. In most areas of the United Kingdom the expectant mother now has a choice of ways in which to deliver her baby, ranging from the full panoply of medical care in a hospital delivery room to a relatively private event in a birthing pool.

Preparing for labour

By the end of pregnancy the baby is ready to be born; its lungs are the last organs to be mature enough to cope outside the womb. Hopefully, you and your partner are psychologically prepared for the process of birth. Through reading and questioning, try to ensure you know in some detail what to expect – the types of pain and what they mean, who will be dealing with you, the role of the midwife and the obstetrician, the equipment and examinations required. Above all, remember that birth is a natural process and that modern obstetric care aims to assist rather than replace nature.

In most cases the baby lies head down, facing the mother's left or right side. In a first pregnancy the baby should engage at around 36 weeks; the baby's head settles low in the womb in a fixed position. As this relieves pressure at the top of the womb this is also called lightening. In later pregnancies engaging occurs just before birth.

Thanks to the hormone progesterone, the cervix is soft and can dilate easily; the joints between the pelvic bones are relaxed enough to let the baby's head through. Something as yet unknown then triggers the beginning of labour and the mild Braxton Hicks contractions often felt throughout pregnancy become stronger.

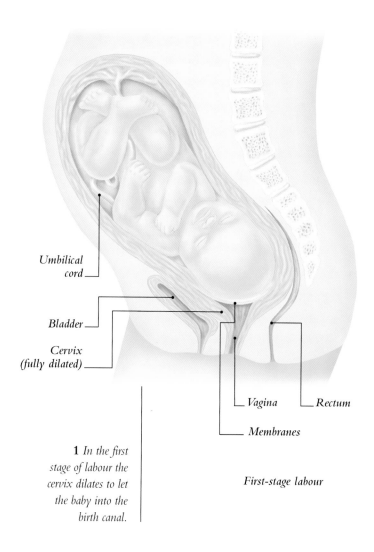

Umbilical cord

Bladder

Cervix (fully dilated)

Vagina   Rectum

Membranes

1 *In the first stage of labour the cervix dilates to let the baby into the birth canal.*

First-stage labour

MONITORING THE BABY

◆

The use of this technique has waned, but it is still important in higher-risk pregnancies. One element involves monitoring the baby's heart rate during contractions. The other is to take a sample of blood from the baby's scalp. These tests show whether the baby is coping with the stress of birth or whether it is being starved of oxygen and therefore needs to be delivered urgently either by forceps or by Caesarean section (see page 141). During labour your attendants will keep checking to see how the baby is coping. The readings are especially important if there are difficulties such as prolonged labour or exhaustion of the mother.

Early (first stage) labour

With each contraction of the womb the cervix is pulled up towards the womb and then dilates (widens). This process takes between four and eight hours and is not especially painful except towards the end of this time. During this process, the baby drops further into the pelvis, often causing backache and bladder discomfort. In the first stage you may be able to walk and relax in between the increasingly strong contractions. Any urge to push must be resisted until the midwife is satisfied that the cervix is fully dilated to 10 cm/ 4 in, otherwise you would be trying to push the baby through too narrow an opening.

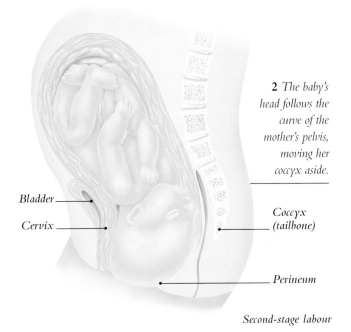

2 The baby's head follows the curve of the mother's pelvis, moving her coccyx aside.

Bladder

Cervix

Coccyx (tailbone)

Perineum

Second-stage labour

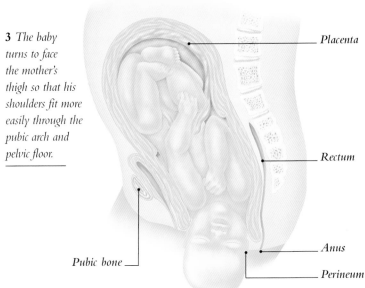

3 The baby turns to face the mother's thigh so that his shoulders fit more easily through the pubic arch and pelvic floor.

Placenta

Rectum

Anus

Perineum

Pubic bone

Third-stage labour

Second-stage labour

Now the active process of birth begins as the womb exerts its maximum effort to expel the baby. It is usually at this stage that the waters break; the amniotic membrane surrounding the baby in the womb ruptures and 500 ml/18 fl oz or so of fluid leaks from the vagina. The urge to push is at a maximum and with each contraction the mother bears down, sending the baby another stage down the birth canal, through the by now fully dilated cervix and into the vagina.

Most babies travel initially looking to one side, a position giving maximum head clearance. Further down the canal, the anatomy alters so that the baby's head should naturally turn to look towards the mother's back, a process called rotation. The midwife may urge you to resist pushing while this takes place.

The head is now visible and the lips of the vagina are fully dilated. This is when the perineum may tear, and a planned cut (episiotomy) may be made. With more efforts the head is pushed out and you will be asked to resist pushing while the baby's body rotates to one side. This allows the shoulders to emerge more easily. With more pushes the whole baby emerges: a moment of exhilaration for the mother, her partner and all her attendants, and one that never loses its magic.

The umbilical cord Within moments of birth the baby's heart and circulation undergo complicated changes so that the baby no longer relies on the blood coming from the placenta. This process is set off by the baby drawing breath and crying; at that moment the lungs expand and blood begins to flow through them. This is why it is so important for the baby to begin breathing immediately. Once that has happened, blood flow through the umbilical cord ceases, so it can be safely cut and tied.

Third-stage labour

Now all that remains is to expel the placenta, which detaches as a result of the womb's vigorous contractions. It is usually pulled out by gentle tugging on the umbilical cord. There is a risk of bleeding from the raw surface where the placenta was attached. To reduce this risk it is normal to inject a drug called syntometrine to speed up the contraction of the womb.

Afterbirth This is usually a time of rushed activity as the attendants check the baby, examine the mother for tears that need stitching and monitor for excessive blood loss. These initial essential checks finished, the baby is given to the mother

PAIN CONTROL

◆

Women have a choice of using natural methods of pain control such as relaxation techniques or of accepting pain-relieving drugs. Pain control can be given by injection, usually pethidine, or an anaesthetic gas, usually nitrous oxide, under the mother's control. Increasing numbers of women opt for epidural anaesthesia. A tiny tube is introduced by needle into the fluid space around the spinal cord. A continuous infusion of anaesthetic is dripped in, making the mother numb from that point down. An epidural also numbs the desire to push, so the birth has to be more closely monitored and managed by the attendants.

The best preparation for childbirth is to read as much as possible on the subject, to learn some relaxation techniques and to discuss beforehand what pain relief is available.

(ideally with her partner) for a moment of peace in which to gaze at her baby, fondle her then give a first breast feed. Many women are so exhausted physically and emotionally by this stage that they will doze off for a few minutes.

Modern childbirth

Completely natural childbirth can be hazardous. In the underdeveloped world, the physical damage that most often affects women is tears of the vagina and perineum that do not heal properly and lead to constant urinary **incontinence**.

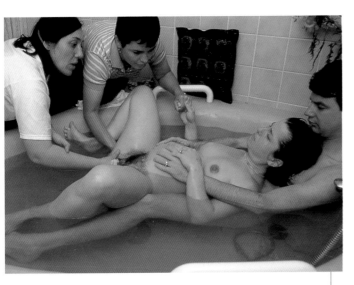

Above: Giving birth in a birthing pool may reduce the mother's pain and allows her partner to be more involved.

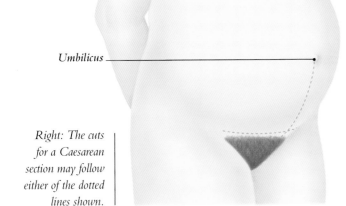

Umbilicus

Right: The cuts for a Caesarean section may follow either of the dotted lines shown.

In the United Kingdom, as recently as the 1930s one in every two hundred women died in childbirth from blood loss, high blood pressure or infection. Now the death rate is less than one in seventeen thousand. Although much of the improvement is due to better general health and more sophisticated anaesthetics, a large measure is as a result of obstetric care. However, many health professionals now accept that managed childbirth went too far in the 1970s and welcome the return to childbirth in an environment with less emphasis on 'high tech' and more on making the experience emotionally rewarding for all involved, while keeping the high-tech equipment available in case it is needed.

Complications in childbirth This vast subject cannot be adequately covered here. It includes multiple pregnancy, poor growth of the baby and maternal ill health, especially **diabetes** and **high blood pressure**; everything that can go wrong during delivery such as the baby getting stuck, the mother getting exhausted or torrential bleeding; and interventions such as forceps and Caesarean section. Fortunately, at least 97 out of every 100 births go normally but the situation during childbirth can change very rapidly. It is with this knowledge that many health professionals are cautious about the current move towards more home births.

CAESAREAN SECTION

◆

This operation removes the baby directly from the womb through a cut just above the bikini line. After the baby and placenta have been removed, the walls of the womb are stitched back together and the abdominal cut is repaired. The wound takes ten to fourteen days to heal.

Caesarean section is an extremely safe operation, and is done when the risk of vaginal birth, to either mother or baby, appears unacceptable. Some risk factors are clear before labour begins, for example if the mother is carrying triplets or more, or if she has a very small pelvis or high blood pressure. In such a case Caesarean section is a planned procedure for which the mother is prepared.

Often, however, the decision to deliver the baby by Caesarean section is only made once labour has begun, if it is not progressing normally for some reason – for example, the baby may be distressed or stuck, or there may be sudden heavy bleeding. Most obstetricians will recommend Caesarean section at any sign of labour going wrong.

POST-DELIVERY PROBLEMS

Problems for mothers following childbirth – mostly of a minor and easily treatable nature.

CAUSES

There are various kinds of post-delivery problems. To give birth, the vagina has to dilate enough to allow the 10 cm/4 in diameter of the baby's head to pass. During this process tears of the vagina are almost inevitable. An episiotomy, a planned cut at the lower part of the vagina, may be performed to avoid large uncontrolled tears from the vagina to the rectum.

There is always some bleeding at the time of delivery, small amounts of which continue for days if not weeks afterwards.

A Caesarean section (see page 141) involves a cut across the lower abdomen into the womb. Although it heals rapidly, pains are common at the site of incision for several weeks.

Many women who have an epidural anaesthetic to reduce pain during labour suffer headaches and backache for a week or so after. After birth it takes a few days for the hormones that make the breasts secrete milk to build up. For women who are not breastfeeding this engorgement can become intensely painful. Mild infections of the breasts are common, occasionally worsening into a breast abscess. Lastly, whether through hormonal changes or the psychological stress of childbirth, new mothers may have emotional problems.

SYMPTOMS

It is usual to feel tender, especially at the site of an episiotomy. Abdominal tenderness that gets worse and is associated with sweating or shivers suggests infection. Similarly, a bloody vaginal discharge will continue but should gradually lessen as the womb returns to its non-pregnant state over the next eight weeks. An increase in blood flow together with lower abdominal pains and sweats suggests infection of the womb.

If remnants of the afterbirth remain within the womb there will be persistent heavy loss of fresh blood as the womb is unable to contract fully. If the bleeding is severe you may need a curettage, to scrape the walls of the womb clean of any debris. Otherwise minor bleeding can be left for nature to deal with, which is why the first couple of periods after childbirth are often heavy and contain clots.

Breasts

There is often an extra flow of blood from the womb whenever a woman breastfeeds. This is because suckling stimulates the release of the hormone oxytocin, which makes muscles around the milk glands contract and so let down milk. At the same time oxytocin also makes the muscles of the womb contract and so expel blood. This is nature's way of getting the womb back to its usual size as soon as possible.

A breast infection is recognized by increasing pain in the breast, which becomes firm and red over the area of infection. You feel very unwell with shivers and sweats. If you are not breastfeeding the breasts become engorged with milk and very hard and painful for several days.

Psychological symptoms

The elation of birth almost invariably gives way to mild **depression** after a few days. This coincides with going home, getting into the relentless routine of a new baby and coping with all the other domestic responsibilities, too. For the great majority of women this is just a passing phase but about ten per cent of women become more persistently depressed, either immediately after childbirth or within the first three months. They find it difficult to care for the baby, are irritable and cry easily. More extreme, although rare, is puerperal psychosis, which is a very serious depressive illness often accompanied by thoughts of harming the baby.

TREATMENT

The system of postnatal care provided by midwives, health visitors and doctors is intended to pick up problems at an early stage. Many of the above-mentioned problems are dealt

---

SOME WARNING SYMPTOMS AFTER CHILDBIRTH, AND WHAT THEY MAY MEAN

- *Pain and swelling in one calf (deep vein thrombosis, see page 53)*
- *Heavy, fresh red vaginal bleeding (retained portions of the placenta or infection of the womb)*
- *Abdominal or perineal pain, an offensive discharge with or without fever (infection of the womb or perineum)*
- *Tender and red breast area with or without fever (breast abscess)*
- *Burning sensation on passing urine and a need to go frequently (urinary infection)*
- *Sudden breathlessness or sharp chest pain (a blood clot on the lung – a pulmonary embolus, see page 69)*
- *Persistent, deepening depression and neglect of the baby (puerperal depression or psychosis)*

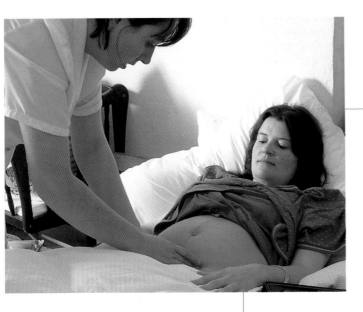

Above: Examining whether the womb has fully contracted, which is one important check after delivery.

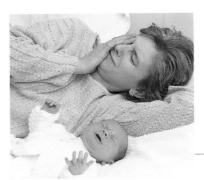

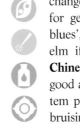

Left: The stresses of a demanding baby can occasionally end in severe depression.

with in this way, perhaps with an antibiotic if appropriate. Hospital intervention is rarely needed unless an episiotomy wound breaks down, there is persistent heavy bleeding that requires curettage or a breast abscess is unresponsive to an antibiotic and needs surgical drainage.

Indigestion, **haemorrhoids** and **constipation** rapidly disappear after birth with the loss of intra-abdominal pressure. Backache is common during pregnancy but should go over a few weeks as the joints and ligaments of the spine and pelvis, which become lax during pregnancy, return to normal.

Psychological treatment

The best and often the only medicine required is the opportunity to discuss worries with the postnatal team. Common queries revolve around feeding schedules, babies who appear demanding and cry all the time, and mild depression. Many women feel inadequate for the heavy demands of motherhood. There is no easy answer to these concerns, which are an inevitable part of the burden of having a new baby.

Women who are isolated from their family, who have unsupportive partners or who live in difficult socio-economic circumstances may especially have problems. Some babies are genuinely difficult and the mother needs help in coping with this. Many mothers find they gain important support from mother-and-baby groups during this demanding time.

Persistent depression that leads the mother to neglect herself and the baby may require treatment with an antidepressant for a few months. Those few women who suffer from puerperal psychosis are best treated in a psychiatric mother-and-baby unit where they can be closely supervised and have intensive medical and psychological therapy.

Sex

It is usually several weeks before sexual relationships are restarted after childbirth, simply because of physical discomfort, tiredness and true lack of sexual desire thanks to the constant demands of a baby. Some men have difficulty seeing their partner in both maternal and sexual roles.

By the routine postnatal check at six to eight weeks the body should be almost back to its non-pregnant state. Contraception and psychosexual queries can be discussed and vaginal pain checked, but there is no need to wait for this to resume sex, which can start as soon as you both feel ready.

In women not breastfeeding periods restart between six and ten weeks after delivery and they are fertile from that time. Breastfeeding suppresses the menstrual cycle so periods do not usually begin in this case for four to six months, but this cannot be relied upon as a method of contraception.

Complementary Treatment

Bach flower remedies – walnut for adjustment to change, star of Bethlehem for shock, Rescue Remedy for general restoration of calm, mustard for 'baby blues', cherry plum for fear of doing the baby harm, elm if you feel overwhelmed with responsibility. **Chinese herbalism** and **acupuncture** are especially good at retuning and rebalancing your hormonal system post-delivery. **Homeopathy** – arnica is good for bruising and soreness, ignatia can help for baby blues. **Chakra balancing** offers energy balancing and relaxation effects. **Aromatherapy** oils can help heal stitches and, in conjunction with **massage**, alleviate the baby blues. **Chiropractic** treatment for backache is common post-delivery, and aims to restore normal joint and muscular function to ease pain and discomfort. **Yoga** can help your body return to normal after pregnancy and delivery. *Other therapies to try: shiatsu-do.*

BREASTFEEDING

◆

This is a natural activity but there may be problems and women will benefit from advice passed on by others.

BACKGROUND
◆

Each breast is made up of 15–25 lobes, each of which is a complete milk-secreting unit. The milk from a lobe drains via tubules, ending in a milk duct in the nipple. Fatty tissue surrounds each lobe, giving the breast its shape. In pregnancy the lobe system enlarges ready to secrete milk. However, milk production only begins in earnest after childbirth, under the influence of the hormone prolactin from the pituitary gland. As long as the baby is regularly suckled, prolactin production is maintained and the breasts continue to secrete milk.

What is breast milk?
Breast milk is a complex mixture of water plus sugar (lactose), protein, fat, sodium, iron, vitamin C, vitamin D and calcium. It has less protein than cow's milk, but 50% of its energy is in the form of fat, a much higher percentage than in cow's milk. Breast milk also contains immunoglobulins – antibodies from the mother – so the breast-fed infant has some protection from infectious illness in the first few months.

In addition, breast milk is on tap at no cost and delivered conveniently at the correct temperature and hygienically.

How does it get out?
Thanks to prolactin, the breasts store milk ready for release whenever the baby suckles. Another hormone, oxytocin, makes muscle surrounding the milk glands contract, so squeezing out the milk. This is called the 'let-down' reflex. The release of oxytocin is controlled by a number of factors. Simply thinking about breastfeeding will stimulate its release, as will hearing the baby cry with hunger and preparing to feed. This is why the breasts start to leak even before feeding begins. Suckling further stimulates the release of oxytocin.

Conversely, **anxiety** and **stress** affect oxytocin and lead to difficulties in let-down, which are easily misinterpreted as an inability to breastfeed. Oxytocin has an additional action in making the womb contract, which is why women may get abdominal cramps and bleeding when breastfeeding.

DIFFICULTIES
◆

Probably the main difficulties that many mothers experience with breastfeeding are getting started, inadequate milk flow, breast infections and pain.

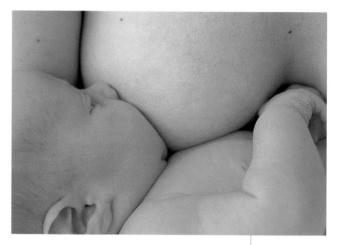

Above: Patience and correct technique should make breastfeeding a pleasure for both mother and baby.

Getting started
It helps to prepare the breasts for feeding before delivery. Some authorities recommend massaging the breasts in the last few weeks of pregnancy, squeezing them towards the nipple. This way you will see some milk expressed. The nipples should be kept soft using moisturizing creams.

After birth it takes two to four days for milk production to get going fully. During this time the breasts secrete a thick yellow type of milk called colostrum, which is adequate for the baby at this time. Thereafter, the more you feed the more you stimulate prolactin and the more milk will be produced.

The technique of breastfeeding is not simply to let the baby latch on to the nipple – by biting on the nipple the baby bites down on to the milk ducts, obstructing them and reducing the flow. The baby needs to suck on the areola, the coloured skin surrounding the nipple, which contains little reservoirs of milk. This way there is no obstruction to the flow of milk through the nipple.

Inadequate milk flow
Rarely a true milk deficiency, this is more likely a result of giving up too soon, which by reflex diminishes the quantity of milk produced; as well, anxiety about feeding inhibits the release of oxytocin. In the first two weeks you can ensure complete emptying of the breasts by manually expressing the milk, which also stimulates maximum secretion of prolactin.

Probably most milk is taken during the first five minutes on each breast; after that the baby continues to get some milk but sucks mainly for pleasure. Time spent on the breast is therefore not an accurate measure of how much milk the baby has actually taken. A better way of judging is whether the baby appears content and comes off the breast without irritation. The most objective measure is obviously whether the baby gains weight at the correct rate of about 175 g/6 oz a week, i.e. doubling its weight in the first three months.

It is tempting to top up breast feeds with bottle feeds 'just in case' but if this is done too much it will have the effect of reducing breast milk production and lead to a vicious circle of diminishing milk production and additional 'topping up'.

Painful breasts and infection

When the milk first comes in the breasts often feel engorged, swollen and tender. This is relieved once the baby suckles. It varies as to how much milk women make and some may have to express some milk initially to relieve discomfort. Those who do not wish to breastfeed will have painful breasts for a few days until prolactin levels diminish. The drug bromocriptine accelerates this process when taken for ten days.

Tender, cracked nipples are common; the cause is not clear. It may be that the technique is at fault, allowing the baby to chew on the nipple rather than the areola. Suckling for too long will lead to sore nipples. Most cases respond to a lanolin cream which is harmless for the baby.

It is easy for infection to enter a lobe of the breast through its duct on the nipple. Once inside, bacteria find the milk an ideal environment in which to grow. The typical breast infection, mastitis, is therefore of one lobe. The symptoms are a red, painful area of one breast and the mother feeling feverish and shivery. Treatment with an antibiotic cures most cases.

A little antibiotic passes across to the baby but it is harmless. It is unusual to require the more extreme measure of draining pus from the breast by a surgical incision. Breastfeeding should continue in mild cases. If severe, stop feeding from that breast but continue to express milk.

Reluctance to breastfeed

Not every woman wishes to breastfeed despite the undoubted benefits for her baby – protection from infection, less chance of **eczema** and fewer episodes of gastroenteritis. Breastfeeding has disadvantages such as tying the mother who wants to work. Other reasons may be lack of success in the past, sheer embarrassment about feeding, the smells and the stains on clothing, and lack of encouragement from family and partner. If it is not for you, do not feel guilty about it but enjoy the warmth and closeness of you baby while you bottle-feed.

QUESTIONS

Does size matter?
Exceptionally small breasts may not produce enough milk; exceptionally large breasts may make it difficult for the baby to grasp the areola without suffocating. These extremes aside there is no evidence to show that size matters.

Do inverted nipples prevent breastfeeding?
Most inverted nipples become sufficiently erect during breastfeeding to be adequate. Massaging or using breast shields to encourage inverted nipples to evert does not work nor is it necessary.

Is breastfeeding a contraceptive?
Breastfeeding suppresses periods for about six months. Although this reduces the chances of conceiving, it is not foolproof. For greater certainty use additional contraception such as the progesterone-only Pill or condoms.

How do I know when to stop breastfeeding?
You could breastfeed for a year or more, but most Western women stop sooner, often on return to work. You may need to supplement breast feeds if the baby is not growing satisfactorily. Your breast milk will diminish naturally as you introduce solids.

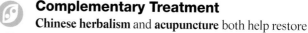

Complementary Treatment

Chinese herbalism and **acupuncture** both help restore and maintain your hormonal balance; an experienced practitioner could advise. **Western herbalism** can help increase both the quantity and quality of breast milk: try infusions of nettle or raspberry leaves. When you want to stop breastfeeding, red sage tea will help reduce the milk flow. **Homeopathy** – use calendula cream for sore or cracked nipples. In conjunction with orthodox treatment, **aromatherapy** might be able to help alleviate mastitis – consult an experienced practitioner. **Yoga** can help by promoting relaxation and enhancing confidence. **Hypnotherapy** – hypnotic suggestion can help increase milk flow, and alleviate mastitis. Many **Ayurvedic** preparations are available to improve the quality and quantity of breast milk. General self-help – chilled cabbage leaves or grated carrot can be placed on engorged breasts to reduce discomfort. *Other therapies to try: Bach flower remedies; shiatsu-do; chakra balancing.*

MISCARRIAGE

◆

A pregnancy that ends prematurely with the loss of the foetus.

CAUSES

◆

Early miscarriages, up to about 14 weeks' gestation, are usually due to fundamental abnormality with the foetus or placenta. The baby may be seriously malformed; the placenta may be unhealthy or poorly attached to the womb. These factors affect at least one pregnancy in six. The risk of two consecutive miscarriages is about one in thirty-six – uncommon but not rare and may happen through pure and sad chance. Fewer than one in two hundred women have three miscarriages in a row. Although this may still be through chance, such mothers may have Hughes' syndrome (see below).

Late miscarriage means a miscarriage between 14 and 26 weeks. (From 26 weeks the baby may survive, so technically it is premature labour.) Late miscarriage is still usually because of abnormality of the baby or placenta. Additional possibilities are infection such as toxoplasmosis, trauma to the abdomen or serious maternal disease. The cervix may be too lax to retain the contents of the womb, a condition called cervical incompetence.

SYMPTOMS

◆

There is vaginal bleeding, slight initially and often brown (from altered blood) rather than bright red. There is a 50% hope of these symptoms stopping (threatened miscarriage). Later there are abdominal cramps, increased bleeding and backache (signs of inevitable miscarriage). The symptoms of complete miscarriage are passing large clots and jelly-like material. Late miscarriages resemble labour.

Abdominal pains on one side as opposed to mid-line warn of an ectopic pregnancy (see PREGNANCY PROBLEMS).

TREATMENT

◆

It is likely that many very early miscarriages are experienced as a slightly delayed, heavier-than-usual period. No treatment is required in these cases. There is about a 50% hope of a threatened miscarriage settling down. Although no treatment has been shown to influence this, it seems both sensible and kind to rest. An internal examination may show that the neck of the womb is open; this means that miscarriage has occurred or is inevitable. Where there is doubt, an ultrasound scan of the womb shows whether the pregnancy is still there and whether the baby is still alive (see page 317).

After definite miscarriage or where a scan shows the foetus has died, the contents of the womb should be removed by curettage to avoid any possible infection of the womb.

The treatment of cervical incompetence involves a purse string stitch around the cervix, called a Shirodkar suture, which is removed in later pregnancy. In cases of recurrent miscarriage investigations are necessary. These may show an abnormal anatomy of the womb or Fallopian tube that interferes with the implantation of the egg. Latest research has shown that some women having recurrent miscarriages have antibodies to a protein called cardiolipin (Hughes' syndrome) and can be helped by taking aspirin during early pregnancy.

In the hurried physical treatment of miscarriage it is easy to overlook the psychological consequences. Miscarriage means the loss of a baby and parents may need to mourn as much as after losing a full-term infant. It may help to reflect that miscarriage will usually have been nature acting for the best.

QUESTIONS

Does a threatened miscarriage affect the pregnancy?
Be reassured that the pregnancy will be unaffected and that there is no more risk of abnormality than in any uncomplicated pregnancy.

Is it important to wait before falling pregnant again?
It is reasonable to allow one normal period; this is often heavy as it carries away any remaining debris from the womb. There is no need to wait three months as used to be advised.

Does physical activity lead to miscarriage?
There is no evidence that ordinary sport, sex or stress affect the overall chances of miscarriage at all. Women who have recently had a miscarriage would be sensible to avoid excessive physical activity during the first 12 weeks of their next pregnancy.

       Complementary Treatment
Complementary therapies cannot halt a miscarriage once it has begun, but they can help while you are recuperating. **Chakra balancing** and **healing** can help you through both emotional and physical pain and can also help with reactions such as insomnia, tension, guilt and anxiety. **Hypnotherapy** can be used to lessen anxiety in future pregnancies. **Ayurveda** can offer help in preparing your body for the next pregnancy, as can **acupuncture** and **Chinese herbalism**.

BREAST PROBLEMS

Pain, skin changes and discharge from the breasts – problems for which there are many innocent reasons.

CAUSES

The desirability of large or small breasts varies with all the fickleness of fashion. Very large breasts can cause back and neck pain. Many women suffer breast pain during the second half of the menstrual cycle, when the breasts enlarge under the influence of hormones. This is usually just a mild inconvenience, although some women actually suffer severe pain for two to three weeks every month.

Localized pain

The breasts are easily bruised so localized pain often follows an overlooked injury. It is less likely that pain is due to disease but a new or persistent pain should be assessed. There is absolutely no evidence that breast injuries lead to cancer.

Sore skin or discharging nipples

The skin of the nipples is subject to any of the afflictions of skin suffered elsewhere, for example **eczema** or infection. A sweat rash under the breasts is extremely common, especially if they are full. It is sensible to have these diagnoses confirmed by a doctor the first time they happen.

An abnormal secretion of prolactin (the hormone that stimulates the breasts to produce milk) from a (benign) growth in the pituitary gland may result in a milky discharge. A green or yellow discharge is usually harmless and comes from glands within the breast.

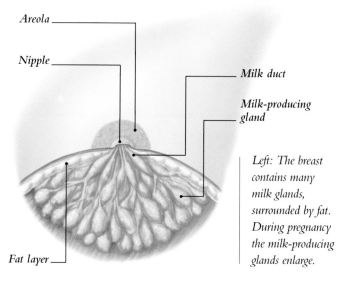

Areola
Nipple
Milk duct
Milk-producing gland
Fat layer

Left: The breast contains many milk glands, surrounded by fat. During pregnancy the milk-producing glands enlarge.

SYMPTOMS

Pain that is definitely cyclical is usually benign, especially if associated with firm glandular tissue within the breast. Pain localized to one portion of the breast is potentially more serious and should be brought to medical attention. The common sweat rash under the breasts is sore, red and itchy.

Any persistent discharges call for a careful medical assessment, possibly including measurement of prolactin in the blood. Bleeding from a nipple is a very important symptom that should always be investigated as it may be the first symptom of cancer within a duct of the nipple. The general rule is to seek medical advice if you notice any unusual change in your breasts, be it a lump, discharge, tenderness of the breast or of the nipples, or an altered appearance such as dimpling.

TREATMENT

A well-fitting and supportive bra helps mild cyclical pain and reduces discomfort caused by very large breasts. Breast reduction surgery might be a sensible option for extreme cases.

Oil of evening primrose is a therapy for cyclical breast pain; it has to be taken continuously for three months for full effect. Of course if there is anything unusual to feel in the breast you may require mammography or biopsy of a suspicious area (see page 321). Danazol and bromocriptine are drugs for severe breast pain, but have many side effects (see PMS).

Many skin problems respond to a mild steroid cream such as hydrocortisone, often combined with an antibiotic cream and antifungal agent.

Persistent pain and especially a bloody discharge need full assessment by a breast specialist. The treatment for abnormal prolactin depends on the cause.

See also BREAST CANCER.

Complementary Treatment

Chinese herbalism and **acupuncture** have much to offer – consult a reputable practitioner in Chinese medicine. **Homeopathy** – arnica cream is useful if breasts are bruised following an injury, calendula cream is useful for general soreness. **Nutritional therapy** – coffee, tea and chocolate have all been linked with increased risk of breast lumps and cysts. **Yoga** promotes relaxation and enhances confidence. **Ayurveda** offers detoxification and *marma* therapy. *Other therapies to try: naturopathy; chakra balancing.*

BREAST CANCER

The most common cancer among women, affecting about one in fourteen women. With treatment, about 50% of patients survive 10 years or more.

CAUSES

Cancer happens when cells grow independently of the body's control. A breast remains a breast because all the millions of cells that make it – skin, blood vessels, muscles – continue to do their jobs as skin cells, muscle cells and so on, maturing and dying as determined by their position in the breast. Cancer begins when a cell breaks free of that control and duplicates itself endlessly. What the trigger for this escape may be is the main concern in cancer studies. In breast cancer a number of factors increase the risk of that happening.

Heredity
Women with a mother or sister with breast cancer are two or three times more likely to get it themselves, having a one-in-five risk. However, there is no single gene that causes cancer. Rather it appears that inheriting a number of genes that control cell growth determines the risk in any one individual. These genes are called either oncogenes or tumour suppressor genes. A woman may inherit such defective genes or they may be mutated by radiation. Women with a family history of breast cancer should be medically examined annually.

Hormones
Being born female is the greatest risk for breast cancer. Men do get it but very rarely. Female hormones are involved in most, though not all, cases and the longer women are exposed to their female hormones, the greater their risk. Thus breast cancer is rare below the age of 30 and becomes more common upward of 40. Women are at greater risk the earlier their periods began, or if they have few or no children, or if they have a late **menopause**. These factors all increase the length of time their breasts are exposed to oestrogen.

Hormone replacement therapy (HRT) slightly increases the risk of breast cancer. This has to be weighed against the protective effects of HRT on heart disease and **osteoporosis**. The risks from the Pill are debatable: it possibly increases the risk slightly in women who start it in their teens.

Environment
The incidence varies greatly from country to country. The United Kingdom and United States have some of the highest rates whereas, for unknown reasons, it is uncommon in Japan.

SYMPTOMS

Most cancers are diagnosed after finding a lump in the breast. It is a good idea to examine your breasts regularly – the best time is midway between periods. There is no set time interval; just be aware of your breasts in order to detect early changes.

Bear in mind that breast lumps are common and only about one in ten proves to be cancerous, even fewer in women under thirty. The normal glandular tissues of the breast feel firm and slightly irregular but in a continuous sheet through the breast, whereas a lump feels firm but separate from the rest of the breast tissue. Most breast lumps are benign overgrowths of the normal milk-secreting glandular tissue of the breast. Cysts, fluid-filled lumps, are also common. Breast pain is usually innocuous, but it is suspicious to have pain over a breast lump.

FEATURES OF A POSSIBLY CANCEROUS LUMP

- *Hard and irregular as opposed to smooth*
- *Feeling tethered to one place as opposed to mobile*
- *Associated with inversion of a previously normal nipple*
- *With puckered skin over it*
- *Associated with bleeding from the nipple*

Discharge from the nipple
This always needs to be medically examined. Bleeding from a nipple has to be regarded as coming from breast cancer until proven otherwise, and is not to be ignored. Green or yellow discharges, however, are usually benign.

Further investigation
Mammography is a specialized X-ray of the breast which distinguishes between benign and cancerous lumps. In the United Kingdom this is offered every three years to women between the ages of 50 and 65, which is the time of greatest risk. The benefit from breast screening is controversial and not all authorities agree that it makes a difference to survival rates as opposed to early detection rates.

A biopsy can be taken through a special needle as an outpatient procedure (see page 321) and allows the direct microscopic analysis of a suspicious area of tissue. Sometimes the only way of being sure is to remove the lump under anaesthetic for full analysis.

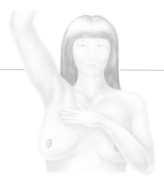

1 *Check each breast for lumps, differences in skin texture and changes around the nipple. Feel right into each armpit.*

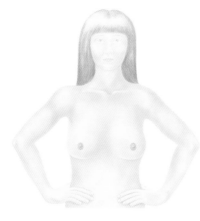

2 *Repeat the checks in several positions – lying, sitting and with different arm postures.*

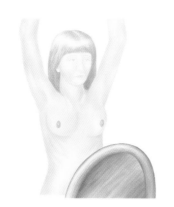

3 *Standing in front of a mirror helps you to become familiar with the usual appearance of your breasts.*

Above: It is important to learn how to examine your breasts yourself.

TREATMENT
◆

The aims are to remove the cancer itself and to detect and treat any spread (metastases or secondaries) to bones, liver and the brain. In planning treatment it is essential to know if and where there are metastases. Examination of the liver and armpits is the first step but only detects large secondaries. To detect small secondaries without symptoms it requires a bone scan and a CT scan of the liver, lungs and brain.

In the case of localized disease, the cancerous lump plus any glands within the armpit that may be involved are removed. After the wound has healed a course of radiotherapy (see page 338) is given to the armpit and breast in order to kill any remaining cancerous cells.

Hormone therapy
Hormone therapy is used if the disease has spread. Commonly used is tamoxifen, which is an anti-oestrogen. A similar effect is achieved by removing the ovaries, which immediately decreases the amount of oestrogen in the body. There are additional drugs if the woman is post-menopausal, for example anastrazole. Tumours vary in their responsiveness to oestrogen; this is discovered by analysing the tumour and helps predict how likely it is to respond to hormonal treatment. Tamoxifen is widely used even for localized disease and may be taken for several years.

Chemotherapy
Formerly reserved for women whose disease recurred after initial surgery, strong evidence now points to the value of giving chemotherapy (see page 339) at the same time as the initial surgery. American results suggest that this improves survival by about 25%. The drugs are given by tablet or injection every week or two – commonly methotrexate, cyclophosphamide and 5-fluorouracil. In addition, steroid drugs shrink secondaries and reduce the effects in, for example, the brain.

Prevention
There are a few women whose family history of breast cancer is so poor that their chances of getting cancer are extremely high. After suitable counselling these women may opt to have both breasts removed. Although this sounds extreme, the logic behind it is scientifically sound and understandable.

Complementary Treatment

No woman should spurn conventional assessment or approaches of her condition. However, many complementary therapies have a role during treatment. Check that your chosen practitioner is experienced in treating breast cancer. **Chakra balancing** helps with symptom control and energy balance, aids relaxation during orthodox treatment and offers support during rehabilitation programmes. **Massage** can help promote self-esteem and a positive body image, especially after surgery. **Aromatherapy** massage with scented oils can reduce stress and tension associated with this disease. **Reflexology** can offer support during orthodox treatment. Diet is extremely important and a **nutritional therapist** or **naturopath** would tailor a diet to suit your particular needs and circumstances – any diet is likely to feature plenty of wholefoods and fresh fruit and vegetables. *Other therapies to try: see STRESS.*

CERVICAL CANCER

◆

Cancer of the neck of the womb, which is treatable and often curable if detected early enough.

CAUSES

◆

Since the cervix projects into the vagina, the cells of the cervix are exposed to any infection within the vagina and to sperm; both may be involved in causing cervical cancer. The cancer is slow growing and alters the microscopic appearance of the cells of the cervix in its early stages. This is why the cervical smear screening programme is valuable. Untreated cancer spreads through the cervix and eventually invades the surrounding tissues. The disease is more common in smokers, although it is not known why.

Viruses and sexual activity

The human papilloma virus can be detected in the cervix in many cases of cancer. The same virus causes genital warts and can therefore be sexually transmitted. Cervical cancer is less common in women whose partners use condoms, supporting the notion of a viral cause. However the virus is also commonly found in women (and men) who are perfectly well.

Evidence suggests that the women at greater risk of cervical cancer are those who began sexual activity early and who have had many partners. This further supports the theory that a sexually transmitted agent contributes to the condition.

SYMPTOMS

◆

Early cervical cancer does not cause any symptoms at all. Symptoms only appear once the cancer is fairly well established, causing a raw area on the cervix. Possible symptoms then include a heavier-than-usual vaginal discharge, intermenstrual bleeding and bleeding after intercourse (from rubbing of the cervix). Pain is not a feature of the condition unless the cancer has spread into surrounding tissue. There are, however, many innocent causes of these same symptoms.

Cervical smears

Scraping the cervix with a spatula painlessly gathers cells for microscopic examination, so as to detect any early changes. The spatula is usually a wooden stick specially shaped to allow it to pass into the cervix; the scrapings are transferred on to a glass slide. Smears are graded on the appearance of the cells from normal, through possible early malignancy to frank cancer. Sexually active women should have regular smears, normally every three years, until the age of 65.

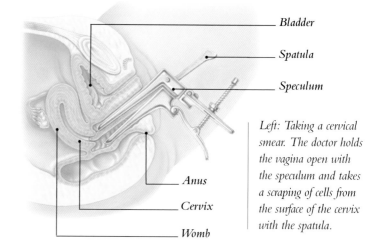

Bladder

Spatula

Speculum

Anus

Cervix

Womb

Left: Taking a cervical smear. The doctor holds the vagina open with the speculum and takes a scraping of cells from the surface of the cervix with the spatula.

TREATMENT

◆

Suspicion that areas of the cervix contain pre-cancerous cells can be confirmed using a colposcope, an instrument that gives a magnified view of the cervix. The surgeon looks through this while applying acetic acid to the cervix; abnormal areas turn white and biopsies are taken for more detailed analysis. Pre-malignant or early cancer cells are destroyed by laser beam or by cauterizing or by freezing (cryotherapy). These modern techniques can be used to perform a cone biopsy, whereby if problem areas are numerous, a whole cylinder of abnormal cells can be cut out, without causing any significant damage or affecting future fertility. More advanced disease is treated by removal of the cervix in a **hysterectomy**, followed by radiotherapy (see page 338) to the pelvis.

In theory, regular cervical screening should make cancer of the cervix an avoidable disease. Treatment of early disease virtually guarantees cure. Of the women who have advanced disease (i.e. invasive) at least 80% will survive 5 years.

Complementary Treatment

Keep up regular screening. If cancer is diagnosed, do not spurn conventional approaches – complementary therapies cannot cure cancer. However, many therapies have a role during treatment. **Chakra balancing** can help with symptom control and energy balance, and aid relaxation during orthodox treatment. **Reflexology** can offer support during orthodox treatment. **Aromatherapy** reduces stress and tension associated with this disease, especially when linked with **massage**. *Other therapies to try: see* STRESS.

CANCER OF THE WOMB

Uterine cancer accounts for about 3000 deaths per annum in the United Kingdom, making it the second most common cancer in women after breast cancer.

CAUSES

The cancer arises in the cells in the lining of the womb, the endometrium. These are influenced by the hormones oestrogen and progestogen, which regulate the menstrual cycle. It appears to be this regular pattern of hormonal stimulation that predisposes to malignancy. Growing slowly, the cancer eventually spreads through the womb (uterus) to surrounding pelvic tissues and finally to the lungs, liver and bones.

Some women are at greater risk of cancer of the womb than others by virtue of an increased lifetime exposure to oestrogen. This means women who began their periods at an early age, who have a late **menopause** or who have no children. The risk is also higher in those women who are overweight because fat tissues produce oestrogen.

Early types of hormone replacement therapy (HRT), when it was given as oestrogen alone, caused an increased risk. Now, in the United Kingdom, women with a womb have HRT containing progesterone for ten to twelve days each month which is sufficient protection.

SYMPTOMS

The alerting symptom of womb cancer is unusual vaginal bleeding, especially after the menopause. In fact any vaginal bleeding after the menopause is suspicious, even if the bleeding is occasional or just enough to cause a blood-tinged vaginal discharge. This does not mean that all post-menopausal bleeding is from cancer. Far from it; mostly it is caused by innocent post-menopausal thinning of the walls of the vagina or by benign changes within the womb.

Cancer of the womb is less common before the menopause (25% of cases) and less likely to be suspected. This is because the symptoms – irregular bleeding or heavier-than-usual bleeding – are common from the late 30s onward anyway. The best advice is to take account of any uncharacteristic and persistent change in your menstrual pattern.

Pain is not a feature of this cancer unless it is advanced.

Diagnosis
The diagnosis is established by ultrasound scan of the womb (see page 317) to detect areas of unusual thickness in the walls. An essential further investigation is endometrial biopsy, which means sampling cells from the lining of the womb. This can be done as an outpatient procedure in the gynaecology clinic in contrast with the older dilation and curettage (D&C) (see PERIOD PROBLEMS), which required a general anaesthetic.

TREATMENT

In almost all cases the womb must be removed (a **hysterectomy**), together with the ovaries, because these produce oestrogen, which would encourage the spread of the cancer elsewhere. It is usual to have a course of radiotherapy to the pelvis (see page 338) to destroy any cells remaining within the pelvis and the lymph nodes. Because of its side effects, chemotherapy (see page 339) is reserved for those with advanced disease that has spread widely within the pelvis or elsewhere.

The chances of cure are excellent if the cancer of the womb is diagnosed early. At least 85 of every 100 women treated will survive 5 years or more.

QUESTIONS

Can womb cancer be screened for?
There are no blood tests currently available. Women taking HRT should have a regular pelvic examination to detect any enlargement of the womb. This can be combined with having a smear (see CERVICAL CANCER).

Is every change in menstrual pattern significant?
All women experience variations, especially as they get older, the vast majority of which are innocent in nature. Therefore minor month-to-month changes are not likely to be important. You should take notice of any persistent change that involves periods getting heavier or irregular. In the case of post-menopausal bleeding, you should report even the tiniest episode to your doctor.

Complementary Treatment
You should not spurn conventional approaches – complementary treatments cannot cure cancer. However, many therapies have a role during treatment. **Chakra balancing** will help with symptom control and energy balance, and aid relaxation during orthodox treatment. **Reflexology** can offer support during orthodox treatment. **Aromatherapy** is excellent at reducing the stress and tension associated with disease. *Other therapies to try: see STRESS.*

OVARIAN CANCER

Malignant growths of the ovary are among the most common cancers in women.

CAUSES

Cancer of the ovary is a particularly complex subject, because there are many different types of growth, each with its own natural history, progression, response to therapy and outlook.

The ovary produces a number of cysts every month, each containing an egg. It is therefore not surprising that many cancers begin as cysts: fluid-filled growths that can reach a large size before causing any problems. The diagnosis is complicated because ovarian cysts are common and what appears to be a benign cyst may become malignant over time.

As with **breast cancer** and **cancer of the womb**, ovarian cancer seems stimulated by the female hormone oestrogen and so the women at higher risk are those who have been longest exposed to oestrogen: those who began to have periods early, experience a late **menopause** and have few or no children. Having a close relative with the condition increases the risk several times over.

Taking the contraceptive Pill reduces the incidence of ovarian cancer by about 40% – a much under-publicized benefit of this contraceptive. Ovarian cancer is mainly a disease of women who are in their 50s upwards, but cases of the cancer in younger women or even children are not rare.

SYMPTOMS

Unfortunately, ovarian growths may reach a considerable size without causing any suspicious symptoms. Even with a growth several centimetres in diameter there may be no features. In cases where symptoms are present they manifest as lower abdominal swelling, discomfort and urinary frequency, caused by pressure on the bladder. Periods may or may not be affected. Advanced tumours lead to swelling of the legs and gross abdominal swelling.

It is possible to feel the ovary on a vaginal examination, but it is not possible to tell by examination alone whether or not an enlarged ovary is malignant or caused by an innocent cyst.

TREATMENT

An ultrasound scan of the ovaries (see page 317) is a useful aid for confirming an ovarian swelling but this diagnostic tool alone cannot tell if the swelling is malignant or benign. For this, laparoscopic surgery is required (see page 340) so

that the swelling can be inspected by the gynaecologist.

Once diagnosis is certain, treatment is always removal of the affected ovary and often of the womb as well, if it looks as if the tumour has spread. After this, it is usual to direct radiotherapy at the pelvis. Chemotherapy is used to try to eradicate any remaining cells and any that may have spread (metastasized) elsewhere in the body. (See pages 338 and 339.)

Very recently, the drug taxol, from the bark of the Western yew, has offered new hope in treating the condition.

Some ovarian cancers produce a biochemical marker in the blood stream called Ca 125, which can be used to measure response to treatment and is an early indication of recurrence.

QUESTIONS

How curable is the condition?
This depends very much on the exact type of tumour, varying from a 95% 5-year survival to just 10%. In general ovarian cancer carries a poor prognosis because it tends not to be diagnosed until the cancer is well established.

Is there any screening test?
The only recognized test is to have a pelvic examination of your ovaries every year. This should also be done whenever you have a cervical smear test. With the discovery of Ca 125 it was thought that this could be extended to general screening of the population but so far the scientific evidence warranting general screening of women is lacking.

How serious are ovarian cysts?
Small cysts are more common than once thought. In young women they are nearly always benign. A gynaecologist will perform a laparoscopy if in doubt or if cysts are detected in older women.

Complementary Treatment

No complementary therapy can cure ovarian cancer. However, many have a role during conventional treatment. **Chakra balancing** will help with symptom control and energy balance, and aid relaxation during orthodox treatment. **Reflexology** offers support during orthodox treatment. **Aromatherapy** is excellent for reducing stress and tension, especially when combined with **massage**. There are **homeopathic** treatments for benign ovarian cysts, if the diagnosis is certain. *Other therapies to try: see* STRESS.

PREMENSTRUAL SYNDROME (PMS)

◆

Various symptoms as a consequence of the effects of hormone changes during the menstrual cycle.

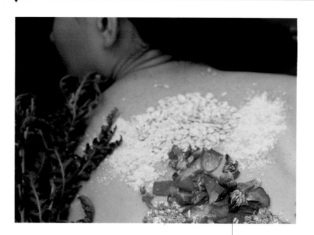

Above: Many women with PMS find that herbal remedies are helpful. It may be worth trying them for yourself.

CAUSES

◆

While it seems self-evident that it is the cycle of hormones that causes PMS, it has proved difficult to pinpoint just what is responsible for what. Most women experience tension and irritability during the second half of their menstrual cycle, which coincides with rising levels of oestrogen and progesterone. If fertilization does not happen the levels of these hormones fall until menstruation occurs. Numerous studies have tried to relate concentrations of hormones to symptoms but without reaching generally accepted conclusions. Such evidence as is agreed increasingly suggests that the level of oestrogen is more important than those of other hormones.

In addition, women vary as to how well they tolerate these changes; it may be that swings in mood that would normally be coped with become intolerable for women who have other stresses in their life such as children, marital or money problems. Surveys show that women aged in their 30s and 40s are most affected by PMS.

SYMPTOMS

◆

To make the diagnosis it is essential to show that symptoms fluctuate in a regular cycle. Certain symptoms are especially frequent: feeling bloated, depressed, irritable and anxious and getting headaches. Cravings for sweet things is common.

These symptoms should begin from mid-cycle onward, reach a maximum just before menstruation and disappear within a couple of days of the onset of menstruation. The severity of symptoms often varies from cycle to cycle.

Despite PMS being a probably universal experience for women, most cope well. An estimated ten per cent suffer more severely; for perhaps one to three per cent of women PMS is a major problem each month, disrupting relationships and family and work responsibilities.

TREATMENT

◆

The treatment for PMS is as controversial as the explanations offered. Women must be prepared to try a variety of treatments to find one that works well for them.

One scientifically validated treatment is vitamin B$_6$, essential for enzymes that form the neurotransmitters serotonin and dopamine, important in depression. There is no agreed reason why women should become cyclically deficient in B$_6$ but many women do benefit from taking a small dose.

Diuretics reduce fluid retention, relieving bloating and breast tenderness, but should be taken for only a few days each time. Danazol is a drug that suppresses oestrogen and progestogens. It is an effective treatment for some women but its side effects such as nausea and weight gain make it unacceptable for many. The same goes for bromocriptine, which is good for breast tenderness but causes nausea.

Oil of evening primrose is a rich source of gamma linoleic acid. This theoretically reduces prolactin levels, which some researchers believe are a cause of the breast tenderness and mood changes. Oestrogen in tablet form helps some women.

Tranquillizers or antidepressants are not recommended for PMS except for those few women who experience overwhelmingly bad symptoms at very specific times. Otherwise the drawbacks and side effects outweigh their value.

Complementary Treatment

Western herbalism can encourage hormone regulation before periods and help with specific symptoms. In **Chinese herbalism** a useful remedy is *Xiao Yao Wan* (free-and-easy wonder formula). **Bach flower remedies** – mustard for depression for no reason, cherry plum for loss of control, beech for intolerance, impatiens for impatience and irritability, and willow for self-pity. Useful **aromatherapy** oils include chamomile, geranium, rose, bergamot and clary sage. *Other therapies to try: most therapies have something to offer.*

PERIOD PROBLEMS

◆

Upset of the delicately balanced menstrual cycle – caused by emotion, dieting, medication or hormonal fluctuations.

BACKGROUND

◆

During the menstrual cycle changing concentrations of hormones prepare the ovaries and womb for pregnancy. This cycle reaches a peak on average 14 days after the first day of the previous period. Up to this stage the ovaries are stimulated by follicle-stimulating hormone (FSH), a hormone which comes from the hypothalamus, and which makes a few eggs mature. A pituitary hormone, luteinizing hormone (LH), then induces the release of one egg.

Meanwhile, the maturing eggs themselves release oestrogen, which makes blood vessels grow within the lining of the womb, ready to supply nutrients to a fertilized egg. The ovary also begins secreting progesterone, the hormone of pregnancy, which further prepares the womb to receive an egg.

By mid-cycle the woman's body is in an optimal state for successful fertilization. If this fails to occur concentrations of progesterone and oestrogen fall; the rich blood supply of the lining of the womb degenerates to a point where the lining dies and is shed as the menstrual flow. This, as it were, wipes the lining clean ready for the next cycle.

It is only by convention that 28 days is considered the 'normal' length of a cycle. It is perfectly normal to have a cycle of 21 days or of 35 or more days.

TYPES OF PROBLEMS

◆

Periods may be absent or infrequent, or prolonged. They may be scanty or heavy, painless or painful. Many period problems are the result of fluctuations of the interplay of hormones, so hormones play a useful role in dealing with them.

Absent or infrequent periods

Causes: When periods first begin and towards the **menopause**, the ovaries often fail to produce an egg. The resulting lack of oestrogen and progesterone makes for menstrual irregularities – and often for heavy periods, too.

Absent or scanty periods are also common for several months after stopping the contraceptive Pill. Alternatively, periods may be made irregular by emotional problems, dieting (in anorexia nervosa they stop altogether) or heavy athletic training. Much less likely is the failure of hormone production by the pituitary gland. Another possibility, and more common than once thought, are polycystic ovaries –

causing an excess secretion of male hormones, suggested by a combination of absent periods, hairiness, acne and obesity.

Pregnancy always has to be borne in mind, too. In women past the age of 30 with previously regular periods, the abrupt cessation of periods could be due to an early menopause.

Symptoms: These can range from total lack of periods to infrequent scanty periods, which may or may not be painful.

Treatment: A girl who has reached 16 and not begun menstruation should have a full gynaecological assessment, looking for hypothalamic failure, hormone disorders and abnormal anatomical or genetic make-up. Otherwise, if infrequent periods are not a source of worry treatment is not essential.

Infrequent periods can leave a niggling doubt about pregnancy, allayed only by pregnancy tests. If treatment is desired, the contraceptive Pill will give a regular cycle.

Older women with a previously regular cycle should have a full hormonal assessment looking especially for premature menopause and hyperprolactinaemia, the abnormal secretion of prolactin from the pituitary gland. During pregnancy prolactin stimulates the breasts to make milk but can be secreted at other times by disease of the pituitary gland. Treatment is with bromocriptine, which blocks production, or removal of a pituitary tumour by surgery or radiotherapy.

Treatment for polycystic ovaries includes the Pill, steroids or clomiphene to stimulate egg production and improve fertility.

Heavy or painful periods

Causes: Painful periods are common in the first few years of menstruation. If occurring later the combination suggests **fibroids**, **pelvic inflammatory disease** or **endometriosis**. The contraceptive coil causes heavier periods, too. A rarer reason is **cancer of the womb**, a possibility in women over 40 with significant changes in their menstrual pattern.

Symptoms: What is a heavy period for one woman is considered normal by another. The average blood loss of the whole period is 30–80 ml. Symptoms that are suggestive of truly heavy periods are becoming anaemic, flooding or clots, or high use of tampons or sanitary towels. Pain on intercourse plus heavy, painful periods suggests disease of the womb as opposed to benign hormone disorders.

Treatment: Assuming other disease is excluded, the treatment is with hormones. The contraceptive Pill gives a regular moderate period. Progestogen tablets, such as norethisterone or dydrogesterone, are helpful taken for several days each month. Effective non-hormone treatments include mefenamic acid and tranexamic acid, both of which reduce bleeding and pain if they are taken in the first few days of the period.

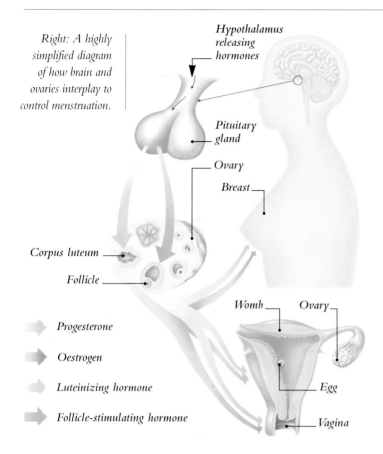

Right: A highly simplified diagram of how brain and ovaries interplay to control menstruation.

Hypothalamus releasing hormones

Pituitary gland

Ovary

Breast

Corpus luteum

Follicle

Womb

Ovary

Egg

Vagina

Progesterone

Oestrogen

Luteinizing hormone

Follicle-stimulating hormone

At one time a D&C was both routine investigation and treatment in older women; this is a scraping (curettage) of the womb via the widened (dilated) cervix and was used to exclude cancer of the womb. The operation is becoming obsolete thanks to smaller sampling syringes, which give just as reliable results but do not require a general anaesthetic.

If these strategies fail, a recent option is ablation (destruction) of the lining of the womb using a laser or similar heat source (see page 333). Although this is a safe and effective treatment, symptoms tend to recur after a year or so.

Finally, there is **hysterectomy** – removal of the womb. Many gynaecologists favour this, since it removes a possible site of future cancer. In younger women the ovaries are kept, to avoid an abrupt, early menopause.

Irregular periods

This refers to bleeding without any regular pattern.

Causes: Most cases are due to fluctuations of hormones. This is common in women who are approaching the menopause or who are in the first few years after starting to menstruate, and it is unlikely to be serious.

It is important to distinguish irregular, which means unpredictable, from intermenstrual bleeding. The latter means bleeding in between an otherwise normal menstrual cycle; it may be spotting mid-cycle or bleeding after intercourse. Intermenstrual bleeding is important since it may be caused by erosion on the cervix, **cervical cancer**, polyps in the womb or cancer of the womb.

Bleeding after the menopause is never ever 'normal' and it is essential to have investigation for even the slightest blood loss, to exclude cancer of the womb.

Symptoms: The menstrual cycle may be completely irregular, or there may be a relatively regular cycle with additional episodes of blood loss mid-cycle, i.e. intermenstrual bleeding.

Treatment: In younger women, as long as health and a physical examination are normal, it is not necessary to treat irregular periods other than to provide the convenience of having a predictable cycle. This is achieved with the contraceptive Pill.

Innocent hormonal fluctuations are still the likeliest explanation for irregular periods in older women but it is advisable to have further investigation because disease of the cervix or the womb is more common than in younger women. This is all the more important if the bleeding is intermenstrual. The treatment for a cervical erosion, as for polyps, is cauterization (burning it away). A sample of the lining of the womb should be taken either by a D&C or by an outpatient procedure, to exclude cancer.

Complementary Treatment

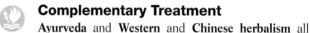

Ayurveda and **Western** and **Chinese herbalism** all offer preparations to reduce pain and spasm and regulate both the menstrual cycle and the severity of bleeding. In **acupuncture** an important point is Spleen 6, above the ankle, at the meeting point of three energy channels that all connect to the womb. In **auricular therapy** needling points on the ear is thought to influence the hormonal system, so this is of great value in treating period problems. **Chiropractic** treatment can provide relief, back pain being frequently associated with period problems. **Yoga** can cure period problems if practised regularly. **Healing** helps regulate the menstrual cycle and restore a balanced hormonal picture. **Hypnotherapy** visualization and suggestion therapy can help if the problems are linked to negative conditioning about periods. *Other therapies to try: homeopathy; tai chi/chi kung; shiatsu-do; nutritional therapy; naturopathy; chakra balancing.*

MENOPAUSE

The cessation of menstrual periods, which affects all women by the time they are in their mid-50s.

CAUSES

Most women menstruate from the menarche (the time of first menstruation) for the next 35–45 years. This is controlled by an elegant system of hormones in the hypothalamus and pituitary glands, which act on the ovaries and womb (see PERIOD PROBLEMS), becoming erratic as the 'biological clock' ticks on.

By the mid-40s, the number of immature eggs within the ovaries has diminished and those remaining are relatively unresponsive to the hormones that should bring them to maturity. As a consequence oestrogen levels fall, while levels of other hormones rise. Eventually menstruation ceases, which occurs on average when women are in the early 50s.

From this point the ovaries no longer produce eggs but they continue to secrete some oestrogen. Oestrogen is also formed within fatty tissue and the skin so that it does not completely disappear after the menopause but, except in the obese, it decreases to pre-pubertal levels.

It is not known why the menopause happens when it does, nor why some women experience an early menopause and others a late one. A fair guide to when to expect the menopause is the age your mother or sisters reached it. Menopause occurring in women in their 30s is premature. There is rarely any serious reason for this, although it may be distressing, meaning as it does the end of the woman's childbearing days.

Any woman who has to have her ovaries removed will experience an abnormally abrupt menopause with correspondingly severe symptoms. This might be required as treatment for **cancer of the womb**, **ovarian cancer**, **breast cancer**, **endometriosis** or **pelvic inflammatory disease**.

SYMPTOMS

By convention the menopause is taken to be definite when periods have finished for a year. Before then periods might occur just every couple of months until ceasing. Some women experience clear menopausal symptoms such as hot flushes while continuing to menstruate, presumably because of falling levels of oestrogen. Where there is doubt, blood tests can confirm that you are entering the menopause by measuring the levels of stimulating hormones which rise at the menopause.

The following symptoms last for two to five years. Although all women experience some symptoms, for only about one-third of women are they a serious inconvenience.

Hot flushes

There is a feeling of heat that sweeps across the body within seconds and is accompanied by sweating, especially at night. They are the result of instability of the circulatory system, which usually controls the dilation of blood vessels in response to emotions, changes of temperature and tension.

Physical changes

With the fall in oestrogen, the parts of the body sensitive to oestrogen return to a pre-pubertal state. The breasts diminish in size with reabsorption of fatty tissue, becoming thinner and shapeless. The walls of the vagina depend on oestrogen to remain thick and supple; after the menopause these become thin and drier. This leads to discomfort during intercourse and, not uncommonly, slight bleeding from the vagina's walls, which look dry and shiny, and also to recurrent cystitis.

Heart disease

Women are relatively protected from this before the menopause, perhaps because of a positive protective effect from oestrogen. It may also be that oestrogen shields against the harmful effects of women's natural male hormones (androgens) until the menopause, after which falling oestrogen levels remove this buffer. After the menopause the risk of heart disease for women rises rapidly to equal that of men.

Osteoporosis

After the menopause women lose bone mass, which becomes thin and lighter (see OSTEOPOROSIS). This process continues for decades after the menopause but the loss is especially rapid at the time of the menopause and for a couple of years afterwards. Accompanying the bone thinning it is common for post-menopausal women to notice a general stiffening of their joints and aches all over. This is partly the effect of ageing, but some of it is due to oestrogen deficiency.

Mood changes and psychological adjustment

Symptoms often recounted are irritability, emotional instability, worsening memory, **depression** and tiredness. It is hard to decide which of these are from hormonal changes as opposed to being coincidental effects from psychological adjustments.

TREATMENT

It is vital to bear in mind that the menopause is a natural and inevitable event. However inconvenient its symptoms and however distressing the psychological effects, it is not a med-

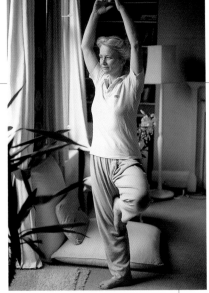

Below: HRT is popular as pills or patches, as well as implants or gels.

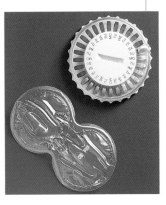

Above: Exercise, relaxation and a good diet are all important strategies for post-menopausal health.

ical abnormality. Indeed, many women welcome the end of menstruation. What is important is to reduce the impact of the most upsetting symptoms and to deal with those aspects of the menopause that may have long-term health implications – essentially osteoporosis and cardiovascular disease.

Hormone replacement therapy (HRT)

HRT reliably alleviates many of the most distressing symptoms of the menopause. The hormone being replaced is oestrogen and it can be supplied as a tablet, a pellet implanted into the lower abdomen, a patch worn on the hip or a gel rubbed into the arm. A woman who has had a **hysterectomy** can take just oestrogen daily (known as unopposed oestrogen). A woman who still has her womb has to take additional tablets containing progestogen for ten to twelve days each month; this is to counteract the effect of pure oestrogen on the womb, which otherwise increases the risk of womb cancer. The effect of the additional tablet is to cause a light menstrual bleed each month; there are some recent formulations that reduce the bleeding to just once every three months or not at all.

Advantages: It gives a sense of wellbeing, improves skin texture and reduces aches in the joints. Hot flushes are virtually abolished, it reduces vaginal dryness or soreness and often relieves **cystitis** due to drying of the urethra. It prevents osteoporosis and, combined with an appropriate diet, may actually reverse it. While on HRT women continue to enjoy the relative protection from heart disease they had before the menopause.

Drawbacks: Weight gain, breast tenderness and nausea are all common side effects in the first few months but usually disappear. HRT carries a slightly increased risk of thrombosis

(see DEEP VEIN THROMBOSIS and PULMONARY EMBOLISM). Evidence suggests that HRT slightly increases the risk of breast cancer the longer it is taken.

Conclusion: On balance, if HRT is taken for two to five years its benefits outweigh its disadvantages. Thereafter the balance is still overall in favour of HRT because its continuing protection against heart disease and osteoporosis outweigh the risks of breast cancer. However, the individual woman must consider the pros and cons herself. It is a personal decision that needs thorough discussion with her medical advisor, and the picture will change as more research is done.

Other treatments

Vaginal dryness alone can be treated with an oestrogen cream but this should not be used for more than a few years. Many women find a non-hormone lubricating gel is sufficient. (Regular sexual intercourse after the menopause reduces vaginal dryness without the need for hormones. As many women find their sexual interest is the same or greater after the menopause as those who lose interest.)

Hot flushes can be reduced by taking blood pressure medication (clonidine). Osteoporosis is delayed by giving up smoking, maintaining a high calcium and vitamin D intake and regular weight-bearing exercise.

See also WOMEN: THE MENOPAUSE AND AFTER, page 22.

Complementary Treatment

Chinese and **Western herbalism** both offer herbs to reduce the severity of a range of problems such as hot flushes and fatigue. **Chakra balancing** – often psychological balancing is needed here and this can definitely help. **Auricular therapy** – needling points on the ear is thought to influence the hormonal system, so it is of great value during menopause. For severe symptoms such as hot flushes, treatment should be daily initially, but the severity should lessen within days. **Aromatherapy** can help adjustment to change by balancing nerves and hormones; oils to try include chamomile, cypress, rose, geranium, fennel and juniper. **Nutritional therapy** – supplements of vitamins B, D and E often alleviate menopausal symptoms. Cut out coffee. **Yoga** can be useful. **Hypnotherapy** can help, especially cell regeneration therapy. **Ayurveda** offers detoxification, oral treatments, and yoga meditation. *Other treatments to try: tai chi/chi kung; acupuncture; homeopathy; healing; shiatsu-do; Bach flower remedies.*

PELVIC INFLAMMATORY DISEASE

Infection of the womb and ovaries, which can start and progress with minimal symptoms. Abbreviated to PID.

CAUSES

The female genital tract is especially liable to infection, because germs easily gain access from the outside. They ascend through the vagina into the womb, then to the Fallopian tubes and ovaries. They can then gain entry to the interior of the abdomen. Infections lead to scar tissue and bands of fibres which tether the womb or block the Fallopian tubes or ovaries, reducing their normal function and leading to chronic pain and **female subfertility**.

Sources of infection

Sexually transmitted diseases are the most important causes of infection and include gonorrhoea and chlamydia.

Following a **miscarriage** or a termination of pregnancy, not uncommonly fragments of the placenta remain in the womb. In the majority of cases these will be expelled with the next menstrual cycle, otherwise the dead tissue is a fertile breeding ground for bacteria. This is why it is recommended to have a D&C (see PERIOD PROBLEMS) after a miscarriage to clear the womb thoroughly.

The contraceptive coil carries a risk of pelvic inflammatory disease in women who have had PID before.

As with any part of the body with a rich blood supply, the womb and tubes can be subject to infection purely by chance, although this is a relatively uncommon cause of PID.

SYMPTOMS

The diagnosis of pelvic inflammatory disease is suggested by a combination of aching over the lower abdomen and an offensive yellow or green vaginal discharge. The woman may feel ill with fever and shivering. The diagnosis is straightforward with such symptoms but PID can follow a much less obvious course with just a transiently abnormal vaginal discharge and other symptoms emerging over several months. These are increasingly heavy and painful periods and pain on intercourse, felt deep inside.

One possible consequence of pelvic inflammatory disease is subfertility, because the ovaries cannot release their eggs properly or sperm cannot reach the egg because the Fallopian tubes are blocked. The disease may be first detected on investigation for subfertility, when special X-ray studies of the womb and Fallopian tubes reveal the blockages.

TREATMENT

The first step in treatment is to identify the infection responsible by taking a swab of vaginal secretions. This gives guidance as to the most appropriate antibiotics to use. These are then given in high dosages for at least ten days. Tests will also identify any sexually transmitted infection. Sometimes the infection is so severe that the woman needs intravenous antibiotic therapy in hospital.

The same approach is used if the disease is chronic. In addition, it may be possible to release the ovaries surgically from any fibrous bands or to reopen the Fallopian tubes in order to restore the woman's fertility. Where pain and discomfort on intercourse is persistent, **hysterectomy** may be the woman's only option.

QUESTIONS

Is the diagnosis of PID straightforward?
Given classic acute symptoms it should be easy. The diagnosis is more difficult if there is just slight abdominal discomfort and a mildly abnormal discharge. In such cases the diagnosis should be confirmed by a laparoscopy, which means looking inside the pelvis to see if the internal organs are inflamed.

Is PID invariably due to sexually transmitted disease?
There is a great deal of overlap between pelvic inflammatory disease and sexually transmitted disease (see page 164) but it would be wrong to regard them as identical since PID can arise simply through chance.

What are the risks of subfertility?
There should be no problem with promptly and vigorously treated acute pelvic inflammatory disease. The risks increase with more chronic or repeated episodes of PID.

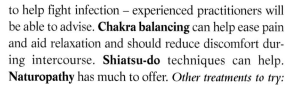

Complementary Treatment

If PID is diagnosed, antibiotics should not be shunned. **Chinese** and **Western herbalism** can both offer herbs to help fight infection – experienced practitioners will be able to advise. **Chakra balancing** can help ease pain and aid relaxation and should reduce discomfort during intercourse. **Shiatsu-do** techniques can help. **Naturopathy** has much to offer. *Other treatments to try: homeopathy; aromatherapy; Bach flower remedies.*

ENDOMETRIOSIS

◆

Deposits of cells from the womb that seed within the pelvic organs and elsewhere, causing pain and subfertility.

CAUSES

◆

Endometriosis is being increasingly recognized. The lining of the womb, the endometrium, consists of cells sensitive to oestrogen and progesterone, which regulate the menstrual cycle. Towards the end of the cycle these cells degenerate and bleed, forming the menstrual flow. For unknown reasons, these same endometrial cells can lodge elsewhere in the body and still go through a menstrual cycle, including bleeding.

There are many theories to account for this. One theory is that some cells escape during menstruation and, instead of leaving in the menstrual flow, ascend the Fallopian tubes into the pelvis. There they lodge on the ovaries, the outside of the womb or the intestines. The collections of cells are often very small, but endometriosis can spread across the pelvic organs, forming large cysts.

SYMPTOMS

◆

Minor endometriosis is quite common and asymptomatic. If the deposits are large they give rise to pain at the time of menstruation, because the blood they produce accumulates as a painful cyst. In more extensive disease, there is the formation of scar tissue which binds the womb and ovaries in a way similar to **pelvic inflammatory disease**. There is pain felt deep inside on intercourse, and periods become painful and heavier. There is a risk of **female subfertility** through blockage of the Fallopian tubes by scar tissue.

Deposits can be felt on internal examination but more often the diagnosis is established by laparoscopy, which gives a full idea of the extent of the condition.

Although most cysts lodge within the pelvis, endometrial deposits can turn up anywhere in the body; they have been known to cause such bizarre symptoms as a belly button that bleeds in exact sequence with the menstrual cycle.

TREATMENT

◆

Until recently, there was no treatment to reverse the condition and the woman could be offered only **hysterectomy** and removal of the Fallopian tubes to relieve pain. Now hormone treatment is available with drugs that block oestrogen. The first was danazol, taken by mouth but with many side effects. There are now injectable drugs with fewer side effects such as

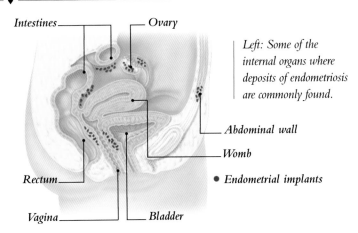

Left: Some of the internal organs where deposits of endometriosis are commonly found.

Intestines — Ovary
Abdominal wall
Womb
Rectum
Vagina — Bladder
● *Endometrial implants*

goserelin, which shrink the endometrial deposits so they no longer cause symptoms. In addition, large deposits can be destroyed by laser under laparoscopy. It may be possible to reopen blocked Fallopian tubes, with improvement in fertility.

QUESTIONS

How common is endometriosis?
Up to 20% of women who need a laparoscopy because of gynaecological symptoms prove to have endometriosis. It is the cause of subfertility in about 10–15% of subfertile women.

How serious is it?
Often an unexpected, incidental finding, it is not dangerous in itself but is important because of the pain and subfertility it may cause. Treatment is not necessary if it is not causing symptoms.

Is endometriosis becoming more common?
Endometriosis used to be diagnosed by the combination of symptoms plus feeling cysts on internal examination. The increased use of laparoscopy is revealing how common endometrial cysts are that are too small to be felt on internal examination alone.

Complementary Treatment

Traditional Chinese medicine (**herbs, acupuncture and tai chi/chi kung**) can have a good effect, especially in lessening pain. **Homeopathy** can help but treatment depends on what brings on the pain, how it presents, what makes it better or worse, and so on. **Chakra balancing** helps ease pain, aids relaxation and reduces discomfort during intercourse. **Hypnotherapy** can be used in pain control, and to lessen anxiety.

FIBROIDS

Benign overgrowth of muscle in the womb that can reach an enormous size.

CAUSES

The walls of the womb are mostly composed of tough muscle, which enlarges during pregnancy. It is this muscle that gives rise to minor contractions during pregnancy and eventually expels the baby during labour. A fibroid begins when a number of muscle cells start to expand and grow into a tumour within surrounding healthy muscle. This is not a cancerous process; the tumour is entirely benign. Fibroids grow very slowly and can reach the size of a small melon before causing any symptoms. Untreated they can continue to grow up to 20 kg/44 lb in weight. It is common to have several fibroids in the womb of varying sizes; the larger they are the more they distort the shape of the womb and the more they project into the cavity of the womb, giving rise to symptoms.

Just what sets off the process is unknown, but fibroids are more common in women who have had no children or who have delayed having children until after 30 (which remarkably now includes the majority of women in the United Kingdom). This suggests that prolonged exposure to oestrogen has something to do with it, in support of which is the fact that fibroids tend to shrink after the **menopause**, when oestrogen levels diminish. Nor are they that rare: about 20% of women will have them.

SYMPTOMS

Small fibroids do not cause any symptoms and are a chance finding on gynaecological examination or on a scan of the womb. If larger, the most common symptoms are heavy and irregular periods (see PERIOD PROBLEMS). Pain is not a feature of fibroids except in the uncommon instances of the fibroid degenerating through outgrowing its blood supply. The largest fibroids will cause abdominal swelling and put pressure on the bladder leading to a constant desire to pass urine.

There is no agreement as to whether fibroids can affect fertility. A large fibroid might prevent implantation, affect the growth of the baby or prevent normal delivery.

TREATMENT

Treatment is only needed if fibroids are causing symptoms or if they might interfere with a future pregnancy. It is difficult but possible to cut out each individual fibroid in an operation

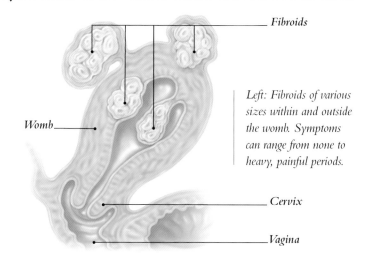

Fibroids

Womb

Cervix

Vagina

Left: Fibroids of various sizes within and outside the womb. Symptoms can range from none to heavy, painful periods.

called myomectomy. Many fibroids can be removed at the one operation. Myomectomy is suitable for women who contemplate a future pregnancy or who do not want a **hysterectomy**.

Many women do opt for a hysterectomy, to avoid the ten to fifteen per cent chance of fibroids regrowing.

It may be possible in the future to make fibroids shrink using the same drugs used in **endometriosis**, for example goserelin, which reduce oestrogen levels.

QUESTIONS

Can the diagnosis be made on examination only?
There is a typical feel to most fibroids that allows gynaecologists to be confident about the diagnosis simply on internal examination. If in doubt they can order an ultrasound scan of the womb or, if there is pain, perform a laparoscopy.

Do fibroids cause pain on intercourse?
This is not a recognized symptom of fibroids; if you are experiencing this, other diagnoses such as endometriosis or pelvic inflammatory disease must be considered.

Complementary Treatment

Chinese medicine (**herbs**, **acupuncture** and **tai chi/chi kung**) – an experienced practitioner might be able to reduce the size of small fibroids, otherwise it would still be possible to reduce bleeding. **Cymatics** can help by focusing corrective sound waves at your womb. **Hypnotherapy**, especially visualization techniques, can be effective – consult an experienced therapist.

HYSTERECTOMY

An operation to remove the womb – necessary for various reasons and one of the most commonly performed operations on women.

CAUSES

Hysterectomy is almost always a planned operation; there are few situations that call for an emergency hysterectomy. The operation is performed when there is a problem within the womb which cannot be isolated. Probably the most frequent reason is persistent heavy periods, resistant to medical treatment or to radio-frequency ablation – a procedure to burn the lining of the womb (see PERIOD PROBLEMS). The next most common reason is probably large **fibroids**, where again the periods are heavy.

Women are prone to urinary **incontinence** due to anatomical drooping of the outlet from the bladder. Although operations to correct this do not necessarily require a hysterectomy, it often makes technical sense to do this at the same time.

Cancer of the womb of course requires hysterectomy, as does **cervical cancer** if it is invading tissues outside the cervix itself. **Endometriosis** and **pelvic inflammatory disease** are conditions in which the womb becomes chronically inflamed or tethered and it is sometimes best to remove it.

A pre-menopausal woman considering hysterectomy must be convinced that it is the necessary treatment for her, in the understanding that it brings her childbearing days to an end.

SYMPTOMS

The conditions described above usually produce heavy, painful or irregular periods or else the symptoms of cancer of the womb or cervix.

TREATMENT

The womb can be removed either by abdominal surgery or via the vagina. The abdominal approach is technically easier, because the field of view is greater. It involves an incision just above the bikini line. The Fallopian tubes are cut where they join the womb and the vault of the vagina is stitched closed where it meets the womb. Vaginal hysterectomy is technically more complicated but is a preferred method if the woman is also having the walls of the vagina tightened for prolapse. Also, there is no external scar.

In both cases recovery takes a couple of weeks. Hysterectomy can be a debilitating operation and it may take eight to twelve weeks to recover completely from the operation.

The ovaries

Usually the ovaries are left in pre-menopausal women so as to allow them to continue to produce oestrogen. To do otherwise would start an abrupt menopause. If removal is unavoidable, for example if they are caught up with endometriosis or pelvic inflammatory disease, hormone replacement therapy (HRT) would be given at or about the time of surgery.

Complications

Serious complications after hysterectomy are uncommon. Possible minor complications include urinary infections, wound infections and loss of belly muscle tone. Several important structures, for example the bladder, lie near the womb and could be damaged by surgery. However, such problems are exceptionally rare.

QUESTIONS

Does hysterectomy affect sex?
Many women fear it will, imagining that they are in some way less female or more delicate. This is not at all the case and a normal sex life can resume within a month or so.

Is hysterectomy done for trivial reasons?
Removal of the womb takes with it all future problems of menstruation and cancer of the womb or cervix; many women find that an unalloyed blessing. However, you must feel comfortable that the gynaecologist has covered all non-surgical options.

Will I still have a menopause?
When your ovaries fail, you will get symptoms such as hot flushes. Because you no longer have periods, it can only be confirmed with blood tests to detect levels of relevant hormones.

Complementary Treatment

Many therapies can help postoperatively. **Chakra balancing** can help with pain control and aid healing of wounds. **Homeopathy** uses arnica to reduce bleeding and bruising, staphisagria if healing is slow. In **aromatherapy** bergamot and sandalwood are both useful for alleviating postoperative fatigue. **Bach flower remedies** – for emotional aftercare, star of Bethlehem for shock and grief, willow for weepy introspection. After recovery, **yoga** can be beneficial – tell your teacher you have had a hysterectomy.

FEMALE SUBFERTILITY

This means difficulty in becoming pregnant. In cases of couples who appear subfertile about 40% are the result of problems within the woman.

BACKGROUND

A successful pregnancy is the end result of a process of extraordinary complexity. The ovaries have to bring a normal egg to maturation under the influence of hormones from the brain and from the ovaries themselves. This egg has to be picked up by the Fallopian tubes and swept along towards the womb. At some point in this journey a sperm, one of a hundred million that began the journey, will meet the egg and enter it, merging the genetic material from both parents.

The fertilized egg has to implant in the womb, and will gain its nutrition and blood supply from the placenta, whose growth and efficiency has to keep pace with the baby's development for the next nine months. Problems can arise at every step of the way.

Before embarking on the uncomfortable and often disappointing trail of subfertility investigations, it is important to make sure about the fundamentals: that intercourse is taking place regularly and with a correct technique and at mid-cycle, when the egg has been released. **Male subfertility** is a factor in about 30–40% of all couples experiencing problems with conception. Not all subfertility is understood – in at least 20% of cases no convincing reason can be found to explain subfertility yet the couple fail to conceive.

Subfertility must be distinguished from repeated early **miscarriage**, which has its own investigations and treatment.

REASONS FOR SUBFERTILITY

Failure to release eggs (ovulate)
Causes: Failure to ovulate is quite common and means that the woman has all the right hormones but that an egg is not reaching maturity. The problem is recognized by measuring the hormone progesterone in the second half of the menstrual cycle. Any serious generalized illness, for example **diabetes**, **stress** or abnormal dieting, might cause ovulation to fail.

The ovaries might be malformed or might even be absent, as a result of the chromosome abnormality of Turner's syndrome. More common are polycystic ovaries, where the ovaries are covered in small cysts containing immature eggs which do not progress to full maturity. Women with polycystic ovaries have an excess of male hormone, leading to acne and hairiness as well as irregular periods and subfertility.

Symptoms: Congenital problems are suspected if a woman fails to begin menstruating and has poor breast development. The diagnosis is confirmed by blood tests showing low levels of female hormones and by making a chromosome analysis, using cells scraped from the inside of the cheek. Abnormalities of the ovary might be to blame if menstruation is irregular or absent and can be confirmed by ultrasound imaging of the ovaries or by examining them via a laparoscope.

Treatment: Ovulation can be improved by using drugs such as clomiphene which stimulate the release of more eggs. This has to be done very carefully, however, to avoid stimulating too many eggs at once, leading to multiple pregnancy. The treatment of polycystic ovaries also uses clomiphene plus steroids to enhance egg production.

If the problem is a congenital absence or malformation of ovaries, unfortunately nothing can be done.

Barriers to eggs implanting
Causes: Essentially this means a physical barrier within the Fallopian tube or the ovary so that the egg cannot reach the womb. The likeliest reasons for this are chronic **pelvic inflammatory disease** or **endometriosis**, both of which tether the Fallopian tubes with fibrous material that blocks them. Much less commonly, the barrier to implantation lies within the womb, which might be misshapen, for example with an abnormal division up the middle – a bicornuate womb.

Symptoms: The woman fails to become pregnant despite having a normal menstrual cycle. There is a history of pelvic infection, periods are heavy and painful and she suffers internal pain during intercourse.

A malformed womb is undetectable without a specialized dye test to show the outline, called a hystero-salpingogram. A dye that shows on X-ray is injected into the womb and outlines the shape of the womb. The dye should emerge from each Fallopian tube. This test is sometimes combined with laparoscopy to inspect the Fallopian tubes carefully.

Treatment: It is sometimes possible to release the tethered tubes or to enlarge the channels through them. A malformed womb might also be surgically correctable. Otherwise such cases are best handled by artificial fertilization techniques (see below).

Other factors
Some women appear to develop antibodies to their partner's sperm, which are destroyed. This is diagnosed by a post-coital test, which samples semen from the vagina several hours after intercourse and analyses how many sperm are still alive and

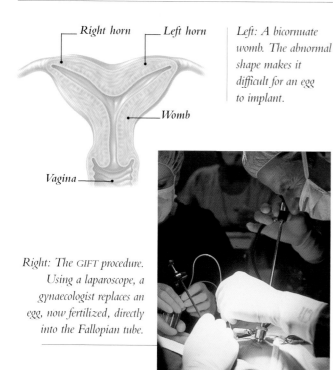

Right horn — Left horn

Left: A bicornuate womb. The abnormal shape makes it difficult for an egg to implant.

Womb

Vagina

Right: The GIFT procedure. Using a laparoscope, a gynaecologist replaces an egg, now fertilized, directly into the Fallopian tube.

hope to many couples. The technology is still new and, like all new technologies, is imperfect but continually improving. The success rate is still quite low – a 15–20% success rate is considered good. The procedure is expensive and the whole process can seem mechanical. This makes it particularly important that couples embarking on this route should ensure they are attending properly accredited clinics where their treatment is supervised by doctors who, as well as being technically proficient, offer the combination of optimism and realism required by subfertility treatment.

QUESTIONS

How common is subfertility?
After one year 90% of all couples will have achieved a pregnancy. Of the remaining 10% just under half will eventually conceive, either through chance or through treatment. One in thirteen couples will remain infertile.

For how long is it worth trying treatment?
After five years, whatever the treatment, the chances of success are very low. Moreover, most couples find that the emotional and financial stresses of subfertility treatment are too much to bear after that length of time. Unexpected pregnancies have been known to happen years after all hope and treatment have been abandoned.

active. At present there are no treatments to improve this situation other than some experimental techniques.

If a woman has irregular or prolonged menstrual cycles it can be difficult to judge the most fertile time for intercourse. Urine-based tests are now available that indicate ovulation and therefore the best time to have intercourse.

Age affects fertility: there is a marked decline in a woman's natural fertility from the age of 35 onward. Whatever the economic and personal reasons for wishing to postpone conceiving, it is important to bear in mind that the older you get the more likely it is you will have difficulty conceiving.

IN VITRO FERTILIZATION
◆

Artificial fertilization techniques go by a variety of names, for example GIFT. The process involves harvesting an egg via laparoscopy. This egg is fertilized by the man's sperm within a test tube, hence *in vitro* fertilization. The fertilized egg is returned to the woman and reimplanted within her womb or within the Fallopian tubes.

The development of *in vitro* fertilization and other similar techniques has been a tremendous advance in dealing with subfertility and, despite the ethical problems, they offer new

Complementary Treatment
You may feel that it is worth trying gentle complementary approaches, which can be very effective, before resorting to disruptive, and possibly expensive, conventional interventions. A qualified practitioner of traditional Chinese medicine (**herbs**, **acupuncture**, **tai chi/chi kung**) may be able to help. **Chakra balancing** may make you more likely to conceive by relaxing you, and could help by balancing energy from your hormones and enzymes. **Healing** – an experienced practitioner may be able to help you come to terms with the emotional implications. Diet – nutritional deficiencies such as zinc and vitamin A may be implicated in subfertility and a **nutritional therapist** would be able to advise on supplementation. **Hypnotherapy** – hypnotic regression and suggestion can help if the subfertility is caused by subconscious fears of birth or motherhood. *Other therapies to try: homeopathy; naturopathy; Ayurveda; see also STRESS.*

Sexually transmitted diseases in women

Diseases spread by sexual contact, known as STDs.

Background

Although many sexually transmitted diseases in women are more inconvenient than serious, a significant number do pose an important threat to health. Unfortunately those with long-term health consequences are the ones that usually produce the least symptoms, for example gonorrhoea and chlamydia. Therefore there is an onus on men with STDs to alert their partners to the possibility that they too may be infected. This is also why genito-urinary clinics put so much emphasis on tracing the contacts of men or women with STDs. (See SEXUALLY TRANSMITTED DISEASES IN MEN.)

Different types of STD

Trichomonas

Causes: This is a single-celled organism that is usually, but not always, spread venereally.

Symptoms: The symptoms are **vaginitis** – pain and inflammation of the vagina – plus a green or yellow and often frothy vaginal discharge.

Treatment: Treatment is with the antibiotic metronidazole.

Herpes simplex

Causes: The herpes virus responsible is a type of herpes virus that causes cold sores on the lips. The virus is spread by sexual contact with someone with active genital herpes or by oral sex with someone with cold sores. As with other herpes viruses, it is able to live for many years within the nervous system and can be reactivated from time to time, meaning that symptoms can recur several times a year for several years.

Symptoms: After a few days of burning discomfort, a very tender group of blisters appears on the genitalia. The blisters take seven to ten days to dry and disappear; they are infectious during this time and for a few days after disappearing. The blisters recur at times of stress or simply at random, each time being preceded by a few days of warning painful irritation that sufferers come to recognize with foreboding.

Treatment: Antiviral drugs, if taken early enough, reduce the severity of each appearance. The best-known drug is acyclovir, used as a cream applied to the skin or as tablets. Fortunately, with time attacks become less frequent and less severe. If a pregnant woman has active herpes at the time of delivery the baby must be delivered by Caesarean section to avoid the serious consequences of infecting him with herpes.

Thrush

Causes: This is one of the most common causes of vaginal symptoms (see THRUSH). By no means all cases are via sexual contact because the fungus responsible is a natural inhabitant of the body. In cases of recurrent infection, sexual transmission may be to blame.

Symptoms: The symptoms are vaginal itch and a vaginal discharge containing white curd-like deposits.

Treatment: Treatment is with antifungal agents in the form of creams or pessaries, for example clotrimazole, and, for resistant cases, tablets such as fluconazole.

Gonorrhoea

Causes: Whereas gonorrhoea in men produces discharge from the penis and burning on passing urine, in women infection can persist in a low-key manner. The gonococcus lives within the female genital tract, so that the first the woman may know of infection is when she develops **pelvic inflammatory disease** (PID) or is found to be subfertile.

Symptoms: There may be an infected vaginal discharge plus **urethritis**. If there is PID there will be pelvic pain and a high fever. Unfortunately in about 70% of women infected with gonorrhoea there are no specific symptoms.

Treatment: This is with a single dose of amoxycillin with probenecid as tablets. The cure rate is very high. If the disease becomes chronic with PID it is difficult to eradicate. The effects on fertility are irreversible, although all the treatments given for subfertility are available (see FEMALE SUBFERTILITY).

Syphilis

Causes: The initial infection is even less likely to produce symptoms than gonorrhoea. The organism responsible, *Treponema pallidum*, causes long-term damage to the nervous system and will infect the baby of any future pregnancy.

Symptoms: There is a small sore on the lips of the vagina, which occurs one to three months after infection. There may be a sparse generalized skin rash, which lasts for several weeks, then warts appear around the genitalia and there is enlargement of lymph nodes in the armpits and the groin. There are often no further problems for many years but eventually there may be difficulty with walking, generalized body pains and, ultimately, dementia. This is called tertiary syphilis. The diagnosis is made by blood tests.

Treatment: Treatment of early syphilis requires injections of penicillin for two weeks. Even the established disease can be cured by the same treatment but the effects on the nervous system are irreversible.

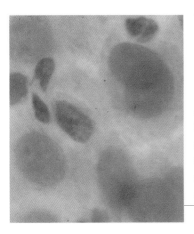

Left: Abnormal cells that have been affected by chlamydia, an organism responsible for pelvic inflammatory disease and subfertility.

Chlamydia

Causes: This small micro-organism has in recent years been increasingly recognized as one of the most common causes of PID and sterility. Estimates suggest that up to 30% of sexually active women have had it, while 1–5% are at serious risk of active chlamydial infection and its consequences.

Symptoms: The organism can cause urethritis, with burning on passing water and a discharge, but only in a minority of infected women. Otherwise it goes on to cause inflammation of the cervix, then inflammation of the womb and Fallopian tubes. All this takes place silently, with no warning symptoms. There may eventually be chronic pelvic pain.

Chlamydial infection appears to increase the risks of ectopic pregnancy (see PREGNANCY PROBLEMS). There is an estimated ten per cent chance of subfertility. The diagnosis is difficult to make even using specialized swabs. Blood tests are becoming available to assist in diagnosis.

Treatment: Chlamydia responds well to antibiotics such as tetracycline and erythromycin, taken for seven to twenty-one days. The disease is so widespread that there are moves to introduce screening for it on the basis that it is common, carries a high risk of causing ill health and is readily treatable.

Genital warts

Causes: These extremely common STDs are caused by the wart virus and arise spontaneously. (Syphilis can cause multiple genital wart-like lesions.)

Symptoms: There are collections of flat warts around the genitalia. Warts cluster around the anus in those who practise ano-genital intercourse. The warts vary from just a few in number to enormous quantities.

Treatment: You must be screened for other STDs. Although most warts can be distinguished from those of syphilis by appearance alone, blood tests should be done. Treatment is

with paints containing the drug podophyllin; if there are large numbers they may have to be cauterized (burnt off). The wart virus can invade the cervix and predispose to **cervical cancer**, so it is important to have regular cervical smears.

See also AIDS.

QUESTIONS

How can I avoid sexually transmitted disease?
Know the sexual habits of your partners. Anyone who has several sexual partners in a short period of time is at significant risk of getting an STD. Use condoms unless you are in a stable long-term relationship. Report any unusual vaginal discharge.

What if I have an STD?
You should seek help as soon as possible from a genito-urinary diseases clinic. Such clinics are completely confidential, will check for any coincidental STDs and, crucially, will trace contacts.

Can STDs affect pregnancy?
Apart from reducing fertility some may have serious consequences for the foetus. It is important to inform your doctor if you have genital herpes and if there is any risk of syphilis or HIV/AIDS.

Complementary Treatment

There are serious consequences from the inadequate treatment of STDs, so always seek a conventional opinion. Complementary therapies can both boost the immune system to help the body resist further attack and alter the acidity of the vaginal secretions so they become hostile to harmful organisms. **Western herbalism** – echinacea boosts the immune system, and herbal douches can change the environment of the vagina. Traditional Chinese medicine (a combination of **herbs**, **acupuncture** and **tai chi/chi kung**) could help. **Ayurvedic** treatment might involve a combination of detoxification, oil massage and yoga. Various **aromatherapy** douches are available, and this therapy may have some effect on herpes – an experienced practitioner could advise. In some instances, **homeopathy** can be helpful, especially for genital warts, where useful remedies include thuja, medorrhinum, nitric ac and sabina. *Other therapies to try: nutritional therapy; naturopathy; Alexander Technique.*

VAGINITIS

Inflammation of the vagina, most often caused by infection of the walls of the vagina.

CAUSES

Trichomonas is a micro-organism that causes vaginitis; bacterial vaginosis is the term for infection by one of several other non-specific bacteria that cause inflammation. Another common infectious cause is **thrush**. Many irritants can inflame the vagina, such as vaginal deodorants, bubble baths or even condoms.

SYMPTOMS

There is itchy discomfort, often with a vaginal discharge. There may be internal discomfort from inflammation of the cervix, called cervicitis. The colour of the discharge provides a clue: a frothy yellow-green discharge suggests trichomonas; a grey smelly discharge bacterial vaginosis and a thick white discharge thrush. The diagnosis is confirmed by a swab.

TREATMENT

The antibiotic metronidazole is effective against both trichomonas and bacterial vaginosis; clindamycin vaginal cream is a more specific treatment for bacterial vaginosis. Treatment is continued for a few days and recurrences are common. Obviously any irritants such as bubble baths and vaginal deodorants should be avoided.

Treatment is essential. Even asymptomatic trichomonas should be treated or it will eventually provoke symptoms. Bacterial vaginosis may affect the unborn baby and complicate gynaecological surgery so should be treated in those circumstances, but otherwise not unless it is causing symptoms.

Complementary Treatment
Chakra balancing can help ease pain and aid relaxation, and should reduce discomfort during intercourse. **Naturopathy** – dietary changes might be recommended, along with fasting, **yoga** and hydrotherapy. **Hypnotherapy** can help.

VAGINISMUS

Spasm of the vagina, associated with psychosexual problems.

CAUSES

Apprehension about having sexual intercourse normally underlies this fairly common problem. There may be logical reasons: a woman may be rejecting intercourse with a man she has mixed feelings about or worrying about pregnancy. There is spasm of the muscles around the vagina, preventing entry or making entry very uncomfortable. This should be distinguished from normal entry followed by pain felt deep inside during intercourse, which suggests a pelvic problem such as **endometriosis** or **pelvic inflammatory disease**.

SYMPTOMS

Nothing appears out of the ordinary until intercourse is attempted and entry has to be abandoned. The muscles around the vagina are seen to be in spasm. This is sometimes noticed during routine gynaecological examination, for example taking a smear, when the vagina goes into spasm when the doctor tries to examine internally or to pass an instrument.

TREATMENT

It is important to exclude causes of localized pain such as unhealed tears from childbirth, herpes or **vaginitis**. Otherwise it is a matter of discussing the psychological factors that might contribute to the condition. These could be ignorance and therefore apprehension about sex, previous pain or rape, or lack of foreplay leading to inadequate lubrication.

Treatment involves the woman getting used to feeling her own anatomy, using vaginal dilators of graduated size, plus explanation of sexual technique for both partners.

Psychological therapy helps by diverting attention away from intercourse, substituting other sexual activity such as manual stimulation or cunnilingus. The couple return to sexual intercourse once they have mutual trust.

Complementary Treatment
Acupuncture relaxes your muscles and calms your mind. **Chakra balancing** eases pain, aids relaxation and reduces discomfort during intercourse. **Hypnotherapy** – suggestion and regression techniques can find the cause, and deal with the symptoms.

THRUSH

♦

A widely found fungal organism that commonly affects women.

CAUSES

♦

Thrush is caused by a member of the yeast family of fungi, called *Candida albicans*. Candida thrives in warm, moist conditions with the food supply those areas provide and grows by putting out filaments on which new bodies bud.

Candida is a normal inhabitant of the intestinal tract and of the mouth. It is not an infection 'picked up' from somewhere, nor is it a typical sexually transmitted disease (STD), although it often goes to and fro between sexual partners.

Candida is but one of hordes of micro-organisms found on the body and which compete for available food sources. Its moment of glory comes if other organisms are reduced in number, for example following antibiotic treatment. Antibiotics destroy susceptible organisms all over the body and not just in the infection targeted. This is why vaginal (and oral) thrush is so common after an antibiotic, although women vary greatly in how liable they are to this side effect.

Thrush will overgrow if there is a superabundant food supply, as when someone has excess sugar in the body – **diabetes**.

Finally, the damper and warmer the body's climate the more thrush thrives. This applies particularly to the areas under the breasts, in skin folds of the upper thigh and in the vagina.

SYMPTOMS

♦

There is an itchy red rash under the breasts or on the inner thighs. Vaginal thrush causes an itchy discharge, with white curd-like deposits. The diagnosis is confirmed by taking a swab of the vaginal discharge. Thrush can actually live within the vagina without causing symptoms, and only be discovered if a smear or swab is taken for some other reason.

TREATMENT

♦

Thrush on the skin is treated with drugs called imidazoles, which kill the fungus. Drug names are clotrimazole and imidazole and are often combined with stronger antiseptic agents and with hydrocortisone to reduce itching.

Vaginal thrush is treated with pessaries containing an imidazole. Pessaries are inserted at night for one to six nights. Often an antifungal cream needs to be applied to the vagina, too. Thrush resistant to these methods can be eradicated with an antifungal agent taken by mouth, such as fluconazole. This may be taken as a single large dose or spread over several

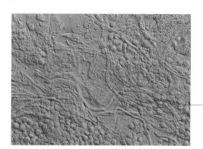

Left: The fungus causing thrush, showing the filaments on which new buds eventually form.

days. Sexual partners should use an antifungal cream on the penis. Anyone, female or male, who keeps getting thrush should be tested for diabetes.

Wearing loose-fitting clothing helps reduce heat and sweating in skin folds. Since candida lives in the intestinal tract, after opening the bowels a woman should wipe from front to back, otherwise she may self-infect the vagina.

QUESTIONS

Do antithrush treatments lose effect?
In general they do not; the organism does not develop resistance in most cases. Recurrent problems are more likely a result of reinfection rather than of resistance.

Why don't antibiotics kill thrush too?
Antibiotics are very specific in their targets and those that kill bacteria do not have antifungal effects. The same is not quite true in reverse: antifungal drugs often have a weak antibacterial activity.

Is self-treatment a good idea?
Certainly for women who get occasional, typical thrush. Anyone getting frequent or apparently resistant thrush should see a doctor to consider diabetes or other rarer causes of recurrent thrush.

Complementary Treatment

Chinese and **Western herbalism** both offer remedies with antifungal effects. Western herbalism offers a range of teas to be used as effective washes: try lavender, marigold, rosemary or thyme. **Aromatherapy** – try tea tree oil in pessary form, or one of the following in a daily sitz bath (six drops): frankincense, myrrh, lavender, tea tree. **Nutritional therapy** might suggest cutting out sugar, fermented foods and yeast. Garlic and live yogurt have antifungal properties. *Other therapies to try: naturopathy; homeopathy; hypnotherapy.*

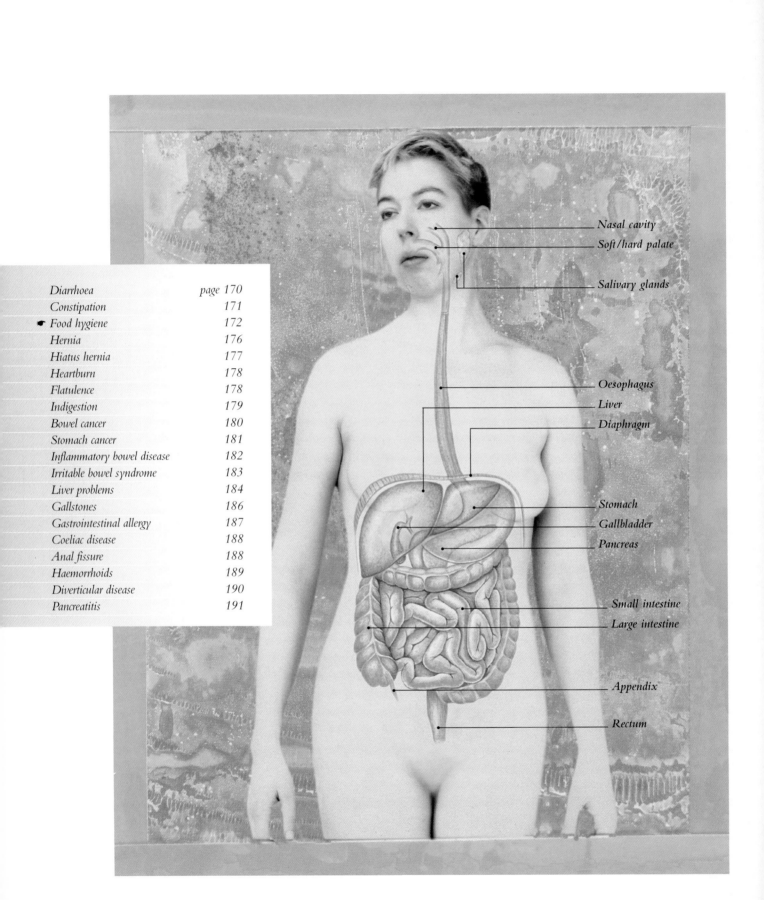

Nasal cavity

Soft/hard palate

Salivary glands

Oesophagus

Liver

Diaphragm

Stomach

Gallbladder

Pancreas

Small intestine

Large intestine

Appendix

Rectum

All the ingenuity of food presentation and the inventiveness of cooks is reduced by the digestive processes to certain fundamental materials. These are carbohydrates, fats, proteins, minerals and vitamins.

DIGESTIVE SYSTEM

THE BASIC MATERIALS we need to function are carbohydrates, fats, proteins, minerals and vitamins. *Carbohydrates* (starchy foods) are large molecules that can be turned into sugar (glucose) to provide the main energy source of the body. Glucose can also be transformed into fat and protein.

Fat is a very high energy source used throughout the body.

Proteins are found in, for example, meat, pulses and grains. They are complex molecules formed from amino acids. Amino acids are like building bricks that, once digested, become available to make all the other body structures, such as muscles, nerves, organs, blood and skin.

Minerals include calcium, potassium, sodium, iron and many more. Each mineral has an important role to play in the body's metabolism, so there are specialized digestive processes that harvest them from food.

Vitamins are biochemicals of a particular type which the body cannot, on the whole, make for itself, but which are essential to cell metabolism. Even though tiny amounts are required, they are vital for making blood, bones, skin, the nervous system, energy production and much more.

The digestive process

Enzymes break the raw food molecules into smaller fragments, which are absorbed and transported all around the body. This begins in the mouth, where saliva starts the breakdown of starch. Digestion begins in earnest in the stomach, where food plunges into a warm highly acidic bath of hydrochloric acid mixed with enzymes.

The liquid mass now passes into the small intestine, the site of the bulk of both digestion and absorption. Yet more enzymes from the pancreas attack the food, breaking down protein. Bile from the liver dissolves fat molecules.

The lining of the small intestine is composed of billions of frond-like outgrowths, which vastly increase the surface area. The outer layer of each frond contains specialized cells that actively transport molecules from the food slurry into the blood stream. Within the blood stream yet more specialized proteins pick up the newly digested food and carry it mainly to the liver for further processing.

The digestive process is by and large complete by the time that material reaches the large intestine – called the colon. Huge quantities of bacteria live in the large intestine and complete the digestion of tough carbohydrate fibres. Water and minerals are also reabsorbed there.

Control

The process of digestion is under an array of biochemical and nerve controls, which are far from fully understood. These cause the right enzymes to appear at the right times and regulate acid and bile production. They influence the complicated muscle layers in the walls of the bowels, which sweep food through the system and which expel it at the end.

Digestive disorders

Many bowel problems revolve around the production of excess acid (ulcers, **indigestion** and **heartburn**), the upward escape of acid (**hiatus hernia**) and disordered movements of the intestine (**constipation**, **diarrhoea** and **irritable bowel syndrome**). The rapid turnover of cells within the digestive tract predisposes to cancer, especially of the stomach and large intestine.

Left: The chemical resources of the digestive system break food down within hours into usable components.

DIARRHOEA

Liquid motions that occur if the bowel fails to reabsorb fluid.

CAUSES

For much of its passage through the intestinal tract food moves as a liquid slurry, totalling about 8 litres/1¾ gallons a day. Water is reabsorbed in the large intestine until the motions are solid or semi-solid. This process is affected by infection, inflammation or growths in the bowel. The overwhelming majority of cases of diarrhoea are caused by minor and self-limiting infection.

Infection and inflammation

Many germs can cause a temporary inflammation of the bowel, which interferes with fluid absorption. Even the common cold viruses do this, especially in children. More serious infections such as cholera or typhoid are unusual in the developed world. These lead to dangerously high fluid loss in a very short period of time.

Food poisoning may be caused by a definite germ or by poisons (toxins) within the food that do not infect the bowel but cause it to be overactive. The terms gastroenteritis and food poisoning largely overlap. Chronic diarrhoea is a feature of **inflammatory bowel disease**.

Growths

Growths, benign or cancerous, in the bowel cause diarrhoea by interfering with its normal function. Much less common than gastroenteritis, these bear consideration if an older person has diarrhoea lasting more than a couple of weeks.

Miscellaneous causes

Less common reasons include worry ('my bowels turned to water'), malabsorption (as in **coeliac disease**) or an overactive thyroid gland (see THYROID PROBLEMS). In the elderly diarrhoea often coexists with **constipation**.

SYMPTOMS

The motions are semi-formed if not pure liquid. Abdominal cramps are relieved by opening the bowels urgently many times a day. Blood is not uncommon with gastroenteritis; recurrent blood loss or mucus in the motions suggests inflammatory bowel disease or a growth, as does persistent diarrhoea, diarrhoea at night, abdominal pains and weight loss. Thirst and tiredness with prolonged diarrhoea suggest serious fluid and mineral loss and require medical attention.

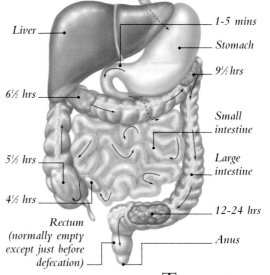

Oesophagus (gullet)
Delay of 3 secs
Liver
1-5 mins
Stomach
9½ hrs
6½ hrs
Small intestine
5½ hrs
Large intestine
4½ hrs
12-24 hrs
Rectum (normally empty except just before defecation)
Anus

Left: Timed progress of the first part of a meal through the digestive system, after leaving the mouth. (The latter part of the meal takes 3–5 hours to leave the stomach.) Food reaches the large intestine as liquid. If water is not properly absorbed there, diarrhoea results.

TREATMENT

The vast majority of cases of diarrhoea settle without any medication over a few days. The individual should simply drink 2–3 litres/3½–5 pints a day of bland drinks such as water, tea, or fizzy drinks gone flat. It is best to avoid milk and sweet drinks, which can make diarrhoea worse. It is especially important for both the elderly and children to take extra fluids containing the minerals lost in diarrhoea, such as potassium.

Various antidiarrhoea remedies work on the nervous system, which controls the bowels, slowing it down. They are useful for short-term control but see a doctor for diarrhoea lasting more than a few days. Drugs include loperamide and codeine. Analysing a stool sample may reveal infection treatable by an antibiotic. Antibiotics such as ciprofloxacin are helpful if diarrhoea acquired abroad is persistent and severe.

See also page 296 for diarrhoea in children and babies.

Complementary Treatment

Most complementary therapists will offer dietary advice along with treatment: **nutritional therapists** and **naturopaths** can be especially helpful. Commonly used **acupuncture** points are Stomach 25, on the abdomen, and Stomach 36, below the knee. **Chinese herbalism** remedies to strengthen a weak digestive system include *Dang Shen* and *Bai Zhu*, both part of the formula called *Si Jun Zi Tang* (four noble formulae). *Other therapies to try: homeopathy; Western herbalism; shiatsu-do; cymatics; hypnotherapy; auricular therapy; Ayurveda; chakra balancing.*

CONSTIPATION

Bowels that open infrequently with hard, uncomfortable motions.

CAUSES

Whereas **diarrhoea** results from excess fluid in the large intestine, constipation is quite the opposite. The contents of the bowel stay so long that excess fluid is absorbed, leaving the motions so hard that they are difficult to pass. Constipation also occurs if something obstructs the passage of motions or reduces the normal rhythmic contractions of the intestines.

Delayed transit time

This extremely common cause affects everyone at some time and the elderly more than most. There is a reduction in the bowel's rhythmic contractions that normally push food through the system. Faeces accumulate within the large intestine; the longer they stay the more water is extracted and the harder they become. Eventually the bowels open through sheer weight of material, although it can be painful and leaves the individual feeling that the bowel is incompletely emptied.

Children often deliberately withhold opening their bowels for reasons clear to Sigmund Freud but unclear to everyone else. The resulting pain on defecation leads to a vicious circle of further retaining of motions.

Obstruction and other factors

In an older person, persistent change of bowel habit to constipation (or diarrhoea) could indicate a growth in the large bowel, especially if the change in bowel habit is accompanied by pain or bleeding. Rarely, children are born with congenital malformations of the bowel which interfere with defecation.

Constipation is a feature of both severe **depression** and an underactive thyroid gland (see THYROID PROBLEMS). Most powerful painkillers also cause constipation, for example codeine, morphine and co-proxamol. This can be a problem for those individuals who need to take such painkillers for chronic pain. Constipation is a feature of **irritable bowel syndrome** and is common during pregnancy (see PREGNANCY PROBLEMS). Constipation can also be an indicator of inadequate dietary fibre.

SYMPTOMS

There is no definition of constipation in the sense of how much, how often. People vary from having a bowel action twice a day to having one once a week. Therefore constipation is defined by reference to your usual bowel habit and not by reference to any rules. If the bowels are opened only infrequently but without straining there is no reason for concern, whereas a daily struggle may indicate a problem.

Constipation plus blood in older people needs full investigation. Sudden constipation plus abdominal pain and distension is typical of a bowel obstruction needing emergency care.

TREATMENT

Temporary constipation responds to increased fluid or a laxative. Some laxatives, for example senna, stimulate the muscle of the bowel to move faeces faster and can lead to uncomfortable cramps. Others, such as lactulose or fibre drinks, draw water back into the motions. If necessary a suppository will stimulate the bowel quickly; an enema literally washes out the bowel. Sometimes children with constipation resistant to mild laxatives may have emotional problems that need unravelling. All cases benefit by increasing the amount of fibre in the diet.

Techniques for investigating possible **bowel cancer** include sigmoidoscopy, colonoscopy to look at the lining of the bowels (see page 323) or a barium enema (see page 316).

QUESTIONS

Are regular laxatives harmful?
Stimulant laxatives such as senna lead to reduced muscular activity of the bowel and are not advisable. Those that retain fluid and fibre drinks are safe for long-term use.

Why is constipation so common in the elderly?
Older people eat less and often take less bulky foods. They exercise less (immobility is constipating) and may be on painkillers that have constipation as a side effect.

Complementary Treatment

Consult a **nutritional therapist** or **naturopath**; boost your fibre intake. **Acupuncture** and **Chinese herbalism** – see DIARRHOEA. **Chakra balancing** reduces pain and relaxes the abdominal wall, stimulating defecation. **Aromatherapy** oils to stimulate digestion are black pepper, marjoram and rosemary. **Hypnotherapy** can get the bowel moving regularly. **Ayurveda** offers bowel cleansing with various enemas and laxatives. *Other therapies to try: homeopathy; tai chi/chi kung; auricular therapy; cymatics; shiatsu-do; yoga.*

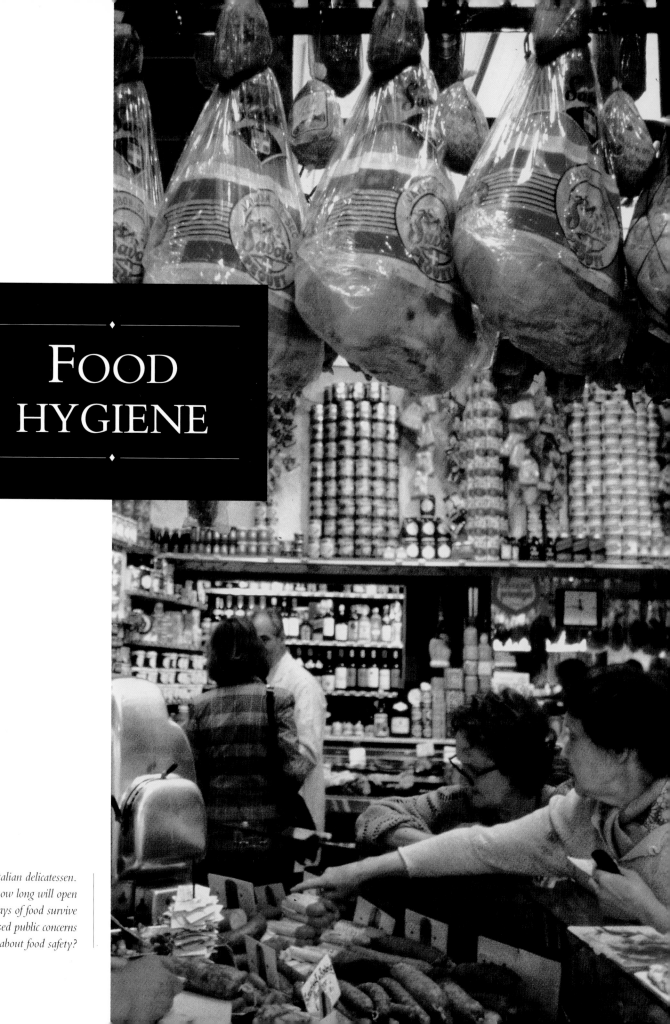

FOOD HYGIENE

*An Italian delicatessen.
For how long will open
displays of food survive
increased public concerns
about food safety?*

THE INCIDENCE OF FOOD POISONING has soared in recent years. Responsibility for food hygiene is shared between producers and consumers. While high-profile problems occur in institutions such as hospitals or old peoples' homes, most episodes occur within the home. Despite this, food poisoning is still rare in relation to the millions of meals prepared each day.

What is hygienic food?

What is food for you is just as much food for micro-organisms like bacteria and moulds. Much food technology and advice on food preparation is directed at reducing the risk from such organisms to a minimum. This is done by harvesting or rearing food in hygienic circumstances, processing it rapidly and cleanly, storing it safely, cooking it thoroughly and serving it promptly. However, the possibility of lapses in hygiene accompanies each step of this food chain.

Hygienic farming In the United Kingdom in recent years there have been scares about salmonella in eggs and chickens, BSE in cattle and *E. coli* in meat products. The true level of risk from these problems is extremely hard to calculate.

They have, however, served to focus attention on making farming methods safer. In the case of BSE this means not giving animal-based feeds to cattle, tracking outbreaks of BSE and culling herds where it occurs. In the case of *E. coli* it has led to an examination of the cleanliness of slaughtered cattle so as to reduce their contamination with faecal material.

Intensive farming of animals in crowded conditions increases the risk of outbreaks of disease and therefore antibiotics are often used to try to control such problems. These conditions are probably the reason why salmonella infection in meat and poultry has soared in the last 20 years as resistant, aggressive strains of salmonella have spread.

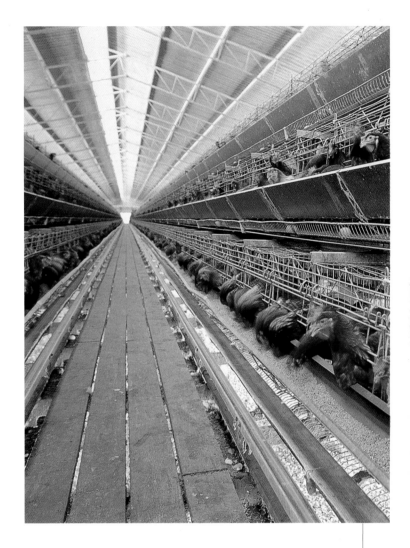

Above: Inexpensive food may cost much in animal suffering and hygiene problems. We can choose alternatives, but must be prepared to pay more.

Processing food Strict regulations govern industrial food handling in order to keep the risk of contamination to a minimum. Most modern food companies have an impressive record in processing food rapidly at low temperatures and preserving the food by many means, such as canning, freezing and drying. These companies use standardized systems called hazard analysis and critical control point systems to control possible risks.

Fresh food has a limited life and to overcome this preservatives are often added. These are chemicals that kill or retard the growth of micro-organisms. You may not like the idea of additives or irradiation of food but without it many foods will have a far shorter shelf life. There are also the traditional methods of preservation such as smoking, pickling and jam-making, which have been employed for centuries.

Storing food Most food now comes with storage information, giving the temperature at which to keep it, the length of time it can be kept (the shelf life or 'best before' date) and what to do once the packaging has been opened. These recommendations are cautious and they do not necessarily mean food immediately goes off, but they are an important guide.

Most uncooked foods such as meat, fish and fruit cannot be stored for long.

HYGIENIC FOOD HANDLING

Do . . .

♦ *Wash hands and utensils often*
♦ *Use a fridge thermometer*
♦ *Either chill raw food rapidly or cook it*
♦ *Keep raw and cooked food separate*
♦ *Cook food to the recommended temperature and time*
♦ *Eat or chill cooked food rapidly*
♦ *Reheat leftovers thoroughly*
♦ *Thaw food completely before cooking, ensuring it is hot right through*
♦ *Keep work surfaces clean*
♦ *Look at food and smell it; if in doubt discard*
♦ *Throw away milk from damaged containers*

Don't . . .

♦ *Use the same utensils on raw and cooked food without washing them in between*
♦ *Leave cooked food out*
♦ *Refreeze food after it has thawed*
♦ *Eat raw eggs if pregnant*
♦ *Eat soft/blue cheeses or meat pâté if pregnant*
♦ *Let pets near food*

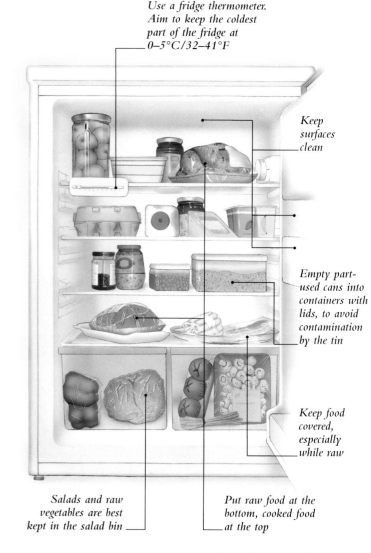

Use a fridge thermometer. Aim to keep the coldest part of the fridge at 0–5°C/32–41°F

Keep surfaces clean

Empty part-used cans into containers with lids, to avoid contamination by the tin

Keep food covered, especially while raw

Salads and raw vegetables are best kept in the salad bin

Put raw food at the bottom, cooked food at the top

Above: Organizing your fridge with food hygiene in mind is important.

Safe food preparation and cooking

Once food enters the home there is the risk of contamination through poor hygiene, micro-organisms from other foods and inadequate cooking. Poor hygiene includes dirty work surfaces and utensils and the lack of attention to basic precautions such as frequent washing of the hands. However, most infections, including salmonella, will be eradicated by cooking the food properly. This means taking the food to a correct and evenly high temperature so that it cooks right through, killing the bacteria.

Cooked food is immediately at risk of renewed contamination, so it must be stored under cover, chilled as appropriate or eaten immediately. Nothing is more likely to guarantee

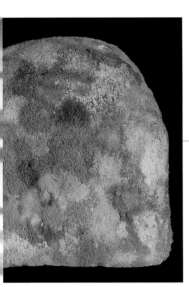

Left: Bread contaminated by moulds, which thrive on humidity and warmth. Such moulds, however, also yielded penicillin.

the food responsible, although reheated food, takeaway food and shellfish are likely culprits.

The diagnosis of food poisoning is usually obvious. The organism responsible can be identified by analysing faeces, although it is often difficult to link this up with a specific food unless a number of people are affected at one event or in one institution.

Treatment rarely requires anything more than fluids (avoid milk), sugar and salt solutions available from pharmacists and bland food like rice or pasta. In severe cases a doctor may give an antibiotic, especially in the elderly.

Some common organisms infecting food

Salmonella This is a family of bacteria found in poultry and eggs. It should be eradicated by proper cooking, which means reaching 70°C/158°F for at least two minutes. It causes symptoms within 12–24 hours, occasionally longer. The diarrhoea and vomiting reaction it causes is rarely dangerous except for the very young, the frail and elderly. However, it can be carried for two to three months after infection. It is therefore important that people who handle food must be shown to be clear before they can return to work. The main risk is from eating raw egg (for example in mayonnaise and meringues) and poultry.

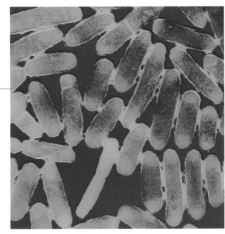

Right: E. coli bacteria cause urinary infections. Ingested in food they cause diarrhoea or occasionally very severe food poisoning. Proper heating kills them.

E. coli These bacteria naturally inhabit the bowels; certain varieties produce highly poisonous toxins that cause diarrhoea, vomiting and stomach pains within two to three days of infection. In the elderly and frail there is a risk of blood poisoning, which is very dangerous. E. coli spreads through beef, especially minced beef and beefburgers, cheese and contaminated water or milk. However, proper cooking to a high temperature eradicates it.

Campylobacter This is now the most common identified reason for food poisoning in the United Kingdom. The microorganism lives especially in contaminated milk and poultry. The diarrhoea it causes often includes blood, appears three to four days after infection and may last two to three weeks. Again, cooking eradicates it.

Listeria This is a widespread naturally occurring bacterium that rarely causes problems but is capable of causing a flu-like illness. It is found especially in soft cheeses, blue cheeses and meat pâtés. As it may cause miscarriage or premature labour, such foods should not be eaten by pregnant women. Listeria is destroyed by cooking; it can continue to grow at temperatures as low as -1°C/30°F.

contamination than leaving out warm food, uncovered, for hours on end and cutting freshly cooked food with utensils that have also been used on old food.

Consider, too, that meat heated on barbecues may not be thoroughly cooked – something especially important to remember with meat burgers and poultry.

Food poisoning

The symptoms are **diarrhoea**, nausea, often griping abdominal pains and a **fever**. Many cases recover within a day or two, but others can last over a week. Symptoms usually begin at least six hours after infection so it can be difficult to pinpoint

HERNIA

Protrusion of an internal organ through muscle wall covering it.

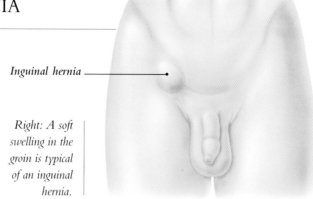

Inguinal hernia ——————

Right: A soft swelling in the groin is typical of an inguinal hernia.

CAUSES

The common types of hernia occur in the groin, where there is always a weakness of the muscle wall. A hernia here is called an inguinal hernia. In men the testicles descend from the abdomen into the scrotum a few weeks before birth or shortly afterward. They descend along a path called the inguinal canal, which always remains a little weak. Anything that increases abdominal pressure pushes away at that potential weakness, for example **chronic bronchitis** with its persistent cough, or constant heavy lifting. Eventually the muscle weakens so much that a loop of intestine gets inside and appears as a bulge. Women do get inguinal hernias but much less often.

For similar reasons the other common sites for hernias are the umbilicus (belly button), which passes through the muscles of the abdominal wall, and at the site of surgery over a muscle – an incisional hernia.

SYMPTOMS

An inguinal hernia begins as a small uncomfortable bulge in the groin, which steadily increases in size. It aches when the person is standing, becoming particularly uncomfortable if he is straining, but disappears when he is lying flat and relaxing.

A hernia is termed incarcerated if a loop of intestine becomes stuck, unable to retract back inside the abdomen: the lump is firm and feels tender. More serious again is a strangulated hernia, when the loop of intestine is not only stuck but its blood supply has become obstructed; the lump is then extremely painful and hard. This is a surgical emergency, marked by severe pain then vomiting from bowel obstruction. In theory hernias elsewhere can become incarcerated or obstructed, but this is much less common.

Inguinal hernias are quite common in baby boys and often grow smaller without treatment or even disappear.

TREATMENT

Once an inguinal hernia has appeared in an adult it is only a matter of time before it gets bigger and needs repairing. Although trusses were once the vogue treatment, most doctors now regard them as obsolete and recommend surgery. In surgery the weakness in the muscle layer is repaired either by stitching it together or using an artificial plastic or metal mesh. Laparoscopic (key hole) surgery (see page 340) now

allows this with just a tiny incision and internal stitching.

An incarcerated hernia can be treated by a whiff of general anaesthetic which makes the surrounding muscles relax. A strangulated hernia has to be dealt with as an emergency before the bowel dies through lack of blood flow. There is a chance of a hernia recurring in people who are constantly coughing or who are overweight, although improved surgical techniques are making this less likely.

Hernias elsewhere are in general less likely to run into problems of pain or obstruction so surgical repair is not essential.

QUESTIONS

What are the advantages of key-hole surgery?
It is as strong as conventional repair, less painful and recovery is much quicker – a matter of days if not hours. Technically far more complicated than open surgery, it is still under judgement.

Must hernias be repaired?
Other than in cases of incarceration or strangulation, there is no medical need for repair except for the knowledge that you may eventually have too much discomfort to bear. This is bound to happen at the most inconvenient time for you.

Complementary Treatment

Alexander Technique – hernias can be helped by improved postural balance and a decrease in contractions along the spinal column. **Reflexology** treatment is aimed at reflex points associated with the adrenal glands and the affected area. **Homeopathy** – depending on circumstances, suggested remedies might include nux or aesculus. **Hypnotherapy** can lessen anxiety and hence help reduce problems. **General self-help** – avoid lifting heavy objects.

HIATUS HERNIA

A weakness in the diaphragm that allows stomach contents to wash upward into the gullet.

CAUSES

This extremely common condition follows from the inevitable weakening of the diaphragm as people get older.

The diaphragm stretches across the upper abdomen, roughly in line with the lower ribs. It is a sheet of tough muscular fibres, which marks the boundary between the chest and the abdominal contents. One important function of the diaphragm is in breathing: as the diaphragm moves up and down it draws air into the lungs.

Certain structures have to pass from the chest into the abdomen, notably major blood vessels, nerves and the gullet. The junction between the gullet and the stomach is especially important since without a tight seal, the contents of the stomach will wash up into the gullet, the walls of which are not designed to withstand the powerful stomach acid.

A hiatus hernia alone does not necessarily lead to symptoms unless other factors increase the chances of acid washing back up, known as reflux. These include **obesity**, smoking and high alcohol intake (see ALCOHOL AND ALCOHOLISM).

SYMPTOMS

Acid in the lower gullet produces **heartburn** with belching and pain localized behind the breastbone. It is typical that the symptoms are worse when you are lying flat or bending over, circumstances in which the stomach contents can more easily reflux. Having a hiatus hernia does not inevitably mean that you will get symptoms; nor is it necessary to have a hiatus hernia to get symptoms from reflux, although having one does make reflux for any other reason worse.

A hiatus hernia is diagnosed on a barium swallow, which shows a characteristic appearance. The constant irritation of the gullet can lead to inflammation and oozing of blood which can, in turn, lead to **anaemia**. Endoscopy (see page 323) is necessary to establish how inflamed the lower gullet is and to look for complications such as ulceration or constriction.

TREATMENT

This can be as straightforward as avoiding wearing tight clothes around the waist, reducing smoking and raising the head of the bed slightly, all of which reduce the chances of acid refluxing through the hiatus hernia. Otherwise treatment is similar to that for **indigestion** or heartburn. Initially there are antacids, especially those containing alginate, which form an insulating layer on the acid, reducing the chances of reflux. Next steps include acid-reducing drugs such as H2 blockers (cimetidine and ranitidine) and proton pump inhibitors (lansoprazole and omeprazole). Other drugs increase the rate at which food passes through the stomach, again reducing the chances of reflux; these include cisapride and metoclopramide.

Surgery

It is possible to repair the weakness of the diaphragm and restore the normal anatomy. This is not surgery to be lightly undertaken without tests to make quite sure that the hiatus hernia is the cause of the symptoms and that all medical avenues have been explored. Recent developments mean the repair can now be done laparoscopically (key-hole surgery) (see page 340), avoiding the previous extensive surgery that required opening both the chest and the abdomen.

QUESTIONS

How important is reflux?
Symptomatically reflux is greatly annoying by interfering with the enjoyment of food. Constant irritation can lead to narrowing of the gullet and difficulty in swallowing. This has been shown to be more common than once thought, stimulating research into improving diagnosis and treatment.

Are there other risks?
Constant irritation of the gullet by acid may predispose the cells to become cancerous. A great deal of research is currently addressing the problem as to which people should have endoscopy to detect these changes and how often.

Complementary Treatment

In **cymatics** corrective soundwaves will be focused on your abdomen, thus rebalancing its energy to promote healing. **Alexander Technique** – hernias can be helped by improved postural balance and a decrease in contractions along the spinal column. **Reflexology** treatment is aimed at reflex points associated with the adrenal glands and the affected area. You will find that a **nutritional therapist** or a **naturopath** could tailor a diet to help you reduce acidity. *Other therapies to try: homeopathy; Chinese herbalism.*

HEARTBURN

◆

Raw feeling behind the breastbone from an inflamed gullet.

CAUSES

◆

Swallowed food progresses down the gullet to the stomach. There is a muscular system that should prevent stomach contents from escaping back into the gullet, but this mechanism frequently fails. Strong stomach acid then irritates the walls of the gullet and is felt as heartburn. It can happen that the gullet becomes inflamed spontaneously, called oesophagitis, when the mere act of swallowing causes discomfort.

SYMPTOMS

◆

Soon after eating a burning sensation spreads across the front of the chest. Belching often accompanies the pain; acid may rise into the mouth. It is important to distinguish it from chest pain arising from exertion, which may come from the heart.

TREATMENT

◆

Often it is enough simply to avoid the foods you find cause your heartburn, for example acidic foods and alcohol. Simple antacids are the next step in treatment. These work by neutralizing the stomach acid and providing the walls of the gullet with a protective coating. Acid-blocking drugs such as ranitidine may be needed for the most severe symptoms.

See also INDIGESTION and HIATUS HERNIA.

QUESTION

How easy is the diagnosis?
The close relationship to eating normally clinches the diagnosis. Heartburn in older people for the first time can be indistinguishable from angina (see page 43) and doctors may order heart checks.

If you vomit blood or have difficulty in swallowing your doctor will arrange for endoscopy of the gullet in case the symptoms are caused by a growth in the gullet.

 Complementary Treatment
Western herbalism – the following herbs improve digestion and reduce acid production and inflammation: meadowsweet; caraway; dill; aniseed; ginger; chamomile and peppermint. *Other therapies to try: most have something to offer.*

FLATULENCE

◆

A common problem of excess intestinal gas and its consequences.

CAUSES

◆

Gas is formed during the digestion of food: within the large intestine bacteria complete the digestive process with gas as a byproduct. The gas is methane, with a little hydrogen sulphide, nitrogen and carbon dioxide. Eating a high-fibre diet predisposes to excess gas and abdominal distension. Another source of wind, said to be important, is from swallowed air that accumulates within the intestines.

SYMPTOMS

◆

The abdomen feels swollen; relief is obtained by belching and by passing wind through the rectum. People become aware of what appears to be excessive amounts of both – as judged by the reaction of others. General health is normal.

TREATMENT

◆

Reducing the amount of vegetable fibre in the diet helps to relieve the problem of flatus, although reducing too much may lead to **constipation**. It is really a matter of trial and error, eliminating high-fibre foods.

Try to eat without talking, since you may be swallowing large amounts of air unconsciously. In terms of medication, peppermint is a natural deflatulent and aid to digestion; charcoal tablets are used on the basis that charcoal absorbs gases.

Antacids containing alginates reduce stomach wind, limiting the quantity of wind entering the intestines.

 Complementary Treatment
Nutritional therapy – steer clear of pulses, onions and cabbage. Helpful **aromatherapy** oils include peppermint, fennel, chamomile, cardamom and basil. *Other therapies to try: most have something to offer.*

INDIGESTION

Problems from excess acid production, including peptic ulcers.

CAUSES

Indigestion is very common and progresses in only a fraction of cases to ulceration and on to stomach and duodenal ulcers.

The stomach secretes highly concentrated hydrochloric acid, which begins the process of digestion and sterilizes the food. Thick mucus coats the walls of the stomach, protecting it from this acid. Good as this protection is, it commonly breaks down where there are persistently high levels of acid production. Anything that further irritates the lining of the stomach, like alcohol and acidic foods, adds to this. The gullet has less protection against acid, so any acid there causes **heartburn**. Similarly, acid in the duodenum irritates its walls.

For many years the organism *Helicobacter pylori* was thought to be an innocent inhabitant of the stomach and duodenum but it is now recognized as a potent source of gastric irritation, peptic ulcers and possibly even of **stomach cancer**.

Certain drugs irritate the stomach – most commonly anti-inflammatories such as aspirin and ibuprofen – and vary in how irritant they are. Stress, alcohol and smoking all greatly increase the risks of indigestion and peptic ulcers.

SYMPTOMS

At its mildest there is a burning, gnawing sensation in the pit of the stomach. There may be heartburn. The sensation may be provoked or relieved by eating.

Symptoms suggesting a peptic ulcer are more persistent pain, especially one that wakes you at night and seems to gnaw into the back. However, it is now known that the symptoms bear a poor relationship to the severity of the condition. The diagnosis requires endoscopy, a breath test to detect *H. pylori*, which gives off a characteristic gas, or biopsy of an ulcer, which is to exclude malignancy and is one reason why endoscopy has replaced barium studies. Duodenal ulcers are almost certainly benign; a stomach ulcer may be malignant.

If an ulcer erodes through a blood vessel in the lining of the stomach or duodenum, there may be vomiting of blood or the passage of blood in the stools, colouring them jet black. If the bleeding is seen at endoscopy to be slight, treatment with tablets alone will be sufficient. If it is more severe, urgent surgery will be required. Potentially, a peptic ulcer can erode through the stomach or duodenal wall, to become a perforated peptic ulcer. This surgical emergency causes sudden severe upper abdominal pain and peritonitis.

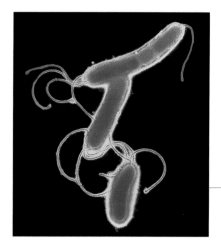

Left: Helicobacter pylori. These common micro-organisms probably cause chronic indigestion, peptic ulcers and possibly some stomach cancers.

It is easy to dismiss the importance of indigestion. The symptoms of stomach cancer exactly mimic it. Anyone over 40 with unusual or persistent indigestion should see a doctor.

TREATMENT

Remedies for mild indigestion neutralize the acidity of the acid, reducing burning. Often they are sufficient. It is essential to reduce smoking, alcohol and **stress**, which is also a factor.

A more efficient way to reduce acid is to block its production with drugs called H2 blockers, such as ranitidine or cimetidine. Newer and even more potent are the rapidly acting proton pump inhibitors like omeprazole and lansoprazole.

There is much research at present looking into the best way of destroying *H. pylori*. Current regimes combine antibiotics (amoxycillin or metronidazole) with a powerful antacid such as omeprazole. Eradicating *H. pylori* cures peptic ulcers.

Surgery is now a rarity for peptic ulcers. It involves severing the vagal nerve, which controls the secretion of acid by the stomach. Surgery is essential for the emergency of a perforated peptic ulcer.

Complementary Treatment

Western herbalism – try peppermint or psyllium. See a **nutritional therapist** or a **naturopath** for dietary advice. **Chiropractic** – mid-upper back pain can come with indigestion; treating the spinal irritation and muscle spasm in the mid-thoracic area with manipulation helps ease pain and settle the indigestion. *Other therapies to try: homeopathy; tai chi/chi kung; chakra balancing; cymatics; hypnotherapy; Ayurveda; acupuncture; Chinese herbalism; auricular therapy.*

BOWEL CANCER

Malignant growths within the intestines are common in the West and are curable if detected early.

CAUSES

The small intestine is where the bulk of digestion takes place; despite its great activity it is unusual to develop cancer here. Cancer is far more common in the large bowel, even though it is a less energetic environment. Most growths arise in the final part of the large bowel, called the descending colon, the rectum and just inside the anus itself.

Bowel cancer, the second most common cancer in the United Kingdom, is rare in Africa and Asia, which suggests that environmental factors are involved. Possibly the Western low-fibre diet means that faeces remain in the large intestine for longer so that any cancer-producing agents in the diet have longer to influence the cells of the bowel wall.

There is a genetic tendency to bowel cancer: people with a close relative who has it have a two to four times increased risk themselves. People with ulcerative colitis (see INFLAMMATORY BOWEL DISEASE) have as much as a 40 times increased chance of bowel cancer once they have had colitis for more than 15 years.

SYMPTOMS

The disease is most common after the age of 60, and is rare below 40 except in the high-risk groups above.

Change of bowel habit is the prime symptom to be aware of, whether it is towards **diarrhoea** or towards **constipation**. Temporary changes of this sort are extremely common; changes lasting more than a couple of weeks need investigating. Bleeding from the bowel is another 'must investigate' symptom, even though there are plenty of benign causes.

Anaemia in an otherwise healthy adult with a good diet is a possible indication of internal bleeding from a silent growth and investigation would be recommended. Other symptoms may include weight loss and abdominal pains, although these are features of more advanced disease.

A rectal examination picks up about one-third of all bowel tumours. Other bowel investigations include checking the stools for traces of blood, sigmoidoscopy, colonoscopy (see page 323) and barium enema (see page 316).

TREATMENT

If caught early, when the cancer is confined to the surface layer of the bowel, bowel cancer is virtually curable – there is a better than 95% 5-year survival. Treatment involves an abdominal operation to cut out the tumour with part of the bowel and to rejoin the healthy bowel. Modern surgical techniques mean that it is now uncommon to need a colostomy, other than as a temporary measure, except for tumours that are sited very close to the anus.

Once the cancer has spread deeper inside the wall of the bowel or into the surrounding tissue, the chances of a cure are less, there being a 30–65% 5-year survival. Radiotherapy and chemotherapy (see pages 338 and 339) are slowly improving these figures, however.

QUESTIONS

Is screening worthwhile?
Evidence is gradually supporting regular screening of people after the age of 50. This is done by testing a stool sample for blood. Some specialists go further, recommending sigmoidoscopy every five to ten years. People at high risk of bowel cancer should have regular colonoscopy of their bowel in order to detect early disease – every three years at least.

What happens with untreated cancer?
It erodes into surrounding tissue, causing pain and bleeding, and may obstruct the bowel. It spreads to the liver, causing liver failure.

Complementary Treatment
See STOMACH CANCER

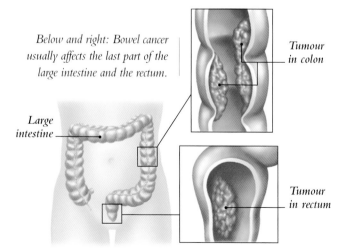

Below and right: Bowel cancer usually affects the last part of the large intestine and the rectum.

Large intestine

Tumour in colon

Tumour in rectum

STOMACH CANCER

A common cancer, although becoming less common worldwide.

CAUSES

Wide international variations in how common stomach cancer is have led to a search for triggers. Diet has been closely studied and factors under suspicion include preservatives in food and alcohol intake. The evidence for these, however, is currently slim and controversial.

There is a hereditary tendency but not as much as with **bowel cancer**. People with type A blood group have a slightly increased risk, as do people with pernicious **anaemia**.

The trigger that has been receiving most attention in recent years is the *Helicobacter pylori* infection. This organism is found in people with gastric irritation; indeed it has become recognized as a major cause of peptic ulcer (see INDIGESTION). Researchers believe that inflammation induced by *H. pylori* increases the risk of malignant change in cells.

SYMPTOMS

Early cancers are silent but eventually there is indigestion and later actual stomach pain. Stomach cancers tend to ooze blood, so that anaemia may be the first symptom of disease. Later in the illness there is persistent pain over the stomach, and loss of appetite and weight.

Indigestion is such a common symptom that it is understandably difficult for a doctor to decide whether or not to investigate. As a rule, an individual over 40 who develops indigestion for the first time or whose indigestion is unusually persistent or intense should have further investigation. The preferred investigation is endoscopy (see page 323) for a thorough inspection of the gullet, stomach and duodenum; samples can be taken from any suspicious areas. Endoscopy is replacing barium meal as the investigation of choice.

TREATMENT

In early disease it is possible to remove the part of the stomach containing the cancer, preserving the function of the rest of the stomach reasonably well. In more advanced disease it is possible to remove the whole stomach (a gastrectomy). This serious and risky operation offers a chance of cure, providing the cancer has not spread outside the stomach, for example to the liver. If cancer has spread it will recur despite gastrectomy, making it hard to justify exposing a patient to risk and discomfort for no gain. Sometimes this decision can only be

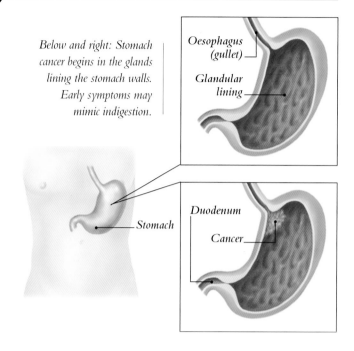

Below and right: Stomach cancer begins in the glands lining the stomach walls. Early symptoms may mimic indigestion.

made after opening the abdomen to explore the cancer.

Even if the cancer is inoperable, surgery can divert the flow of food past the diseased part of the stomach. This gives relief from vomiting and obstruction, which are otherwise such distressing symptoms of advanced disease. Chemotherapy (see page 339) has been found to improve the survival by a few months but at the cost of severe side effects.

The outlook for early stomach cancer is about 90% 5-year survival; this falls to about 30% in people who have more advanced disease but where surgery still appears justified. Overall, there is a 10% 5-year survival, which is a grim outlook. For this reason many surgeons advocate aggressive investigation of older people who have symptoms that are suggestive of early stomach cancer.

      Complementary Treatment

No complementary therapy can cure cancer, but many have a role during orthodox treatment. **Chakra balancing** will help with symptom control, energy balance and relaxation, and offer support during rehabilitation programmes. **Reflexology** can offer support during orthodox treatment. **Aromatherapy**, especially when linked with **massage**, can be excellent at lessening the stress and tension associated with disease. Diet – a **naturopath** or **nutritional therapist** should be consulted. *Other therapies to try: see* STRESS.

INFLAMMATORY BOWEL DISEASE

Illnesses that are characterized by pain, diarrhoea and bleeding from the lining of the intestines.

CAUSES

The two recognized forms of inflammatory bowel disease are Crohn's disease and ulcerative colitis. Crohn's disease can affect any part of the digestive tract from the mouth to the anus; ulcerative colitis affects only the large intestine. Some specialists believe that these are related diseases differing in severity. It is possible that both are caused by an auto-immune condition. Many sufferers lead mainly normal lives in between flare-ups, although severe flare-ups are potentially dangerous. Life expectancy is little affected by ulcerative colitis, whereas people with Crohn's disease are twice as likely as the general population to die prematurely.

Crohn's disease

Crohn's disease has become more common during the 20th century, leading to a search for a causative factor such as a virus. Currently the measles virus is suspected but there is no definite proof. There is a strong family tendency in white racial groups, less so in black groups. It is four to six times more common in smokers, whereas smoking appears to have a protective effect against ulcerative colitis. The peak incidence is between 20 and 40 years of age.

Ulcerative colitis

Ulcerative colitis is also more common in families and certain racial groups, for example Jews. Smokers are half as likely to get the condition. (See LUNG CANCER, however, for the great dangers of smoking.)

SYMPTOMS

Abdominal pains and **diarrhoea** are prominent features of both conditions, although these tend to be worse in ulcerative colitis. Bleeding and the passage of mucus with diarrhoea are particular symptoms of ulcerative colitis. In both diseases there are periods of ill health, weight loss and **anaemia** interspersed with remissions when you feel quite normal. People may also have inflammation of their joints and eyes.

The diagnosis is confirmed by blood tests, which show inflammation, and by colonoscopy whereby the bowel can be inspected and biopsies taken. As Crohn's disease can extend outside the large intestine, barium studies are useful to show the extent of the condition (see page 316).

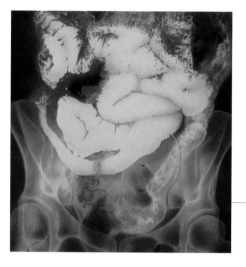

Left: A barium enema of the intestines. The narrow intestine on the left is typical of Crohn's disease.

TREATMENT

In acute attacks antidiarrhoea compounds such as loperamide or codeine are needed, plus steroids to reduce inflammation and drugs like mesalazine or salazopyrin to reduce overall bowel inflammation. Disease confined to the rectum can be treated with enemas containing steroids. People can become very ill very quickly through dehydration, bleeding and the bowel rupturing, so hospital treatment is often needed. Many people find that taking mesalazine or similar daily reduces the frequency and severity of the condition. Such drugs are more effective for ulcerative colitis than for Crohn's disease.

Surgery is avoided if possible because the bowel does not heal well, but it may be a last resort for severe persistent ulcerative colitis. The whole large bowel and rectum are removed, leaving an ileostomy – a bag worn on the abdomen into which the small intestine empties. For Crohn's disease it may suffice to cut out areas of localized disease.

Ulcerative colitis has a greatly increased risk of **bowel cancer** after 15–20 years, so that regular screening is advisable.

Complementary Treatment

      Useful **acupuncture** points are Stomach 25, on the abdomen, and Stomach 36, below the knee. In **Chinese herbalism** helpful herbs include *Dang Shen* and *Bai Zhu*, both part of the formula called *Si Jun Zi Tang* (four noble formulae.) **Chakra balancing** can help reduce inflammation of the gut and aid healing of the gut wall surface. Diet – consult a **naturopath** or **nutritional therapist**. *Other therapies you could try: homeopathy; healing; shiatsu-do; chiropractic.*

IRRITABLE BOWEL SYNDROME

A blanket term for many abdominal disturbances for which no other cause can be found.

CAUSES

There are no agreed causes for the condition of irritable bowel. The general medical thinking is that it is a disorder of the system that controls mobility of the bowel – the nerve layer within the walls of the bowel that makes the muscle of the bowel contract.

Many sufferers appear to be under **stress**, if not definitely suffering **depression**. Since irritable bowel syndrome is what is wrong with the majority of patients seen by gastroenterologists worldwide, it is unlikely that some simple cause such as candida has been overlooked. More likely it is a non-specific, humble part of the human condition.

SYMPTOMS

Most people with irritable bowel are young women. The core symptoms are recurrent abdominal pains, often with minor changes in bowel habit from **constipation** to **diarrhoea**. A consistent finding is that pain is relieved by defecation and made worse by stress. There is a feeling of abdominal distension and bloating. The motions may be pellet-like and individuals need to keep opening their bowels.

The symptoms are experienced for months, if not years, despite which the individual looks well, does not lose weight and there are no abnormalities to be found on examination apart from non-specific abdominal tenderness.

TREATMENT

It is important to have some basic investigations, not only to exclude other disease, but to reassure individuals that their symptoms are being taken seriously, since no one doubts that they do experience pain.

The main differential diagnosis is **inflammatory bowel disease**; in such cases the individual usually feels ill and loses weight. Investigations involve blood tests, which show inflammation, and sigmoidoscopy to inspect the lower bowel and perhaps take biopsies from the bowel wall.

The older the individual the more extensive the testing, as the risk of cancer grows, but with average individuals in their teens or twenties the diagnosis can be made with reasonable confidence and minimal investigations.

Treating the condition can be difficult. For many people simple reassurance is enough. Others might try more or less fibre in their diet. Numerous drugs, for example mebeverine, are said to relax the muscles of the bowel; some people derive benefit from such drugs, others do not. Recently, specialists have been subdividing irritable bowel into separate syndromes, which may lead to more focused treatment. If there are symptoms of depression or stress a course of anti-depressants can be helpful.

One of the pitfalls with the condition, of which surgeons are well aware, is to indulge in ever more extensive investigations. Their reluctance to do more should not be interpreted as being uncaring; operations carry hazards and can lead to abdominal pains themselves. With reassurance many people find the condition decreases over a few years.

SYMPTOMS TO BE TAKEN SERIOUSLY

The following symptoms should be taken seriously, even if a diagnosis of irritable bowel syndrome has previously been given. (Possible diagnoses are given in brackets – these are not fully comprehensive.)

♦ *Abdominal pain unrelieved for more than about six hours, especially if accompanied by fever, loss of appetite and vomiting (peritonitis)*
♦ *Abdominal pain with the passage of blood or mucus from the rectum (inflammatory bowel disease below the age of 40, cancer of the bowel above 40)*
♦ *Lower abdominal pain after missing a period or having an unusual period (ectopic pregnancy)*
♦ *Pain with fever, vaginal discharge (pelvic inflammatory disease)*
♦ *Abdominal pain accompanied by weight loss (inflammatory bowel disease, cancer)*

Complementary Treatment

Diet – consult a **nutritional therapist** or **naturopath**. **Auricular therapy** relieves anxiety and regulates digestion, in conjunction with dietary changes following traditional Chinese principles. **Chiropractic** can help if the condition is accompanied by low back pain. **Ayurveda** offers oral preparations, *panchakarma* detoxification, yoga meditation and *marma* therapy. *Other therapies to try: homeopathy; tai chi/chi kung; cymatics; hypnotherapy; acupuncture; Chinese and Western herbalism; autogenic training; chakra balancing.*

LIVER PROBLEMS

◆

Disease of the liver caused mostly by infection, alcohol and cancers.

CAUSES
◆

The largest internal organ of the body, the liver is a power-house of activity. It is a storage site for glucose, the fuel of the body, and can synthesize it rapidly if stores are insufficient. It makes bile, later kept in the gall bladder. Bile is necessary for the absorption of fat from food. The liver also makes the fats needed for cell metabolism, including triglycerides and cho-lesterol. The bulk of protein synthesis takes place in the liver and, crucially, it makes the proteins needed for blood clotting such as fibrinogen.

Also, the liver contains cells that catch and destroy bacteria and viruses from the intestine and so prevent them gaining access to the rest of the body. Lastly, the liver inactivates many hormones once they have done their jobs and this caretaking function extends to the destruction of drugs, alcohol and old blood cells. These are the main source of the pigment biliru-bin, which is responsible for the jaundice of liver disease and which eventually makes the motions and urine brown.

With its huge blood supply and never-ending activity, it is to be expected that the liver is prone to disease. Many infections and drugs cause temporary effects on the liver, which may be felt simply as a vague discomfort over the liver or detected on monitoring of liver function blood tests.

Infections

Many infections, including the common **glandular fever** virus, cause a mild hepatitis – inflammation of the liver. Some spe-cific viruses cause a more severe hepatitis. New hepatitis viruses are occasionally discovered and now range from A to G. Some are acquired through pure chance; others such as B and C are transmitted by sexual contact (especially male homosexual activity) in semen or saliva or through blood products and intravenous drug abuse. Internationally, hepati-tis B is a huge cause of chronic hepatitis, cirrhosis and liver cancer, affecting hundreds of millions of people mainly in the Far East and Africa. It carries a one per cent risk of death from liver failure and a permanent risk of future cirrhosis (up to fifty per cent) and liver cancer. Mothers positive for hepati-tis B almost always pass on the virus to their unborn baby.

Alcohol, drugs and immune conditions

These can all lead to cirrhosis of the liver. Cirrhosis is a degen-eration of the active cells of the liver, being replaced by fibrous tissue, which is of course non-functioning. Although

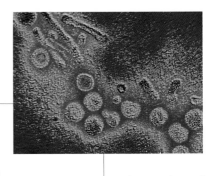

Above: A cluster of the viruses that cause hepatitis B. After invading cells, they reproduce in enormous numbers.

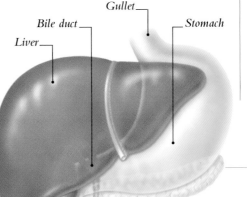

Gullet

Bile duct

Stomach

Liver

Pancreas

Gallbladder

Duodenum

Left: The liver occupies the right upper abdomen. It is vital for digestion, blood formation and handling toxins.

early cirrhosis may be reversible, established cirrhosis is per-manent. In the case of paracetamol poisoning the effects may be fatal rapidly. Chronic cirrhosis is a risk for people regularly drinking more than about 30 units of alcohol per week, i.e. 15 pints of beer or 5 bottles of wine.

Tumours

In the West the majority of tumours within the liver have spread there via the rich blood supply from cancers else-where, especially bowel tumours. This so-called secondary liver cancer is often the way in which people with cancer finally die. Worldwide, primary cancer of the liver is common and often follows previous infection with the hepatitis B virus.

SYMPTOMS
◆

Viral infections produce hepatitis of rapid onset. There is an incubation period from the time of infection with the virus. In the case of the common hepatitis A this is two to three weeks; in the cases of hepatitis B, four to twenty weeks. There is a week or so of nausea, vague ill health, **fever** and upper abdominal discomfort, after which the individual becomes jaundiced (yellow) from the deposit of pigments that the liver would ordinarily handle. In most cases the illness settles over another week or so. It is rare for people suffering from hepatitis A to have other problems.

Alcohol, drugs, immune conditions and tumours

The immediate effects on the liver of a serious drug or alcohol overdose are nausea, jaundice and itching, followed by bleeding because blood-clotting factors are no longer being made. As toxins build up in the blood stream there may be confusion and a slide into unconsciousness.

Chronic poisoning has more subtle and widespread effects. Itching is common and there may be a hint of jaundice. Men notice breast development and may suffer from impotence (see ERECTILE DYSFUNCTION) because female hormones normally broken down by the liver are at higher than usual levels. The palms become red – also related to female hormones.

Tiny dilated veins appear on the hands, face and chest, called spider naevi. As the cirrhosis worsens, there is accumulation of fluid in the abdomen called ascites and in the ankles. There is a risk of bleeding, leading to widespread bruising and possibly bleeding into the gullet. Eventually the liver fails, with increasing jaundice, confusion, then unconsciousness.

Means used to confirm and measure liver disease are blood tests of the chemicals produced by the liver and markers of any viruses responsible. An ultrasound scan (see page 317) can show typical features of cirrhosis. A liver biopsy (see page 321) is the best way of establishing the exact diagnosis.

TREATMENT

♦

Acute liver damage is usually due to viral infection or drug damage, especially overdose of paracetamol. The drug itself is neutralized by biochemical means in a drip. Patients then have to be nursed in intensive care, receiving correction of the widespread biochemical changes in the blood stream that accompany acute liver failure. They need infusion of clotting factors to prevent internal bleeding and measures to reduce swelling of the brain, which is the main reason for death. Liver transplantation may be the final hope (see below).

Acute liver failure is a very serious condition, with a high mortality rate even in the best centres. If the liver disease is caused by spread of a cancer, there is little that can be done other than general supportive care.

Chronic damage (cirrhosis)

You must stop any behaviour contributing to the cirrhosis, i.e. give up alcohol. This will not reverse the changes in the liver, but will reduce the load it has to bear. Outlook is poor: a 50% 5-year survival. A major risk from chronic cirrhosis is bleeding from dilated veins in the gullet called oesophageal varices, which may bleed torrentially and need emergency repair.

Liver transplantation

This now offers hope to those facing inevitable liver failure, from many causes. It is not suitable in cases of liver failure caused by spread of cancer, which will invariably spread into the new liver, but it can be done in cases of people with primary liver cancer.

The risk from the actual surgery is low; the major risk is from rejection of the liver. The results now offer a remarkable 90% survival to 1 year and better than 70% 5-year survival, figures that are improving all the time. (See also page 331.)

QUESTIONS

What is a dangerous dose of paracetamol?
As little as 10 g (20 standard tablets) can be enough to cause serious liver damage. Just 15 g (30 tablets) can be a fatal dose. Urgent treatment is needed within hours of a suspected overdose.

What vaccination is there against hepatitis?
Hepatitis A vaccination is for travellers who might eat shellfish and poorly washed salads, and protects for up to ten years. Vaccination against hepatitis B is for healthcare workers who face exposure to contaminated blood, needles and body fluids.

Are women's livers weaker?
They have to handle the breakdown of the female hormone oestrogen, and therefore have less capacity to cope with alcohol or drugs.

 ### Complementary Treatment

No complementary therapies can prevent or cure hepatitis in its various forms. **Chinese herbalism** can be very helpful, but note a reputable practitioner will insist on regular blood tests to monitor liver function. **Shiatsu-do** strengthens the blood quality through improved organ functioning and toxin discharge. In **nutritional therapy** the liver is considered to be stressed by an excess of saturated fat in the diet; a number of foods and herbs could be used to help drain these fats, for example beetroot and dandelion. **Hypnotherapy** – anxiety interrupts the free flow of enzymes; hypnotherapy can lessen anxiety, and hence help reduce problems. **Ayurveda** – liver tonics and special preparations for inflammatory liver disease are available; detoxification is an essential part of healing. *Other therapies to try: acupuncture; tai chi/chi kung.*

GALLSTONES

Greasy stones within the gall bladder, sometimes causing pain.

CAUSES

Gallstones form within the gall bladder as a result of precipitation of cholesterol and bile salts from the bile. Women are twice as likely as men to get them, but in later life there is a roughly equal chance of gallstones.

Most bile is formed by the liver from cholesterol. It mixes with yellow and green pigments derived from the breakdown within the liver of old blood cells. Bile makes fat soluble, which is an important step in the absorption of fat from the intestinal tract. The liver secretes a remarkable 1 litre/1¼ pints a day of bile, half of which is stored temporarily in the gall bladder, the rest going directly into the duodenum via a network of ducts from the liver.

There are a few rare conditions where an excessive load of bile pigments increases the risk of gallstones, for example certain types of **anaemia**. Gallstones are extremely common: ten to twenty per cent of the adult population have them, and only a fraction cause symptoms.

SYMPTOMS

Many gallstones are silent. They lie within the gall bladder and are simply a chance finding on investigation for other abdominal symptoms.

A stone obstructing the gall bladder causes severe upper right-sided abdominal pain, which comes and goes in waves as strong muscular contractions try to overcome the obstruction. Other classic symptoms are mild intermittent pain under the right ribs, which is worse after eating – especially after fatty foods because fat in the diet provokes a reflex contraction of the gall bladder. The pain is from partial obstruction of the flow of bile from the gall bladder into the duodenum.

If there is complete obstruction, infection of the gall bladder invariably results after 24 hours, causing **fever** and jaundice (see LIVER PROBLEMS).

TREATMENT

Fewer than 20% of silent gallstones will cause problems, even over 15 years, and treatment is unnecessary. By contrast if you are getting pains, most surgeons recommend removal because there is a much higher chance of eventual obstruction.

During an acute attack, you will need powerful analgesics to deaden the pain until the gallstone falls away from the bile

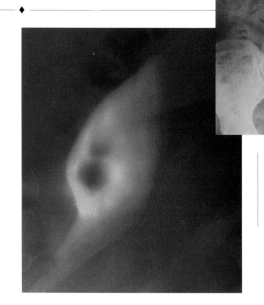

Gallstones are seen as dark shadows under the ribs (above) and in X-ray (left).

duct. This usually takes a few hours. If there is infection an antibiotic is given. Mild episodes of pain can be left to settle themselves. Meanwhile the diagnosis is confirmed by an ultrasound scan (see page 317) of the gall bladder, showing stones.

Surgical opinion differs as to whether to remove the gall bladder immediately the acute attack has settled or to defer surgery for a few months. Both attitudes are widespread.

Dissolving gallstones was popular when drugs for this were first found. It takes up to two years of continuous treatment with a fifty per cent chance of recurrence once treatment is stopped, so they are rarely used now that surgery is so safe.

Surgery for gallstones

The usual procedure is laparoscopic removal of the gall bladder (see page 340). Occasionally the older-type operation has to be performed, which involves a long incision under the ribs and from which it takes several weeks to recover.

Gallstones lodged in the duct between the gall bladder and duodenum can be removed by endoscopy (see page 323).

Complementary Treatment

Diet – gallstones are linked with the consumption of too much fat and sugar; a **nutritional therapist** or **naturopath** will be able to provide a diet programme. **Chakra balancing** helps reduce pain attacks and supports orthodox therapies; postoperatively it aids relaxation and promotes healing of wounds. **Hypnotherapy** can lessen anxiety and so promote the free flow of enzymes, reducing problems. *Other therapies to try: tai chi/chi kung; see also* STRESS.

GASTROINTESTINAL ALLERGY

Adverse reaction to certain foods, although the conventional view is that true gastrointestinal allergy is rare.

CAUSES

It is a matter of common experience that certain foods make other conditions worse, for example **eczema**, **asthma** and migraine (see HEADACHES AND MIGRAINE). Beyond that, the subject is bedevilled by lack of agreement as to what else constitutes a reaction and the possible mechanisms whereby the food alleged to be responsible has that effect.

Certain people clearly experience a true allergic reaction; others have more of an intolerance of certain foods. Acute gastroenteritis with **diarrhoea** leaves the lining of the intestine unable to handle the absorption of milk for a few days and the resulting persistent diarrhoea can be misinterpreted as allergy.

Coeliac disease is a true allergic reaction to gluten in the diet. Allergy to peanuts has for unknown reasons become more common in recent years. Other substances identified as possible causes of gastrointestinal allergy are tyramine in cheese, tartrazine (a food additive), egg protein and histamine in strawberries. The widespread concern about E numbers has not been scientifically substantiated.

SYMPTOMS

There may be a true allergic reaction: within minutes there is a blotchy skin rash, tingling in the mouth, swelling of the lips and throat and wheezing. At its most severe there may be collapse through a fall in blood pressure, called anaphylaxis.

Food intolerance would be suspected by the appearance within hours or days of diarrhoea, bloating, or a worsening of asthma or of eczema. The diagnosis is supported by showing regular and repeated reactions to the foods in question. Individuals can be tested by exposure to dilute samples of the foods to which they might be intolerant.

A child who is suspected of cow's milk or lactose intolerance with accompanying poor growth and diarrhoea should show catch-up growth and loss of bowel symptoms when a substitute is given. Lactose intolerance can also happen in adults, causing diarrhoea and **flatulence**.

There is no scientifically proven link between the many other symptoms, such as headaches and behavioural disturbances, that people complain of and true sensitivity to certain foods. For example, in double-blind trials individuals have unknowingly had foods they say they are allergic to, yet they have not shown the expected reaction.

TREATMENT

Where there is a definite association with a particular food, avoid the offending substance. The more severe the reaction the more scrupulously this must be done, for example people with an acute anaphylactic reaction to eggs or nuts must be obsessive about avoiding them. Such people should wear a bracelet with medical details. There are self-injection devices containing adrenaline for immediate treatment. Lesser degrees of allergy are treated with antihistamine tablets or steroids for stronger reactions.

There is little orthodox medical support for diets that exclude a wide range of common foods on the basis that they cause arthritis, malaise, tiredness, hyperactivity and so on.

QUESTIONS

What is an exclusion diet?
It is a very simple diet with just a few foods. The idea is to see whether symptoms disappear, then to introduce a single food from fortnight to fortnight until one provokes the symptoms.

What is wrong with this?
Few people manage to do it properly for the many weeks that are necessary. The interpretation is difficult as the symptoms are often vague and not easily objectively assessed. Extreme exclusion diets may not be nutritionally complete if followed for long periods.

Are other tests available?
Blood tests may show abnormal reactions, but their interpretation is controversial. Scientific studies of hair analysis and many other complementary and alternative procedures do not support the faith some therapists have in them.

Complementary Treatment

A registered **homeopath** could greatly reduce, or even eradicate, your food sensitivity. **Nutritional therapy** can help you identify food intolerance; if you have multiple allergies they could be linked to toxic overload and you will need to undertake work to improve your bowel, liver and digestive system. **Hypnotherapy** can be used in conjunction with a desensitizing programme. **Ayurveda** treats gastrointestinal allergy through detoxification, and oral preparations and *marma* therapy are also important.

COELIAC DISEASE

A hypersensitivity to gluten leading to destruction of the food-absorbing surface of the small intestine.

CAUSES

Coeliac disease is an allergy to gluten, a protein found in most cereals, but principally wheat and rye. The disease was confirmed in The Netherlands during the starvation conditions of the Second World War. The health of certain children improved because bread was scarce and they were therefore no longer exposed to gluten.

The surface of the lining of the small intestine is made of innumerable finger-like outgrowths called villi, which greatly increase the surface area for absorption of food. Gluten makes these villi disappear, leading to malabsorption of food.

SYMPTOMS

In children there is failure to grow, which coincides with the introduction of cereals. Adults, usually women, become tired, and have abdominal pains and **diarrhoea**. On investigation there is **anaemia** and often **mouth ulcers**. The diagnosis is confirmed by taking a biopsy of the small intestine through an endoscope (see pages 321 and 323).

TREATMENT

Gluten is excluded from the diet and replaced by any of the wide range of gluten-free foods now available. Within three to four months the surface of the small intestine will have recovered. This gluten-free diet has to be lifelong.

QUESTION

How common is coeliac disease?
Rare in non-Caucasians, the disease affects one in fifteen hundred to two thousand of a Caucasian population. In some areas it is far more common, for example affecting one in three hundred Irish people. There is a strong family association, suggesting a genetic tendency. However, the exact mechanism whereby gluten affects the villi is not known.

Complementary Treatment
Nutritional therapists use a number of products to help heal the gut. **Naturopathy** is helpful. *Other therapies to try: acupuncture; Chinese and Western herbalism.*

ANAL FISSURE

A tear of the back passage, usually through straining.

CAUSES

The anus is held closed by muscular tissue, which distends to allow motions out of the rectum. Passing a large hard motion may be too much, with the result that the canal tears. Recurrent or multiple tears may be caused through bowel disease, in particular Crohn's disease (see INFLAMMATORY BOWEL DISEASE).

SYMPTOMS

There is pain after passing a large motion and bleeding is visible on cleaning. The pain recurs each time the bowels are opened. The tear can be seen as a raw area in the anus and it is extremely tender if the doctor examining it attempts to pass a finger inside the rectum.

TREATMENT

Small tears are common and heal spontaneously, maybe with an anaesthetic gel to reduce pain on defecation. It is important to keep the motions soft with a bulk-forming laxative.

Large tears that show no signs of healing are dealt with by dilating the anus under anaesthetic. This reduces the extent to which the fissure stretches on defecation, and so allows it to heal over a couple of weeks. It is unusual to have to resort to more than this, but it may be necessary to stitch up a chronic fissure. Never ignore rectal bleeding, although benign causes are common.

Complementary Treatment
Nutritional therapy would reccomend boosting fibre intake and adding natural laxatives to your diet for a while until regular bowel habits are established. These include linseed products and blackstrap molasses.

HAEMORRHOIDS

Swollen veins, popularly known as piles, are the most common cause of bleeding from the back passage.

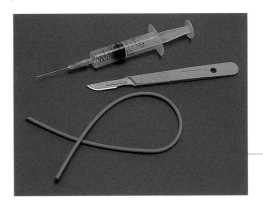

Left: Injections, scalpel and rubber band – all are treatments for haemorrhoids.

CAUSES

There are two types, internal and external piles. The causes are the same. External piles are visible as swellings around the back passage and can be felt. They are veins that have become dilated and varicose, similar to varicose veins on the legs. Internal piles are a little more complicated. They are pillars of cushioning tissue supporting the rectum and cannot usually be felt unless they prolapse (drop) through the anus.

Anything that increases the pressure of blood within the abdomen increases the chances of piles, for example spending much time standing, pregnancy (see PREGNANCY PROBLEMS) and chronic **constipation** with accompanying straining.

Piles are more often a nuisance than anything else, unless they prolapse. When this happens to internal piles the piles become trapped by the muscles of the anus and remain as large painful swellings that cannot be pushed back inside. External piles can thrombose – meaning that the blood inside them clots.

SYMPTOMS

Often there is slight discomfort around the back passage, itching and occasional bleeding after defecation. Prolapsed piles are felt and seen as large tender swellings at the anus.

TREATMENT

Mild piles are common and cause little by way of symptoms. Even though they occasionally prolapse they are easily pushed back inside. No treatment is needed apart from avoiding constipation and straining, by increasing fibre and fluid intake. It may be possible to spend less time standing. Piles appearing during pregnancy will go after birth.

If the pile has prolapsed and is tender, treatment is with painkillers and creams containing a local anaesthetic rubbed into the pile. It will shrink over a few days. Occasionally, a pile causes so much pain that a surgeon will need to cut it open to let out the blood, but this does prolong the healing process.

Various treatments for piles that give recurrent problems all cause the blood to clot inside the pile, which will then shrink away. Piles can be burnt, gripped with tough rubber bands, frozen or injected. Whatever is done, piles tend to recur after a few years and haemorrhoidectomy, offering a good chance

of permanent cure, may be necessary. This involves cutting a portion of the rectal lining, taking the pile with it. The operation has a reputation for being painful, as has the first opening of the bowels afterwards. Good anaesthetic technique avoids this by blocking the pain nerves at the time of surgery.

QUESTIONS

Should I worry that I often get bleeding from piles?
It is tempting to ascribe rectal bleeding to piles. While this is safe in young people with obvious piles, older people should have further checks to exclude other causes of bleeding.

Are piles dangerous?
Theoretically there is a risk of anaemia through constant blood loss but this is very unusual unless significant bleeding is neglected.

Is there any harm in self-treatment?
If you know you have piles and if the symptoms are familiar, there is little harm. The older you are the more seriously you should take any change in the amount or pattern of bleeding or discomfort.

Complementary Treatment

Homeopathy – paeonia ointment for external piles, or paeonia suppositories for internal piles. **Chakra balancing** aids pain control and healing; the relaxation effect eases defecation. **Aromatherapy** – try a daily sitz bath with one of the following oils (six drops): cypress, chamomile, lavender. A **nutritional therapist** would suggest boosting your fibre intake. **Ayurveda** – oral preparations are given, plus dietary advice. **Yoga** is especially helpful, together with pelvic floor exercises. *Other therapies to try: shiatsu-do.*

DIVERTICULAR DISEASE

Weakening of muscle of the walls of the large intestine, allowing the formation of small stagnant pockets.

CAUSES

This appears to be a disease of the West, almost certainly caused by a lack of fibre in the diet. The theory is that high fibre leads to bulky, soft stools, which are expelled by the colon with little effort, whereas the small hard stools of a low-fibre diet require strong muscular effort for the same result.

The walls of the large intestine contain muscle which does the propelling and churning of the faecal material, prior to defecation. Under pressure, the wall weakens and a pouch may form. It is more common in older people because the walls of the colon naturally weaken with age.

Most people over the age of 50 have a few of these pouches of just 1 cm/½ in diameter. In diverticulitis there are dozens if not hundreds. For much of the time these diverticulae are asymptomatic. They are a potentially stagnant area – if faeces lodge in them it is only a matter of time before infection occurs, when symptoms and possible complications arise.

SYMPTOMS

Few with diverticular disease have symptoms. Mild effects may be pains in the left lower abdomen of a colicky nature that come and go over a few hours, and there may be rectal bleeding. These symptoms are from mild irritation of diverticulae. If there is a serious infection, then there is much more pain plus **fever**. The lower left side of the abdomen is tender.

Considering how common the condition is complications are rare. One is peritonitis with very severe stomach pains and collapse. This only happens if one of the diverticulae has burst (perforated), allowing faeces to spill into the abdomen, and is

a surgical emergency. The other complication is obstruction with colicky pains, vomiting and loss of bowel action.

A barium enema shows up the diverticulae (see page 316); symptoms should also be investigated by sigmoidoscopy and colonoscopy (see page 323) as this is the same age group risk as for **bowel cancer** and the symptoms can be very similar.

TREATMENT

Mild attacks need only painkillers and an antibiotic. Once the diagnosis is established, doctors recommend a high-fibre diet and an antispasmodic such as mebeverine to relieve any occasional colicky pains. Usually nothing more is necessary. Only in patients with severe and persistent problems is it necessary to remove the diseased portion of colon – a colectomy.

In cases of sudden severe pain hospital admission may be necessary for intravenous antibiotics and to exclude obstruction or the dangerous complication of perforation and peritonitis, needing emergency surgery.

QUESTIONS

Diverticulitis/diverticular disease – what are they?
Diverticular disease means simply having multiple diverticulae, but without experiencing symptoms, the condition being discovered while investigating other abdominal symptoms such as rectal bleeding. Diverticulitis is inflammation of one of those diverticulae, giving rise to symptoms as above.

What are the risks?
It is estimated that of the 50% of over 50s who have it, only 10% will get any symptoms at all and only 1% will run into serious complications requiring surgery or intensive treatment. Asymptomatic disease is best left alone.

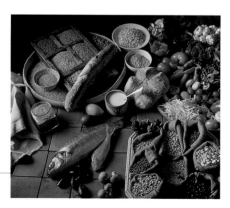

Right: High-fibre foods protect against constipation and therefore diverticular disease.

Complementary Treatment

Diet – consult a **nutritional therapist** or **naturopath**. Useful **acupuncture** points are Stomach 25, on the abdomen, and Stomach 36, below the knee. **Chinese herbalism** remedies include *Dang Shen* and *Bai Zhu*. If the condition is accompanied by low back pain, **chiropractic** can help. **Ayurveda** – *panchakarma* detoxification, oil laxatives and enemas are used, often with oral medicines. *Other therapies to try: chakra balancing; Western herbalism; homeopathy.*

PANCREATITIS

Inflammation of the pancreatic gland, which is always serious.

CAUSES

The pancreas lies behind the stomach at the back of the abdomen. It secretes insulin, which is of fundamental importance in the handling of glucose. It also secretes pancreatic enzymes into the small intestine which are important in digesting protein and fat. These are powerful juices; the seriousness of pancreatitis lies in the fact that the release of these juices leads to auto-digestion of whatever they come into contact with, for example the lining of the abdomen, the liver, the intestines and other internal organs. Pancreatitis is divided into acute and chronic.

Acute pancreatitis

Sudden inflammation of the pancreas is thought to be related to liver or gall bladder problems. This may be because the ducts through which pancreatic juices flow lie close to these structures and become blocked or irritated by bile. A few drugs can cause pancreatitis and it can be a rare consequence of viral infections including **mumps**.

Chronic pancreatitis

This is nearly always associated with alcoholic liver disease (see LIVER PROBLEMS), when the pancreatic gland becomes converted to fibrous tissue.

SYMPTOMS

In the case of acute pancreatitis the illness begins with upper abdominal pain, which appears to radiate into the back. It is impossible at this stage to distinguish it from the condition of severe **indigestion** without investigations. The pain may be mild but persistent or it may be excruciating, accompanied by collapse of blood pressure and nausea, and so severe that peritonitis is suspected.

The diagnosis is very difficult to make without measuring enzymes released by the inflamed pancreas into the blood stream. The most useful one is amylase, which should be measured in all cases of severe upper abdominal pain.

Chronic pancreatitis is characterized by recurrent upper abdominal pain in a heavy drinker (see ALCOHOL AND ALCOHOLISM). As the gland deteriorates there is weight loss because the juices are no longer available to digest food. **Diabetes** develops through lack of insulin. The diagnosis is difficult to make without a CT scan (see page 318).

TREATMENT

Acute pancreatitis is a very dangerous condition, with mortality at best one per cent, and in severe cases fifty per cent or higher. Treatment is with drip feeding to maintain blood pressure and energetic treatment of any internal infections, which are common. Sometimes fluid-filled cysts within the abdomen need be surgically drained. Recovery takes weeks or months.

To treat chronic pancreatitis, it is essential that the individual stops drinking alcohol to avoid further progression of the disease, although this will not reverse the damage done. Diabetes is treated with insulin, drugs or diet depending on how bad it is. Capsules are available containing the digestive enzymes no longer being produced by the pancreas. Painkillers are needed for persistent pain, which can also be helped by surgically removing diseased parts of the pancreas. The pain of chronic pancreatitis can be intense – a painkiller as strong as morphine may be required at times. The outlook is quite good as long as the individual gives up alcohol.

QUESTIONS

Is pancreatitis related to cancer of the pancreas?
There is no evidence for this; cancer of the pancreas is steadily increasing in frequency for unknown reasons, but there has been no such increase in the incidence of pancreatitis.

How risky are gallstones?
Considering how common gallstones are (see page 186) – affecting 20% of an adult population – very few actually cause pancreatitis. However, anyone with gallstones who has even mild pancreatitis would be well advised to have the gall bladder removed as soon as possible. Investigations for gallstones are routine in anyone presenting with pancreatitis.

Complementary Treatment

Acute pancreatitis is a medical emergency, and should be treated by a conventional practitioner. **Chakra balancing** helps reduce pain attacks and supports orthodox treatment; postoperatively it aids relaxation and promotes healing of wounds. **Cymatics** could help for chronic, long-term pancreatitis. You should use all means of support to give up alcohol, and **hypnotherapy** can have a role here, too. *Other therapies to try: see ALCOHOL AND ALCOHOLISM.*

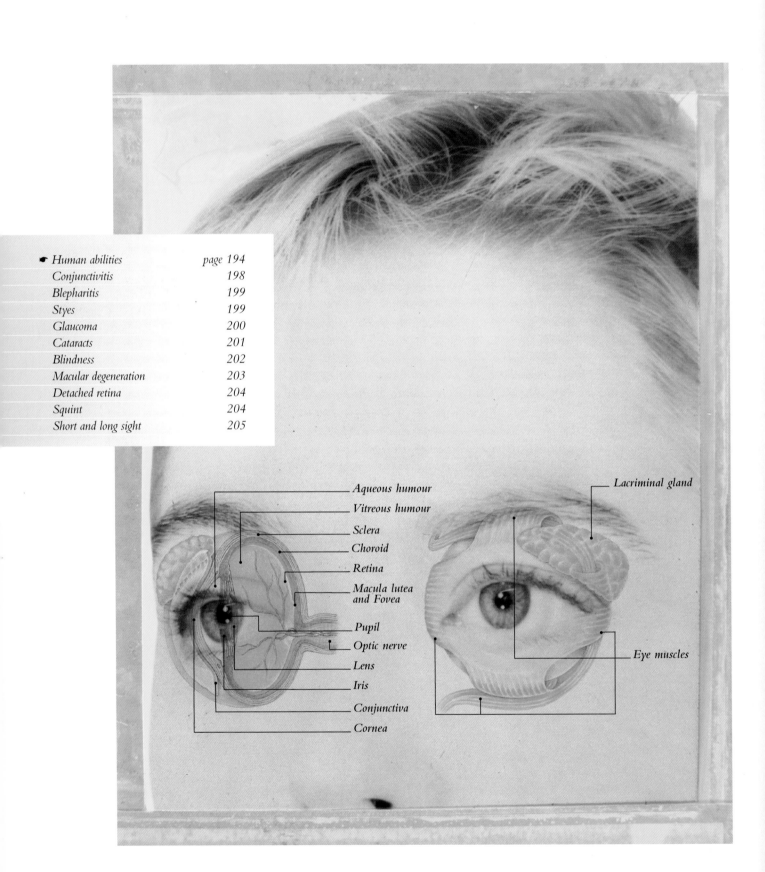

Aqueous humour

Vitreous humour

Sclera

Choroid

Retina

Macula lutea and Fovea

Pupil

Optic nerve

Lens

Iris

Conjunctiva

Cornea

Lacriminal gland

Eye muscles

The visual system is rightly seen as one of the wonders of the human body. As more is known about it, our sense of astonishment grows at its complexity. But eyes are fragile organs, subject to disorders and injuries that can cause the loss or curtailment of vision. This makes their care vital.

EYES

THE EYES ORIGINATE as outgrowths from the brain, and are specialized to detect light. Each is a fluid-filled globe of intricate design. Light enters through the transparent cornea; it strikes the lens, which focuses light on to the retina, the light-sensitive surface at the back of the eye. From there electrical signals leave via the optic nerve which goes to the brain.

The retina

Within the retina there are two types of receptor called rods and cones – this refers to their shape. Each receptor is a single cell that contains a pigment that reacts to light by firing an electrical impulse. The pigment in the rods is called rhodopsin and is derived from vitamin A.

Rods give black and white vision. Bright light reduces the amount of rhodopsin in the rods: when you go into the dark it takes 20 minutes for quantities of rhodopsin to rise to a maximum. This explains why it takes time for eyes to adapt to the dark. The fully dark-adapted eye is about 100,000 times more sensitive to light than the light-adapted eye.

Cones are responsible for colour vision and for detailed vision. It is believed that there are three types of cone, each one containing pigments that respond best to a particular colour. Colour vision is the result of the integration of the output of all three types of cone.

Each eye contains about 120 million rods and 6 million cones. The electrical output flows through nerve cells within the retina, which begin the process of analysing vision by sharpening up the output from the receptors. However, the great bulk of analysis of information takes place in the brain by processes that are still far from well understood. There are specialized collections of cells that deal with visual output all the way from where the optic nerves enter the brain to the visual cortex, which is at the back of the brain. Some centres appear to coordinate eye movements, while others seem to deal with the interpretation of images.

Other parts of the eye

The eye contains many structures other than the retina, although all structures are designed to maintain efficient vision. The cornea is crystal clear; there are no blood vessels in it. Its cells are unique because they gain their nutrition and oxygen from the fluid beneath them. The lens is a semi-liquid structure surrounded by muscles that change its shape and so alter the focus of light. The amount of light entering the eye is varied by the iris, which is another sheet of muscle; the pupils are the aperture through the iris. The surface of the eyes is bathed constantly by tears, which are antiseptic. Six muscles control the movements of each eyeball.

Eye problems

Most eye problems result from degeneration with age of the structures of the eye, especially the lens – causing **cataracts**, and the retina – causing **macular degeneration**. The increased pressure of fluid within the eye causes **glaucoma**. The eyes and eyelids are prone to infections and allergies.

Left: No computers can yet remotely match how eyes and brain interpret patterns of light.

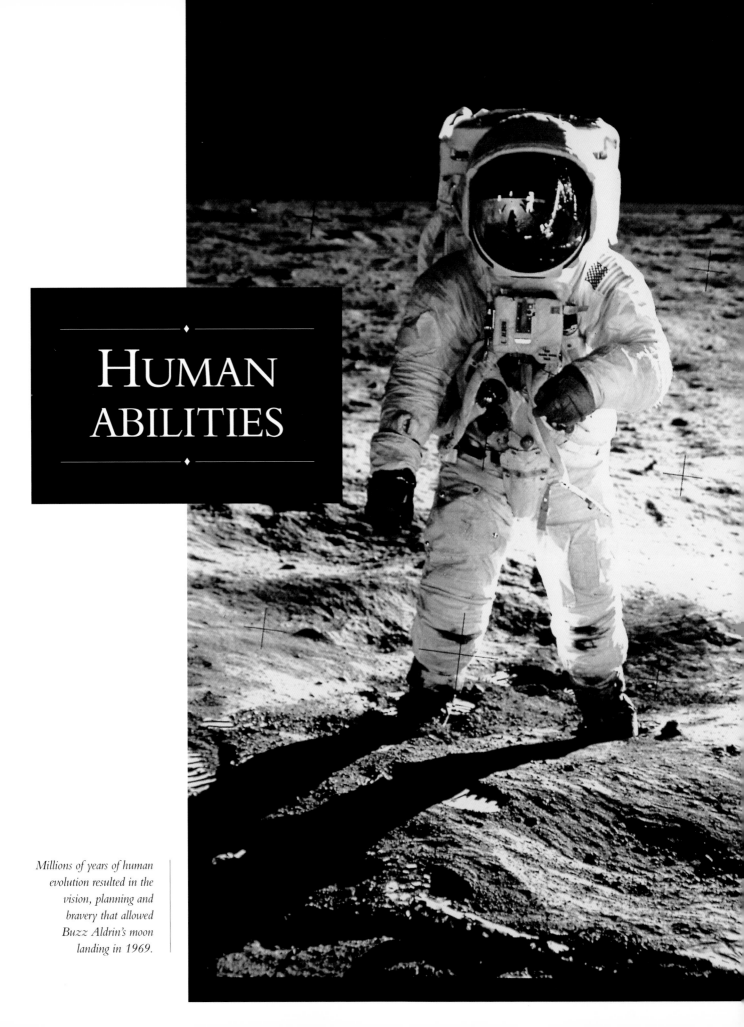

HUMAN ABILITIES

Millions of years of human evolution resulted in the vision, planning and bravery that allowed Buzz Aldrin's moon landing in 1969.

W E HUMANS ARE NOT the most distinguished when it comes to physical abilities. A rabbit can outrun us, a flea (proportional to size) can outjump us, and a monkey can out-shriek us. What we do have in our favour is exceptional brain capacity and powers of understanding. As a result we can use our intellectual abilities to outwit our would-be predators and to dominate our environment.

The senses

Vision The eye detects light with extraordinary efficiency, all the more remarkable since only ten per cent reaches the light-sensitive retina. The rest is lost in passage through the eye. More remarkable again, the light receptors face away from the incoming light as a quirk of the evolutionary development of the eye. In its most sensitive parts there are 150,000 colour-detecting cones per mm^2 of retina and 160,000 rods.

Night vision is 100,000 times more sensitive than day vision, although it lacks the capability of discerning colour and fine detail. It takes 20 minutes for the eyes to adapt fully to the dark, by which time they can detect just a few photons of light energy as a flash. The fully dilated pupil lets 32 times more light into the eye than when constricted.

The eyes can detect shifts of position with impressive accuracy – an object moving a few centimetres/inches can be seen from a distance of 1.6 km/1 mile.

The brain analyses the signals from the eyes and this is how we learn to recognize things under different conditions of light and position. So important is this that ten per cent of the brain is devoted to processing information from the eyes.

Our eyes produce a binocular, stereoscopic image of what we see, because when we look at something the image falls on approximately the same part of each eye. However, this reduces our field of vision. Many animals and insects have eyes that each see a different scene, giving the impression of having eyes at the back of the head – and some almost do.

The skin The skin contains nerve receptors that detect temperatures up to 45°C/113°F and down to 10°C/50°F. Pain is recorded by nerve endings scattered through the skin and internal organs, although there are none in the brain itself. Touch varies greatly over the body. On sensitive regions such as the fingertips you can distinguish between objects just 2 mm/$^1/_{16}$ in apart, whereas on the back of the hand they must be 50 mm/2 in apart before they are identifiable as more than one object. The fingertips can detect vibration of as little as one ten-millionth of a metre.

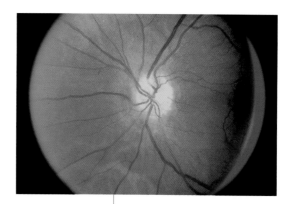

Above: The retina of the eye. Blood vessels and the optic nerve emerge from the yellowish optic cup.

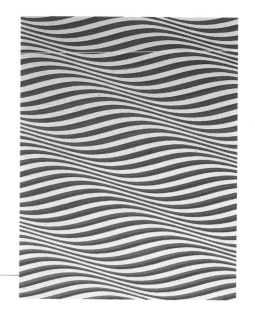

Right: Optical illusions make the brain misinterpret visual information. Here, flat wavy lines give the illusion of three-dimensional depth.

Smell and taste Specialized cells in the nose transmit straight to the brain, into a system also involved with emotions. Humans can detect up to ten thousand different smells, sometimes recognizing just one single molecule of an odour. One of the smelliest substances is mercaptan, a sulphurous compound smelling of sewage and rotting fish, which is detectable at just one part in over four hundred million parts of air.

Taste alone detects only sweet, bitter, salt and sour, relying on smell for all the subtleties. This is why you lose your sense of taste when you have a cold.

Hearing The human ear detects sounds in the range of 20–20,000 waves per second, sometimes higher. The quietest detectable sound moves the eardrum by just one-millionth of a millimetre. The trained ear can tell the difference in sounds that differ by just 0.3% in frequency (pitch) and can detect the loudness of sounds from barely audible to sounds billions of times louder. We can tell where sound comes from: by analysing the difference in the way a sound strikes both ears, we can tell the direction of sounds to within a few degrees.

Thought

A Japanese man has memorized Pi to forty thousand places, which he can recite. Others can calculate multi-digit numbers in seconds. These feats seem extraordinary, but remember that we nearly all pick up language with its complex rules and tens of thousands of words and most of us can recognize thousands of different objects instantly.

Structure Neurones are nerve cells that run from the spinal cord and brain around the body. They transmit impulses along an axon, which is like an electrical wire, to other cells. The shortest axons are under 1 mm/³/₆₄ in, the longest over 1 m/39 in. Electrical current flows at between 1 m/3¹/₄ ft per second, for example in the fibres which make the pupil contract, to 100 m/328 ft per second in the knee-jerk reflex. The electrical flow depends on chemical pumps in the cell wall, which exchange electrically charged atoms – ions – of sodium and potassium. A typical neurone has a million of these pumps; nerves may fire up to 300 electrical impulses per second, the pumps exchanging 200 million ions per second.

Jumping gaps Nerves meet at junctions called synapses, or on muscles at end plates. How does electricity jump that gap? Nearly always it is by chemical transmission with minute globules of a transmitter. Some ten thousand are released with each signal down the nerve; they cross the gap in about ¹/₂₀₀₀ of a second, setting off the electrical wave in the next fibre. Many drugs work by affecting transmitters.

The average brain weighs 1.3–1.6 kg/3–3¹/₂ lb. This is about two per cent of total body weight, but it gets twenty per cent of the heart's output of blood. The brain contains a hundred thousand million neurones with billions of additional supporting cells. You are born with all the neurones you will ever have. From the time of birth ten thousand a day die – two hundred and fifty million over a seventy-year lifetime. It sounds enormous, yet that still leaves you with over 99.9% of all those you began with.

The number of interconnections is beyond comprehension – about a hundred million million. It is within these interconnections that we experience emotion, thought and memory, expressed as electrical brain waves at a frequency of 4–25 cycles per second.

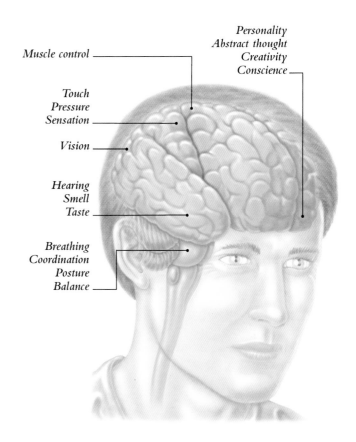

Muscle control

Touch
Pressure
Sensation

Vision

Hearing
Smell
Taste

Breathing
Coordination
Posture
Balance

Personality
Abstract thought
Creativity
Conscience

Above: A very general map of the brain showing where it handles various senses, activities and abilities.

Circulation

At rest, the heart pumps 5 litres/8 pints of blood every minute through an estimated 96,500 km/60,000 miles of blood vessels, comprising arteries, veins and capillaries. The total surface area for exchange of blood and fluid in an adult is 2600 km²/1000 sq miles.

In each cubic millimetre of blood there are over 5 million red blood cells, thousands of white cells and 250,000–450,000 platelets for blood clotting, quite apart from a horde of biochemicals, hormones, proteins, cholesterol, fats and glucose. Every second 2.5 million new red blood cells are released from the bone marrow, replacing a similar number that are destroyed or damaged.

Per day the heart pumps 7000–8000 litres/12,300–14,000 pints, which increases greatly on exertion. Normally 20% of blood flow goes to the brain, 25% to the intestines and liver, 20% through the muscles and 4% through the heart itself. The rate of blood flow to the heart increases fivefold during exercise.

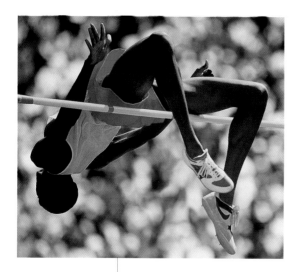

Above: A purely human feat – a demanding, unnatural target, elegantly achieved through sheer determination. Right: The competitive urge spurs us on.

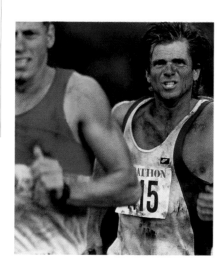

Exercise and muscles

During heavy exertion the heart beats harder and faster, increasing the flow of blood to 25 litres/44 pints per minute. The heart gets a fivefold increase, but blood flow to the main muscles increases by 20 times. Most of the increased output is through the heart beating faster but there is a limit to this, which decreases with age. Regular exercise increases the volume the heart can pump with each beat, which is why trained athletes can pump high volumes of blood without having very high heart rates.

Muscles Muscles comprise thousands of muscle fibres, organized into bundles that are controlled by nerve fibres.

How do muscles move? The process is very complex and not entirely certain but seems to involve the ultra-rapid formation of chemical bridges between proteins within muscle fibres that pull one strand of protein along another, so shortening the muscle fibre. This movement is triggered by the electrical activity of the nerves.

WHAT GOES IN TO THE BODY AND WHAT COMES OUT

◆

What goes in . . .

◆ *Adults need 1200–5000 calories of energy a day, depending on the physical work they do. An average is 2000–2800 calories*

◆ *At rest you need 250 ml per minute of oxygen, obtained by breathing 6 litres per minute of air. On exertion this increases to 100–200 litres of air per minute, absorbed through 40–80 m²/430–860 sq ft of lung surface*

◆ *Your kidneys filter the whole blood volume every 40 minutes, equivalent to filtering 180 litres/315 pints of blood a day*

◆ *You digest food with 7–9 litres/12–16 pints a day of saliva and digestive juices, passing through 4 m/13 ft of short intestine and 1.5 m/5 ft of large intestine, totalling 200 m²/2150 sq ft of absorptive surface*

◆ *You need about 150 g/5 oz a day of carbohydrate, 80 g/3 oz of fat, 40–50 g/1½–1¾ oz of protein and minute amounts of vitamins and minerals*

◆ *You have over seven billion billion defensive cells ready to act against invading germs*

What comes out . . .

◆ *You use energy at the rate of 2–10 calories a minute. A brisk walk uses 5 calories a minute, gardening 6, aerobic dancing 6.5, jogging 10 and competitive football 15*

◆ *You expend this energy via some 600 muscles acting on some 206 bones*

◆ *You produce 1.5 litres/2¾ pints of urine a day on average but this can be varied from 23 litres/40 pints a day to just 400 ml/14 fl oz a day depending on fluid intake and loss through sweating. Your bladder can hold 700–800 ml/1¼–1½ pints of fluid. You produce 200 ml/7 fl oz of fluid a day in motions*

◆ *Other fluid is lost through the lungs and the 19,350 cm²/3000 sq in of skin*

◆ *Your eye muscles move 100,000 times a day*

◆ *You have more thoughts, plans and dreams than we can possibly measure*

CONJUNCTIVITIS

Inflammation of the eyes as a result of an infection or allergy.

CAUSES

An inflammation of the outer surface of the eye, conjunctivitis may be bacterial, viral or allergic, or caused by a foreign body. Bacterial infections are common in children and often spread rapidly in schools and nurseries. They also occur after a foreign body – even a speck of dust – gets into the eyes. Babies often have sticky eyes after birth, having been infected via the birth canal. Viral conjunctivitis often arises in local outbreaks. It is resistant to standard antibiotics but is often self-limiting.

An allergy and an infection produce a similar appearance in the eye – the clue is the seasonal nature of the redness and its persistence. Sources of allergy are pollens, fumes and dust (see HAY FEVER).

SYMPTOMS

The eyes feel prickly and uncomfortable. Redness then spreads over the whites of the eyes as a result of the dilation of normally invisible blood vessels. The greatest redness is at the eye's margins – this pattern is important in confirming diagnosis. Redness concentrated around the iris of the eye (the coloured portion) may be due to different diseases – iritis or an ulcer on the cornea. A yellow or green discharge sticks the eyelids together, which have to be gently bathed open.

Viral conjunctivitis causes similar symptoms but lasts for weeks rather than the few days of bacterial infection. Allergic conjunctivitis leads to persistent irritation as well as redness. The eyes stream tears and the person keeps sneezing or has a persistent runny nose. In all types of conjunctivitis the under surface of the eyelids, seen by flicking down the eyelid, is red and inflamed. In allergic conjunctivitis the under surface has many small cysts that give a 'cobblestoned' appearance.

TREATMENT

Tears contain a natural antiseptic that cures most minor infections within a day or two. Where there is a lot of discharge and redness, an antibiotic is used in the form of drops or an ointment. Drops need to be used four to six times a day, ointments two to four times a day – the choice is a matter of personal preference and convenience. Drops are easier for treating children, because they are simply dripped on to the eyelids and allowed to soak through on to the eyeball.

Viral conjunctivitis will not respond to antibiotic drops and

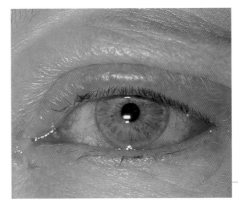

Left: In conjunctivitis, the redness gets worse further away from the iris.

will take several weeks to settle down. Treatment for allergic conjunctivitis depends on its severity and the associated symptoms. Use antiallergic eye drops or ointments such as cromoglycate three to five times a day. Try an antihistamine first; it is often enough to relieve itching and redness as well as any other symptoms of hay fever. The sticky eyes in newborn babies respond to bathing with salt water or antibiotic drops; a swab should be taken first to confirm diagnosis.

WARNING SIGNS ABOUT RED EYES

Seek medical opinion if, as well as redness, the following occurs:
- *Only one eye is red*
- *The redness is concentrated around the coloured part of the eye*
- *There is blurred vision*
- *The eye feels painful, rather than itchy*
- *The redness follows any injury to the eye*
- *There is profuse watering of the eye and light irritates intensely*

Such features could indicate iritis, an ulcer of the cornea, injury of the cornea or glaucoma.

Complementary Treatment

WARNING: Never use aromatherapy oils near the eyes. **Western** and **Chinese herbalism** – anti-inflammatory herbs can supplement, not replace, orthodox treatments. **Homeopathy** – make an eyewash using a level teaspoon of salt and ten drops of euphrasia mother tincture in 300 ml/½ pint boiled, cooled water. **Nutritional therapy** – zinc supplements may help; seek advice. **Ayurveda** – try herbal eyewashes and drops. *Other therapies to try: acupuncture; chakra balancing.*

BLEPHARITIS

Inflammation at the roots of the eyelashes that spreads into the eyelids.

CAUSES

Blepharitis is caused by infections that enter the eyelids through the base of the eyelashes. It can occur at all ages and the condition can become chronic.

People who have **eczema** and dandruff may get blepharitis, because of their general skin sensitivity. Any cosmetic preparations that reach the eyelids, for example moisturizing creams, perfumes and nail varnish may cause eczematous blepharitis, but people with eczema may get blepharitis without any obvious irritant. Similarly, blepharitis can be caused by an allergic reaction to eye make-up or skin preparations. However, often the cause is obscure.

SYMPTOMS

The edges of the eyelids are swollen, red, scaly and itchy. There may be crusting of the eyelids but, unlike **conjunctivitis**, this crusting tends to spare the eyes themselves. They are rarely affected and are therefore neither red nor sticky. There may be eczema elsewhere – dry, irritant flaking skin and scalp, or dandruff. In severe cases small ulcers may develop at the root of the eyelashes and the lashes may fall out.

TREATMENT

Work antibiotic eye drops or ointments into the eyelashes. For severe infection an antibiotic is given by mouth. If the cause is eczema, it can be very hard to treat. Consider irritants that have transferred to the lids; mild steroid creams on the lids should cure the condition. If there is dandruff, the blepharitis may be helped by using an antidandruff shampoo on the scalp.

Good eyelid hygiene is important. Clean the eyelids twice daily with a cotton-wool bud and warm water to remove all crusts, especially before applying any ointment. Removing the crusts reduces the risk of reinfection.

 Complementary Treatment
WARNING: Never use aromatherapy oils near the eyes. **Homeopathy** – bathe your eyes with saline solution and lightly apply calendula ointment. *Other therapies to try: Western and Chinese herbalism; nutritional therapy; naturopathy; chakra balancing; Ayurveda.*

STYES

Infections of eyelash roots, similar to skin infections elsewhere.

CAUSES

Eyelash roots are a convenient entrance site for bacteria, as are any hair-bearing parts of the body. The bacteria proliferate into a small abscess called a stye, which people often get as a result of rubbing at their irritated eyelids.

SYMPTOMS

The base of one eyelash feels uncomfortable. In a few hours it swells into a visible abscess with a yellow head on it; the lid is often a little swollen, too.

TREATMENT

Pull out the eyelash to allow the pus to drain. Antibiotic eye drops or eye ointment help deal with the infection, as does irrigating the eye with salty water. The great majority of styes settle with this treatment within three to five days. Only very occasionally does the infection spread deeper within the eyelid, causing greater swelling. In these cases an antibiotic by mouth is required.

QUESTION

Are styes infectious?
They are only mildly infectious and much less so than conjunctivitis. Thorough and regular handwashing greatly reduces the risk of spreading the infection.

 Complementary Treatment
WARNING: Never use aromatherapy oils near the eyes. **Bach flower remedies** – try a dilution of crab apple and Rescue Remedy in water, or apply Rescue Remedy to the affected area as a cream. *Other therapies to try: homeopathy; chakra balancing; naturopathy.*

GLAUCOMA

Raised pressure of fluid within the eye that affects vision and can end in blindness. It occurs in one per cent of the population.

CAUSES

There is a circulation of fluid, called aqueous humour, within the eyes, between the cornea and the lens. This fluid is continually being produced and normally drains through channels at the edge of the iris – the coloured portion of the eye. In many people this drainage system deteriorates with age, ultimately resulting in increased pressure of fluid. This is chronic glaucoma. Acute glaucoma is a type of glaucoma where the drainage is abruptly obstructed, causing sudden symptoms; fortunately acute glaucoma is rare.

Glaucoma affects vision by damaging the optic nerve where it leaves the back of the eyeball. This causes a loss of the outer (peripheral) field of vision. Unless it is treated, deterioration continues until blindness occurs.

People who use steroid eye drops for long periods of time may develop glaucoma. Some drugs, for example anti-depressants and certain drugs prescribed for **Parkinson's disease,** worsen pre-existing glaucoma by widening the iris, thereby reducing drainage of fluid. There is also a strong family tendency to glaucoma.

SYMPTOMS

Early glaucoma does not produce any noticeable symptoms. Even though peripheral vision is being lost, the brain compensates as long as central vision remains good. However, at night, when pupils are dilated to a maximum, fluid drainage is reduced. People may notice haloes around lights and there may be slight discomfort in the eye.

Acute glaucoma causes dramatic symptoms – sudden blindness or extremely hazy vision, the eyeball is intensely painful and red and the normally clear cornea becomes cloudy. Increased pressure within the eyeball makes it feel very hard.

Screening

The best way to detect early glaucoma is with regular tests of the field of vision using special charts. There is a screening test where air is directed at the eyeball, depressing it briefly; pressure within the eye is calculated from the degree of depression. A more accurate measure is by applying a pressure gauge to the eyeball under local anaesthetic. Glaucoma causes characteristic appearances at the back of the eye as seen through an ophthalmoscope.

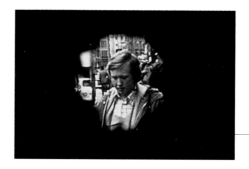

Left: Tunnel vision in advanced glaucoma. Outer vision has been lost.

TREATMENT

Chronic glaucoma is controlled with eye drops that reduce the pressure within the eye. Some drugs reduce the rate of production of the aqueous humour fluid, thereby keeping pressure low. Other drugs keep the pupil constricted and drainage at a maximum. Similar treatment is used for acute glaucoma, with higher doses and sometimes using drugs taken by mouth. When surgery is required, it involves cutting the edge of the iris with a small scalpel or laser to improve drainage.

QUESTIONS

When should people be screened?
If you have a close relative (for instance a parent or a sibling) with glaucoma you should be screened every three years from the age of forty onwards – the condition runs in families. Everyone else should see their optician for an eye check specifically for glaucoma when they reach sixty.

Can glaucoma be cured?
There is no permanent cure for glaucoma, but drugs can help to control the condition. Even after surgery you will need to see an ophthalmologist regularly.

 Complementary Treatment
WARNING: Never use aromatherapy oils near the eyes. Acute glaucoma is a medical emergency – see your doctor immediately. Complementary therapies provide options for long-term glaucoma. A **nutritional therapist** might recommend cutting down on protein and/or supplementing vitamins A, B_1 and C, and the minerals chromium and zinc. *Other therapies to try: homeopathy; reflexology; naturopathy; yoga.*

CATARACTS

❖

The normally clear lens of the eye becomes opaque, causing hazy and indistinct vision. It affects 20% of people by the age of 60.

CAUSES

Light passes through the cornea, lens and fluid in the eyes with great efficiency, but eventually the clarity of the lens deteriorates. Exposure to daylight over many decades may be the main cause of the condition, probably because ultraviolet light changes the protein within the lens.

Diabetics are at greater risk of cataracts, developing them ten to fifteen years earlier than otherwise expected (see DIABETES). Those who take steroids by mouth, for example for **rheumatoid arthritis**, run a significant risk – perhaps up to 75% – of developing cataracts. They should be checked regularly by a doctor to detect cataracts early.

Injury that has penetrated to the lens will leave scarring. There are a few rare congenital or biochemical causes of cataracts that might be suspected if cataracts appear at an unusually early age.

SYMPTOMS

The effect of a cataract is similar to looking through frosted glass. Light is scattered so that the edges of objects look blurred. Bright light causes a glare and objects are indistinct unless brought very close to the eyes, and even then may be fuzzy. As well as loss of clarity there is deterioration of colour vision, which again can be reproduced by looking through frosted glass. Lesser degrees of cataract can be indicated by a non-specific change in vision and difficulties with close work. Changing the prescription of glasses makes no difference.

Cataracts seen through an ophthalmoscope appear as a white opacity to the bright light. The usual tests of visual acuity will show how much vision has been affected in order to judge how urgently surgery might be required.

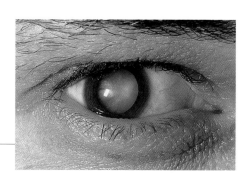

Right: An advanced cataract. The lens is hazy and white, vision is greatly reduced.

TREATMENT

❖

Cataract surgery is a highly developed and delicate branch of ophthalmology that can, in most cases, restore good vision. Surgery involves removing the opaque lens, usually by very fine dissection, from its attachments. Increasingly, surgeons do this by a technique that liquefies the lens so it can be sucked out, causing less disruption to surrounding structures. An artificial lens is replaced within the capsule that contained the natural lens (a lens implant).

Unlike the natural lens, which can of course vary focus, the replacement lens is a fixed focus. Therefore you may need glasses in order to deal with distant or close vision, but you will notice that your overall vision will be restored to its normal clarity and normal colour.

Cataract surgery is a relatively safe procedure that is usually done under local anaesthetic. Any surgery carries a risk of infection or bleeding. For this reason, if you have cataracts in both eyes, surgeons will normally defer dealing with the second eye until after full recovery from the first operation.

QUESTIONS

What are 'ripe cataracts'?
This was a term that meant cataracts bad enough to justify surgery and the heavy cataract glasses that were inevitably necessary following surgery.

Will I need thick-lensed glasses?
These date from when cataract surgery removed the lens and did not replace it. Therefore the only way to achieve focusing was by using very thick lenses. Thanks to lens implants, these type of glasses are now rarely required.

Complementary Treatment

WARNING: Never use aromatherapy oils near the eyes. Eye surgery is the only effective treatment for cataracts, although complementary therapies do play a supportive role. **Chakra balancing** – there is evidence that cataracts may become less opaque for a few days following treatment but this is not yet proven. **Nutritional therapy** – boosting the intake of antioxidant vitamins (A, C and E) can aid prevention. **Yoga** and **massage** are both therapies that are beneficial postoperatively. *Other therapies to try: see STRESS.*

BLINDNESS

While some loss of vision is fairly common, complete loss of vision is relatively unusual.

CAUSES

Blindness can result from disease anywhere along the visual pathways from the eyes to the brain. Causes therefore include not only diseases of the eyes but brain disorders as well.

Retinal damage
Most blindness in the developed world results from damage to the retina, which is the light-receiving surface at the back of the eye. This is a densely packed structure where specialized light receptors – the rods and cones – react to light. Much of the initial processing of information takes place in complex nerve interconnections within the retina that begin the recognition of shape, movement and position. The retina needs a good blood supply to function, and interference with it underlies much acquired blindness.

The major causes of blindness are **glaucoma**, diabetic eye disease (see DIABETES) and **macular degeneration**. These all affect blood supply to the critical receptors through disease of the blood vessels.

Trauma
Direct injury to the eye will cause blindness if it damages the lens or destroys the eyeball. This includes **detached retina**.

Brain disease
The information from the eyes reaches the brain through the optic nerve and is finally analysed in specialized regions of the brain. A **stroke** may damage some of those fibres. This is unlikely to produce total blindness but it can destroy part of the field of vision. A tumour of the pituitary gland also causes gradual loss of part of the field of vision.

Other causes
Other important causes are parasite infection of the eye and deficiency of vitamin A, required to make the visual receptors.

SYMPTOMS

Abrupt blindness is immediately recognized but a slower onset blindness can be easily overlooked. This is especially true if only one eye is affected because the brain compensates. This happens with glaucoma, diabetic eye disease and also a slow-growing **brain tumour**.

Blindness after a stroke typically affects only part of the field of vision – one-half or one-quarter – and this too can be overlooked unless specifically tested for. This is done by measuring the whole field of vision with special charts.

The reflexes of the pupils of the eye and the appearance of the back of the eye viewed through an ophthalmoscope give some clue as to the likely cause of blindness.

TREATMENT

Emergency treatment may help when the cause is a detached retina or blockage of blood flow to the retina. Blindness as a result of strokes in the brain cannot be treated but there is a high probability of improvement with time and as the brain compensates. The treatment of trauma, brain tumours and parasitic infections varies from case to case. Early treatment is essential for glaucoma and diabetic eye changes to reduce the risk of deteriorating vision.

QUESTIONS

How common is blindness?
In the United Kingdom about 140,000 people are registered totally blind; many more are registered as severely visually impaired. Such individuals can often cope well if they are given input from specialized advisers. Similar percentages of blindness apply elsewhere in the developed world.

When can temporary blindness occur?
Migraine can cause loss of vision, usually in one eye, accompanied by headache and nausea. Vision returns after an hour or two. Sudden painless loss of vision that recovers within hours is almost certainly due to a stroke. Since this may herald a larger stroke, it is important to have an urgent medical assessment.

Complementary Treatment
WARNING: Never use aromatherapy oils near the eyes. No specific therapy is recommended as treatment, but some can ease the stress associated with increasing blindness and help you come to terms with your deteriorating vision – **aromatherapy massage** to the body can be beneficial in promoting positive acceptance; **arts therapies**, **chakra balancing**, **healing** and **hypnotherapy** also have a role here. *Other therapies to try: see STRESS.*

MACULAR DEGENERATION

Progressively poor vision due to disease of the fovea, the most light-sensitive part of the retina.

CAUSES

The whole of the retina is a light-sensing surface, the most sensitive part of which is the fovea. This is a tiny pit in the retina, which is surrounded by a reddish area called the macula. Macular degeneration is caused by disease of the fovea and the surrounding macula.

Within each fovea there are only about 4,000 cones, but each one is individually wired into the optic nerve. This makes the fovea the area of the most precise vision and with the highest visual acuity. Paradoxically, this part of the eye is the least sensitive to light and needs bright light to work properly.

So important is the fovea that it has its own dedicated blood supply. Age is the usual reason for the blood supply to degenerate, through leakages or blockages. This leads to the death of a number of cones which are irreplaceable. Age-related macular degeneration may run in families.

Conditions that weaken blood vessels increase the risk of macular degeneration. The most common one is **diabetes**, the other is **high blood pressure**.

SYMPTOMS

There is usually a gradual loss of visual acuity – the sharpness and clarity of vision. This cannot be corrected by new prescription glasses, because the problem is not one of focusing light but rather of the light receptor itself.

Vision outside the macula is unaffected so you can still walk along a crowded street or take in a whole visual scene. Awareness of movement at the corner of the eye also remains efficient because this does not rely on the macula. However, as soon as you try to focus on something there is difficulty, because you are focusing light on to the macula.

A way of demonstrating retinal changes is with fluorescein angiography, where fluorescent dye is injected into a vein and photographed passing through the retina. Blood vessels show up as bright strands and the circulation around the macula is visible. (Leaking vessels can be treated by laser – see below.)

TREATMENT

It is not possible to restore blood flow to the macula once it has been damaged. Efforts have to be directed instead at preventing poor blood flow in the first place.

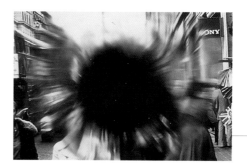

Left: Macular degeneration affects central vision but peripheral vision remains normal.

Because there are no warning signs with macular degeneration, it is vital for diabetics to have annual eye checks in order to see whether diseased blood vessels are encroaching on the macula. If this is so, it can be arrested with laser treatment. This entails placing a very precise burn directly on to the diseased blood vessel that is threatening the macula.

People with macular degeneration should have treatment for any high blood pressure and also stop smoking, since both of these increase the risks of progression of the condition.

QUESTIONS

I have been diagnosed with macular degeneration; will it make me blind?
Rest assured that this will not happen, because you will still retain all the rest of the retina outside the fovea. However, you will find that you will have problems in fine work and in reading.

How can I best cope with this condition?
It is important to have good light for reading and also magnifying devices. Over time you will learn how to look at things slightly off centre so that the image is focused off the macula and on to a part of the retina which still has efficient vision.

Complementary Treatment

WARNING: Never use aromatherapy oils near the eyes, although **aromatherapy massage** to the body can be beneficial. You must follow the advice and treatment programme put forward by your orthodox practitioners. Complementary therapies have a supportive role. **Hellerwork** relaxes the facial muscles and helps to reduce eyestrain. **Chakra balancing** has a deep relaxation effect and rebalances energy. *Other therapies to try: see* STRESS.

DETACHED RETINA

Occurs when the retina loses its adherence to the back of the eye.

CAUSES

The retina – the light-sensitive inner layer – rests on the back of the eye and is mainly held in place by the pressure of fluid in the eye. The usual reason for detachment is a hole in the retina through which the fluid of the eye enters and forces the retina off the back of the eye. Short-sighted people are at greater risk of holes, because their retina is thinner.

A sudden blow to the head could also detach the retina and it is a recognized hazard of bungee jumping and boxing.

SYMPTOMS

When the retina becomes detached, you see flashing lights as it tears away from the eyeball. People talk of a curtain falling across part of their field of vision; the remaining vision is distorted because of ripples in the retina. Detachment is often preceded by an increased numbers of 'floaters', those otherwise innocent objects that drift across the field of vision and are in fact cells shed into the fluid of the eye.

TREATMENT

A detached retina is a surgical emergency: the retina will need to be repositioned on the back of the eye by an operation. Early treatment has a high chance of success.

QUESTION

How quickly should a detached retina be dealt with?
Unless reattached within hours, the detached part of the retina will suffer irreversible damage from lack of blood supply. Therefore seek an urgent opinion if you experience flashing lights or sudden distortion of vision. The unaffected eye will need careful assessment, as there is an increased risk of detachment on this side as well.

Complementary Treatment

Seek immediate orthodox treatment. Complementary treatment is not appropriate for a detached retina but post-operatively any stress-reducing therapy could help you to overcome the trauma.

SQUINT

Imbalance of the muscles that move the eyeballs, leading to misalignment. The condition runs in families.

CAUSES

Each eye is moved by six muscles that swivel it in all directions. Squint happens if, through an imbalance of muscles, one eye fails to move precisely in line with the other. The other main cause of squint is poor vision in one eye as the brain will tend to favour the better focused eye.

Temporary squints are normal in newborn babies but after three months they should be taken seriously, as should a newly appearing squint which may signal brain or eye disease.

SYMPTOMS

One eye turns in or out more than the other and does not move in coordination with the other. Double vision is rare.

Gross squints are obvious, but minor squints are difficult to quantify without specialist assessment.

TREATMENT

Children do not grow out of a squint, and if the condition is left untreated, the vision will be permanently affected.

If the cause is poor vision, the good eye is patched (covered over) and glasses are worn to correct the weaker eye. Patching forces the brain to accept signals from the poorer eye and to learn to control its muscles better. If the cause of squint is muscle imbalance, this can be corrected by surgically shortening or lengthening the muscles responsible.

Squints occurring in adults will need to be investigated for a brain disorder. Any double vision will require special glasses or surgery.

Complementary Treatment

WARNING: Never use aromatherapy oils near the eyes. **Hellerwork** will help to relax the facial muscles and reduce eyestrain. There is some evidence of the power of traditional Chinese medicine but more research needs to be done in this area.

SHORT AND LONG SIGHT

Variations in the shape of the eyeball are the cause of these extremely common problems.

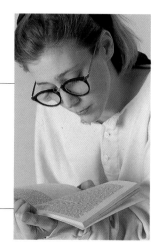

Right: Glasses can effectively compensate for changes in the focusing ability of the eyes.

CAUSES

The eyeball is a slightly elongated globe, the size of which should match the focusing power of the lens. Ideally the lens of the eye will focus light precisely on the retina, regardless of the distance of the object being looked at. It does this by using muscles that alter the thickness of the lens and therefore its focusing power.

In the case of long sight the eyeball is slightly too short. Despite maximum power the lens cannot focus objects on the retina; the point of focus actually lies behind the eyeball.

Short sight, or myopia, is where the eyeball is too long, so that light is focused in front of the retina except when objects are held very close to the eye. In both cases the lens mechanism of the eye tries to compensate as best as possible.

The focusing ability of the eye changes over time, as the lens becomes less elastic. This is illustrated by measuring the near point of vision: the closest position on which the eye can focus. At age eight this is about 8 cm/3 in, by age twenty this is 10 cm/4 in, and by age sixty, 83 cm/33 in. This is why children can read with the book pressed up to their face while their parents, anxious to know if this is normal, have to consult their book of child development at arm's length!

SYMPTOMS

The vision is blurred looking either at distant or close objects (myopia or long sight respectively). There may be discomfort in the eyes as well as headaches, through overwork of the muscles in the eye that are trying to pull the lens into the best shape for focusing.

In children, a **squint** may be the first clue to poor vision, whether through long or short sight.

Eye charts will define the precise degree of the problem.

TREATMENT

Glasses and contact lenses are still the most widely used and tested methods for dealing with poor vision. The artificial lens is shaped to bend light enough to compensate for the visual problem, bringing the image to focus precisely on the retina. Treatment is especially important in children in order to avoid the brain disregarding the information from a poorly focusing eye. Rapid changes in vision also need investigation.

Photo-refractive keratectomy

This new surgical technique to correct short sight has superseded that of radial kerotomy, in which a series of slashes was made in the cornea, resulting in a change in focal length and reducing the need for glasses. In photo-refractive keratectomy a laser is used to shave a disk off the cornea and effectively shorten the eye. It is a novel and promising technique that offers an alternative to wearing glasses or contact lenses.

QUESTIONS

Does a lot of studying weaken the eyes?

This is a controversial question. In surveys, children who are of above-average intelligence tend to be short sighted more often than others. This observation has not been explained. It is thought unlikely that their eyes have become weakened by studying.

How safe is photo-refractive keratectomy?

In skilled hands the technique has a good success rate for mild short sight but results are unpredictable. The risks are infection, subsequently finding bright light dazzling and failure to provide sufficient correction and in any case it will not obviate the need for reading glasses as people grow older. The technique will probably become more widely used as the laser technology improves.

Complementary Treatment

WARNING: Never use aromatherapy oils near the eyes. The **Alexander Technique** teaches you to unlearn habits of overstraining, which can have a beneficial effect on the neck and facial muscles, helping reduce problems associated with eyestrain. With **autogenic training** improved short sight has been reported, but more research is needed. **Hellerwork** relaxes the facial muscles and reduces eyestrain. *Other therapies to try: rolfing; naturopathy; nutritional therapy.*

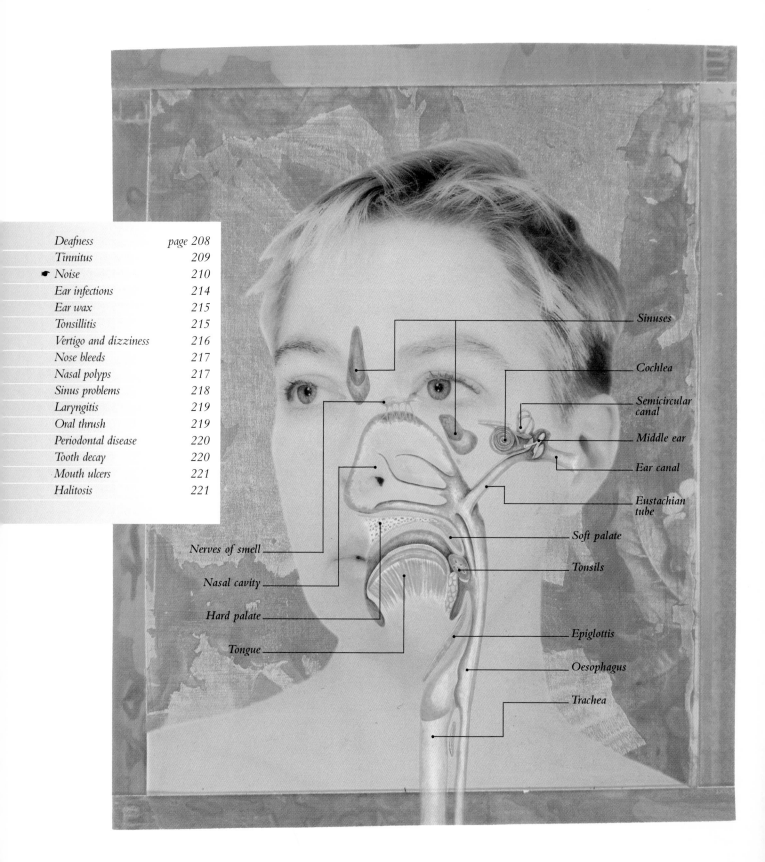

Sinuses

Cochlea

Semicircular canal

Middle ear

Ear canal

Eustachian tube

Soft palate

Tonsils

Epiglottis

Oesophagus

Trachea

Nerves of smell

Nasal cavity

Hard palate

Tongue

*Shared embryonic development and shared connections
mean that problems in one of these structures frequently
affect the others. Hence* ENT *(ear, nose and throat) specialists
deal with all three areas.*

EAR, NOSE AND THROAT

THESE STRUCTURES ARE GROUPED together because they are so closely interconnected that diseases in one part often influence other parts – for example, nasal congestion leading to ear infection. The most common ENT problems are those to which all hollow organs are liable – namely infections and blockage. The following pages concentrate on infections of these structures, rather than malformations or cancers.

The ears

These miracles of micro-engineering turn sound waves into nerve impulses for interpretation by the brain. Sound waves make the eardrum vibrate. A tiny bone, the stapes, lies against the eardrum and moves as the drum vibrates. Through a series of joints with two other bones those vibrations are amplified and finally applied to the inner ear, the cochlea, a bony organ that looks like a snail shell.

The cochlea is filled with fluid that picks up the amplified vibrations. What happens next is complicated and still not completely understood. The cochlea has a lining of specialized nerve tissue covered in hairs, called the organ of Corti. Sounds of different frequency set up waves in the fluid which bend the hairs at different sites of the organ of Corti; the site stimulated is interpreted by the brain as pitch. The degree of bending of the hairs is interpreted as loudness. The electrical output goes to the brain for this sophisticated analysis.

Close to the cochlea are the semi-circular canals, three more fluid-filled structures and, oddly, a number of tiny crystals.

Head movements cause movements of the fluid and crystals to be sensed by yet more specialized cells and turned into nerve impulses. These are interpreted to give us our sense of position and direction of movement.

The nose

Inhaled air passes over the blood-rich lining of the nose, which warms it and extracts odours for the sense of smell. Tiny hairs in the nose trap larger dust particles, while other particles are absorbed on to the moist surface of the back of the nose and throat. The sense of smell is provided by cells in the roof of the nose which respond to just a few molecules in the air. The resulting nerve impulses go straight to a part of the brain also involved with mood and emotion for analysis, which explains why smells can have such an evocative or disturbing effect.

The throat

Here channels from the mouth, nose and sinuses meet before dividing up into the trachea leading to the lungs, and the gullet going to the stomach. Some slick muscular coordination takes place during swallowing to keep airways and food intake separate: food in the lungs is dangerous. Being a first port of call for bacteria and viruses, the throat is not surprisingly the place where many infections begin.

Speech is produced as exhaled air makes the vocal cords vibrate and is given power and resonance by the shape of the nose, throat, mouth and sinuses.

*Left: These related structures handle
hearing, balance, breathing, speech
and swallowing, via amazingly clever
muscle and brain control.*

DEAFNESS

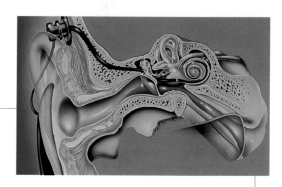

Loss of hearing through natural decline or disease.

CAUSES

Hearing, like other systems, is subject to deterioration with age. Hearing relies on the conversion of sound into electrical impulses. Sound waves cause minute movements of the eardrum, amplified by a chain of bones (the ossicles) which transmit movements to the cochlea. Deafness from problems with the ossicles or eardrum is called conductive. The cochlea turns sounds into nerve impulses; diseases from this region onward cause sensori-neural deafness.

Conductive deafness
In otosclerosis, joints between the ossicles stiffen with age. The eardrum and bones may be damaged by severe infection or trauma. Accumulated **ear wax**, middle ear infections and glue ear (see EAR INFECTIONS) decrease hearing temporarily.

Sensori-neural deafness
The most common cause is presbyacusis, the hearing loss from ageing, due to the degeneration of nerves within the cochlea. An accelerated form of this is from acoustic trauma – constant exposure to loud noises. Ménières disease is a disorder of blood flow to the ear associated with **tinnitus**. Several drugs affect the nerves of hearing, for example gentamicin. Tumours of the auditory nerve are uncommon. Some children are born deaf as a result of malformation of the inner ear. **Rubella** is one cause, although unusual. At any age infection can destroy the nerve pathways, for example **mumps**, **shingles** and meningitis (see BACTERIAL and VIRAL MENINGITIS).

SYMPTOMS

Within a few weeks of birth a child should be startled by sudden loud noises and by three to four months he should turn to interesting sounds. Children should be babbling by about nine months and saying a few words by one year. If these milestones are not met or if the child's speech starts to deteriorate, immediate investigation is needed. Modern techniques can confirm hearing problems in babies as young as three to six months, especially if their hearing might be at risk from premature birth. Immediate investigation is needed so that the child can begin a programme to acquire skills. Older children can say if their hearing is indistinct. Certain children are at high risk of hearing difficulties and should be screened, for example following an illness such as meningitis.

Above: A cochlear implant, showing the microphone and wiring going to the cochlea.

In adults sudden hearing loss is obvious. A more gradual loss, for example presbyacusis, is easily overlooked and is as likely to be picked up by others as by yourself. Presbyacusis reduces sensitivity for high tones, the ones important in conversation and telephone listening. Deafness that is associated with pain or discharge should never be ignored.

TREATMENT

Conductive deafness is more likely to be treatable than sensori-neural deafness. With the former there are operations to replace diseased ossicles, repair the eardrum and remove fluid from within the ear caused by infections.

Sensori-neural deafness is treated with hearing aids (both behind-the-ear and within-the-ear devices) that amplify sound. However, these are limited by the efficiency of the remaining nerve pathways, which cannot be repaired. Cochlear implants (see page 330) may help to overcome this.

QUESTIONS

When should a deaf child be treated?
The sooner the child gets into a deafness programme, the better it is for language acquisition, performance and social skills.

What is a cochlear implant?
A microphone leading to electrodes implanted in the cochlea, stimulates the nerves directly. These ever-more sophisticated devices may one day become standard treatment for the totally deaf.

 ### Complementary Treatment
Always seek orthodox medical advice for any kind of deafness. **Hellerwork** can help improve hearing although results, as with other therapies, depend on the level of deafness; it cannot restore hearing to someone who is profoundly deaf. *Other therapies to try: auricular therapy; reflexology; osteopathy.*

TINNITUS

◆

Ringing in the ears – a common problem and difficult to treat.

CAUSES

Tinnitus appears to be somewhat similar to the feedback noises of other types of amplification system. It can accompany any other ear disorders, such as presbyacusis – the deterioration of hearing with age. Other common associations are with otosclerosis, where the chain of bones transmitting sounds gets stiff. Tinnitus after noise trauma is common – think of the ringing in your ears after some loud noise such as an explosion or a pop concert, which may take a day to disappear. Ringing in the ears can become permanent in people constantly exposed to noise, for example gunnery officers.

Ménières disease

This poorly understood disease, thought to come from deterioration of blood flow to the ear, causes **deafness** together with tinnitus and vertigo (see VERTIGO AND DIZZINESS).

Other causes

Drugs can cause tinnitus, the most common being aspirin and alcohol. Even **ear wax** and **ear infections** may also provoke it.

SYMPTOMS

◆

Ringing affects both ears, one usually more than another. It is frequently a high-pitched ringing noise that varies in intensity but rarely disappears. People with severe tinnitus often get depressed for understandable reasons. Tinnitus plus deafness and vertigo suggest Ménières disease. Tinnitus affecting only one ear is uncommon and may be a feature of disease of the nerve in that ear, especially if accompanied by deafness.

There are no objective ways to measure tinnitus; doctors must rely on what the patient reports.

TREATMENT

◆

It is worthwhile removing ear wax and any other source of irritation within the ear. Hearing tests can be done and will determine whether the tinnitus is a consequence of conductive deafness or of sensori-neural deafness. Treating deafness with a hearing aid may relieve the tinnitus.

One-sided tinnitus should be investigated for the rare cases caused by a tumour on the nerve of hearing, called an acoustic neuroma. This search, once extremely difficult, is now straightforward with a brain scan.

After investigation there will remain many people for whom no definite cause can be found and for whom treatment is unlikely to be curative. Nevertheless, there are a number of ways in which people with tinnitus can be helped.

In people who suffer **high blood pressure** this should be treated. It is worth trying a number of drugs that reduce pressure within the ear, such as betahistine and cinnarizine; however, these drugs do not work for everyone.

If a hearing aid has not helped, then a masking device might be able to. This looks like a hearing aid and is worn behind the ear. It generates white noise, which is noise that has neither pattern nor content. The idea behind this is to find a pitch and loudness that will cancel out the tinnitus. It may seem odd to attack one noise with another, but it is a form of treatment that does work.

Finally, a few very unfortunate people, usually with Ménières disease, have so much upset from tinnitus and vertigo that they are willing to have the hearing nerve destroyed on that side; this is a drastic, very carefully considered last resort that is rarely needed.

QUESTIONS

What should I do if I hear other constant noises?
Various sounds bear medical consideration if the noise heard is unusual. For example, a rushing noise may be transmitted from the carotid arteries in the neck or from a heart murmur.

Are antidepressants helpful if you have tinnitus?
Depression often accompanies severe tinnitus, for obvious reasons. Treatment helps reduce the mental burden of the constant noise, but people should also consider self-help organizations.

Complementary Treatment

Auricular therapy treatment can be effective at weekly intervals, but once it stops the symptoms may return. **Nutritional therapy** might suggest supplementing B vitamins, magnesium, manganese and potassium, and essential fatty acids. **Chiropractic** – treating the neck using manipulation and soft tissue massage cannot clear tinnitus, but it can help to make your life more bearable. **Hypnotherapy** has worked when all other methods have failed: you learn to turn down, and turn off, the ringing. *Other therapies to try: tai chi/chi kung; healing; acupuncture; chakra balancing.*

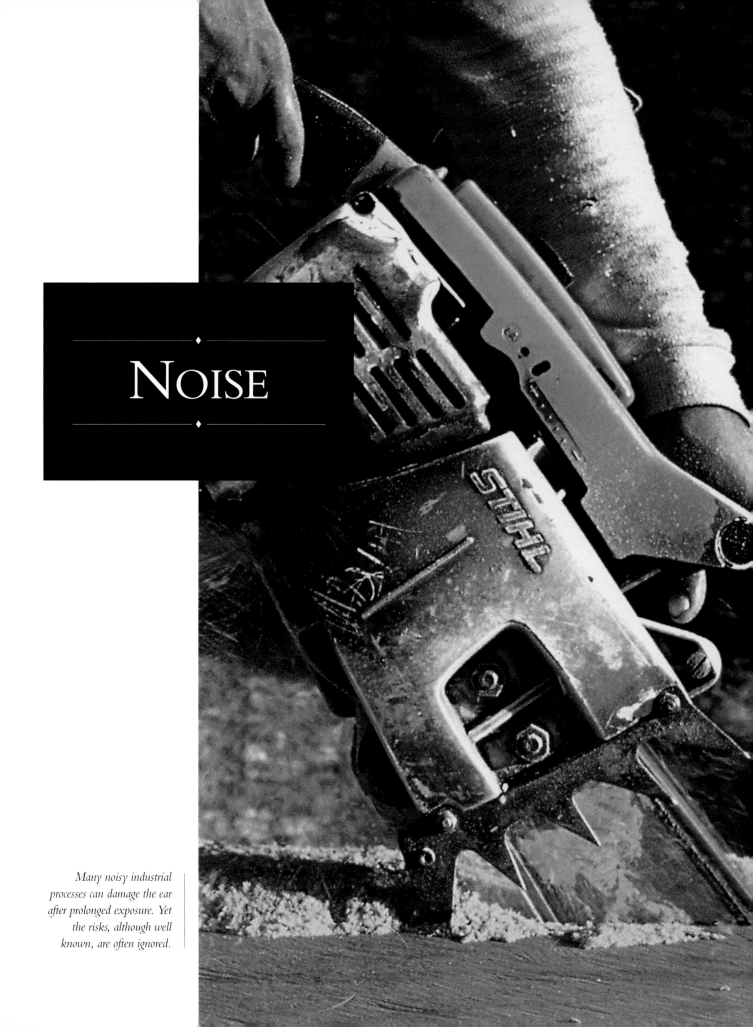

NOISE

Many noisy industrial processes can damage the ear after prolonged exposure. Yet the risks, although well known, are often ignored.

NOISE HAS BECOME A POLLUTANT of our society and an increasingly recognized form of urban stress. Even minor noises are irritating, whether from radios or TVs, personal stereos or mobile phones. And while no one would voluntarily expose themselves to the noise of a screaming jet, many young people accept similar noise levels in concerts, discos and clubs. There are real worries about the long-term effects on their hearing.

Sound and intensity

Sound is wave vibration carried in air or other materials. The range of audible vibration is from about 20 waves per second to about 20,000 per second. Our ears are most sensitive to sounds in the range of 500–5000 waves per second, which is the range within which most speech takes place.

Frequencies above 20,000 per second (abbreviated to 20 kilohertz) are termed 'ultrasound'. Although we cannot hear such frequencies many animals can, especially dogs. Bats use a highly sophisticated ultrasound system as a means of navigation, emitting frequencies from 20 to 150 kilohertz. Although they are very loud, they are mostly inaudible to us.

Measuring noise The intensity of noise reflects the pressure the vibrations make in the air. This can cover an enormously wide range and is expressed as decibels, a rather complicated physical concept. Every increase of 10 decibels is heard by the ear roughly as a doubling of sound. Therefore a 90-decibel noise sounds twice as loud as an 80-decibel noise and four times as loud as a 70-decibel noise. Continuous exposure to noise above 85 decibels carries a risk of damage to hearing, depending also on the maximum noise level, the average noise level and how long it persists.

What does noise do? We hear thanks to a system of tiny bones in the ear that conduct the vibrations of air. They pass these vibrations on to the inner ear, where they are turned into electrical impulses that go to the brain. (For more details see pages 206 and 208.)

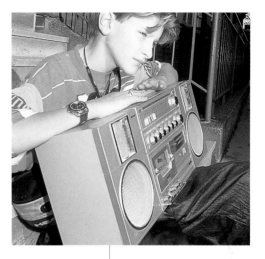

Above: Stereo systems and loud discos are potential health hazards, as well as irritants to others.

A SCALE OF NOISE AND ITS EFFECTS

20–30 decibels	*A whisper*
50–60 decibels	*Normal conversational speech*
80 decibels	*Heavy traffic, as heard in the street*
85 decibels	*Point at which permanent damage occurs*
100 decibels	*The noise of an underground train*
120 decibels	*Noise begins to cause physical discomfort*
140 decibels	*Noise causes physical pain*
160 decibels	*The noise from a military jet engine at maximum thrust★*

★ The jet engine sounds (subjectively) over 16,000 times louder than a whisper.

When first exposed to noise, the ear reacts with a protective reflex. More prolonged noise damages the cells which translate vibration into electrical impulses. Initially this causes a loss of hearing which is temporary, assuming the noise source disappears. Even so, it can take two weeks to recover fully from serious exposure and the main hearing loss is in the sensitive range that is essential for hearing human speech. Often accompanying such hearing loss is **tinnitus**, or ringing in the ears.

If noise lasts long enough, it causes permanent damage to hearing; it is permanent because the affected cells die and cannot be replaced. Just how and why this happens is not well understood. Over and above actual hearing loss, noise damage can distort what hearing remains.

Noise and annoyance It is not just the sheer volume of noise that can irritate, but the mix of frequencies of noise. We all recognize this as the difference between listening to the loud but melodious and complex sounds of a concert orchestra as opposed to quieter but discordant sounds from a squeaking door. And of course everyone has their own psychological thresholds for what they deem to be an unacceptable noise level, irrespective of the actual decibel level.

Then again the ear rapidly adapts to a certain level of sound, thanks to tiny muscles that alter the tension on the bones within the inner ear. Therefore it can be more annoying to hear a relatively quiet noise that keeps changing, compared to a louder but constant noise. This is why people can sleep with a background drone of traffic yet awaken on hearing a quiet whimper from a baby.

Other effects of noise Noise above 50 decibels is enough to disturb sleep in most people. Constant noise causes irritability and interferes with concentration. How important this is varies according to the jobs people are doing. There is some evidence that constant noise causes psychological illness and increases blood pressure.

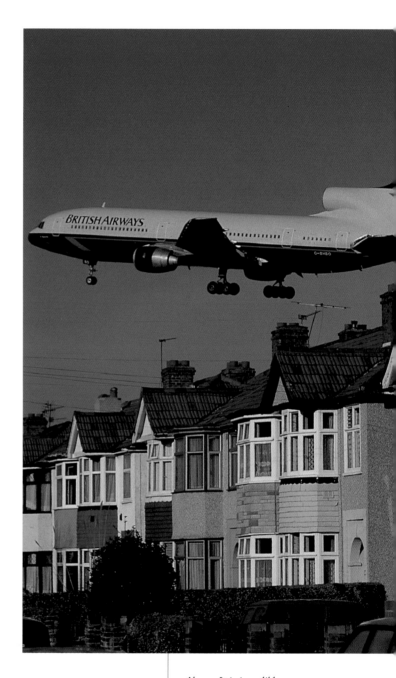

Above: It is incredible the noise that people can put up with if they are forced to.

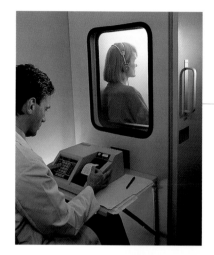

Left: Playing sounds of varying loudness and pitch to the woman in the booth in order to check her hearing.

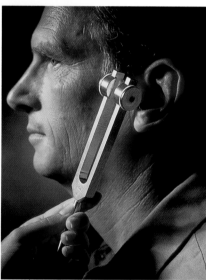

Above: Tuning forks allow the medical practitioner to make a quick check of someone's range of hearing.

Loss of hearing

This is measured with equipment known as an audiometer, which generates noise of known frequency and loudness. The individual listens through earphones and says when sound appears or disappears. The result is a graph showing how sensitive the hearing is across the range of frequencies. Hearing loss that has been caused by noise damage gives characteristic tracings.

In certain occupations employees have regular screening of their hearing if they may be at risk of noise damage caused by their job. People particularly at risk are military personnel using firearms (in whom damage is virtually certain without ear protection), those who must use grinding and sanding equipment, workers in sawmills, quarries and mines, builders using air or pneumatic drills and musicians.

One problem with hearing loss is that it creeps up on the individual and is more likely to be noticed by others than by the person experiencing it. In addition, workers together in one industry may all be suffering hearing loss so that it takes an outsider to recognize what is happening.

Protecting against and reducing noise Many millions of workers are potentially exposed to excessive noise. Laws are in place in many countries to try to control the problem. People vary greatly as to how much noise affects them, so there will always be some individuals who feel a fuss is being made about nothing. Since hearing loss is likely to be permanent, this is an unacceptable attitude. There is also interaction with previous ear trouble such as recurrent **ear infection**.

The ideal way of reducing noise is by changing the procedures or muffling the noisiest parts of a process. However, much industry is inherently noisy and little can be done to reduce the noise. More practical steps, therefore, are to limit exposure and to ensure employees wear ear protection. This means ear muffs. It is recognized that these will only be used if they are comfortable so considerable effort goes into making muffs acceptable to the people who have to wear them.

Failing ear muffs, ear plugs are not too bad an alternative; cotton wool stuffed into the ear is useless.

Ultrasound and infrasound

There is much interest in the possible effects of sounds that lie outside the range of normal hearing but might even so stimulate the ears. Infrasound (very low frequency sound) can arise from engine rooms and from driving in a car with windows open. Although infrasound is annoying there is little evidence that it has any physical effect.

People might be exposed to ultrasound from ultrasound equipment. Some do complain of a feeling of fullness in the ears and may experience nausea. Ear muffs are adequate protection against this rather unusual hazard.

EAR INFECTIONS

These comprise internal infections and external skin complaints.

CAUSES

Although ear infections are a common childhood problem, treatment is still controversial. Adults are less frequently subject to infection, but commonly suffer **eczema** of the outer ear.

Middle ear infections (otitis media)

The inner ear communicates to the outside world via the Eustachian tube, a channel that ends at the back of the throat. Each time you swallow this tube opens, allowing air to enter or leave the inner ear. A child's narrow tube predisposes to the stagnation of secretion and infections of the eardrum.

Outer ear infections (otitis externa)

The outer ear skin can suffer from eczema, boils (see BOILS, SPOTS AND ABCESSES) and **fungal infections**. Over-vigorous cleaning of the ear with cotton-wool buds increases the chances of infection by scratching the skin of the canal.

SYMPTOMS

With middle ear infection, pain is the prime symptom, typically in a child who has a cold. It begins abruptly and is very distressing, and is due to the pressure of fluid within the middle ear. A severe infection may lead to rupture of the eardrum, with discharge of pus and blood but also relief of pain.

With outer ear infections there is itching and a watery discharge; scaling may spread from the ear canal on to the ear. A boil in the canal is painful out of all proportion to its tiny size.

TREATMENT

Treatment for middle ear infections ranges from painkillers and time to an appropriate antibiotic. If the eardrum has burst, letting out pus, a follow-up check-up is necessary to ensure that the eardrum perforation has healed up. This should take a few weeks. In the rare cases of failure to heal an operation may be needed to put a graft in place.

Many children experience infections every few weeks during childhood. As long as each infection resolves entirely it is best to wait for the child to outgrow these naturally as the air passages of the ears and nose enlarge. However, some children are so much affected that they merit having their adenoids (glands at the back of the nose that can obstruct the air passages of the ears) removed and grommets inserted in their

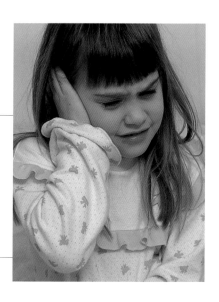

Right: Children with distressing earache should have painkillers sooner than antibiotics.

eardrums. Some children have persistent mucus within the ears, termed a glue ear, which reduces hearing. If it persists for several months, involves both ears and causes significant hearing loss then most ENT surgeons would once again perform an adenoidectomy and insert grommets.

With outer ear infections it can be difficult getting the medication to where it is needed. Medicated drops containing an antibiotic and an antifungal settle most minor infections or eczema. Any but the most minor infections need an antibiotic by mouth, especially boils in the canal. Chronic infections or eczema need specialized ENT treatment to remove debris from the ear canal and to pack it with antiseptic gauze.

QUESTIONS

Can acute ear infections be avoided?
These are more common where the parents smoke, although the precise relationship is uncertain. While courses of antibiotics or decongestants are often prescribed, they may have little value.

What are grommets?
These are tiny tubes placed in the eardrum to let air into the middle ear and to let secretions out. Although ENT surgeons tend to disagree on the use of grommets, there is agreement on their value in selected cases of chronic ear disease.

Complementary Treatment

Chinese and **Western herbalism** can be very effective in helping the body fight infections: seek professional advice for specific remedies. **Homeopathy** can be extremely effective but treatment depends on what brings the problem on, how it presents, what makes it better or worse and so on. **Chakra balancing** can help with pain control and healing. *Other therapies to try: naturopathy; acupuncture.*

EAR WAX

Discharge of wax is normal, but sometimes causes difficulties.

CAUSES

Glands within the ear canal continuously secrete wax, which keeps the eardrum supple. Wax is swept towards the ear opening where its bitter taste repels insects and traps any that get into the ear. Some people produce more wax than others. In dusty or dry conditions it may become hard and accumulate.

SYMPTOMS

Wax may be to blame if hearing becomes muffled or if, after a shower or swimming, the ear feels blocked, due to water trapped behind wax. Nearby wax melted by the warmth of **ear infections** can be mistaken for an infected discharge.

TREATMENT

Wax should only be treated if it is causing a problem, for example muffled hearing. Avoid removing wax with cotton-wool buds, which can push wax into a firm plug over the eardrum and make hearing worse. Buds often scratch the ear canal and introduce infection, leading to chronic irritation or **eczema**. Wax softens in warm water; letting water into the ears when washing may keep levels down. There are many eardrops that dissolve it. Syringing should be a last resort.

QUESTION

Does wax cause pain?
This is unlikely; more often pain signifies an infection of the eardrum or in the ear canal. Doctors avoid syringing a painful ear, even if there is a clear plug of wax, until antibiotics have settled any infection. Similarly they will not syringe a discharging ear.

 Complementary Treatment
Auricular therapy – needling the ear to treat any condition will often produce sensations of warmth and increase local blood circulation; treatment focused specifically on the ear can lead to improvements. *Other therapies to try: reflexology.*

TONSILLITIS

An infection of the tonsils, which can be very painful.

CAUSES

The tonsils and adenoids are part of a ring of specialized tissues surrounding the throat and nasal passages, that trap infection before it gets further into the lungs or gullet. The frequent sore throats of childhood are this system mopping up germs. Sometimes this leads to severe inflammation of the tonsils. In teenagers, **glandular fever** is a common cause of tonsillitis; generally, sore throats are caused by viruses, but full-blown tonsillitis may be the result of bacterial infection.

SYMPTOMS

A mild sore throat rapidly becomes severely painful, with the feeling of a lump in the throat and difficulty swallowing. Often pain is felt in the ears and breath smells bad (see HALITOSIS). White spots or a white slough are all over the tonsils, but appearances do not always correlate with the severity.

TREATMENT

If the cause is a bacterial infection treatment is with penicillin. Painkillers and throat sweets give relief. For a run of bad throats or an unusually inflamed one a blood test could exclude glandular fever or a blood disorder.

QUESTION

When is removal of tonsils advisable?
If you have more than six attacks of tonsillitis a year with severe symptoms and are losing time from school or work.

 Complementary Treatment
Aromatherapy – try a gargle of sage, myrrh or thyme (two drops in half a glass of water). *Other therapies to try: naturopathy; nutritional therapy; Western and Chinese herbalism; acupuncture; homeopathy; healing.*

VERTIGO AND DIZZINESS

Sensations most commonly experienced by older people.

CAUSES

True vertigo means a sensation of spinning. Dizziness is a much vaguer term, which includes light-headedness and feeling faint. There are many possible causes but experience shows that the great majority result from a few conditions which, although inconvenient, are not dangerous.

A viral infection, labyrinthitis, causes abrupt vertigo with nausea. Similarly, vertigo may accompany an ear infection or congestion of the ear. Deterioration of blood flow to the ears is believed to account for many cases of vertigo. An acute **stroke** may cause vertigo and unsteadiness, along with other symptoms. The long list of less likely causes of vertigo includes drugs affecting the ear, tumours on the auditory nerve and neurological disease.

Osteoarthritis of the neck, universal in older people, can squeeze the major arteries to the brain in certain neck positions and the resulting fall in blood flow causes dizziness. In many older people postural hypotension (see below) results in light-headedness. Vague dizziness is a frequent complaint of people under **stress** or with **depression**.

SYMPTOMS

The pattern of symptoms is the best clue to the likely cause. Most diagnoses can be made after assessing the patient's ears, blood pressure, heart sounds, neck and limb movements and psychological status. Brain scan and specialized tests of the organs of balance within the ear are available for puzzling disabling vertigo or dizziness but are of little help in diagnosing most acute cases. Acute vertigo with nausea and no ear inflammation is probably viral in origin. Acute vertigo with slurred speech or limb weakness may be a result of stroke or brain disease. Osteoarthritis of the neck can cause dizziness when looking up, which goes on looking level again. Light-headedness on standing, with a measurable drop in blood pressure, suggests postural hypotension or anaemia. Vertigo plus **tinnitus** and **deafness** is the triad of Ménières disease.

TREATMENT

Medication to relieve the giddiness and nausea of an acute attack of vertigo includes prochlorperazine and domperidone. These drugs are available as tablet, injection or by pellet that dissolves in the mouth. Treatment continues for as long as

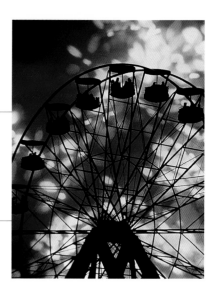

Right: Providing the thrill of vertigo is the basis of a section of the leisure industry.

necessary, but most acute vertigo passes after a week or two.

The problems associated with postural hypotension and osteoarthritis of the neck are difficult to treat effectively. Strategies include learning to stand up slowly and to wait a few seconds for blood pressure to adjust, wearing support stockings to keep blood pressure up when standing and having adjusted any medication for **high blood pressure**, which may be contributing to the problem. People with osteoarthritis of the neck need to learn to avoid sudden neck movements.

Psychological causes may respond to counselling or anti-depressants.

QUESTIONS

Why is it so important to differentiate between the terms 'vertigo' and 'light-headedness'?
It is necessary for the doctor to first work out what a patient mean by these terms in order to avoid diagnostic blind alleys for what may simply be a problem of stress or tension.

Is low blood pressure bad?
British and American doctors consider it a good thing unless it causes dizziness. European doctors blame it for widespread ill health and treat it. There is no common ground on this intriguing cultural difference.

 Complementary Treatment
See your doctor if you have recurrent vertigo. **Chiropractic** may help since vertigo can be aggravated by neck stiffness and muscle spasm. Vertigo responds particularly well to **hypnotherapy** regression and suggestion therapy. **Western herbalism** – ginkgo may help dizziness caused by poor blood flow to the brain. *Other therapies to try: tai chi/chi kung; acupuncture; homeopathy; cymatics.*

NOSE BLEEDS

A common occurrence, which only rarely has a serious cause.

CAUSES

Several arteries run very close to the surface near the front of the nose and bleed readily if irritated through inflammation or trauma – typically when having a cold or picking at the nose.

Nose bleeds are more common in children, and in the elderly. Every adult with a nose bleed without an obvious cause should have their blood pressure checked, although in fact most people with **high blood pressure** do not get nose bleeds. People who have profuse or recurrent nose bleeds should be tested to ensure their blood is clotting normally.

SYMPTOMS

Blood drips painlessly for several minutes and there may be a blood-tinged ooze which lasts for a day or two.

TREATMENT

The first aid treatment (see page 362) is to pinch the soft part of the nose, just below the bridge, hard enough to close the blood vessel for about ten minutes. Most bleeding will stop

provided that probing fingers are kept away from the scab.

A profuse nose bleed will require the nose to be packed tightly with a long ribbon of gauze to put pressure on the blood vessels. It is removed after 48 hours. The curative treatment for nose bleeds is to burn the offending blood vessel with silver nitrate or an electric cautery.

QUESTION

Is a nose bleed dangerous?

Bleeding for more than a few hours causes significant blood loss – it may be due to the rare cases of poor blood clotting and must be dealt with appropriately. High blood pressure (probably coincidental) should be handled in the standard way. The majority of nose bleeds are otherwise merely inconvenient rather than dangerous.

Complementary Treatment

Acupuncture can rectify intolerance causing bleeding.

Homeopathy – treatment depends on circumstances, for example take arnica if bleeding follows injury, ipecac where blood is bright red and phosphorus if bleeding follows nose-blowing.

NASAL POLYPS

Fleshy benign growths in the nose that cause obstruction.

CAUSES

The surface lining of the nose reacts naturally to dust or fumes by secreting mucus. Often the surface overgrows into a polyp in people who are continuously exposed to irritant atmospheres, or in those with **hay fever** who have a perpetually overactive mucus surface. Each polyp has a 0.5–1 cm/¼–½ in diameter, is pinkish-grey, hangs on a stalk and blocks the nasal passage. Where there is one there are often several.

SYMPTOMS

Someone whose nose keeps running or who is forever sneezing eventually finds that their nose constantly feels blocked. Often one side is worse affected than the other. An ENT specialist can see how many polyps there are and plan treatment.

TREATMENT

If the nasal polyps are small, there is a fair chance that a steroid nasal spray such as fluticasone or beclomethasone will make them shrink. Some people have so many polyps that sprays are unlikely to work sufficiently. If medical treatment with steroid sprays fails or you are simply fed up with having to use the spray daily surgery is possible. The polyps can be removed under a local anaesthetic. Each one is snared and cut off. If necessary, this can be repeated every few years.

The mucus surface of the nose can also be removed for a permanent cure, although this quite extensive operation is less commonly performed.

Complementary Treatment

Aromatherapy inhalations could help ease symptoms: try eucalyptus, thyme or myrrh (two to four drops in a bowl of hot water or on a handkerchief).

SINUS PROBLEMS

Disorders of these cavities in the skull, mostly caused by infection.

CAUSES

There are three main sinuses: the maxillary in the cheekbones, the frontal sinus above the eyes and the ethmoidal behind the bridge of the nose. The linings of the sinuses produce a mucus secretion, which carries away any infection and dust that have penetrated the sinuses. The secretions drain through ducts into the posterior part of the nose.

Sinusitis often follows a cold which has obstructed the drainage ducts. The roots of the upper molar and premolar teeth end very close to the floor of the maxillary sinus and inflammation may spread into it from the teeth. In addition, jumping or diving into water can force water up the nose and into the sinuses.

The function of the sinuses is unclear. It may be to make the skull lighter or to add resonance to the voice. During sinusitis a person may sound like Donald Duck.

Chronic sinusitis

Chronic sinusitis may be congenital, for example unusually narrow ducts, or it may be provoked by allergies such as **hay fever**, which thicken the mucus surface around the drainage channel, or by **nasal polyps**, which block the channel.

SYMPTOMS

In the case of acute sinusitis, a few days after a cold, pain increases over one of the sinuses, most often the maxillary sinus. Pressure is felt in the skull, and there are aching teeth and pain behind the eyes. On bending forward you feel a rush of fluid within the sinus and increased pain. The nasal discharge becomes particularly offensive and yellow and drips down the back of the nose to the throat, creating a foul taste.

Pain that occurs at the top of the nose or deep behind the eyes suggests an infection of one of the deeper sinuses. If there is pain and swelling of the eye, then this will point to a very serious internal infection.

In chronic sinusitis there is persistent nasal obstruction and discharge of infected mucus, plus the pressure symptoms mentioned above. Often the individual is a smoker, has allergies or is under some degree of tension (see STRESS).

The diagnosis of sinusitis on clinical grounds alone is not terribly accurate. The definitive test is a CT scan (see page 318) to demonstrate fluid; these show that many presumed diagnoses of sinusitis are wrong.

TREATMENT

For acute sinusitis an antibiotic is used to penetrate the pus in the sinus. This requires a high dosage over ten days of, for example, amoxycillin or doxycycline. Decongestant nose drops and tablets are helpful, as are steam and menthol inhalations to improve the effectiveness of medication.

Infection of the frontal sinuses or ethmoidal sinuses is treated similarly but with higher doses of antibiotic and with drainage of the sinus if infection worsens.

Chronic sinusitis

Scans first prove the diagnosis and exclude an underlying cause such as allergy or **tooth decay**. The treatment is as for acute sinusitis but given for longer. If this fails, you will need a wash out of the sinus with a hollow needle under local or general anaesthetic. Failing this, a more permanent drainage channel can be made through the nose or via the upper gum.

Endoscopic instruments allow the surgeon to inspect the interior of the sinus, remove polyps or to enlarge the drainage channels. Similar techniques can be used to drain the frontal or ethmoidal sinuses in cases resistant to antibiotics.

QUESTIONS

Do children get sinusitis?
The sinuses do not begin to form until about five years of age and are not fully formed until about twelve. Thus sinusitis is impossible below the age of five and unusual before the age of twelve.

Is sinusitis dangerous?
Prompt treatment with antibiotics makes complications unusual, but in theory infection could spread into surrounding bone or into the brain. A bloody discharge should not be attributed to sinusitis without investigation for a possible tumour.

Complementary Treatment

Aromatherapy – try inhaling cajeput or eucalyptus oil (two to four drops in a bowl of hot water, or on a handkerchief). **Nutritional therapy** – food allergy might be the underlying cause: seek advice. **Chiropractic** helps alleviate pain and tension as part of the overall treatment plan. **Ayurveda** offers herbal steam inhalations, oral preparations and dietary advice. *Other therapies to try: most have something to offer.*

LARYNGITIS

Inflammation of the larynx, the part of the tube through which air passes to the lungs, which contains the voice box.

CAUSES

The upper airways bear the brunt of what the atmosphere can throw at them – smoke from cigarettes, fumes from pollution, pollen in the air, bacteria or viruses such as the common cold. Some people find that dry or air-conditioned atmospheres give them persistent discomfort in the larynx. Using the voice a lot will also lead to inflammation of the airways. Laryngitis can be acute or chronic and is more common in smokers.

SYMPTOMS

There may be pain of a burning nature that is felt all the way from the back of the throat down behind the breastbone. The voice of someone with laryngitis varies from hoarse through every type of squeak to even complete loss.

Children, whose airways are narrower than adults, may cough more and feel more unwell.

Hoarseness lasting more than three weeks may be caused by cancer of the larynx and you should see your doctor.

TREATMENT

Stop smoking. Most cases are due to viral infections, so antibiotics are of little use. It is better to rest your voice, keep the throat moist with drinks or lozenges and avoid smoky or dry atmospheres. Children benefit from being in a steamy room. The rare cases of airways obstruction need hospital treatment.

QUESTION

Is whispering a good idea when you have laryngitis?
Whispering actually puts a similar strain on the voice as talking normally and arguably more if you have to keep repeating yourself! Reconcile yourself to pointing, gesturing or holding up signs during the three to five days that it takes for the condition to improve.

Complementary Treatment
Western herbalism – helpful astringent and antiseptic herbs include myrrh and thyme. **Aromatherapy** – see SINUS PROBLEMS. *Other therapies to try: naturopathy; acupuncture; homeopathy; Chinese herbalism.*

ORAL THRUSH

A common fungal infection affecting all age groups.

CAUSES

The organism that causes oral thrush, candida, also causes vaginal **thrush** and **nappy rash**. Some cross-infection may occur in these cases. Babies are especially prone to oral thrush by transfer from their mother's skin. It is common after taking an antibiotic, which kills germs that compete for the food supply, and affects asthmatics using steroid inhalers. Persistent or recurrent oral thrush may be a warning of **diabetes** or, less commonly, a deficiency in the immune system.

SYMPTOMS

The inside of the mouth is coated with small white deposits, which are the thrush organisms. If they are scraped off, the underlying surface bleeds. The mouth feels sore; babies may be reluctant to feed because of this.

TREATMENT

Babies are treated with mouth drops and adults with lozenges; resistant cases require antithrush tablets. Thrush elsewhere is treated to avoid reinfection. Severe cases need investigation.

QUESTION

How contagious is oral thrush?
There is no risk of spread as long as cups and glasses are kept clean and not shared. Babies' teats should be sterilized.

Complementary Treatment
Homeopathy – try an aloe vera mouthwash. **Aromatherapy** – gargle myrrh or tea tree (two drops in half a glass of water). *Other therapies to try: naturopathy; Western and Chinese herbalism; acupuncture.*

PERIODONTAL DISEASE

◆

Disease of the gums around the teeth, leading to teeth loosening.

CAUSES

◆

Teeth make a special joint with the bone of the jaw called a gomphosis, meaning a nail or bolt. Fibres grow from the bone into the tooth, securing it in place. Periodontal disease begins when food debris accumulates around the tooth, allowing in chronic bacterial infection, which works its way down the root and loosens the tooth fastening. Eventually it involves the tooth, the gum and the bone of the jaw, resulting in ever looser teeth and increased risk of infection.

SYMPTOMS

◆

The gums feel tender through an inflammation called gingivitis. They bleed easily, even on brushing, and the teeth feel loose. Persistent infection causes **halitosis**. There may be pus around the teeth, but only in totally neglected conditions.

TREATMENT

◆

Unfortunately, the damage from chronic infection cannot be repaired. Teeth loosened by infection cannot be tightened up and the same goes for loose gums around the teeth or erosion of the jaw bone. Dental hygiene can, however, help to prevent progression of the process, which would otherwise end in loss of teeth or chronic gingivitis.

Since periodontal disease cannot be reversed, prevention is the best step. Remove food residue every day, using a toothbrush and floss to remove debris from between teeth. Tartar (accumulated food debris) should be regularly removed by a dental hygienist. Antiseptic mouthwashes may help.

Complementary Treatment

A **nutritional therapist** might recommend boosting your intake of vitamin C. **Bach flower remedies** – try Rescue Remedy. *Other therapies to try: Western herbalism; homeopathy.*

TOOTH DECAY

◆

Destruction of the teeth caused by enamel erosion and infection.

CAUSES

◆

The basic cause of tooth decay (dental caries) is acid that dissolves the hard enamel coating teeth. Acid comes from bacteria growing in plaque around the teeth, which feed on sugar. Once enamel erosion has occurred, bacteria invade deeper into the tooth, eventually reaching the pulp. The resulting inflammation destroys the pulp, leaving the tooth fragile.

SYMPTOMS

◆

Decay does not cause pain until it inflames the nerve-rich pulp. Throbbing pain may worsen into the excruciating pain of an abscess and swelling of that part of the face. The diagnosis is confirmed by examination and X-ray.

TREATMENT

◆

Antibiotics can reduce the degree of infection, but almost certainly the tooth will need drilling in order to let out the pus. In less severe cases, filling the tooth should stop further decay.

With more serious decay, the tooth can be capped. In very severe cases, prompt root canal work can save the tooth even though the pulp has died; extraction is the only sensible option for a badly decayed tooth.

QUESTION

How can decay be prevented?
You should avoid sweets, sugar, starch and sugary drinks on which bacteria thrive. Daily careful brushing with a fluoridated paste is very worthwhile in preventing tooth decay. Plaque should be removed regularly by a dental hygienist. Fluoridated water is a highly effective public health measure and worries about its safety have little scientific support.

Complementary Treatment

There are no alternatives to conventional dentistry. Aim for prevention by cutting out sugary foods and drinks, and maintaining good dental hygiene with regular flossing and cleaning of teeth. A variety of herbal toothpastes is available.

MOUTH ULCERS

Open sores, most of which, though irritating, are benign.

CAUSES

The majority of mouth ulcers are caused by viral infections or by scratches, whether from a toothbrush, hard food or sharp teeth. Common viral causes include herpes and Coxsackie. Rarely, the mouth may ulcerate because of disease elsewhere in the gastrointestinal system, for example Crohn's disease (see INFLAMMATORY BOWEL DISEASE), Behçet's disease, **coeliac disease** or **systemic lupus erythematosus**.

SYMPTOMS

Crops of tiny painful ulcers appear over the walls of the mouth and tongue. Ulcers clustered over the soft palate and back of the mouth are probably caused by a herpes virus. Mouth ulcers with itchy spots on the palms and feet are typical of the alarming sounding but benign **hand, foot and mouth disease**, caused by the Coxsackie virus. Mouth ulcers can last for up to seven to fourteen days. Recurrent or large ulcers associated with ill health or abdominal pains need investigating for an unusual bowel or immune cause.

TREATMENT

Mouth ulcers are treated with a steroid gel or pellet held in contact with the ulcer. Children badly hurt by mouth ulcers may stop eating until the pain subsides, after about three days.

QUESTION

When should you see a doctor about changes in the mouth?
Any ulceration of the mouth, white patch or area of irritation that lasts more than about a fortnight should be seen by a doctor or dentist. This is to pick up the rare serious ulcers caused by cancer or to consider the unusual bowel or immune diagnoses.

Complementary Treatment

Aromatherapy – see ORAL THRUSH. A **nutritional therapist** may suggest avoiding citrus fruits. **Ayurveda** – cleansing medications would be prescribed, along with dietary advice. *Other therapies to try: homeopathy; chakra balancing; naturopathy; hypnotherapy.*

HALITOSIS

Bad-smelling breath with many causes – several preventable.

CAUSES

The mouth has an effective self-cleansing mechanism in the antiseptic properties of saliva. If it breaks down then poor dental hygiene is the number one cause (see PERIODONTAL DISEASE) – the smell comes from bacteria around the teeth. Bacterial colonization is also the reason for halitosis in people with chronic nasal discharges, **tonsillitis**, sinusitis (see SINUS PROBLEMS) and chronic lung infections. Less likely is halitosis from stomach disease or peptic ulcers. Diet, alcohol and smoking may also contribute.

SYMPTOMS

These may be those of periodontitis, gingivitis, sinusitis or indigestion. You might be aware of your own halitosis. Some people imagine they have halitosis when others say this is not the case; this may be a self-image problem. However, people are mostly unaware of their own halitosis because the nose rapidly becomes accustomed to ever-present odours, including the smell of one's own breath, which is why it takes an outsider to point out the problem.

TREATMENT

Good oral hygiene is the key, plus treatment for any focus of infection whether in the teeth, sinuses or lungs. It may take reassurance or other psychological treatment to help someone who imagines they have halitosis; they may need the reassurance of mouthwashes and oral deodorants to allay their fears.

Complementary Treatment

Homeopathy – treatment will depend on the specific details of your case; useful remedies include nux, mercurius, pulsatilla, quercus and arnica. *Other therapies to try: hypnotherapy; nutritional therapy; naturopathy.*

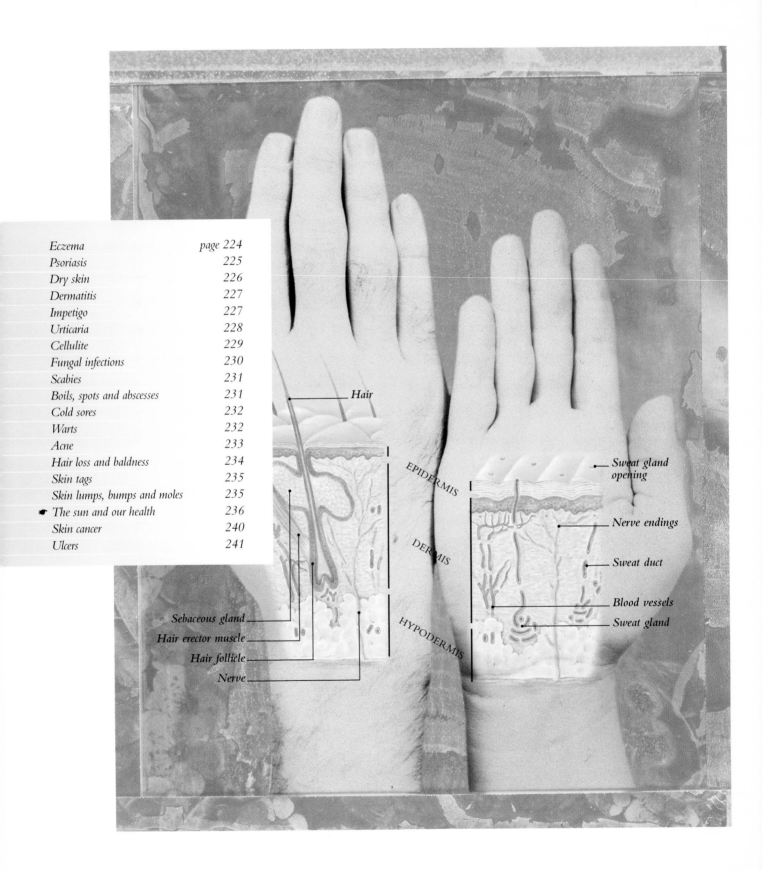

Hair

EPIDERMIS

DERMIS

HYPODERMIS

Sebaceous gland

Hair erector muscle

Hair follicle

Nerve

Sweat gland opening

Nerve endings

Sweat duct

Blood vessels

Sweat gland

While the other organs of the body enjoy a high profile, the skin is relatively undervalued, despite it being the largest organ of the body in terms of weight. It performs many vital roles that we rarely think about — from keeping our bodies cool to protecting against infection.

SKIN AND HAIR

SKIN NOT ONLY ACTS as a covering for the body's organs, it also maintains a vital interface between the ever-changing external environment and the relatively more stable internal environment.

The skin is a three-layered and multi-function structure. The outer epidermis comprises cells rich in keratin, which render it waterproof. They migrate from a deeper level, die at the surface and are shed continuously, the process taking about 30 days. In this layer are cells that pigment the skin and cells that mount immune responses to infection.

Below the epidermis is the dermis, a complex layer combining elasticity and flexibility with many other functions as follows. Hair grows from hair follicles in cycles up to three years long (see HAIR LOSS AND BALDNESS). Nails, which are modified keratin, are generated from specialized cells below the nail folds. A greasy secretion called sebum keeps the skin supple; this is derived from the sebaceous glands within the dermis and excreted into hair follicles.

The sweat glands, which are found all over the skin, regulate body temperature and salt balance. A particular variety of sweat gland is found around the armpits, genitalia and breasts and may have a sexual function producing pheromones, the animal equivalent of nectar to a bee.

The deepest layer of skin, the subcutaneous tissues, is made of fat, blood vessels and yet more sweat glands.

In addition, skin also plays an important role in calcium balance (and therefore bone formation), by synthesizing vitamin D using ultraviolet light. Pigmented skin acts as a protection against harsh sun.

Scattered throughout the skin are multitudes of sensory receptors for touch, pressure, movement and pain. The dense blood supply rushes clotting factors and protective cells to any breach in the surface of the skin.

Skin problems

The most common skin diseases arise from the rate of cell formation (which greatly increases in **psoriasis**), immune reactions causing **dermatitis** and **eczema**, and infections leading to boils (see BOILS, SPOTS AND ABSCESSES). Overactivity of certain cells leads to excessive sweating and to the many **skin lumps, bumps and moles** to which skin is prone.

The skin is one organ, even though the delicate skin of the eyelid looks very different from the callused skin of the soles of the feet. This is why an irritation in one part of the skin often causes reactions elsewhere, for example a flare-up of eczema from a skin irritation will bring out a sympathetic eczematous response in more distant parts.

The state of the skin's health is something we notice immediately: its greasiness, dryness, flaking, blushing and weeping. Although few skin diseases are actually infectious, we experience an almost instinctive reaction to both poor and excellent skin health, influencing social isolation or acceptance.

Left: Skin and hair protect, insulate and cool the body, enhance its appearance and give much of our individuality.

ECZEMA

Inflammation of the skin through an inherent hypersensitivity.

CAUSES

In eczema the skin reacts unusually vigorously to external irritation, or it may even react without any external irritation at all. This differentiates eczema from **dermatitis**, where the cause is clearly an external irritant.

People who are most liable to eczema are atopic, meaning they have a heightened immune system, and often also suffer from **hay fever** and **asthma**. Blood tests confirm high levels of proteins involved in immune responses, called IgE, which release inflammation-provoking substances called cytokines and interleukins that cause the skin changes.

There is a large genetic component: if both parents have eczema there is up to a 60% chance of their children having it.

SYMPTOMS

Infant eczema can begin within weeks of birth, with the baby having red and scaly rashes over her cheeks, scalp, chest, groin and eyebrows. The baby appears unsettled and irritable, not surprisingly given the tenderness of the skin. As the baby grows into a child, the skin looks less greasy and more red and dry. The parts of the body that are then most affected are the skin creases of the elbows and knees, with rashes scattered elsewhere. In areas where there is particular irritation the skin becomes thickened and cracked, called lichenification. The eczema will have greatly improved in at least 50% of children by the age of 5 and in 80–95% by adolescence.

Adults who have suffered lifelong eczema will have areas of lichenified skin. There will be the same red, dry patches anywhere on the body or face. These will vary in severity with external influences, such as dry or cold weather and irritant clothing. Adult eczema may involve the palms of the hands and soles of the feet, causing tiny itchy fluid-filled lesions. Eczema can accompany **varicose veins**. Individuals will often have associated asthma and hay fever.

TREATMENT

The aim at all ages is to keep the skin moisturized and to avoid obvious irritants. It is usual to start with moisturizing creams, for example aqueous creams combined with bath lotions, that go all over the body. There are many proprietary brands of varying degrees of greasiness. These help keep the condition under control, but require meticulous application.

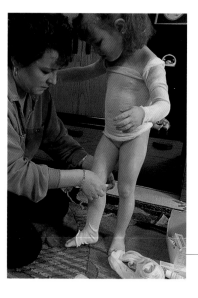

Left: Children with severe eczema need careful daily treatment. Fortunately, eczema often improves with time.

It is also very important to wear materials, such as cotton, that are non-irritating and absorbent.

Since the 1960s steroid preparations, in the form of creams and ointments, have revolutionized the treatment of eczema. However the use of these strong steroids is kept to a minimum because, on the face for example, they will thin the skin and cause pimples. As treatment for acute flare-ups, however, steroids are unsurpassed.

For more regular treatment, mild hydrocortisone preparations are safe for all ages, can be used for months and can be applied to the face. However, preparations of ever-increasing potency may be required – even, rarely, on the face. The strongest of these preparations, for example betamethasone or clobetasol, are reserved for the most resistant cases, especially eczema of the hands. Anti-itch drugs may be needed at all ages, for example chlorpheniramine or terfenadine.

In recent years the role of infection has been recognized in causing flare-ups of eczema, so there is renewed interest in steroid/antibiotic preparations.

Complementary Treatment

Chinese herbalism – see DERMATITIS. **Western herbalism** – your medical herbalist is likely to ask you to drink teas or infusions, as well as applying ointments or pastes to the affected area. **Homeopathy** – use calendula cream as a moisturizer and rub evening primrose oil on to unaffected areas of skin as a preventive measure. **Ayurveda** – see SCABIES. *Other therapies to try: healing; shiatsu-do; naturopathy.*

PSORIASIS

A problem characterized by skin scaling and red patches, affecting about two per cent of the population.

CAUSES

As a result of an increased rate of cell growth in the outer layers of the skin, cells pile up in characteristic plaques. Many people with psoriasis have a genetic tendency to the condition, which makes them up to seven times more likely than average to suffer from it. In susceptible people a streptococcal throat infection can trigger it, as can constant pressure on or rubbing of the skin. Psoriasis may prove to be an auto-immune condition, that is, one where the body reacts against its own tissues. Many people find that emotional upsets will cause a deterioration. Others find that the cold makes it worse by drying out the skin. Certain drugs can bring on psoriasis, notably lithium and beta-blockers. But however bad psoriasis looks, it is not catching and there is no risk to others.

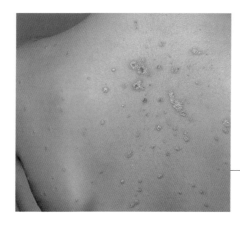

Left: Plaques of psoriasis, showing the typical scaling and redness.

SYMPTOMS

Psoriasis does not begin until late teens or adult life. Silvery plaques of skin accumulate over the elbows, knees and pressure areas such as the base of the spine. Similar plaques form around the hair margins on the scalp. Plaques can affect skin anywhere, from the chest to the palms, soles, groin and the genitalia. People may get joint pains and their nails often have tiny pits in them. In severe psoriasis, where there is chronic scaling and disfigurement, significant loss of protein through the shed skin and disabling joint stiffness, people may become reclusive through psychological and physical distress.

TREATMENT

Unfortunately, psoriasis is not curable. It is difficult to treat well and the treatment has to be tailored to the individual. This calls for trust and patience on the part of patient and doctor.

Steroid creams
These are used where there are just a few small plaques giving little trouble. They are unsuitable on the face or for long use.

Coal tar preparations
A mainstay of treatment, these are applied as pastes, creams, lotions and bath additives to reduce inflammation and the amount of scaling. Pure coal tar is messy and cosmetically unacceptable, so preparations have been made that both smell better and do not stain skin or clothing, for example alphosyl and dithrocream. Cosmetically acceptable scalp preparations are now available.

Calcipotriol
This is a form of vitamin D applied as a cream. It is pleasant to use and effective for small plaques or on the scalp, but it is impractical for widespread psoriasis.

Psoralens with ultraviolet A (PUVA)
This is treatment with ultraviolet light in a special booth; tablets containing psoralens, which increase skin sensitivity, are taken a couple of hours beforehand. Ultraviolet A refers to the wavelength of the light. PUVA, which has excellent results, takes about three months for full effect; thereafter treatment every few weeks should keep the condition under control.

Other forms of treatment
Acitretin is a hospital-only treatment for severe psoriasis but with many side effects, for example dry skin and liver damage. Because it damages the foetus, acitretin must not be taken during pregnancy; this risk persists for two years after treatment. Cytotoxic drugs, as used in certain cancers, may be advisable for otherwise unresponsive psoriasis.

Complementary Treatment

Chinese herbalism – see DERMATITIS. **Shiatsu-do** – skin disorders worsened by stress, including psoriasis, are responsive. **Chakra balancing** can help with skin healing and pain control. **Auricular therapy** could help, especially in conjunction with **acupuncture**. A **nutritional therapist** could recommend a diet to enhance liver function. **Cymatics** could help. **Ayurveda** – see SCABIES. *Other therapies to try: see STRESS.*

DRY SKIN

The natural self-lubricating glands of the skin tend to become inefficient with age.

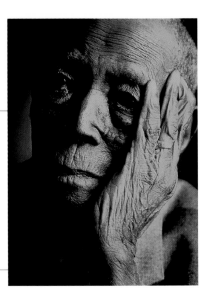

Right: Sun-damaged skin. With care, even aged skin can remain supple and self-repairing.

CAUSES

The skin is kept oiled by slightly greasy secretions of the sebaceous glands. With age, these glands become less efficient and, combined with loss of the skin's natural elasticity and water content, this results in dry skin that cracks easily. Exposure to strong sunlight and harsh weather also accelerates drying of the skin. The skin of smokers ages more rapidly and looks drier and more wrinkled at an earlier age. Many women find that their skin becomes drier after the menopause.

Dry skin is rarely due to disease, with the exception of **eczema**, where there is dryness combined with redness and inflammation. A severely underactive thyroid gland leads to dry skin (see THYROID PROBLEMS).

Anything that degreases the skin inevitably leads to dryness; common degreasants are detergents, washing-up liquids and industrial solvents.

Very occasionally people have congenitally abnormally dry, cracked skin structure, the condition of ichthyosis.

SYMPTOMS

Dry skin feels irritable and cracks easily. It looks flaky and cells may be shed on to clothing. Itch can be a big problem, especially in the elderly, but severe itch and dry skin should trigger a search for an underlying problem such as an underactive thyroid gland, **anaemia** or kidney problems (see KIDNEY DISEASE). Secondary infections can get into large cracks.

TREATMENT

Emollients are preparations to lubricate the skin. Some are medical formulations, others have been developed by cosmetic companies; use whatever you find most effective.

Broadly speaking, there are creams where lubricants are dissolved in water, or ointments where lubricants are dissolved in oil. Creams rub into the skin, leaving no residue, whereas ointments leave a greasy layer that may be inconvenient for people employed in certain occupations, for example those handling paper or film.

These preparations are fine for small areas but difficult for widespread dryness. This is where liquid emollients are helpful, as they are put on immediately after showering or are dissolved in the bath water. These tend to be oil based. You may find you need a combination of preparations: a liquid for all-over lubrication, a cream for your hands and an ointment for your arms or your face.

If you get itch or inflammation after using an emollient, you might be allergic to something in the skin preparation that is causing **dermatitis**. The substances most often responsible are lanolin and perfumed preparations. If you have become allergic to one of these you should avoid other skin preparations containing it by checking the detailed ingredient list. This is easy in the case of medical preparations but it may be more difficult with patented preparations.

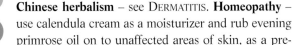

QUESTIONS

Should children routinely use emollients?
These are necessary only for children with eczema whose skin is dry and inflamed.

What is the secret of delaying the ageing of skin?
Moisturizing the skin is a fundamental strategy; avoid excessive exposure to sunlight, wind and cigarettes. If you work with detergents or industrial cleaners, apply emollients liberally; remember that too much washing with soap or bath detergents is degreasing.

Complementary Treatment

Chinese herbalism – see DERMATITIS. **Homeopathy** – use calendula cream as a moisturizer and rub evening primrose oil on to unaffected areas of skin, as a preventive measure. **Aromatherapy** – try a massage oil made up with one of the following: sandalwood, rose or neroli (three drops to 10 ml carrier oil). **Ayurveda** – see SCABIES. Skin disorders that are worsened by stress, including dry skin, are responsive to **shiatsu-do**. *Other therapies to try: Western herbalism; cymatics.*

DERMATITIS

Irritation of the skin through environmental stimuli.

CAUSES

Dermatitis is the general term for an inflammation of the skin caused by some external factor. The most common irritants are oils, greases, soaps and perfumes, metal, plants and ultraviolet radiation. These are all potent sensitizers in some people and once the skin has been sensitized in one area it is likely to show signs of dermatitis elsewhere. It is also the case that people with skin that is sensitive to one agent often prove to be sensitive to several others.

Dermatitis can be cured once the irritant has been identified, unlike **eczema** where there is a congenital tendency to inflamed skin and which is often a permanent problem.

SYMPTOMS

The skin is red and itchy and may flake or ooze tissue fluid. Through repeated scratching the surface of the skin breaks down so that secondary bacterial infection is common, with increased redness and pain.

TREATMENT

Often the offending agent is easily identifiable, for example if hands are raw where gloves end, or the skin is red just underneath a metal watch or the skin improves on holiday and deteriorates on return to work. Skin testing helps identify otherwise obscure agents. Avoidance of the agent is obviously necessary. The symptoms respond to moisturizing creams or steroid creams plus antihistamine tablets to reduce itching.

Complementary Treatment

WARNING: Chinese herbalism – herbs can be extremely effective, but a few people have an adverse reaction that affects the liver. Reputable practitioners insist on regular blood tests to monitor liver function. Formulas are person specific, depending on the skin condition and underlying intolerance, and often change during treatment. **Homeopathy** – use calendula cream as a moisturizer and rub evening primrose oil on to unaffected areas of skin as a preventive measure. *Other therapies to try: naturopathy; healing; chakra balancing; Ayurveda; auricular therapy; shiatsu-do.*

IMPETIGO

A highly contagious infection of the skin.

CAUSES

Impetigo is especially common in children, through the acquisition of skin infections with streptococcus or staphylococcus bacteria. Once these have invaded the skin they cause it to blister and burst, leaving a raw surface that is open to secondary infection. Most cases of impetigo are caught by cross infection from others; hence it spreads fairly easily around schools and homes.

SYMPTOMS

The face is the site that is most commonly affected. What begins as a small spot grows into a cluster of angry-looking lesions within hours. These have a red raw base with a crusted yellow coating and they leak tissue fluid. The infection then spreads easily by direct contact to the hands and arms – in fact anywhere that infected fingers may roam.

TREATMENT

Use an antibiotic cream for a single spot and oral antibiotics for more extensive infection. Do not share a towel and avoid skin-to-skin contact with others. Most cases are cured by a week's worth of antibiotic treatment.

QUESTION

Is impetigo dangerous?
The spots just look unpleasant, and only children with low resistance to infection might become ill. Treatment should be vigorous, however, because it can quickly spread through a community.

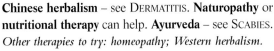

Complementary Treatment

Chinese herbalism – see DERMATITIS. **Naturopathy** or **nutritional therapy** can help. **Ayurveda** – see SCABIES. *Other therapies to try: homeopathy; Western herbalism.*

URTICARIA

Skin rashes that result from an allergic reaction.

CAUSES

Also known as nettle rash or hives, urticaria is the response of the skin to something that triggers an allergic reaction. During the reaction, the skin throws defending cells against a supposed invader and supplements these with chemicals that further affect the skin, for example histamine, prostaglandins and others. This accounts for the skin reactions of swelling and fluid retention.

Often urticaria is an obvious response to a definite substance, either directly on the skin or that has been eaten, for example strawberries or shellfish, irritant plants or aspirin-type drugs. More likely, however, the cause is obscure and remains so even after allergy testing.

Emotion and exercise can cause a particular type of urticaria, called cholinergic urticaria after the nerves involved. Other forms are in reaction to cold, to sunlight and even to water. There are a few uncommon inherited reasons that are important to identify because of the lifelong implications.

Urticaria is most common in children and young adults but occurs at all ages.

SYMPTOMS

The skin reaction usually occurs within minutes of exposure but may take hours, making it harder to identify the cause.

The skin feels itchy and rapidly swells into a weal that is pale in the middle and red around the margins. A sufferer may have a few large weals or multiple small ones of all shapes – more usually called hives. Weals wax and wane within minutes; the whole experience can last minutes, hours or even days.

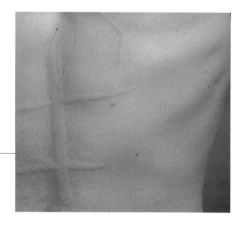

Right: Severe urticaria, showing how even minimum contact with an irritant causes weals.

Soft tissues

It is not unusual for the lips and eyelids to swell. This is called angioedema and is a sign of a widespread allergic response. More severe again, although relatively uncommon, is swelling that may extend to the soft tissues of the throat and trachea, causing difficulty in breathing.

Anaphylaxis

This is the most severe reaction: a collapse of blood pressure through whole-body release of histamine-type substances. Although rare, it most often occurs as a result of insect stings and, more recently recognized, from eating nuts.

TREATMENT

This depends on the severity of the condition. Mild to moderate urticaria is treated with antihistamines by tablet or injection. The older antihistamines such as chlorpheniramine are sedating, which is helpful at night; the modern non-sedating antihistamines are better in the day, for example astemizole. Soothing lotions like calamine are helpful for children.

In the more severe case of angioedema a short course of steroids will rapidly dampen the reaction. The slightest hint of difficulty in breathing or swallowing must be taken seriously and hospital care arranged.

Anaphylaxis

This most serious association with urticaria is a medical emergency. The immediate treatment is to inject adrenaline, which restores blood pressure, after which steroids and antihistamines can be given. People who know they are at risk should wear medical bracelets that alert to the fact and carry an adrenaline self-injection kit.

Many people react to aspirin-type drugs, widely used for arthritis, and it is important to consider whether these might be causing severe urticaria in an adult.

Complementary Treatment

Chinese herbalism – see DERMATITIS. **Homeopathy** – a registered homeopath should be able to help, and will try to find out what triggers your condition, what makes it better or worse, and so on. As a **self-help** measure, urtica ointment relieves itchiness. You can also try applying an ice-pack to the affected area. **Chakra balancing** can help with relaxation and healing. **Ayurveda** – see SCABIES. *Other therapies to try: auricular therapy.*

CELLULITE

A non-medical term for the unwelcome aspect of fat in the body.

CAUSES

At a biochemical level, fat is a highly concentrated means of storing energy (1 g of fat supplies over twice as much energy as 1 g of protein or carbohydrate). It also provides heat, insulation and protection, as well as buffering organs from movement by being distributed under the skin and around many organs. Finally, it forms the external shape of the body and contributes to the texture, as with the hips and the breasts.

But in spite of fat's beneficial roles, people are more concerned about its negative aspect – cellulite. Cellulite is not a medical term but we all know what it means. Medically it refers to the adipose tissue, wherein fat cells hang within a loose connective tissue framework. Each fat cell is a great globule of fat, squeezing the cell nucleus to one side. As we get older the connective tissue framework becomes laxer, while fat tends to accumulate. The result is cellulite.

SYMPTOMS

Cellulite causes a characteristic dimpled appearance over fat-bearing areas, typically the thighs and hips. It is more visible on standing, when the weight of the fat pulls on the connective tissue framework, and from certain angles when light picks out the dimpling. Paradoxically, dieting may actually worsen the appearance, because connective tissue has less fat to support, so the dimpling tends to become deeper.

Cellulite is not the same as **obesity**; even slim people will have plumper parts where cellulite may lurk.

Cellulite is a particularly female phenomenon, because of the way in which the female body is shaped by strategically placed layers of fat.

TREATMENT

It is claimed by some manufacturers that certain creams, when rubbed into the skin, make cellulite disappear. This claim appears improbable: even if you apply something that succeeds in bursting the fat cells, this fat will only be reabsorbed by the surrounding cells. It will *not* slosh around in a liquid form that drips out if you cut yourself!

Dieting to remove cellulite is not an option, as it can actually make it appear more obvious, as mentioned above.

Liposuction is a recent controversial surgical technique to remove cellulite or indeed fat in general. Under anaesthetic a

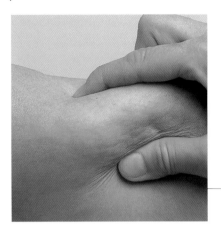

Left: If pinching fat causes dimples like the ones here you may have cellulite.

tube is inserted into the fat-bearing area – the hips, abdomen or thighs – and the fat is literally vacuumed out under suction. The technique carries the risks of bleeding, infection and uneven tissue removal. However, it is becoming a treatment of choice for some and the results in the hands of the very skilled are very impressive.

QUESTIONS

Can early action reduce cellulite?
Evidence suggests that the number of fat cells is determined during foetal development. Possibly, therefore, children born to mothers with a fat-rich diet have more fat cells, which will predispose them to obesity and cellulite in later life.

Why is it relatively difficult to lose fat by dieting?
If you eat less the body turns to using carbohydrate for the energy it needs. The body only begins using fat significantly when these carbohydrate stores are exhausted. This means that you need to follow a very low-calorie diet for this to occur.

Complementary Treatment
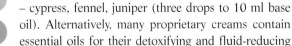
Chinese herbalism – see DERMATITIS. **Aromatherapy** – try making up a massage oil with one of the following – cypress, fennel, juniper (three drops to 10 ml base oil). Alternatively, many proprietary creams contain essential oils for their detoxifying and fluid-reducing properties, and their ability to balance hormones. Diet – a **nutritional therapist** or **naturopath** could help. **Healing** promotes elimination of wastes, which helps keep the skin clear. *Other therapies to try: cymatics.*

FUNGAL INFECTIONS

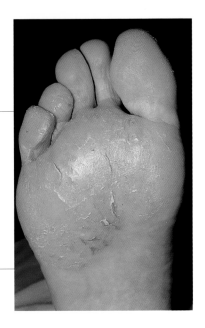

Infections from fungi that can be mild or severe.

CAUSES

Fungal infections can occur in the skin, nails or scalp.

The most common skin infection is caused by candida, a natural skin inhabitant (see THRUSH and ORAL THRUSH). It thrives in warm, moist conditions and where other food competitors are reduced, for example after antibiotic treatment. It grows around the genitalia and groin and under the armpits and breasts. The other common skin fungus is ringworm, which is usually transmitted by close contact with infected animals. Athlete's foot is an infection between the toes caused by yet another family of fungi.

Several different fungi grow in the nails. They are unlikely to spread and are usually caused by self-infection.

Ringworm of the scalp used to be common but it is now found only in cases of gross personal neglect.

Skin and scalp infections are spread by close skin contact. People with unusually widespread or persistent fungal infections should have medical advice, as they may have **diabetes** or an underlying immunity problem.

SYMPTOMS

Fungal skin infections cause an itchy red rash with a definite margin; the margin is the actively growing part of the fungus. Athlete's foot causes intense itching between the toes and flaking of the skin. Fungal infections of the soles or palms can look like **eczema**. The diagnosis of fungal rashes is usually straightforward and confirmed by examining skin scrapings.

With nail infections, the nails thicken, the ends break in a ragged margin and the nail may detach itself slightly from the nail bed. The toenails are more often affected than the fingers. The diagnosis is confirmed by examining nail clippings.

In infections of the scalp, the infected area is itchy and scaly and the hairs break off at the roots. In more severe infection the skin is crusted. Under ultraviolet light the affected scalp fluoresces blue-green, which is a useful confirmatory test.

TREATMENT

Many antifungal creams are available for these skin infections, often combined with a mild antiseptic and a mild steroid to reduce itching. These are very effective for fungal infections of the groin and under the breasts and for athlete's foot. Continuing treatment for at least a week after the rash

Right: Athlete's foot – the fungus makes skin cracked, itchy and inflamed.

has gone ensures complete eradication of the fungus. In really resistant cases, it may be worth taking an antifungal by mouth, such as fluconazole; this treatment is more widely used for vaginal thrush.

Nails are the most difficult to treat, because they are slow growing. If only a few nails are affected, treatment is with an antifungal lacquer containing, for example, tioconazole or amorolfine. This has to be used for at least three months. Otherwise there are oral antifungals such as terbinafine, also taken for at least three months. Recurrence is common and the nails may remain thickened, yellow and unsightly.

Treatment for scalp infections is with an antifungal taken by mouth, such as itraconazole.

QUESTION

How safe is antifungal medication?
Creams and nail lacquers are very unlikely to cause any side effects apart from stinging caused by skin sensitivity. Antifungal tablets are effective but may have significant side effects, especially inflammation of the liver.

Complementary Treatment
Complementary therapies generally attempt to boost the immune system, so treatment is constitutional. **Chinese herbalism** – see DERMATITIS. **Western herbalism** – echinacea boosts the immune system. Unless you are already immune suppressed, **chakra balancing** can promote healing by strengthening the immune system. Diet – either a **naturopath** or a **nutritional therapist** could help. **Ayurveda** –see SCABIES. *Other therapies to try: see THRUSH and ORAL THRUSH.*

SCABIES

◆

A not uncommon insect infestation of the skin, which is highly contagious.

CAUSES

◆

The bug responsible is the scabies mite which, however nasty it looks at a distance, is a thousand times worse in close-up. The female of the species burrows within the skin, laying eggs; the itch of scabies is actually caused by the eggs.

Scabies is spread by close contact and the infection involves just a few mites. A more severe form of scabies involving infection by thousands of mites is associated with a deficient immune system. Scabies is most common in children and young adults, and those who live in an institutional setting where it can spread more easily.

SYMPTOMS

◆

There is intense itching over the skin creases of the wrists and ankles, between the fingers and around the genitalia. The burrows are visible as tiny tracks a few millimetres in length. If you wish you can extract the mite with a needle. Often a generalized sensitivity occurs, leading to widespread itching.

TREATMENT

◆

Treatment is with an antiscabies lotion such as malathion. This is applied all over the body from the neck down and kept on for 24 hours. The standard advice used to be to wash all potentially infected bedding or clothing, but the exact value of this is debatable.

QUESTION

When does the itching stop?
This can take weeks, because it is not just from the eggs but from a hypersensitivity reaction of the body. Similarly, itching only starts a few weeks after infection. Persistent itching should be re-treated.

 Complementary Treatment
Ayurveda treats skin conditions by considering the right diet, right lifestyle and right process for the individual person. Ointments and oral preparations are used. Full *panchakarma* detoxification is effective, especially with yoga meditation and *marma* therapy.

BOILS, SPOTS AND ABSCESSES

◆

All of these are types of skin infection.

CAUSES

◆

Considering how many contaminants occupy the skin, infection is relatively unusual thanks to various protective mechanisms. Fat on the skin surface is a natural antibacterial; 'friendly' germs produce substances which hinder the growth of germs muscling in on the neighbourhood. The dry outer layer of the skin inhibits penetration by bacteria. Yet nicks, cuts and abrasions forever breach these security features while hair shafts offer a direct route into the inner skin. Staphylococci and streptococci are the common invaders.

SYMPTOMS

◆

Infection begins as a small tender swelling. Then a yellow head appears; this is pus, which is a mixture of dead defending cells and bacteria. The more extensive the infection, the larger the collection of pus and surrounding inflamed tissues, forming a boil or abscess. There may also be discomfort or pain at the affected site.

TREATMENT

◆

Small spots and boils respond well to antibiotic creams rubbed over them. Spots and boils that are larger than 1 cm/ ½ in merit treatment with an antibiotic by mouth such as flucloxacillin. An abscess has a large collection of pus that cannot be penetrated by antibiotics. It should be incised and allowed to drain to relieve pain and speed recovery.

 Complementary Treatment
Chinese herbalism – see DERMATITIS. **Western**
 herbalism – try pastes of either slippery elm powder or marshmallow root powder. **Aromatherapy** – tea
 tree oil is effective. *Other therapies to try: homeopathy; auricular therapy; naturopathy; Ayurveda.*

COLD SORES

Skin blisters usually affecting the area around the mouth.

CAUSES

The herpes simplex type 1 virus is the cause of cold sores. After a first infection it continues to live in the nerves in a dormant state until it is reactivated by some external irritant. This may be sunlight or another infection. Cold sores can appear premenstrually. The virus regrows rapidly, leading to the appearance of new sores.

SYMPTOMS

For the first few days you are aware of a tingling sensation typically on one lip, then a rash of small but painful spots appears. Crusts form on these spots and secondary infections may lead to swelling of the lip. It takes ten to fourteen days for the rash to disappear.

TREATMENT

Treatment is typically with acyclovir, a modern antiviral drug that reduces the pain and duration of an attack. It is available as an ointment or as tablets for severe cases. It should be used when the tingling begins, because this is when the viruses are reproducing. A separate antibiotic cream may be necessary if there is a secondary infection. In time the severity of the attacks will diminish until they eventually stop altogether.

QUESTION

Can cold sores lead to genital herpes?
They are both caused by the herpes virus, but genital herpes is more often from a different strain – herpes simplex type 2. It is possible to transmit cold sores to the genitalia although it is not as easy as the transmission of genital herpes to someone else. The treatment of genital herpes is the same as for cold sores.

Complementary Treatment

Chinese herbalism – see DERMATITIS. A **nutritional therapist** might suggest supplementing lysine, an amino acid, vitamin C, zinc and bioflavinoids. Avoid peanuts, chocolate, seeds and cereals. **Aromatherapy** – apply neat lavender oil to the sore with a cotton-wool bud. *Other therapies to try: shiatsu-do; homeopathy; acupuncture; Ayurveda.*

WARTS

Fleshy skin outgrowths of viral origin.

CAUSES

Warts are caused by the many strains of the papilloma virus. The infected skin generates the dense tissue that forms the wart. Warts around the anus and genitalia may be caused by **sexually transmitted diseases** and should be seen by a doctor, although many will prove as innocent as warts elsewhere.

SYMPTOMS

The typical wart is a few millimetres in diameter and height. The surface is rough; the tiny black dots visible in the centre are capillary blood vessels in which blood has clotted. Warts on the face tend to be longer and slimmer, for example the filiform wart, which can grow up to 1 cm/½ in long. A verruca is a wart on the sole that has been flattened by pressure.

TREATMENT

The majority of warts disappear once the body has developed an immunity to the virus responsible. For this reason the treatment should not be worse than the condition itself. Over-the-counter wart preparations destroy the thick skin; they do work but it may take months.

It is possible to freeze warts, including verrucas, with liquid nitrogen, but this is a painful process that is only worth it for particularly unsightly or persistent warts.

Warts on the face may need to be carefully excised in order to avoid scarring.

Complementary Treatment

Homeopathy – apply thuja mother tincture twice daily to the wart and cover with a plaster. **Aromatherapy** – apply neat tea tree oil to the wart with a cotton-wool bud. **Ayurveda** – see SCABIES.

ACNE

There is still uncertainty as to the fundamental cause of these pimples that haunt the teenage years.

CAUSES

Acne results from bacterial colonization of the sebum-producing glands of the skin. The bacteria are emphatically not there through lack of personal hygiene, but rather because increased male hormones (androgens) at puberty stimulate sebum (grease) production, which favours bacterial invasion. This applies to youngsters of both sexes.

Acne may persist into adult life as a result of a continuing excess of androgens. Polycystic ovaries in women cause a combination of acne, hirsutism and absent periods (see PERIOD PROBLEMS). The role of food is debatable: it is really an individual matter as to which foods worsen one person's acne.

SYMPTOMS

The first sign is a blackhead, a dot in the base of a skin pore. This is caused by a colour change in a blocked sebaceous gland. The surrounding area becomes inflamed and swells into the familiar acne pimple: red with a yellow tip. Small spots come and go within days; larger ones may pit and scar the skin. Acne mainly affects the greasier parts of the face, forehead, back and chest. It is not infectious, but infectious secondary bacteria may invade large cysts.

TREATMENT

Although lack of cleanliness is not the cause, the skin should be kept clean with a degreasing agent, and lotions to dissolve the blackheads. Avoid greasy make-up which blocks the pores. Washes containing, for example, benzoyl peroxide induce peeling of a surface layer of skin, taking blackheads with it. Another directly applied preparation is retinoic acid, which reduces the formation of blackheads; this must not, however, be used during pregnancy.

Antibiotics are invaluable for more extensive or resistant acne. That they do work is undeniable, but it cannot be proved they reduce colonization by acne-producing bacteria. For mild to moderate acne antibiotics are applied as a roll-on lotion, for example erythromycin. Otherwise they are taken as tablets. The antibiotics most used are tetracyclines, which are well tolerated and have few side effects. A drawback is that some common foods, for example milk, reduce absorption. Minocycline overcomes this problem, but is more expensive

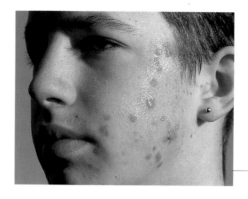

Left: Severe acne should be treated so as to avoid permanent scarring.

and carries a slight risk of arthritis. An antibiotic may lose its effect after a few years, requiring a switch to an alternative.

For women, acne can be greatly reduced with a contraceptive Pill that contains an antiandrogen, called cyproterone. Different types of contraceptive Pill also vary in their natural antiandrogen activity, so changing brands can help.

Where severe acne is causing scars, a final step is treatment with retinoic acid by mouth. A few months' treatment can clear acne for over two years but it has significant side effects of dry skin and liver upsets. It also harms the foetus, so if you are planning to conceive, you should wait a month after finishing treatment with retinoic acid; again it must not be taken during pregnancy.

Acne usually improves in the summer with ultraviolet light, which can also be given as therapy in special light cabinets.

QUESTION

Does chocolate or greasy food make acne worse?
There is no scientific evidence for this but individual experience may suggest otherwise. If you have bad acne and eat a lot of chocolate and/or greasy food, try eating less of it and see what happens.

Complementary Treatment

Chinese herbalism – see DERMATITIS. **Western herbalism** – see ECZEMA. **Auricular therapy** works well in combination with **acupuncture**, especially if some points are bled. **Ayurveda** – see SCABIES. A **nutritional therapist** might suggest supplementation with zinc; other nutritional elements might control excess sebum production. Many therapists offer a cleansing diet, or a course of treatment aimed at expelling toxins from the skin. *Other therapies to try: homeopathy; healing.*

Hair loss and baldness

While partial hair loss is common, complete hair loss is rare.

CAUSES

While a healthy head of hair may appear very stable, hair growth is in fact constantly changing. Each hair follicle goes through phases of growing, shedding and resting. During the growing phase the hair lengthens by about 1 cm/½ in a month; this phase, and therefore the life of an individual hair, is up to three years. Then growth stops, the hair goes into a state of limbo and is soon shed. The follicle rests for three to four months before hair growth recommences. Fortunately these phases are randomly distributed among the 300,000 scalp hair follicles so that only 50–300 hairs are shed each day.

The most common reason for hair loss is the influence of male hormones, which shorten the growing phase and lengthen the resting phase. It is this, plus family tendencies, that accounts for the severity and age of onset of male hair loss.

From the menopause onward, women experience hair loss for similar reasons, as the male hormones become more predominant in their system. Women can also lose a lot of hair after pregnancy, because abnormally large numbers of follicles enter the shedding phase.

Any serious generalized illness may cause hair loss. Other possible causes of a diffuse hair loss are an underactive thyroid gland (see THYROID PROBLEMS), iron deficiency, **eczema** of the scalp, ringworm, **systemic lupus erythematosus** and the side effects of chemotherapy (see page 339).

Hair loss can occur as a result of different types of trauma. This can include chemical damage from perms and hair colouring, heat treatments, brushes that snag the hair, pulling the hair tightly and extreme stress and shock.

Localized hair loss (alopecia areata) is thought to have an auto-immune origin, with a strong family association. Occasionally alopecia extends to complete loss of all body hair.

SYMPTOMS

Male pattern baldness starts at the temples, spreading to involve the rest of the scalp margins and then the crown. It follows a similar pattern in women, although at an older age, and can cause much distress. Alopecia areata is characterized by areas of complete hair loss within otherwise normal hairs. A moth-eaten appearance suggests infection of the scalp.

Except in cases of classic male hair loss or localized alopecia, you should have tests performed in order to exclude thyroid disease, auto-immune conditions and **anaemia**.

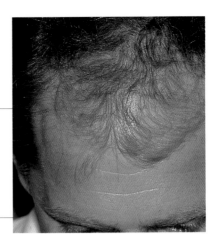

Right: Male pattern baldness: hair recedes from the temples, leaving a fine down.

TREATMENT

Not all hair loss needs treating. If it follows severe illness or pregnancy, regrowth can be expected after the follicles have had their three to four months' rest. Small areas of hair loss may respond to steroid lotions or steroid injections.

Treatment of larger areas is a triumph of hope over evidence although, of course, hormone or iron deficiencies must be dealt with. Steroid lotions may help. Minoxidil, a drug originally used for high blood pressure, stimulates regrowth in about one-third of cases, but has to be used continuously.

Other alternatives include hair transplants, which take hair from the back of the scalp and replant it in the frontal area, as well as wigs and hair pieces.

QUESTIONS

Can hair regrow after alopecia?
It often does after several months or a year. The new hair is initially unpigmented, growing as a white patch. Pigmentation comes in after some months.

Why does shock cause hair loss?
It stimulates loss at one go of all those hairs that have stopped growing but are yet to be shed. This leads to an alarming thinning, but hair can be expected to recover after a few months.

Complementary Treatment

Complementary therapies will not be able to restore lost hair. **Chinese herbalism** – see DERMATITIS. **Aromatherapy** can help if baldness is stress induced. Make up a massage oil for the scalp using the following, alone or in combination: wheatgerm, juniper berry, jojoba, lavender, rosemary or chamomile (three drops in 10 ml carrier oil). **Western herbalism** – herbal shampoos made from catnip, nettle or thyme can stimulate growth.

SKIN TAGS

Tiny growths on the skin that are of cosmetic rather than medical importance.

CAUSES

Constantly irritated skin often responds by forming small growths. These are most common in areas of greatest friction, typically around the collar. By middle age most people have several of these. They are also found in other less obvious sites of friction, such as the armpits, groin and the back.

Babies are sometimes born with small tags on their ears that have been left from the developmental process. These can be removed for cosmetic reasons if parents wish.

SYMPTOMS

Skin tags are more of a cosmetic nuisance than one that causes symptoms. Sometimes they itch. Bleeding may occur if a lesion is torn off, but should stop quickly. Persistent bleeding in a lesion that does not disappear is suspicious and requires further investigation.

TREATMENT

This is only necessary if you are bothered by the lesion or if it is in an awkward place where it keeps getting rubbed. It can be frozen off or surgically excised under local anaesthetic.

QUESTION

Does it hurt to pick off skin tags?
A better remedy is to cut off the blood supply by tying fine thread around the tag – they drop off within days. Be sure that the tag has none of the suspicious features shown by skin cancer and is not where scarring would be unacceptable, for example on the face.

Complementary Treatment
Ayurveda is an excellent therapy for skin problems; even someone with healthy skin should have full detoxification four times a year, with seasonal changes. See SCABIES for further details.

SKIN LUMPS, BUMPS AND MOLES

Most skin lumps and moles are completely harmless and do not need treatment.

CAUSES

Any of the cells of the skin may multiply in benign growths. In general the larger the lump the less likely it is to be malignant. The most common growths are from fat cells, called lipomas, and sebaceous glands, called sebaceous cysts. Many other types of firm lumps can be seen in the skin or felt inside it, for example at sites of previous injury.

Some people have an inherited tendency to lumps, for example neurofibromas from nerve fibres, or lipomas.

SYMPTOMS

There is a smooth nodule in or on the skin. The skin is unbroken and does not bleed or crust. The lesion may be colourless or red from blood vessels in it. If it grows at all it is very slowly. The term mole refers to any coloured skin lump that is not a wart.

TREATMENT

Lumps can be removed, but the size of scar might not make it worthwhile. An exception is for lipomas, which can grow large and unsightly, or sebaceous cysts, which often get infected.

QUESTION

When should a lump be biopsied?
If it grows steadily, itches, is crusted, bleeds or changes colour. Size is no guide – often smaller lesions are more suspicious than larger ones. Biopsy may be warranted for lesions that are unusually hard or have irregular pigmentation.

Complementary Treatment
WARNING: Do not massage directly over the lump or bump. Diet – a **nutritional therapist** or a **naturopath** could advise you if food intolerance is a contributing factor for skin lumps and bumps.

THE SUN AND OUR HEALTH

We need the light provided by the sun but in terms of health there can be too much of a good thing.

MUCH OF THE SUN'S ENERGY hits the earth as heat: part is visible light, part is ultraviolet light. Ultraviolet light causes sunburn on brief intense exposure. Long-term modest exposure ages the skin and predisposes to **skin cancer** in white people. Cloud and humidity are partially protective, otherwise we would risk burning even during the winter.

The fashionable tan

In response to sunlight – or artificial ultraviolet light – the skin tans. Cells called melanocytes produce increased amounts of a pigment known as melanin. Melanin protects against burning from the sun's rays, but does not abolish the risks of long-term damage from sunlight.

Until this century it was actually unfashionable to have a tan. The classic hero or heroine was pale and wan. Even in naturally sunny countries, being pale carried a social cachet by implying that you were wealthy enough not to have to work in the sun.

Now a tan says the complete opposite: not that you have to labour from dawn to dusk but quite the contrary – that you can lounge in the sun at any time of year. And, as a result of foreign travel, we are exposed to sun of an intensity for which many of us are unprepared. The last few decades have also seen a gradual increase in average temperatures, with warmer summers. Because of these factors white skins are exposed to more sun than they can handle (black and brown-skinned people being protected by their natural melanin).

The benefits of sunshine

Humans need light and those who lack daylight suffer. The recently described seasonal affective disorder appears to be a real depression caused by lack of sunshine during the winter months which responds to artificial daylight from light boxes. This treatment works possibly by stimulating the pineal gland in the brain, and/or by increasing serotonin levels.

Sunshine and vitamin D Vitamin D, which is necessary for calcium balance, is formed by the action of sunshine on the skin. Not much exposure is needed – just a few minutes a day to the forearms is sufficient. Without this people are at risk of rickets, especially dark-skinned people having a poor intake of calcium and vitamin D from milk and dairy products.

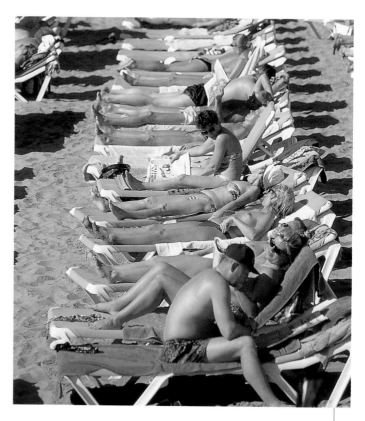

Above: Sunbathing is a fairly recent but enthusiastically followed pastime, which carries a major health risk.

Skin disease Sunlight helps several diseases, especially **psoriasis** and **acne**; some sufferers from **eczema** derive similar benefit. So useful is this that one treatment for psoriasis is to use an ultraviolet light box.

The drawbacks

Sunburn is a true burn, with tissue destruction, and it happens a few hours after exposure to sun. Severe and repeated sunburn in childhood increases the risk of malignant melanoma (see SKIN CANCER).

Sensitivity rashes Many individuals have a sensitivity to ultraviolet light and react with redness, rashes and itch. Unlike sunburn, this reaction occurs after just brief exposure to strong sunshine. Many substances and drugs increase the sensitivity of the skin and worsen this type of reaction, for example perfumes, certain plants (wild parsley being one), drugs such as oxytetracycline and thiazide water tablets. A few rare illnesses are notable for light sensitivity, for example **systemic lupus erythematosus** and porphyria.

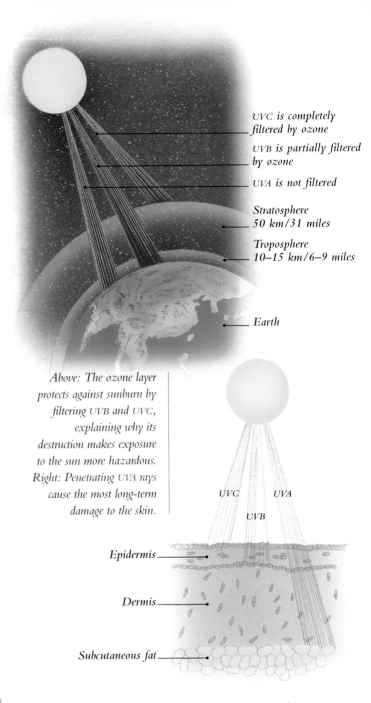

UVC is completely filtered by ozone

UVB is partially filtered by ozone

UVA is not filtered

Stratosphere 50 km/31 miles

Troposphere 10–15 km/6–9 miles

Earth

Above: The ozone layer protects against sunburn by filtering UVB and UVC, explaining why its destruction makes exposure to the sun more hazardous. Right: Penetrating UVA rays cause the most long-term damage to the skin.

UVC   UVA

UVB

Epidermis

Dermis

Subcutaneous fat

SUN AWARENESS

✦

♦ *No sunburn does not mean no damage; it is the non-heat-producing ultraviolet light that does the real damage*

♦ *Altitude heightens damage: the higher you go the more you lose the protective effect of the ozone layer against ultraviolet light. A cool sunny day in the mountains carries more risk than a hot day at sea level*

♦ *Avoid the midday sun when ultraviolet radiation is greatest*

♦ *Glass stops some ultraviolet light and it is protective to be in a car even in hot climates – but you lose the benefit if you hang your arm out of the window*

Ageing skin Relentless exposure to radiation damages collagen and permanently alters the cells of the skin. Eventually the skin is prematurely aged – dry, wrinkled, tough-looking and with colour variations.

Skin cancers The risk of skin cancer is very high for white people living in high-sunshine areas. Fortunately, the majority of cases are relatively benign cancers (squamous or basal cell) and comparatively few are aggressive (malignant melanoma).

The risk of squamous or basal cell cancers reflects the total lifetime exposure to ultraviolet light. They are common in outdoor workers such as farmers and fishermen, appearing on the face and back of the hand as small persistent areas of

rough skin or small ulcers. Although common – skin cancer has reached epidemic proportions in Australia, South Africa and parts of the United States – they are nearly always curable by freezing or surgical removal and serious spread is rare.

Malignant melanoma is a different problem altogether. These dark skin patches are aggressive and infiltrate the skin. Worse, they spread to other parts of the body, especially the liver, and the risk of death is high. Melanomas have become more common due, most specialists believe, to our increased tendency to expose ourselves to sunshine. Another factor may be that raised public awareness sends people to seek help sooner for early suspicious skin change.

Certain people are at a higher risk of melanoma: the fair-skinned and blue-eyed, and those who were severely sunburnt in childhood. People who sunbathe occasionally but inten-

RECOGNIZING SKIN CANCER

✦

♦ *Inspect your skin regularly, concentrating on parts exposed to the sun – your face, ears, chest, back and limbs*

♦ *Take note of persistent patches of rough skin on light-exposed areas*

♦ *Beware spots that bleed or ulcers that do not heal*

♦ *Beware dark-coloured moles or patches that get darker, itch, bleed or spread into the surrounding skin*

♦ *Watch moles! It's boring but protective. Beware any with the above characteristics. If you have more than a hundred moles, it might be worth seeing a dermatologist*

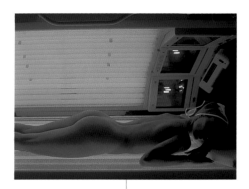

Above: Regular use of sunbeds can pose risks as strong as exposure to tropical sunshine.

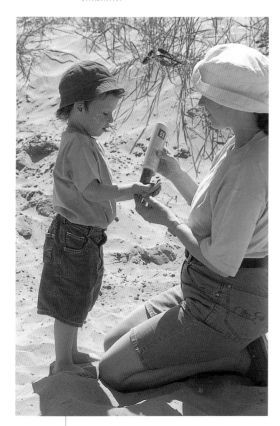

Above: Sensible precautions allow children to play outdoors while reducing later risks of skin cancer.

sively are probably at higher risk than people who are exposed to the sun more regularly. Anyone with more than a hundred moles runs a higher risk, but freckles are not a risk factor.

Sun creams

Sun creams containing titanium reflect or completely block ultraviolet light and do not allow tanning. For tanning as well as protection you need a cream or lotion that only partially absorbs ultraviolet light. The degree of protection is expressed as a factor number. For example, Factor 6 means you could stay exposed for six times longer than the length of time at which unprotected skin would burn. Factor 6 or higher gives reasonable protection but in extreme sunlight you need Factor 25 or higher.

Ordinary sun screens protect against medium-wavelength ultraviolet light (ultraviolet B), which causes sunburn. They do not protect against longer-wavelength ultraviolet light (ultraviolet A) which, while not causing sunburn, does cause long-term skin ageing and cancer. For complete protection either cover up or use sun screens that protect against both UVB and UVA.

SUN PROTECTION – DO'S AND DON'TS
◆

Do . . .

◆ *Encourage your children to enjoy being outdoors, but to wear protective clothing, sun hats and sun screen; the greater their exposure to sun, the greater their risk of skin cancer 20 or more years later*
◆ *Wear cotton or silk; it is a better barrier than looser weaves*
◆ *Cover your limbs or use sun screen*
◆ *Watch your skin and report unusual changes to a doctor*

Don't . . .

◆ *Swim at midday, thinking water protects your back; it does not*
◆ *Have short intensive sunbathing holidays, especially if you are fair-skinned or have more than a hundred moles*
◆ *Forget to renew your sun screen after swimming and after every few hours*
◆ *Use ultraviolet sunbeds all year long. Excessive use is more damaging to the skin than lying under the African sun*

SKIN CANCER

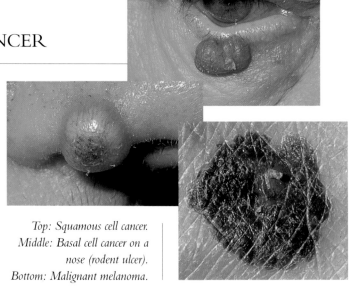

Top: *Squamous cell cancer.*
Middle: *Basal cell cancer on a
nose (rodent ulcer).*
Bottom: *Malignant melanoma.*

CAUSES

The main types of skin cancer are squamous cell, malignant melanoma and basal cell. The first two cancers are stimulated by sunlight or weather beating on the skin; environmental factors are less important with basal cell cancers.

Squamous cell cancer begins in the surface layer of skin in areas of chronic irritation, such as the face, parts of the body previously irradiated for cancer or skin exposed to chemicals. They may arise in skin irritated by **varicose veins** or leg **ulcers**.

A malignant melanoma arises from pigment cells deeper in the skin. Skin that has been severely sunburnt at some time may carry the increased risk of malignancy years later. Certain individuals inherit a tendency to pigmented patches on their body, which carry a small risk of turning malignant.

Basal cell cancer arises from cells in the epidermis for reasons similar to squamous cell cancer. Another type of skin cancer is Kaposi's sarcoma. This is a malignant nodule that was once very rare but is now common in people with **AIDS**.

SYMPTOMS

Basal and squamous cell cancers occur most often by the eyes and on the ears. They are persistently crusted patches a few millimetres in diameter and may stand slightly proud of the skin. They are painless and do not normally bleed.

A malignant melanoma is a deeply pigmented patch in or just proud of the skin. It often itches and may bleed. A malignant melanoma can occur anywhere on the body, including the neck and the soles of the feet. Individuals may have many pigmented spots, but a subtle change in colour or itch may single one out in particular.

Kaposi's sarcoma looks like a bruise that becomes darker and raised; it may occur in several sites at once.

TREATMENT

Basal and squamous cell cancers are treated by surgical removal, irradiation or, most recently, by chemotherapy creams, with very high cure rates. If neglected, they damage local tissues extensively, requiring skin grafting. It is unusual for them to spread distantly (metastasize), but if this happens the metastases are removed or treated with radiotherapy.

A melanoma always has to be cut out for analysis in order to see how deeply it has invaded the skin, because this

WARNING SIGNS OF MALIGNANT SKIN CHANGE

- *Itching, bleeding or colour change in a pre-existing spot*
- *A persistently crusted lesion, especially on the face or the back of the hands*
- *A mole that turns dark and starts to itch*
- *A mole in a position where it keeps getting irritated*
- *A dark, newly appeared spot on the soles of the feet*
- *A patch of dry skin on the face that never goes away*
- *Having multiple moles (more than 100)*

determines the outlook. If it is less than 1 mm/³⁄₆₄ in deep, the cure rate is greater than 90%. The deeper the melanoma invades, the wider the margin around the lesion must be cut out. In more advanced disease chemotherapy is given to the affected limb. Unfortunately generalized radiotherapy or chemotherapy does not appear to be very effective.

Treatment of Kaposi's sarcoma is by radiotherapy or chemotherapy, despite which recurrence is common.

Complementary Treatment

Any changes in the skin must be seen by an orthodox practitioner. Complementary therapies cannot cure cancer, but can have a supportive role during orthodox treatment. **Chakra balancing** helps with symptom control and energy balance, promotes relaxation during orthodox treatment and offers support during rehabilitation programmes. It is especially good at helping the healing of skin grafts. **Massage** can be very supportive, especially when it is combined with **aromatherapy**. *Other therapies to try: see* STRESS.

ULCERS

The outermost surface of an area of skin which has broken down and does not heal within a few days.

CAUSES

There are two broad reasons for this breakdown: problems with venous blood flow or problems with arterial blood flow.

Venous ulcers
The blood returning to the heart through the venous system is depleted of oxygen and carries other waste products from the tissues. Anything interfering with this return of blood predisposes to stagnation, lack of oxygen and tissue breakdown. Common causes are **varicose veins** and previous **deep vein thrombosis** in a limb.

Arterial ulcers
Here the cause is poor flow of fresh arterial blood because of disease of the arterial blood vessels, for example **high blood pressure**, **atherosclerosis** or **diabetes**.

Pressure sores (bed sores)
Constant unrelieved pressure closes the capillary circulation and leads to very rapid breakdown of skin.

Other causes
Several rare auto-immune illnesses cause ulcers and might be suspected because of the unusual appearance of the ulcer or characteristic symptoms elsewhere.

SYMPTOMS

Venous ulcers are found mainly on the lower leg and around the ankle. A central raw core, which can be quite large, is surrounded by an irregular margin; the skin is mottled with white and brown stains from abnormal blood leakage.

Arterial ulcers are also usually found on the legs and feet, although these tend not to be on the ankles. These ulcers are smaller, with more sharply defined edges. The limb has other features of poor blood flow such as absent pulses and thin, hairless skin. If there is doubt, blood flow can be assessed by sound scanning devices called Dopplers.

Pressure sores are found directly over the bony parts of the hips, back and ankles. They can be very deep, even extending into muscles and bone.

The smell of infected ulcers comes from particular bacteria that inhabit the oxygen-starved environment.

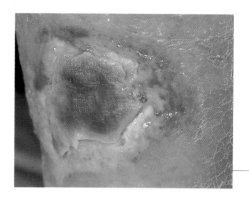

Left: A chronic leg ulcer will take many months to heal.

TREATMENT

Treat a small ulcer with antiseptic cream, but if it persists, see a doctor to exclude other diseases and to have it dressed by a nurse who has particular expertise in ulcer treatment.

An ulcer must be kept clean with antiseptic solutions and treated with an antibiotic if there is resistant infection, suggested by surrounding redness and pus and confirmed with swabs. A dressing should be worn both to allow air to get to the ulcer and to provide a protective cover that soaks up discharge without sticking to the ulcer. This encourages new skin to grow, which is not pulled off when the dressing is changed.

For venous ulcers it is important to improve blood flow by keeping the legs raised and by wearing stockings or bandages which compress the leg. These may have to be worn permanently. Such treatment is inappropriate for arterial ulcers, as compression would reduce blood flow. Where necessary, arterial flow is improved by arterial grafts or varicose veins are surgically removed. It is possible to put skin grafts on to otherwise resistant ulcers. The individual should keep as active as possible and be on a good diet to encourage healing.

Once a bed sore has developed, the pressure must be relieved to help it heal. Change the individual's position every two to three hours, and strategically place cushions and sheepskin on, between or under affected areas.

Complementary Treatment
Chinese herbalism – see DERMATITIS. **Reflexology** is an especially good therapy for leg ulcers. **Naturopathy** treatment would be based on nutrition and dietetics, especially cleansing programmes with fasting. Exercise – after recovery, **yoga** and **tai chi/chi kung** are both gentle forms of exercise which can be beneficial. **Ayurveda** – see SCABIES. *Other therapies to try: Western herbalism; homeopathy.*

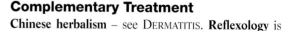

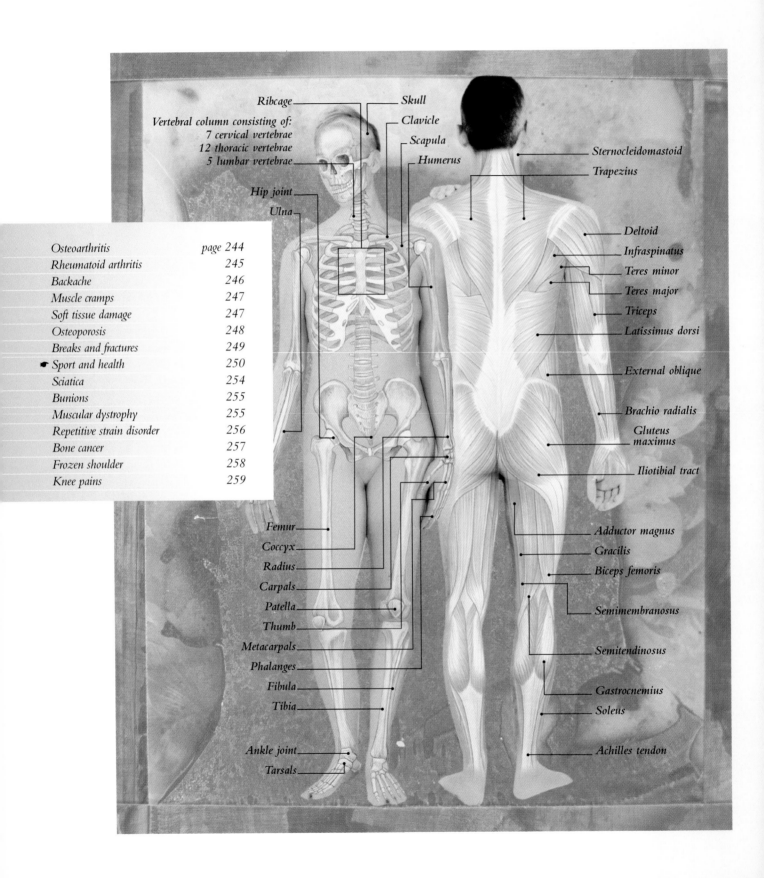

If our sophisticated internal organs, blood vessels, nerves and pipework are not to collapse, something has to keep them supported. This something is the bony skeleton, which is like a building's girders providing support for the walls and floors.

MUSCULO-SKELETAL SYSTEM

A LTHOUGH THE SKELETON can be likened to structural girders, buildings are not noted for walking. Such activity in humans requires another system – that of muscles, tendons and ligaments to convey movement to bones. The nervous system is the interface between brain and body, transmitting the brain's demands for movement to the muscles and thence to bone.

Bone

Bones consist of a tough outer cortex a few millimetres thick and a more sponge-like interior. Most bones end in cartilage, a plastic-like material that lets bone move against bone without grating. Bones seen after death give the impression of being completely inert structures, but this is misleading. Most parts of the bone are actively replacing and remodelling. Bones heal from fractures thanks to cells which throw out fresh material to knit the fracture together, followed by specialized cells which remodel the bone to its correct shape.

Within the hollow interior is the bone marrow, a tremendously active environment where much of the blood is made – the red and white blood cells and the platelets so important in blood clotting. It is this dynamic activity which makes the bone marrow susceptible to disease and poisons. It is where **leukaemia** begins and where drugs that affect bone marrow have their devastating effect.

The two main problems that affect bones and joints (apart from **breaks and fractures**) are **osteoarthritis** and **osteoporosis**. Bone infections are relatively uncommon. **Bone cancer** is also uncommon but secondary cancer frequently spreads from cancer elsewhere. Bone diseases are intimately connected with the metabolism of calcium and phosphate and are affected by several hormones – parathyroid hormone, calcitonin, thyroid, growth hormone and vitamin D, which is necessary for the absorption and deposition of calcium.

Muscle

Muscle is tissue that is specialized for the process of turning energy into movement. There are three types: skeletal muscle, which is considered here, heart muscle and lastly smooth muscle, which is the type of muscle surrounding hollow structures like the intestines and bladder.

Seen under magnification skeletal muscle is made of array after array of fibres, each composed of innumerable microfibres. These in turn are composed of the special proteins actin and myosin, which have the property of contracting when stimulated to do so by an electrical signal. Movement is transmitted from the muscle to bone through tendons, which are fibrous bands that grow from muscle into bone.

Muscle is everywhere in the body, from the minute muscles in the ear to the great back muscles, all of which are under electrical nerve control. The degree of nervous control varies so that, for example, the fine muscles of the eye can be moved more precisely than the thigh muscles. In the case of the latter, power is more important than delicacy of movement. Muscle is a reliable structure and disease of muscle is comparatively uncommon, compared to diseases of the nerve control. However, injury to muscle is very common through accidents or overuse, as are strains or ruptures of tendons.

Left: Muscle power pulls tendons and ligaments, moving the bones and joints which turn thought into action.

OSTEOARTHRITIS

◆

Painful joints caused by 'wear and tear'.

CAUSES

◆

Arthritis, technically called osteoarthritis, is virtually inevitable as people grow older. Although the joints of the body are amazingly resilient, after decades they become worn. The cartilage lining the joint frays, outgrowths of bone form around the joint in an attempt at healing and fragments of bone break off and irritate the joints, which themselves lose their natural lubrication, tending to become stiff and creaky.

Osteoarthritis is hastened by any trauma to a joint, such as accidents, **breaks and fractures** or prolonged overuse through work or exercise such as jogging. There is a strong hereditary tendency, too. Being overweight often hastens osteoarthritis of the weight-bearing joints of the hips and knees. It is a non-inflammatory condition. There is no actual disease process attacking the joint, as is the case with **gout** or **rheumatoid arthritis** (blood tests can be done if these are a possibility).

Although everyone thinks of osteoarthritis as a disease of the bone, it is more a disease of the cartilage that caps bones, which splits and degenerates until eventually bone is rubbing against bone. The deformation of osteoarthritis is caused by overgrowth of bone attempting to repair damaged cartilage. However, research is suggesting that there may be ways in the future to slow down cartilage breakdown, if not reverse it.

SYMPTOMS

◆

The joints most commonly affected are the hips, knees, neck, back and the small joints of the fingers. They become stiff and may creak. It takes time to get them moving each morning and damp weather worsens the pain. As osteoarthritis of the hip progresses, pain in the joint may stop patients sleeping.

The fingers and knees become distorted as bone grows around the joint. It is common to have flare-ups of pain and stiffness from time to time and the joints may swell with fluid.

TREATMENT

◆

Despite mild pain, it it best to keep using the joints, otherwise they stiffen even more. Exercise strengthens the muscles supporting the affected joints, relieving some of the pressure on them. Exercise should be gentle and not put sudden stress on joints such as running. Keeping joints warm also helps reduce pain. Excess weight must be reduced, especially for osteoarthritis of the hips or knees, which take all the body's weight.

Pain relief

It is best to use the mildest painkiller that is effective. For many this will be paracetamol, possibly with some aspirin or codeine. Non-steroidal anti-inflammatory drugs (NSAIDs) are useful for severe pain or to give prolonged relief. Which drug suits which individual is often a matter of trial and error, and previously effective drugs can lose their effect in time.

Heat treatment such as wax baths can be given as part of a physiotherapy programme. Sudden pain in the joint can be helped by a steroid injection.

Surgery

Surgical replacements of the hip and knee can, in selected cases, bring relief of pain and disability. Hip replacement relieves pain and restores mobility in at least 95% of cases. Only in relatively few cases does it make little difference, and rarely makes things worse. At present hip replacements last at least ten years. Less common, but possible, is to replace the shoulder or the small joints of the fingers. These operations are certain to become more routine in the next few years.

QUESTIONS

Is pain a measure of severity?
Severely distorted joints may be relatively pain free and vice versa. *Even X-rays may be misleading – hips that look dreadful on an X-ray can cause no pain. Doctors have to go by what patients report to them in assessing treatment.*

How safe are painkillers?
Paracetamol or co-proxamol are safe at recommended dosages; high dosages damage the liver. Non-steroidal anti-inflammatory drugs (NSAIDs) often cause indigestion, rashes and diarrhoea. The latest ones do this less but still should be taken as little as possible.

Complementary Treatment

Chiropractic manipulation, mobilization and soft tissue techniques are effective in increasing joint mobility and reducing pain. **Aromatherapy** and **massage** with an oil made up of one of the following can help: black pepper, ginger, frankincense, rosemary, lavender, marjoram or juniper oil (three drops in 10 ml carrier oil). **Acupuncture** is very effective in the early stages of the disease. **Alexander Technique** – see BACKACHE. *Other therapies to try: most have something to offer.*

RHEUMATOID ARTHRITIS

An auto-immune condition, with inflammation and distortion of the joints.

CAUSES

Unlike **osteoarthritis**, rheumatoid arthritis is an aggressive disease, which often leads to destruction of joints and considerable disability. Research points to it being an auto-immune condition, one in which the body's protective mechanisms turn against its own tissues. In rheumatoid arthritis the target tissue is called synovium, a membrane that lines joints and provides a lubricating synovial fluid. The synovium is invaded by cells that normally protect against infections. An array of destructive biochemicals is released, causing the synovium to swell. These biochemicals attack nearby cartilage, leading eventually to distortion of the joints.

Three-quarters of sufferers are women in whom the disease starts in their 30s and 40s. It affects 2% of the population worldwide, often those with a family history. About 10% of people end with considerable disability, but by contrast 40% experience only intermittent trouble; the rest have mild to moderate problems. Progression of the disease can take years, and in any case about 25% of cases eventually 'burn out' for reasons not understood.

SYMPTOMS

Rheumatoid arthritis is an illness that is remarkable for affecting not only the joints but many other organs, too. The disease fluctuates in its intensity. It usually begins in an undramatic form, starting with discomfort and swelling of the small joints of the hands or feet; in 25% of cases only a single joint is affected. Eventually the same joints are affected on both sides of the body with pain and stiffness, which is worse in the morning and lasts for several hours. Gradually deformity and weakness of the affected limbs appears. Often people with rheumatoid arthritis feel generally unwell.

Other joints affected may include the knees, shoulders and hips, but not the back. Over time the joints become deformed in a highly characteristic way: the fingers look spindly and fingers or toes distort away from the midline. The distorted and weakened tendons may snap.

Other symptoms include skin nodules and rashes, fluid accumulations in the lungs, **anaemia**, heart, kidney and nervous system problems, and inflamed or dry eyes.

Rheumatoid arthritis is diagnosed on a clinical picture that includes bilateral pain and characteristic deformity of small

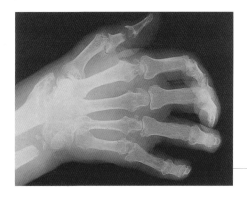

Left: Joints swollen by rheumatoid arthritis, with the fingers displaced to one side.

joints. The disease produces characteristic blood changes – a protein marker (rheumatoid factor) is positive in about 80% of cases, but a negative test does not rule it out.

TREATMENT

Exercise is beneficial at all stages, with physiotherapy encouraging people to use joints and limbs to the maximum.

Non-steroidal anti-inflammatory drugs (NSAIDs) are good for relieving pain and swelling; the choice is a matter of individual preference. Splints are used to support the joints and tendons. Many get by on these methods alone but some people require more powerful medication. In the past the next step was steroids by mouth. These dramatically reduce acute flare-ups but have many potential side effects. The trend now is to use other medication that appears to alter the condition fundamentally and not just damp it down. These drugs, which tend to have more side effects than NSAIDs and need careful monitoring, include gold, penicillamine, cyclosporin and sulphasalazine. The latest is methotrexate, which reduces rheumatoid arthritis activity remarkably.

Orthopaedic surgeons can repair ruptured tendons, inject steroids into joints to reduce inflammation, replace joints, including finger joints, and operate on bones to reduce pain.

Complementary Treatment

In the early stages of the disease **acupuncture** can produce dramatic improvements, partly by helping regulate the immune system. **Nutritional therapy** – extra B complex vitamins, vitamins C and E and zinc are recommended. **Alexander Technique** – see BACKACHE. **Chiropractic** mobilization and soft tissue techniques can help ease pain and stiffness as part of an overall treatment regime. *Other therapies to try: cymatics; tai chi/chi kung; biodynamics; chakra balancing; healing.*

BACKACHE

The causes and treatment of backache are still a matter of controversy.

CAUSES

The high incidence of back problems in humans is probably a reflection of a fundamental design fault that has not entirely adapted the back to an upright position.There is disagreement on where such a fault may lie, and why pain arises in one person but not in another. The bones of the spinal column, the vertebrae, rest on each other, cushioned by fibrous discs, and join with each other via bony projections called pedicles. Tough ligaments surround the bones. The spinal cord runs through an arch of bone; nerves leave the spinal cord snaking past the discs and running close to the bony projections.

Mechanical causes of backache include any pre-existing malformation of the spine leading to unusual curvature, excess weight, pregnancy and physically demanding work – all put extra stress on the spine. In the not uncommon spondylolisthesis, vertebrae are misaligned on one another.

Bone disease accounts for an important minority of cases of backache. **Osteoporosis**, in itself pain free, may lead to the painful collapse of one vertebra. **Bone cancer** causes pain, although there are usually suggestive symptoms elsewhere. Infection of the spine, notoriously from tuberculosis, is now uncommon. The disease ankylosing spondylitis causes a painful, very inflexible back in young men.

In diagnosis, X-rays are over-rated as they can only show osteoporosis, expected changes from **osteoarthritis** and occasionally features of malignancy. The MRI scan is the best procedure for showing the bone, spinal cord and nerves (see page 319). If bone disease is suspected then doctors may order blood tests of inflammation and calcium balance. At least 30% of all cases will remain undiagnosed. Despite psychological strategies and self-help groups, some people remain unable to work and in constant pain for which little can be offered other than variations of painkillers.

SYMPTOMS

Pain is felt on getting up, bending or lifting, and the individual may limp. Pain radiating into the legs suggests **sciatica**. The pain is often sudden in onset and individuals have good and bad days. Pain that was gradual in onset and steadily worsens, is relatively unrelated to movement and present day and night, suggests a secondary cancer or other bone disease. Examination reveals little apart from restricted movement.

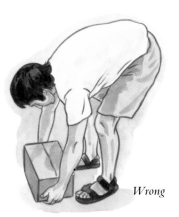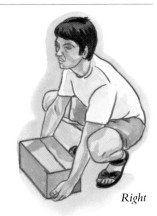

Wrong   *Right*

Above: It is important to lift using the power of your legs and shoulders rather than your back. Keep the object close to your body.

TREATMENT

Severe back pain forces you to rest for a few days but you should start moving again as soon as you can. This replaces the old advice to rest until pain free. Physiotherapy or osteopathy are helpful, encouraging mobilization and showing you correct ways to move. Take the simplest painkillers that give relief – paracetamol alone or with codeine or anti-inflammatories. Muscle spasms can be helped by a relaxant such as diazepam. Do not underestimate the value of a hot bath or a warm pad. Where there is no serious underlying disease, take painkillers for flare-ups and be careful lifting and carrying.

An epidural corticosteroid injection reduces pain and speeds recovery. It is worthwhile in sciatica not responding to routine treatment. Less than one per cent of patients with back pain require surgery; procedures range from the removal of the prolapsed disc (microdiscectomy) to a spinal operation to fuse the vertebrae so they cannot move and cause pain.

 Complementary Treatment
The **Alexander Technique** leads to release of over-contracted muscles, a freeing up of the joints and a lengthening of the spine, all of which reduce mechanical strain. **Chiropractic** manipulation is particularly useful for general, non-specific back pain. **Osteopathy** is effective and one of the least invasive treatments for backache. **Hellerwork** relieves symptoms by organizing the whole body structure with respect to gravity. **Rolfing** improves spinal alignment and posture. *Other therapies to try: acupuncture; aromatherapy.*

MUSCLE CRAMPS

Benign spasms in muscle, usually in the leg.

CAUSES

Cramps follow vigorous exertion when waste products accumulate in muscle. Although this explains the cramps of a marathon runner it does little to illuminate the night cramps that affect the elderly and others, for instance those who have cramps plus restless legs (Ekbom's syndrome).

Some people have particularly sensitive muscles, with points of more exquisite tenderness called trigger points. This condition is called fibromyalgia. This is not a disease, although the condition can certainly be very distressing.

Only rarely are cramps caused by an underlying abnormality; the most important to consider are poor blood circulation and, less often, disorders of calcium balance.

SYMPTOMS

A muscle, usually in the leg, goes into a spasm of contraction; the toes may be pulled over. The cramp lasts just a few minutes. Pain after exertion which recurs when an individual is re-exercising suggests a blood flow problem.

TREATMENT

Quinine tablets at night are widely used and effective; beware taking excessive amounts as they can affect the heartbeat. Muscle relaxants like diazepam are helpful, as are anti-inflammatory gels rubbed on to the muscles. Exercises and massage can also be tried to stretch the affected muscles.

QUESTION

What is Ekbom's syndrome?
This refers to restless legs – legs continuously moving whether or not you want them to, a symptom allied to night cramps. It is sometimes caused by iron-deficiency anaemia. If anaemia has been treated, other medication to use includes diazepam and phenytoin.

Complementary Treatment
Chiropractic – soft tissue techniques are effective with muscular cramps brought on by overuse and sporting injuries. **Western herbalism** – cramp bark is a muscle relaxant. *Other therapies to try: most have something to offer.*

SOFT TISSUE DAMAGE

Injury to muscles, tendons or ligaments, as opposed to bones or joints.

CAUSES

Soft tissues mean muscle, ligaments (the tough strips connecting bone, for example around the knee joint) and tendons (strips where muscle attaches to bone, for example the tendons of the fingers). Injury occurs through overstretching from sport, exercise and awkward movements and direct blows caused by accidents. Occasionally, other pre-existing illness can cause inflammation, for example arthritis.

SYMPTOMS

The affected structure is painful and tender. It swells, often very rapidly, and as a result there is restriction of movement of the affected limb. Complete inability to use a joint or deformity suggest a more serious rupture or tear of soft tissue.

TREATMENT

Most injuries are self-limiting, settling over a few days or weeks; they require only care in use and rubbing in of an anti-inflammatory gel or taking an anti-inflammatory tablet. More chronic problems often respond to a steroid injection into the tender area and physiotherapy with heat treatment or ultrasound, as well as exercises to restrengthen the muscles around the affected soft tissues. You should also consider changes to sports technique and avoid any repetitive strain. (See also the RICE principle for bruises and sprains, page 252.)

Complementary Treatment
Chiropractic is effective in the treatment of injuries anywhere in the body. **Osteopathy** techniques effect a maximum rate of healing. **Hellerwork** – see BACKACHE. **Rolfing** is a therapy that aids mobility; this helps new tissues to build and helps joints to function in appropriate alignment.

OSTEOPOROSIS

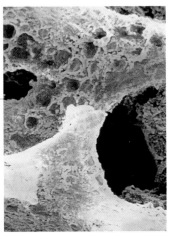

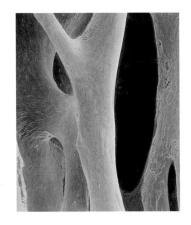

Thinning of bone, with an increased risk of fractures.

CAUSES

Whereas osteoporosis used to be regarded simply as an inevitable result of ageing, increasingly it is being targeted for prevention and treatment. There is now recognition of its consequences in terms of fractures, hospital admissions and deaths. The bulk of bone is calcium and phosphorus regulated by an extremely complex system, including parathyroid hormone and vitamin D, which is necessary to absorb calcium. Large amounts of vitamin D are produced by the action of sunlight on the skin; the rest comes from dairy products.

Above: Osteoporotic bone; the many small, round, dark areas are empty, causing brittleness. Left: Normal bone.

Thin bones
Each year some 20% of the calcium in bone is replaced. For much of adult life this turnover is unimportant, but it becomes a major problem for menopausal women when their oestrogen levels fall. Calcium and phosphorus in bone is lost rapidly up to ten years after the menopause. Men suffer much less from it, but the more it is looked for the more it is also found.

Old age
Bone density, which peaks at the age of 30, continues to fall into the 70s and 80s with immobility contributing to this.

Steroids and other factors
People taking oral steroids for severe **asthma** or **rheumatoid arthritis** risk osteoporosis, a fact that is now more widely recognized. Others are at risk if they have a poor intake of calcium and get little exposure to sunlight. There are also several unusual hormone disorders that predispose to osteoporosis.

SYMPTOMS

Osteoporosis causes neither pain nor tenderness. Often the thin bones are discovered by chance during X-rays for some other reason. Otherwise osteoporosis reveals itself when a weakened bone collapses or fractures. If this happens in the vertebrae there is sudden severe **backache**; the other common sites are a hip or wrist fracture. Gradually, the individual becomes shorter through imperceptible loss of height of the vertebrae and shrinkage of the intervertebral discs, and the back often bends into the so-called dowager's hump.

A bone scan determines the degree of osteoporosis and is helpful in deciding whether treatment is wise. Blood tests may be advisable to exclude the rarer causes of osteoporosis.

TREATMENT

For menopausal women the best treatment is hormone replacement therapy (HRT), which reduces the rate of bone density loss (see page 22). This is even more important for women having an early menopause or who have previously had oral steroids, who are immobile or smoke or drink excessively – all factors further increasing the risks of osteoporosis.

Diet and vitamin D
To build and maintain bones, women should have a diet rich in calcium and vitamin D and stay active throughout their life. Both women and men should take at least 1.5 g a day of calcium, plus vitamin D supplements if they are housebound and getting no sunlight. The same treatment applies to men and women with established osteoporosis of old age.

Medication
Drugs such as etidronate and alendronate improve established osteoporosis by reducing the activity of those cells within the bones which otherwise remodel it.

Complementary Treatment
Nutritional therapy – as well as lack of calcium, magnesium deficiency can be a contributing factor; zinc supplements could be helpful, together with a daily intake of ground sesame seeds and comfrey leaves. **Chiropractic** soft tissue techniques are frequently used to help ease the pain of spinal problems caused by osteoporosis; there is always muscle spasm in the area of the fracture, which causes pain. *Other therapies to try: chakra balancing; cymatics; tai chi/chi kung; shiatsu-do; Alexander Technique.*

BREAKS AND FRACTURES

There are many causes of bone injuries or malformations.

CAUSES

It is easy to think of bones as inert structures acting simply as girders for the body. However, bones are living things with vital roles in calcium metabolism and in forming the cells that circulate in the blood stream. It is because bones are living that fractures do heal, by regeneration of the broken surface.

Accidents account for most fractures, through either direct trauma or some repetitive stress that causes a bone to shear. In theory, any bone in the body can fracture; in practice it is the longer bones of the arm and thigh that are at greater risk through mechanical reasons. There are one or two small bones that fracture readily because of their shape. For example, the scaphoid bone at the base of the thumb can be fractured by a relatively minor fall on the hand.

Anything that weakens the bone increases the chances of it fracturing under normal stresses. **Osteoporosis**, which is the usual reason for this weakening of bone, leads to fractures of the vertebrae of the spine and the hip.

Many types of cancer spread around the body, or metastasize, and bone is a favoured target. The cancerous deposit weakens the bone, causing pain. It then takes just a little extra stress to make the bone fracture. Sites where this occurs most are the vertebrae and the long bones of the arms and the legs (see BONE CANCER).

SYMPTOMS

Following trauma, a bone feels tender and is painful to use. There may be obvious deformity of the limb and bruising over the site of injury. Less commonly, pain occurs spontaneously in the absence of obvious trauma. This most often happens in the case of collapse of a vertebra through osteoporosis or a stress fracture of one of the small bones of the feet.

A spontaneous fracture of a long bone raises suspicion of underlying bone disease or cancerous spread but it must be stressed that these are relatively uncommon.

X-rays confirm most fractures; sometimes subtle fractures need investigation with repeat X-rays or specialized scans.

TREATMENT

This depends on both the site and severity of the fracture. At the most severe, for example fracture of the hip or skull, immediate surgery is required to remove dead tissues and

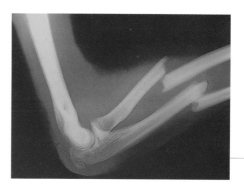

Left: A compound fracture of the forearm, which can be repaired only by surgery.

bone fragments, and to reset bones and fix them in place with screws or artificial replacements, as in the case of a hip joint. More often, bone has fractured in a clean break, requiring only realignment and fixing in position with a plaster cast or firm bandage while healing. Not all fractures need treating: a fractured rib or foot bone can usually be left to heal naturally. Often people need physiotherapy after a fracture in order to recover full use of the muscles around the fracture site.

QUESTIONS

How are fractures categorized?
Simple fractures are partial or complete breaks that just need re-setting without other surgical treatment. Compound fractures are where there are multiple bone fragments, damage to local flesh or opening of overlying skin. These need intensive surgery to reset and in order to avoid infection.

How long does healing take?
Fractures of the upper limbs take three to six weeks to heal; lower limb fractures such as the thigh and tibia take six to twelve weeks. Any fracture may take a year or more to recover full strength.

Complementary Treatment

Alexander Technique – see BACKACHE. A **nutritional therapist** might suggest zinc and vitamin C supplements. **Chiropractic** – soft tissue techniques are often used after a break or fracture has healed to restore movement and help reduce soft tissue swelling, which may remain long after bone damage has healed. **Rolfing** – see SOFT TISSUE DAMAGE. *Other therapies to try: Chinese herbalism; acupuncture; cymatics; healing; Ayurveda; tai chi/chi kung; Western herbalism.*

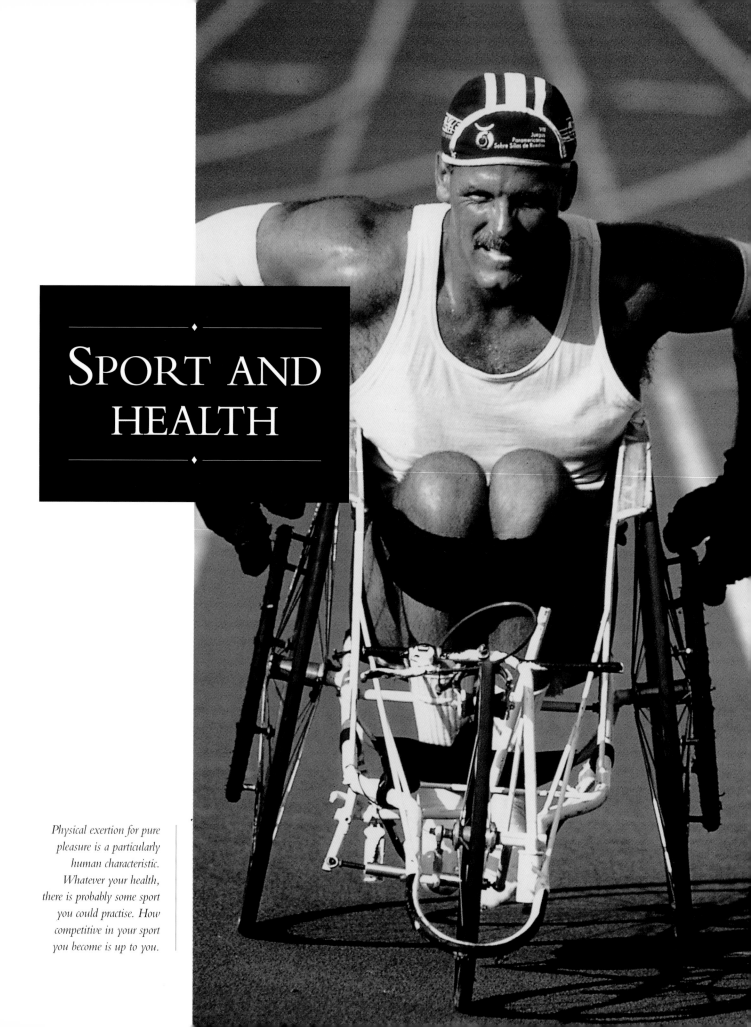

SPORT AND HEALTH

Physical exertion for pure pleasure is a particularly human characteristic. Whatever your health, there is probably some sport you could practise. How competitive in your sport you become is up to you.

Some of our most popular leisure activities involve playing, watching or arguing about sports. This cannot be by chance. Most societies, ancient and modern, have embraced the notion of groups of men or women playing competitive games in a constant search to determine the faster, stronger or more skilful.

Muscle and energy

The body's preferred source of energy is sugar, which is stored as glycogen, but the body can also break down fat or even protein to provide the energy that allows muscle fibres to contract.

Aerobic and anaerobic energy Oxygen is vital to the production of energy by muscles. When the amount of oxygen delivered by the heart and lungs matches the muscles' demands, it allows energy production by aerobic, or oxygen-rich, energy pathways. The body can cope for a while without oxygen by using chemical pathways that avoid the immediate need for oxygen. This is anaerobic exertion.

When you first exercise, more energy comes from anaerobic sources; aerobic pathways start up after a few minutes. However, waste products produced by anaerobic energy production, especially lactic acid, eventually have to be got rid of with oxygen. This is called an oxygen debt and generates heavy breathing.

Training

Our bodies get used to our normal level of activity; by training we aim to enhance that. Training means improving the whole energy-producing system of the body by gradually increasing the level of effort. A little training goes a long way, because it is far easier to improve fitness a little – from, say, poor to modest – than it is to train from excellent to superb. Benefits from training can be felt in just a couple of weeks and significant changes in exercise ability take place within three months.

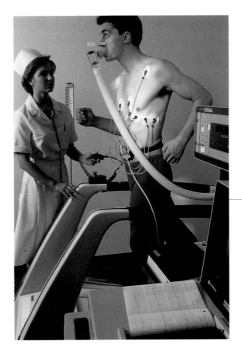

Left: Here an athlete's maximum oxygen consumption is being measured. This knowledge helps a coach to plan a training programme.

What training does Gradually lung capacity rises and the heart muscle becomes larger, beats harder and pumps blood more vigorously round the body. Muscle fibres grow, their blood supply improves and they become more efficient at producing energy.

How training is measured The easiest measure of exertion is heart rate, although specialized units can measure actual work done by the body and oxygen consumption. Everyone has a maximum heart rate reached by a period of steady exertion. For training a programme should keep the heart rate at between 60% and 85% of that maximum for at least 20 minutes, repeated two or three days a week. This can be achieved by brisk walking, jogging, cycling or stepping exercises. Additional exercises will strengthen individual muscle groups in the arms, legs, abdomen and so on.

By gradually increasing the exertion demanded, a training programme forces the body's muscles to adapt and grow, including the heart muscle.

Warming up and warming down

These are important elements whether for sports or for more general exercise. Warming up includes careful stretching of muscles and tendons and gentle jogging. Ten minutes of such exertion shifts up to 70% of blood flow into the muscles (which receive 15–20% in the absence of exertion). The muscles also literally warm up and this improves their efficiency and power output and reduces the likelihood of tearing a muscle or tendon. A warm-up should cause mild sweating.

Why warm down? Gentle exertion after sports or training keeps blood flowing through muscles. This flushes away waste products built up during exertion, preventing the cramps and sudden muscle fatigue that may result from abrupt cessation of activity.

Sport and risk

An element of danger is an essential part of sport – certain sports more than others. Some injuries are pure accident while others are inherent in the sport, such as facial injuries in boxing. Many sports have rules or equipment to reduce the risk of injury, for example penalties for foul play in football and face guards in cricket. Equipment should always be well maintained and properly used. Some people simply may not have the build or flexibility to attempt certain sports and should be advised accordingly.

Sports injuries This encompasses a very wide range of injuries from simple sprains to dislocations of joints, requiring correspondingly skilled assessment and treatment. Many sports injuries are strains and sprains of muscles and tendons. In such injuries fibres are overstretched or torn and there is

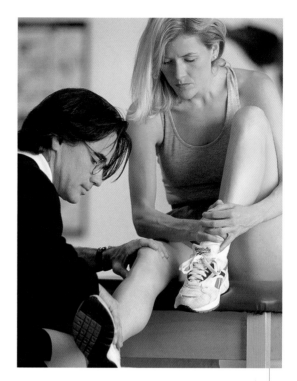

Above: Physiotherapy may be necessary for a sports injury to reduce disability and hasten recovery.

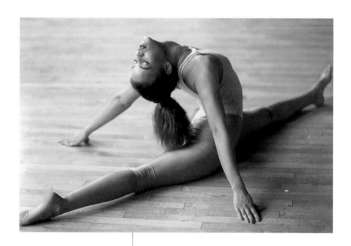

Above: Such remarkable suppleness is achievable only through methodical progressive exercise and care during exertion.

DEALING WITH MINOR INJURIES WITH PAIN AND SWELLING

◆

Remember RICE:

R	*Rest*
I	*Ice to cool the injury and prevent inflammation*
C	*Compression with a bandage to reduce swelling*
E	*Elevation – slightly raising the limb, again to reduce swelling*

Until you are able to obtain a professional opinion, these simple measures will reduce tissue damage and shorten the time for healing. (See also First Aid, pages 350–65.)

SPORTS PHYSIOTHERAPY

Sports physiotherapists are skilled practitioners whose aim is to enhance healing and restore body function. They have many techniques at their disposable. Here are some physiotherapy techniques used in sports injuries:

♦ Mobilization — *Massage, to increase blood flow and to reduce scar tissue formation*

♦ Stretching — *To prevent scarring and shortening of injured ligaments, tendons or muscles and to keep muscles supple*

♦ Exercising — *Maintaining function and preventing bad habits, for example over-protecting an injured limb*

♦ Ultrasound — *Vibrating tissues to break up scars, enhance blood flow and reduce pain*

♦ Megapulse or diathermy — *Electrical or radio-type energy that heats deep tissues, reducing pain and improving blood flow*

♦ Laser — *Reduces inflammation and increases collagen production for healing*

♦ Cooling — *With ice or cold packs to reduce swelling and pain*

♦ TENS — *Electrical stimulation at low frequencies for pain relief. Electrodes are applied to acupuncture points*

often bleeding at the site of injury, with resulting swelling, pain and interference with function. Other injuries are from overuse of muscles and ligaments, bones and joints and may call for a decision on whether a sportsperson is capable of continuing to play.

Myths about sport

'It's dangerous' Death during sport is a rare event but hits the headlines if it occurs during mass exercise such as a marathon. Where thousands of people are participating, statistics suggest that one death can be expected per seven thousand middle-aged people. Studies on middle-aged men suggest that about half of those affected were already known to have some form of heart or cardiovascular disease.

Overall, exercise is definitely good for you, but it should be regular and not intermittent. Statistics show that those people at greatest risk of illness during vigorous exertion are those who are normally inactive.

If you are taking up sport or exercise in middle age, proceed with care. Begin at gentle levels, rest frequently and be alert for unusual breathlessness, faintness or chest pains.

'You're past it' Exercise will benefit you whatever your age, although take care about starting. To be effective, sport or exercise need not be exhausting: simply walking 1.6 km/ 1 mile briskly two or three times a week is excellent activity. Remember, too, that exercise will show a pay-off within a couple of weeks in terms of stamina and breathing, while considerable improvement will take no more than three to four months.

'It will accelerate arthritis' There is some evidence that certain sports cause joints to wear. These are sports involving heavy impact such as jogging, batting or boxing. The evidence is controversial as to whether this accelerates **osteoarthritis**. It seems sensible as you get older to avoid sports such as jogging which put sudden strains on knee and hip joints. Wear well-supporting footwear and try to avoid running on hard surfaces. More suitable alternatives include walking, swimming and golf. If you take care, there is no reason why you should not continue to play tennis or badminton. Weight-bearing exercise is important prevention against **osteoporosis**.

SCIATICA

Pressure on a nerve, leading to backache and pain in the leg.

CAUSES

Sciatica in younger people probably follows partial slippage of a vertebral disc. The intervertebral discs are made up of a jelly-like core within a fibrous ring; a tear in this ring allows the contents to leak out and impinge upon the nerve roots. These coalesce to form the sciatic nerve, which runs down the back of the thigh into the calf and the foot. In older people the cause appears to be osteoarthritic outgrowths of bone that similarly irritate the nerves (see OSTEOARTHRITIS). The sciatic nerve is particularly affected because the vertebrae at the base of the spine – the lumbo-sacral region – are curved to a degree that increases the chances of a disc slipping. Sometimes there is a clear episode that precipitates sciatica; more often a minor exertion seems to bring it on or it appears out of the blue.

SYMPTOMS

The onset is usually acute with sudden severe low back pain, worse on coughing or straining and flexing the back. The pain radiates down the back of the thigh and calf and ends in the sole of the foot. This is classic sciatica but there are variations depending on exactly which nerves are being affected. For example, pain may radiate more over the side and back of the foot. Along with the pain there may be muscular weakness in a pattern that again reflects which nerves are irritated, for example weakness in pressing the foot down or extending the knee. The ritual of tapping out knee and ankle reflexes further determines which nerves are affected. Your doctor will check your straight leg raising, which means lifting your leg to see how high it can go without severe pain. Anything less than about 45° suggests significant pressure on the sciatic nerve.

Investigations are of little benefit at this stage unless examination suggests a serious disc slippage that might need surgery, or any other worrying symptoms of **backache**.

TREATMENT

Treatment overlaps with that of backache. Rest for a few days, then attempt as much movement as you can. Use painkillers, and muscle relaxants if muscle spasms are a problem. Doctors are reluctant to prescribe the most powerful and possibly addictive painkillers for what they know may be a chronic condition. Physiotherapy helps to mobilize the spine and it is also good for boosting confidence.

On this basis most episodes of sciatica will settle, many within a few weeks, but be prepared for full recovery to take three to twelve months. Persistent pain might be helped by a steroid injection into the spinal canal; this requires a general anaesthetic and the effects are often temporary.

In less than one in a hundred cases, symptoms point to a persistently slipped disc: constant pressure on nerves, paralysis of foot movements, interference with urinary control and unremitting pain. Here investigations with an MRI scan (see page 319) may confirm a seriously slipped disc and surgery might be appropriate. This aims to remove the slipped disc by surgically exposing the vertebrae or, as is increasingly done, by guided microdiscectomy, where fine instruments are guided to the disc through a small cut in the back.

QUESTIONS

Why do doctors ask about bladder control?
They want to know about bladder control even if the sciatica seems otherwise routine because you may lose the ability to control your bladder or your bowels and may require emergency disc surgery.

What investigations are available?
The MRI scan is the best for seeing how badly a disc is slipped (see page 319). Back X-rays are of little positive use, although many people find a normal plain X-ray reassuring. If bone disease is suspected, your doctor may suggest blood tests and a bone scan.

Why is surgery done so infrequently?
Since about 80% of episodes of sciatica recover within a few weeks delay is prudent. Although 95% of selected disc surgery is successful, 5% of cases remain the same or get worse.

Complementary Treatment
 Acupuncture is a very powerful treatment. **Alexander Technique** is also useful – see BACKACHE. **Chiropractic** manipulation is an effective and speedy treatment. **Yoga** can be helpful, but must be undertaken only under the guidance of a suitably qualified teacher. **Osteopathy** can help if the cause is a prolapsed intervertebral disc or other spinal condition. **Hellerwork** – see BACKACHE. **Rolfing** corrects imbalances which can compress the sciatic nerve. *Other therapies to try: chakra balancing; shiatsu-do; naturopathy; cymatics; auricular therapy; Ayurveda.*

BUNIONS

A deformity of the big toe, very common to one degree or other.

CAUSES

A bunion is a 'lump' at the base of the big toe, which bends inward, cramping other toes. The lump is caused by outward displacement of the metatarsal bone in the foot itself. Adding to the deformity is a fluid-filled structure, a bursa, where toe and metatarsal meet, plus bony outgrowths. Heredity is thought to play the major part in this. Bunions mainly affect middle-aged people and, occasionally, adolescents.

SYMPTOMS

There may be none at all. Pain is possible from the pressure of footwear. The bursa itself may become inflamed or infected.

TREATMENT

Well-fitting footwear relieves any pain from the bunion and allows many people to put up with bunions if the appearance does not bother them unduly.

Otherwise treatment is surgical correction of the displaced bones, via one of a number of operations to trim different parts of the bones involved. They are quite successful, although they are rather painful at the time.

QUESTION

Do tight shoes cause bunions?
This is a question on which everyone has an opinion and few have a scientifically confirmed answer. Current orthopaedic opinion is that footwear does not play any significant role, even shoes that are narrow and pointed with high heels. Heredity is more likely to blame. Everyone, however, agrees that cramping footwear is best avoided if only for the sake of comfort.

 Complementary Treatment
Chakra balancing promotes relaxation and pain control, and can lessen inflammation and improve healing of damaged tissue. **Cymatics** could help – consult a therapist. *Other therapies to try: chiropractic.*

MUSCULAR DYSTROPHY

Inherited disorders that can affect muscle function.

CAUSES

These disorders alter the way muscle grows, leading to weakness of certain muscles. The most common, Duchenne muscular dystrophy (DMD), affects one in three thousand newborn boys. The genetic defect causes abnormal entry of calcium into the muscle fibres because of lack of dystrophin, a protein in the muscle cell wall. Girls are carriers but are unaffected. DMD can be identified via a heel prick sample of blood from newborn boys. If positive, mothers can be offered screening of subsequent at-risk foetuses and abortion if desired. Female siblings of affected boys should also be tested to see if they carry the gene. There are no easy choices with this disease.

SYMPTOMS

In DMD the boy experiences leg weakness, which hampers normal walking and running; it is usually obvious by the age

of four. The calf muscles often look well developed. Later, other muscles become involved, including the heart muscle. Deterioration is inevitable, ending with heart and breathing problems; survival is unlikely beyond the age of 20. Other types affect the muscles of the shoulders, neck and hands. Most of these, other than DMD, follow a relatively benign path.

TREATMENT

Nothing arrests the progression of DMD, although steroids may slow it down. Physiotherapy helps avoid otherwise inevitable contractures of muscles. It is important to analyse the exact type of muscular dystrophy for an accurate outlook.

 Complementary Treatment
Chiropractic treatment is often used as part of the overall treatment regime to help general joint and muscle movement and flexibility. **Ayurveda** oils are very powerful for improving wasted muscles; specific oil massages are recommended.

REPETITIVE STRAIN DISORDER

Apart from a few accepted syndromes, this problem, sometimes known as repetitive strain injury (RSI), is dogged by controversy.

CAUSES

Many tendons run for part of their course through insulating sheaths, which lubricate and guide them. It is well known that if these tendons swell through excess use, they can 'snag' against the insulating sheath. This is best known in relation to the fingers and thumbs, where it is called tenosynovitis. Different types of tenosynovitis have agreed symptoms and signs and even their own names, for example De Quervain's tenosynovitis of the thumb.

The concept of repetitive strain disorder (RSD) is more controversial, with its combination of non-specific tiredness and discomfort of the limb, especially the hands. This is because, unlike tenosynovitis, there are no identified abnormalities in the limb to account for the symptoms.

Nevertheless, in many countries the law has stepped in where doctors fear to tread and it is now accepted as a condition associated with keyboard workers and assembly workers whose jobs involve repetitive wrist and finger movements.

SYMPTOMS

The pain of tenosynovitis overlies specific tendons, for example those of the fingers, often with red inflammation over them. The patient and doctor may feel a grating sensation on flexing those tendons. At worst the tendon fails to run freely at all through the sheath, moving instead in a series of painful jolts as it catches and breaks free. De Quervain's tenosynovitis involves pain on movement of the base of the thumb.

This contrasts with repetitive strain disorder where there is nothing to find on examination and where the diagnosis rests entirely on individuals, who may have overused their muscles and their tendons, reporting discomfort during work, which disappears on rest.

TREATMENT

Doctors first wish to exclude known treatable syndromes that cause hand and wrist pains, for example carpal tunnel syndrome, which is caused by compression of a nerve at the wrist where pain spreads in a characteristic way across several fingers. It may take electrical tests of nerve function to exclude this kind of problem. Carpal tunnel syndrome is treated by surgical release of the compressing band.

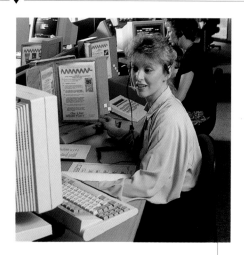

Above: Comfortable working positions are important for everyone, not only people with RSD.

Tenosynovitis responds initially to rest – perhaps aided by a splint on the wrist, the rubbing on of anti-inflammatory gels or taking anti-inflammatory tablets and physiotherapy. The next step is a steroid injection into the point of tenderness. Occasionally there is constant pain and a grating of tendons, for which the treatment is to open up the tendon sheath surgically, although sometimes symptoms recur.

This leaves a number of people with the vaguer complaints of RSD. For these, too, a short period (perhaps a few weeks) off work plus anti-inflammatory treatments may relieve symptoms. Their working practice needs assessing, preferably by a physiotherapist skilled in this area, who will be able to review the timing and length of breaks, and the working position. She might suggest, for example, a better chair or a work desk at a better level, or using a wrist support to help relieve discomfort from typing. Some people, however, still might find they are unable to cope with certain occupations.

       Complementary Treatment

Acupuncture is most helpful in the early stages of the disorder. **Chiropractic** manipulation, mobilization and soft tissue techniques, alongside ergonomic advice, is very effective. **Yoga** is sometimes very effective. **Ayurveda** recommends regular oil massage. **Osteopathy** has achieved excellent results. **Rolfing** eases strain on joints and helps you to move them with less effort. *Other therapies to try: chakra balancing; shiatsu-do; Alexander Technique; cymatics; Hellerwork.*

BONE CANCER

Tumours of bone, usually spread there from cancer in other sites.

CAUSES

Cancers shed cells into the blood stream that are liable to lodge and grow in bones because bones have such a high blood flow. This is called secondary cancer. The cancers most likely to spread in this way are breast, lung and prostate cancer, although many others can do so. Tumours arising from within the bone itself, primary bone tumours, are extremely uncommon; they affect mainly children and young adults. Types include osteosarcoma and chondrosarcoma.

SYMPTOMS

The prime symptom is persistent and gnawing pain, often with tenderness over the site. Cancer pain feels worse at night, so night pain is an ominous symptom. That said, there are certain primary bone tumours that are painful but benign, and also other conditions that can cause bone pain, including injury and infection (osteomyelitis), which can be difficult to differentiate from cancer even after detailed scans.

There may be swelling over the cancer, especially with primary bone tumours. Sometimes the first sign of a cancer is when the weakened bone fractures under modest stress. However, many secondary bone tumours grow with minimal symptoms and are discovered only on investigation of cancers elsewhere following a bone scan. This is a routine test before planning treatment because the options will be different if the cancer has already spread into the bones, liver, lungs or brain.

Bone tumours affect the body's calcium balance and they release enzymes into the blood stream, which in turn can cause other symptoms such as excessive urine production, vomiting and **constipation**.

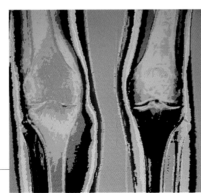

Right: Bone cancer of the tibia (left) glows green in this CT scan.

TREATMENT

In primary bone tumours the exact type of tumour needs to be established by biopsy to plan treatment, which now consists of replacing the diseased bone with metal implants; radiotherapy and chemotherapy are additional treatments (see pages 338 and 339). Secondary tumours are very serious, but something can still be done: radiotherapy can greatly reduce pain and preventive surgery can strengthen a long bone like the femur (thigh bone) that looks as if it might fracture.

Pain relief begins with anti-inflammatory drugs such as diclofenac or ibuprofen, which can be taken together with conventional painkillers such as paracetamol or dihydrocodeine. Eventually it may be necessary to turn to narcotic painkillers. The choice is increasingly wide, with morphine available as a liquid, in tablets and once-a-day preparations.

At the same time, treatment is given to the cancer from which the bone cancer has spread; chemotherapy for the primary may also reduce the pain from the secondary deposits.

The treatment of high calcium may be necessary to relieve excess urine production and constipation. The level of calcium is also a means of monitoring the response to treatment.

QUESTIONS

When should bone pain in children be taken seriously?
Without a clear history of injury, pain persisting for over a week or so should be assessed, especially if a bone appears swollen. Even so, the chances of it being due to a tumour are extremely low.

Why is bone cancer so difficult to cure?
Cure, even if possible, would require high doses of chemotherapy and radiotherapy, which would eradicate the vital bone marrow. Because the cancer is bound to have spread elsewhere, cure would still be improbable.

Complementary Treatment
Complementary therapies cannot cure cancer, but can make a valuable contribution during orthodox treatment. **Chakra balancing** can promote relaxation and pain control, and offer support during orthodox treatment. **Massage** improves self-esteem and encourages a sense of wellbeing. **Reflexology** and **aromatherapy** can both help cope with the stress and tensions generated by this disease. *Other therapies to try: see STRESS.*

FROZEN SHOULDER

A term covering a variety of conditions that cause pain and limit shoulder movements.

CAUSES

The term 'frozen shoulder' is more a description of the effects of shoulder pain than an explanation of the underlying disease process. The joint is literally frozen in position by pain. Uncertainty about the precise cause is mirrored by the many alternative terms for a painful stiff shoulder, for example sub-acromial bursitis, capsulitis and rotator cuff lesions.

The shoulder joint is between the upper arm (the humerus), the collar bone (clavicle) and the shoulder blade (scapula). These are bound together by joint capsules, tendons and muscles in a way that combines strength with a wide flexibility of movement. Usually, movement takes place in the ball-and-socket joint of the upper humerus (the ball) and the shoulder blade (the socket), stabilized by the clavicle. Several of the shorter muscles which move the arm meet in a fused sheath of muscle called the rotator cuff, which overlies the joints. The actions of the rotator cuff are supplemented by those of many other muscles, including the biceps and deltoids. At a rough count there are ten main muscles acting via a number of tendons and cushioned by two large fluid-filled sacs called bursas, which insulate the tendons from bone.

It is clear that there is plenty of opportunity for muscle fibres to tear through excessive force, for tendons to fray, for the fluid-filled sacs to inflame and for bone to rub. It does not take much effort to damage the shoulder and indeed one possible cause is simply disuse of the shoulder. It is fortunate that frozen shoulder usually affects one side only.

SYMPTOMS

The main symptoms are pain and stiffness of shoulder movements, especially those involving rotation of the arm. Symptoms can vary from a twinge when the shoulder reaches a certain position to the situation where any movement of the shoulder is painful, a true frozen shoulder. Specialized examination can pinpoint reasonably precisely which muscles or tendons are involved by seeing which positions provoke pain.

TREATMENT

There is a natural tendency for a frozen shoulder to heal with time, regardless of treatment, taking nine to fifteen months on average. The value of any treatment therefore has to be judged against this natural recovery time. Anti-inflammatory drugs are the logical first choices, but it is important to choose one that is least likely to cause stomach irritation because it will probably need to be taken for several months.

Having early physiotherapy to the shoulder helps prevent the additional stiffness arising from an individual's understandable reluctance to use it. Heat treatment, ultrasound and exercises should relieve pain sufficiently and give back enough confidence to keep the joint in use. A steroid injection into a specifically painful site can be very effective.

In selected cases of frozen shoulder, an orthopaedic surgeon will need to look into the joint with a fibreoptic endoscope, for example if healing is delayed or if a surgical repair of a tendon is thought necessary.

QUESTIONS

Are X-rays helpful?
These are less informative than people think. They are advisable after major trauma which might have broken a bone, but otherwise their value is limited because they do not show up the muscles or tendons. These structures are demonstrated by an MRI scan (see page 319), which is now the preferred investigation.

When is more urgent treatment needed?
If there is severe loss of function, for example inability to lift or rotate the arm. In this case a tendon may have ruptured and will need urgent repair.

How does movement occur if the shoulder joint is locked?
By rotating the shoulder blade and so lifting up the arm. This is similar to overcoming a stiff knee by swinging the leg from the hip.

Complementary Treatment
Acupuncture increases the circulation of blood and energy, reduces inflammation and pain, and stimulates healing of damaged tissues. **Alexander Technique** – see BACKACHE. **Chiropractic** manipulation, mobilization and soft tissue techniques are very effective. **Ayurveda** recommends regular oil massage and yoga. **Osteopathy** can offer highly specific manual treatments. **Rolfing** restores mobility by lengthening the compressed tissues. *Other therapies to try: shiatsu-do; cymatics; yoga; tai chi/chi kung; Hellerwork.*

KNEE PAINS

The causes of knee pain are many and various.

CAUSES

The knee joint is formed by the thigh bone (femur) and the shin bone (tibia). The bones are cushioned by cartilage pads called menisci, which have a curved shape. Tough ligaments tether the bones and the joint is further stabilized by the kneecap and strong thigh muscles.

In children, the cause of pain is almost certainly injury from sport or accidents. The resulting pain is more from strain of tendons and ligaments than any damage to the bone.

Adolescents experience growing pains – they really do exist. In relation to knees the classic condition is Osgood Schlatter's disease, with tenderness where the bone is growing, just below the kneecap. Chondromalacia patellae is a common problem in adolescent girls; it is thought to be caused by irregularity of the back of the patella (kneecap) where it rests against the bones of the thigh and lower leg.

In adults injuries are the most likely cause of knee pain. Sportsmen and women are prone to tear the cartilages in the knee; the torn fragment prevents full movement of the joint. **Rheumatoid arthritis** and **gout** are less common causes of knee pain.

In late adult life and old age, **osteoarthritis** is the cause of most knee pain. It is possible for fragments of bone to break into osteoarthritic knees with an effect like that of throwing sand into a watch movement.

At all ages infection must be considered in any acute pain. Knee pain can reflect disease of the hip joint, as in osteoarthritis, or, in children, a slipped cartilage in the hip joint.

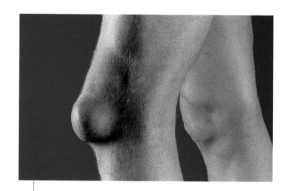

Above: Housemaid's knee – fluid over the kneecap that is caused by constant kneeling.

SYMPTOMS

The knee will be painful and may feel unstable. A locked knee that cannot be bent beyond a certain point is probably caused by a torn cartilage or a fragment of bone in the knee. Torn ligaments cause an unusual laxity of the knee joint. There may be features of osteoarthritis of the knees or hips. Swelling of the knee is common after injury; immediate swelling and bruising means bleeding in the joint.

Knee pains plus fever or joint pains elsewhere suggest infection or more generalized joint disease such as rheumatoid arthritis. A red, hot and swollen joint suggests infection, bleeding or an inflammatory cause such as gout or rheumatoid arthritis. In Osgood Schlatter's disease there is a tender prominent nodule below the kneecap.

TREATMENT

Minor injuries settle with rest, support and an anti-inflammatory preparation in either gel or tablet form. Even torn cartilages and tendons will recover with rest, although it can take months. Physiotherapy is essential in order to maintain the thigh power needed to keep the knee stable.

Knee supports are helpful immediately after an injury to reduce swelling and to prevent swelling on further use of the joint. A knee support must be firm, but not so firm that it cuts into flesh or restricts the blood flow.

Orthopaedic surgeons can look inside the joint with arthroscopy to establish diagnosis of the problem, repair tendons and remove torn cartilages and debris. Any suspicion of infection calls for investigation of the swollen knee and infection requires a prolonged course of antibiotics.

Drawing fluid off a swollen knee joint relieves pressure and restores movement. Analysing the fluid aids the diagnosis of infection and gout.

  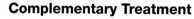

Complementary Treatment

Acupuncture – see FROZEN SHOULDER. **Shiatsu-do** shows excellent results for improving the musculoskeletal system. **Alexander Technique** and **Hellerwork** – see BACKACHE. **Chiropractic** manipulative and mobilization techniques can be very effective, especially if the pain is due to a sporting injury. **Ayurveda** recommends oil massage and yoga. **Osteopathy** offers specific manual treatments. **Rolfing** improves alignment, taking stress off the knee. *Other therapies to try: naturopathy; cymatics; tai chi/chi kung.*

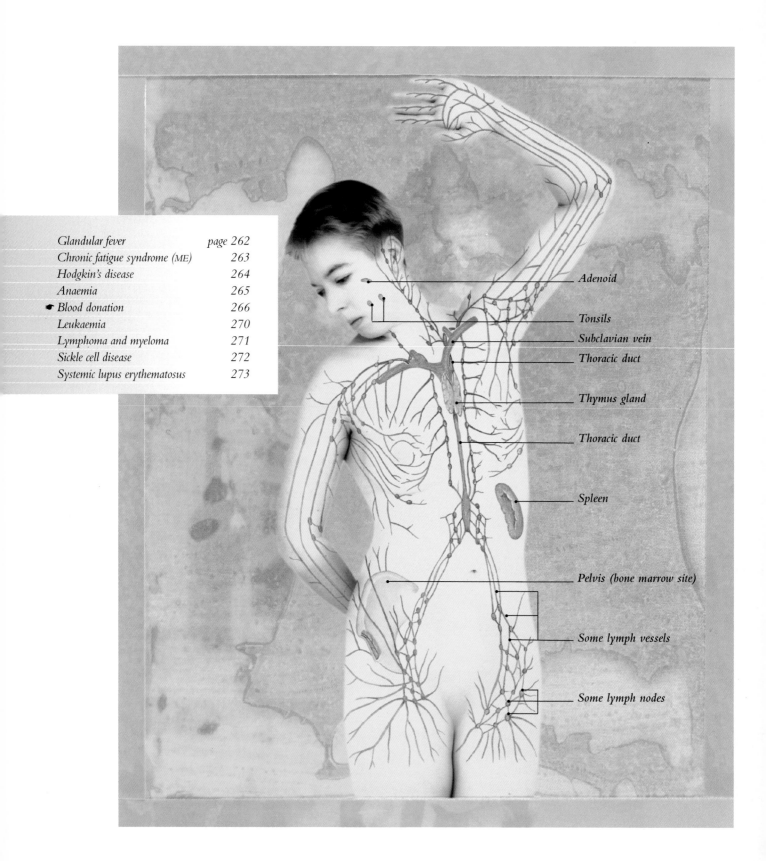

Adenoid

Tonsils

Subclavian vein

Thoracic duct

Thymus gland

Thoracic duct

Spleen

Pelvis (bone marrow site)

Some lymph vessels

Some lymph nodes

*Blood and tissue fluids bathe nearly all parts of the body.
Within them float billions of cells and molecules involved in
oxygen transport and fighting infection. Lymph glands, liver,
spleen and bone marrow play fundamental roles in this system.*

BLOOD, GLANDS AND THE IMMUNE SYSTEM

BLOOD IS THE MEANS by which oxygen and nutrients are taken to every part of the body and carbon dioxide and waste products are returned to the lungs, liver or kidney, for elimination. The main components of blood are red blood cells, which carry oxygen, white cells, which are defence cells, and platelets, which help the blood to clot. There are also hundreds of other components in the blood stream involved in defence, hormone transport, nutrition and much more.

Blood cells are formed within the bone marrow, at least in adults, although the liver and spleen can assist if needed. Adults have about 5 litres/9 pints of blood in their bodies, each drop of which contains millions of these cells.

Glands and the immune system

Throughout the body there are collections of glandular tissues called lymph nodes whose job it is to deal with infection in the body. These glands can be felt around the throat, at the back of the neck, in the groin and in the armpits. There are many more internal lymph nodes within the intestine and following the paths of the major blood vessels.

The siting of these lymph nodes is not random; it provides maximum protection where infection is most likely to enter the body – the various orifices, the lungs and the intestines. Lymph nodes are connected by the lymphatic system, which is similar to the circulatory system of blood. The lymphatic system collects tissue fluid – fluid that has leaked out of the arteries and veins of the blood circulatory system – and returns it to the blood stream via special ducts in the chest.

Other crucial parts of the lymphatic system are the spleen, located below the ribs in the left upper abdomen, and the thymus gland, in the neck below the breastbone. The spleen destroys aged red blood cells and is a kind of filtration plant removing debris from the blood stream. The thymus gland activates lymphocytes, which are attack cells produced in vast quantities by the bone marrow, lymph nodes and spleen.

Defence

The defensive forces of the body are lymphocytes and antibodies – proteins released by lymphocytes which recognize foreign invaders. These primary defences are assisted by a complex array of additional biochemicals such as complement, interferon and cytokines. The cells within the body are continually being challenged to see if they are 'self' or 'foreign', which might include viruses, bacteria and any transplanted tissues. Once foreign matter is detected a cascade of defensive forces swings into action, generating large numbers of lymphocytes from rapidly enlarged lymph nodes, such as the swollen neck glands during tonsillitis, assisted by an assortment of biochemically destructive proteins.

The defence process goes on in the body at a mostly undetectable level but if the system has to meet a major challenge we will experience this as 'feeling ill' with **fever**, sweats, malaise, muscle pains and many enlarged glands.

Potential problems

Considering how complex both the blood and lymphatic systems are, their reliability is high. Where serious problems do arise they are usually due to disease of the bone marrow, cancers of lymph nodes or bone marrow or, commonly, **anaemia**.

*Left: A complex fluid based system,
fighting infection and carrying oxygen,
food and hormones around the body.*

GLANDULAR FEVER

A viral infection causing a sore throat and enlarged lymph glands.

CAUSES

The virus causing glandular fever was first identified in 1964 and named the Epstein Barr virus, after its discoverers. This virus is a variety of herpes virus and is spread through saliva – giving the disease a reputation as the 'kissing disease' – although cases can happen via spread through the air. The medical term for glandular fever is infectious mononucleosis, which refers to certain types of white blood cell appearing during the illness. People of all ages may contract glandular fever, but it is most common in young adults and adolescents. In children the disease is very mild.

SYMPTOMS

Glandular fever begins with a sore throat, which rapidly worsens and often looks indistinguishable from **tonsillitis**. As the name implies, the glands all around the body enlarge, especially the neck glands, and there is the usual malaise and aching that is typical of any viral illness. The virus often affects the liver, causing a hint of jaundice (see LIVER PROBLEMS). Skin rashes are common, too.

The diagnosis can be confirmed by the Monospot blood test. This is useful because it allows prediction about the long course of the illness and reinforces the futility of changing from antibiotic to antibiotic to try to cure the sore throat.

A couple of other viruses, such as cytomegalovirus and toxoplasmosis, can cause a similar picture, and are distinguished by blood tests. Although the list of possible complications from glandular fever is long, for example effects on the heart and pain in the joints, most are rare.

TREATMENT

Many people who present at an early stage with a bad throat or tonsillitis will be prescribed an antibiotic in the reasonable belief that they have a streptococcal sore throat. Once the diagnosis is established, however, antibiotic treatment should be abandoned. The body simply has to develop resistance to the virus, which takes several weeks.

A short course of steroids is helpful in severe cases, for example where there is massive enlargement of the tonsils or inflammation of the liver. Glandular fever may make the spleen enlarge and become fragile, so it is advisable not to play any contact sports for three months after glandular fever. For similar reasons it is advisable to cut out alcohol.

The question of post-glandular fever debility is a much vexed one. Many people experience profound tiredness during the illness, which may persist in a few cases for weeks or months after clinical recovery. A very few fall into the category of **chronic fatigue syndrome**, but far fewer than popular wisdom holds. Because glandular fever does have such a reputation it is best to be positive about the outcome from the start, rather than to assume that you are doomed to a year of lassitude. Immunity to glandular fever is lifelong; you cannot catch it twice and if you think you have had it before chances are one of the diagnoses was wrong.

QUESTIONS

What is the effect of ampicillin on glandular fever?
Ampicillin is an antibiotic used for sore throats. It is a curious fact that taking ampicillin in a case of glandular fever will result in a rash in 90% of patients.

How infectious is it?
Glandular fever is so infectious that nearly all children in the Third World contract it, whereas in the cleaner environment of the developed world children miss catching it until they go to secondary school – hence its frequency in teenagers.

How can the spread of glandular fever be reduced?
Ideally, anyone with glandular fever should not kiss others nor share drinking utensils. Since glandular fever has an incubation period of about 50 days, adherence to such rigid isolation would no doubt devastate teenage social life.

Complementary Treatment
Western herbalism – infusions of yarrow or elderflower induce sweating and keep the temperature stable. Rosemary and yarrow tea alleviate persistent tiredness after glandular fever. Cleavers is specific for the lymphatics. **Chakra balancing** – if you are sensitive to touch, you could benefit from the non-touch techniques employed by this therapy. **Aromatherapy** can boost the immune system and help psychologically too – your practitioner will advise. **Ayurvedic** medicine recommends oral preparations and *panchakarma* detoxification. *Other therapies to try: Chinese herbalism; homeopathy; naturopathy.*

CHRONIC FATIGUE SYNDROME (ME)

Profound tiredness in the absence of definite medical diagnosis.

CAUSES

The term chronic fatigue syndrome (CFS) is preferable to the widespread term ME (myalgic encephalomyelitis), which implies an understanding of the condition unwarranted by current research. It is the enormous publicity given to certain high-profile cases that has helped turn the condition from a curiosity into a research topic. This research has yet to bear any significant fruit. Current thinking is that there is no one cause of CFS, although viral infection may trigger fatigue. The **glandular fever** virus is most often suspected, but its role is completely unproven. Research is currently looking at abnormalities of cell metabolism and the hypothalamic/pituitary axis, but with no firm conclusion as yet.

It is clear that prolonged tiredness acquires psychological overtones long after the virus has left the body. In other words, although it may be a physical event that triggers CFS, it is almost certainly psychological factors that prolong it.

SYMPTOMS

Many healthy people feel tired – some people all of the time. Tiredness alone is not enough to establish the diagnosis. The agreed criteria for CFS are at least six months of fatigue associated with loss of ability to function at work or home; there are often muscle aches and irritability. Tiredness alternates with bursts of activity but these have to be 'paid for' by increased fatigue and muscle pains one to two days later. There are often sleep and mood disturbances but not true **depression**.

The diagnosis of CFS cannot be accepted without first having a full medical examination and comprehensive blood tests, including tests for **diabetes**, thyroid disease (see THYROID PROBLEMS) and hormonal disturbances.

TREATMENT

Probably the first step in treatment of the syndrome is acceptance by both doctor and patient that there is a problem, the cause of which is unknown, but which is not life-threatening. No one dies of CFS. While the cause is still debatable, current thinking is that patients must accept that their own psychological approach to chronic fatigue is their key to overcoming the problem. Treatment starts by identifying any possible contributory psychological factors such as work, relationships or general unhappiness about life.

You must accept that effort will be tiring; this does not mean that you must constantly rest. On the contrary, the more you rest the more tired you will get when you do exert yourself, leading to a vicious circle of rest, frantic effort, tiredness and muscle pains and more rest. You need an agreed level of activity – enough to stimulate you a little but not so much as to exhaust you. This should replace the rest/activity cycles otherwise common in this condition. Do not spend the day sleeping or napping; you will then have restless nights and wake unrefreshed. Antidepressants are widely used and worth trying. Also, the modern serotonin re-uptake inhibitors have a slight stimulant effect which is helpful. Whatever the strategy, you must accept that there is no 'quick-fix' and that improvement may take months rather than weeks.

QUESTIONS

How common is chronic fatigue syndrome?
Surveys suggest that up to one in two hundred of the population has CFS; many more have a CFS-type picture but with features of clinical depression. CFS is most common in women who are aged between twenty and forty.

When is tiredness abnormal?
This is a difficult question because the same surveys show that 20–30% of the population feel tired all the time. Probably the diagnostic criterion is when tiredness is profound enough to interfere with home and work performance, but a great deal rests on your own assessment of your degree of tiredness.

What about recovery?
The picture is still bleak. About 70% of people with CFS remain unwell even after a year. Children recover faster than adults.

Complementary Treatment
WARNING: Do not attempt self-treatment – you are likely to be sensitive to all medication, including natural remedies. **Chinese herbalism** uses herbs to clear 'dampness', which is a kind of clogging of the body's functions, producing lethargy, a muzzy head and poor concentration. **Chiropractic** can help joint and muscle stiffness and improve mobility. *Other therapies to try: Western herbalism; tai chi/chi kung; homeopathy; acupuncture; cymatics; chakra balancing; aromatherapy; Ayurveda; nutritional therapy; naturopathy.*

HODGKIN'S DISEASE

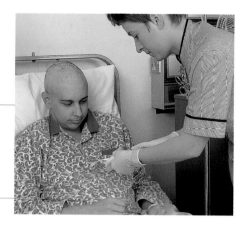

Right: Chemotherapy for Hodgkin's disease may be distressing but cure is highly likely.

A disease of the lymphatic system, the outlook for which has been transformed since the 1960s.

CAUSES

This disease is one of a group of cancers called lymphomas (see LYMPHOMA AND MYELOMA), which involve abnormalities of the lymphoid system, comprising lymph glands, liver and spleen. The trigger for Hodgkin's disease remains unknown. There has been much speculation and research on the possibility of a virus triggering it, especially the Epstein Barr virus which causes **glandular fever**, but the evidence is inconclusive. There is a slightly increased family risk, but it is uncertain whether this implies a genetic risk or whether the family has been exposed to some common hazard or infection.

SYMPTOMS

Peak incidence is in young men, who are affected about twice as often as women. It is more common again in old age. The classic early symptoms are enlarged lymph glands in the neck. These are painless, in contrast to the enlarged glands associated with infection, and have a rubbery feel to them. There are usually other rubbery glands in the armpits and groin and the spleen is frequently enlarged. Additional symptoms include sweating at night, weight loss and generalized itch.

The enlarged glands are highly suggestive of the condition but confirmation has to be made by a biopsy of a gland. As well as confirming the diagnosis, the cells' appearance shows what subtype of Hodgkin's disease is present, which is essential in planning treatment and for predicting the outlook.

Assessment is completed by scans of the interior lymph nodes and spleen. Occasionally an operation might be needed to see how far the disease has spread, but this is increasingly unnecessary thanks to refinements in scanning. The information is put together using an internationally agreed scheme to stage the condition and to decide treatment.

TREATMENT

A choice is made of a combination of radiotherapy (see page 338) and chemotherapy (see page 339), the precise 'cocktail' depending on the type and stage of the illness. The aim is to eradicate the cancerous tissues from all affected sites. The various cocktails are the subject of continuing refinement and increasing sophistication in dosage and in controlling the otherwise unpleasant side effects of therapy such as nausea.

Treatment is given in cycles over several weeks for up to six months, by which time most people are free of active disease. It can normally be given as an outpatient procedure, even though up to eight drugs might be required each time, and some people are able to continue working during part of their therapy. Follow-up has to continue for many years.

The results of treatment have been spectacular. As late as the 1950s fewer than ten per cent of people with Hodgkin's survived more than five years, whereas now over eighty per cent do so. Even if the disease recurs, there is a high probability of getting it back under control and even of curing it.

QUESTIONS

What does treatment do to fertility?
Now that a cure is likely, attention has turned to the side effects of treatment. In men, subfertility invariably follows from the chemotherapy; they are now offered the chance to donate a sperm sample which is kept frozen for later use. Women are most unlikely to suffer any permanent effect on fertility.

Is there a risk of other cancers?
The more that people are surviving, the more it is found that they have an increased risk of other cancers. These are mainly blood disorders like leukaemia. This is a good reason for continued review and regular blood tests.

Complementary Treatment

Complementary therapies cannot cure this cancer. However, they can offer a great deal during diagnosis, treatment and follow-up. **Chakra balancing** can promote relaxation and offer support during orthodox treatment. **Massage** helps to improve self-esteem and encourages a sense of wellbeing. **Hypnotherapy** – hypno-healing could help. **Reflexology** and **aromatherapy** can both help you cope with the stress and tensions generated by this disease. *Other therapies to try: see STRESS.*

ANAEMIA

A condition of below-normal levels of red blood cells.

CAUSES

Anaemia is a symptom and not a definite diagnosis in itself. The causes fall into three main categories: failure of production of red blood cells, excessive loss of blood, or chronic disease leading to abnormal breakdown of cells.

Failure of red blood cell production
The average adult has 5 litres/9 pints of blood made up of billions of cells; the average life of a red blood cell is four months. Red blood cells are produced in vast numbers by the bone marrow, together with the other essential components of blood such as white blood cells and platelets. This frantic production line requires basic raw materials: protein to make the cells and iron to make the haemoglobin molecule. Various trace elements are needed, the best known being vitamin B_{12}. If these are deficient then anaemia inevitably develops. If it is vitamin B_{12} that is deficient, the cause may be pernicious anaemia. Strict vegans may become anaemic through lack of iron, but there is no reason why vegetarians should, as long as they follow a varied diet including eggs.

The cause of anaemia is usually dietary deficiency but it may be failure of absorption through a bowel disorder such as **coeliac disease**. The other production cause is failure of the bone marrow, which occurs in **leukaemia**, or destruction of the marrow after, for example, chemotherapy for cancer.

Excessive blood loss
The spleen destroys worn out old blood cells; a hormone system matches the rate of destruction and the rate of production. This all goes wrong if blood is lost in excessive quantities. The most common reasons for this are heavy menstrual periods, bleeding from ulcers in the stomach or duodenum, cancers of the large intestine or loss in urine. Several drugs cause leakage of blood from the stomach, for example aspirin and anti-inflammatories used for arthritic conditions.

Abnormal breakdown of cells
Some people have inherently fragile blood cells, including those with spherocytosis or **sickle cell disease**. Many chronic illnesses like cancers and kidney disease cause anaemia for reasons not well understood, and are often difficult to treat.

SYMPTOMS

There is a non-specific tiredness. When blood count falls to half the normal count there is profound tiredness and breathlessness through lack of the oxygen carried by red blood cells. Older people may get chest pain. There may be the symptoms of any contributory conditions, for example the weight loss of cancer or malabsorption or heavy periods. Skin colour is not a good measure of anaemia. It is slightly more reliable to judge pallor by turning down the eye lid yet some people may have normal complexions but profound anaemia and *vice versa*.

TREATMENT

It can take some detective work to discover the cause of anaemia: going over diet, checking for blood loss in the bowels or urine and looking for associated diseases such as **hiatus hernia**, **stomach cancer** or **bowel cancer**, especially in older people. If the cause is obvious, as in a poor diet or heavy periods, immediate treatment is with iron and vitamins. Follow-up blood tests are important to ensure response to treatment.

Pernicious anaemia is treated by injections of vitamin B_{12} plus folic acid supplements. Blood transfusion is reserved for profound anaemia causing serious symptoms.

See also PREGNANCY PROBLEMS for anaemia in pregnancy.

Complementary Treatment
Nutritional therapy – besides iron, likely deficiencies include vitamins B_6 and B_{12}, folic acid and zinc. Boost your intake of soya beans, green-leaved vegetables, dried fruit, especially raisins, and red meat and liver (if you are not vegetarian – and not if you are pregnant). A **homeopath** could suggest ways of improving your body's ability to absorb iron. *Other therapies to try: tai chi/chi kung; shiatsu-do; acupuncture; aromatherapy.*

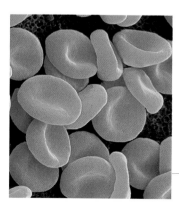

Left: Biconcave red blood cells, packed with haemoglobin. Each drop of blood contains millions of cells.

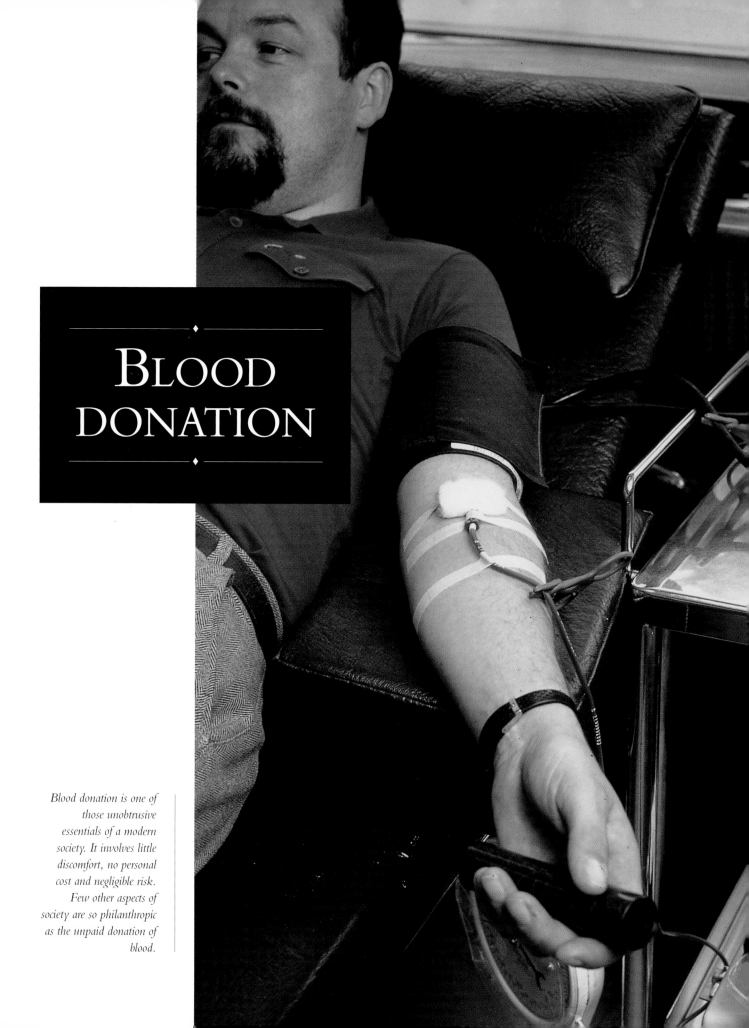

BLOOD DONATION

Blood donation is one of those unobtrusive essentials of a modern society. It involves little discomfort, no personal cost and negligible risk. Few other aspects of society are so philanthropic as the unpaid donation of blood.

B LOOD DONATION IS THE ULTIMATE GIFT: a donation which you can replace within days and which may give life to others. Blood donation and blood transfusion have gone hand in hand with the development of modern medicine, making possible operations that were unthinkable 50 years ago, and enabling the survival of victims of serious injury and disease.

A brief history of blood donation

Transfusions were first carried out experimentally from the 17th century, without any clear understanding of what was being transfused and how it worked. In 1900, the nature of blood groups was recognized, leading to the notion of compatibility of blood. This, plus the impetus of the First World War, greatly increased the transfusion technology, which was tested again in the Second World War.

After the war, blood transfusion became essential to pioneering surgery and the blood donation system was established. In the United Kingdom this is a system based on philanthropy which benefits the 800,000 people in the country who require blood transfusion each year and the many others who make use of blood products.

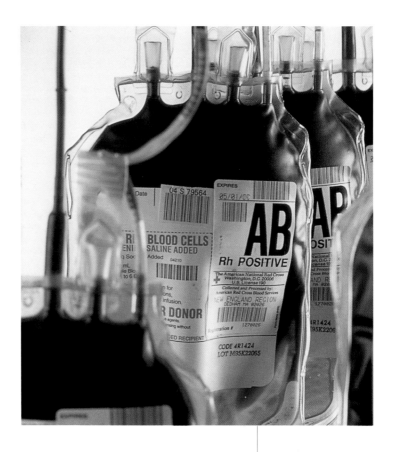

Above: Although whole blood is still necessary, the many components of blood have specialized uses.

Blood groups

Receiving a blood transfusion is similar to receiving an organ transplant. Being a foreign substance, it may provoke an allergic or rejection reaction, just as with kidney or heart transplants. Why does this happen? Each red blood cell has proteins on its surface called antigens, which establish to which blood group it belongs. The most important of these markers form the ABO and the rhesus factor systems. A blood cell may be Group O, Group A, Group B or Group AB and in each case may also be rhesus positive or rhesus negative. These are the major groups, although there are many other lesser antigens that may cause transfusion reactions. Blood groups are inherited characteristics, the frequency of which varies greatly from race to race around the world.

Logical rules govern who can be given what group of blood. For example, Group O blood can be transfused into anyone, but people with Group O blood can only accept Group O blood. People of blood Group AB can accept blood of any group but can only donate to others of Group AB.

Blood grouping This is done by testing a sample from donated blood against blood of known group to see if it causes an antibody reaction. The analysis can be taken to very sophisticated detail, for example if blood is needed for someone who has had serious transfusion problems before.

Cross-matching This is the crucial test undertaken before commencing a transfusion. Even though apparently matching blood has been obtained, there may be subtle antibodies that might cause a transfusion reaction. Therefore samples of the donor blood and the recipient's blood are mixed to check reactivity. Of course in an emergency there may not be time to do so, in which case Group O rhesus negative blood is given until time allows for a full cross-match.

Minor transfusion reactions such as a mild fever, itch and feeling shivery are common. The usual reason is reaction against the white cells in the transfused blood. If there is a reaction against the red blood cells the consequences are much more serious, with falling blood pressure and kidney damage. However, the whole point of cross-matching is to avoid such major reactions, which are very rare.

Blood safety

As well as the need to match blood groups carefully, a possible hazard is transmission of infection. Blood is, after all, a living entity. It is for this reason that blood is screened for the HIV I and HIV I viruses, the viruses of hepatitis B and C and syphilis. In certain parts of the world local hazards such as **malaria** parasites must also be checked.

A donation session

A small pinprick of blood is first tested to make sure you, the potential donor, are not anaemic. You then lie down and a needle is inserted into one of the large veins over the inside of the elbow and connected up to tubing and a collection bag. The usual donation is 450 ml/about ¾ pint and it takes five to ten minutes to collect this quantity. Adults have 5 litres/ 9 pints of blood, so this donation represents under 10% of their blood volume and the healthy body can cope with this blood loss. You should rest for half an hour afterwards to allow your body to adjust. It takes little more than a week for your body to replace the donated blood. You can donate this quantity of blood safely every four to six months.

To give blood you should be in good health and not recovering from any serious infectious illness. You should not donate blood if you are at risk of HIV, for example if you are an intravenous drug user or a practising homosexual, or have been a sexual partner of either of the above. Nor should you give blood if you have had hepatitis B or C.

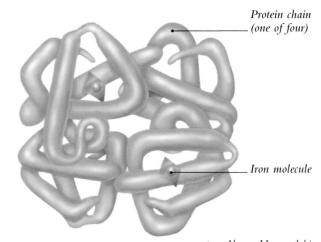

Protein chain (one of four)

Iron molecule

Above: Haemoglobin – iron within the complex structure holds oxygen securely, yet releases it precisely where required within the tissues.

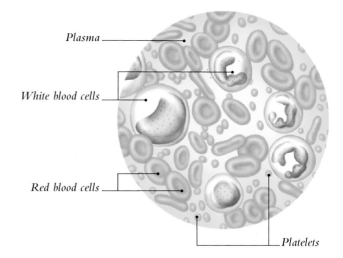

Plasma

White blood cells

Red blood cells

Platelets

Above: Blood, greatly magnified, showing the myriad cells floating in the complex liquid plasma.

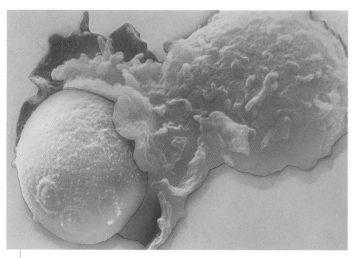

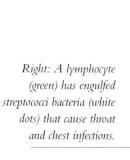

Above: A lymphocyte (white blood cell) engulfing a yeast spore. The constant vigilance of such defensive cells is essential to repel infection.

Right: A lymphocyte (green) has engulfed streptococci bacteria (white dots) that cause throat and chest infections.

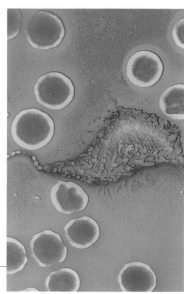

The distribution of donated blood

The red cells, platelets and plasma can be used separately – indeed, it is now unusual to transfuse whole blood except in dire emergencies.

Red cells The red cells are kept for people who need pure transfusion, for example after haemorrhage, accidents and major surgery. These packed red cells keep fresh for up to seven weeks, or longer if frozen, which is done to maintain stocks of rare blood groups.

Platelets Another component of blood is platelets, the tiny fragments involved in blood clotting. These are obtained by

spinning blood in a centrifuge and filtering off the layer containing platelets. Platelets have a short shelf life – only three to five days – and are used for people whose natural clotting mechanism has broken down, for example in bone marrow failure. It is possible to donate platelets alone, using a technique called apheresis, where your blood is cycled through equipment that removes the platelets but returns the rest of the blood to you. The platelets are restored within days.

Plasma and other components This is the fluid in which cells float and is itself a complex mixture of proteins. Whole frozen plasma is used as rapid fluid replacement for severely injured people after burns or heavy blood loss, to replace clotting factors and to restore blood pressure in a way that transfusions of ordinary fluids will not do. Preparations refined from whole plasma are used to restore blood protein levels in such serious conditions as liver failure.

By further purifying plasma, yet other components can be obtained. Clotting factors are proteins essential to prevent bleeding, some of which are lacked by haemophiliacs. Clotting factors are freeze-dried until needed. Other products obtainable are immunoglobulins and the anti-D vaccine used to protect rhesus negative mothers. Immunoglobulins are proteins which give immediate protection against diseases such as **chickenpox** and hepatitis, faster than the body can mount its own immune response.

The future of blood donation

A number of artificial liquids are available that work almost as well as plasma to maintain blood pressure. True artificial blood with an oxygen-carrying capacity still eludes researchers, although recent significant progress has been made in the United States. The goal is a great one – a liquid that would not need the whole array of grouping, cross-matching and screening for infection that real blood entails.

An alternative attracting some interest is autologous blood transfusion, where individuals donate their own blood a few weeks before it will be needed. This has little advantage where there is a reliable blood transfusion service, but is very attractive for planned surgery in those parts of the world where HIV and hepatitis screening is poor. In such countries a blood transfusion may be more dangerous than the operation itself.

For the foreseeable future, the health service in the United Kingdom will continue to rely on the blood donation service and the millions of acts of quiet selflessness that save lives every minute of the day.

LEUKAEMIA

Cancer of the bone marrow with abnormalities in the production of the white cells needed to combat infection.

CAUSES

The term leukaemia covers many related cancers, which vary in their degree of seriousness. The disease affects people of all ages but tends to be more common in children and the elderly, and relatively uncommon in adult life.

White blood cells are produced in the bone marrow and are vital in combating infection by bacteria or viruses. The bone marrow also produces red blood cells and the platelets required for the normal clotting of blood. In the condition of leukaemia the bone marrow switches to producing enormous quantities of white blood cells to the exclusion of the other blood components. Far from enhancing the body's resistance to infection, these white blood cells are inefficient.

In the majority of cases leukaemia arises spontaneously with no agreed pre-existing cause. However, it may be due to previous irradiation of the bone marrow causing a mutation to cancerous cells, for example after exposure to radioactivity or as a result of radiotherapy for **Hodgkin's disease**.

Much research has sought a viral cause since there is a form of leukaemia in Japan caused by a virus, but, in general, results have not supported this view; nor is there any definite conclusion about genetic causes except for a variant of leukaemia called chronic myeloid leukaemia.

SYMPTOMS

Childhood leukaemia tends to be of a swift and dramatic onset, with rapid falls in both red blood cells and platelets. The child becomes lethargic through the onset of **anaemia**, breaks out in bruises and bleeds spontaneously from the teeth or nose. The blood count shows large numbers of the characteristic cells of leukaemia. The most usual types are acute lymphocytic leukaemia or acute myelogenous leukaemia.

Older people tend to get more slowly evolving forms of leukaemia such as chronic myeloid leukaemia or chronic lymphocytic leukaemia. They suffer a period of vague ill health, perhaps increased numbers of infections, enlarged lymph nodes, sweating at night and itching.

In all cases diagnosis is confirmed by taking a sample of bone marrow in order to demonstrate the abnormal production of white cells. Leukaemia, although suspected often, occurs rarely. However, a blood test is advisable for someone with prolonged sore throats, bruising or recurrent infections.

TREATMENT

The outlook for childhood leukaemia or other leukaemia of acute onset is very good. It is essential to remember this during the harrowing periods of treatment with radiotherapy and chemotherapy (see pages 338 and 339) with their attendant hair loss, nausea, constant drips and intensive nursing. Out of this comes recovery in at least 90% of cases and ever-increasing numbers remain cured. Prospects have improved even more with the discovery that cells taken from the umbilical cord can be transplanted into leukaemia patients with a high success rate and without needing powerful anti-rejection medication, as is normally needed for transplants.

The prospects in the more chronic adult leukaemia are less good but by no means hopeless. Chronic myeloid leukaemia is treated with a drug called busulphan and increasingly with bone marrow transplantation (see page 331). The average survival is about five years. Chronic lymphocytic leukaemia is an even more benign form, often found incidentally when taking a blood test for some other reason. Even without treatment people can expect many years without problems. Treatment is with chemotherapy such as chlorambucil.

QUESTIONS

How common is leukaemia?
Despite its high public profile, childhood leukaemia is rare. There are under 500 cases a year in the whole of the United Kingdom and about 7,000 adult cases.

Why is the treatment so difficult?
Cancerous cells in bone marrow cannot be eradicated without eradicating other cells made by the marrow, with great risks of infection and bleeding during therapy. Cancerous cells linger within the brain and spinal cord; radiotherapy to these regions is hazardous.

Complementary Treatment

Complementary therapies cannot cure leukaemia and should be used only to support conventional treatment. Any stress-reducing therapy will help both the patient and the family deal with the strains following diagnosis. Many complementary therapies can help the body cope with the effects of aggressive orthodox treatment, particularly **massage**, **aromatherapy** and **reflexology**. *Other therapies to try: see* STRESS.

LYMPHOMA AND MYELOMA

Lymphoma is a cancer of the lymph nodes. Myeloma is a specific type of cancer of the bone marrow.

CAUSES

Lymphoid tissues defend us against invading bacteria and viruses. The system comprises lymph nodes around the head, neck and groin, many internal lymph nodes and the spleen. It responds to infection by releasing lymphocytes, white cells that recognize invading organisms. How do they do this?

Virtually all cells in the body have a protein marker in their cell wall, which in effect says, 'I'm family, back off'. Lacking these markers, germs are recognized as 'non-family' and trigger attack by white cells and antibodies. Antibodies are complex proteins released by lymphocytes, which recognize germs met previously. They latch on to the germs and destroy them directly or release biochemical markers that rally more white cells to help. It is a wonderfully efficient system but the very rapidity of cell turnover paradoxically carries a risk of cancerous transformation, resulting in lymphoma or myeloma.

Lymphoma

It is believed that lymphomas begin when a single cell mutates and proliferates uncontrollably, replacing healthy lymphoid tissues. They are more likely in late adult life but can occur at any age. (**Hodgkin's disease** is a type of lymphoma, considered separately because it is usually confined to a few tissues, rather than spread throughout the body.)

Myeloma

This is a disease of the bone marrow in cells that produce antibodies. It is almost always a disease of the elderly. Again, it appears that a single cell goes out of control and proliferates. The cell continues to produce fragments of antibody, but not complete antibody molecules. Eventually the blood stream is awash with fragments, but short of the useful antibodies – like a factory that changed from producing complete cars to churning out huge numbers of half-finished hub-caps instead.

SYMPTOMS

With lymphoma, as the cancerous cells spread, lymph nodes all around the body enlarge – those in the neck, groin and armpits the most obvious. The individual feels generally unwell and is prone to infections and **anaemia**. Often the diagnosis is suspected purely on examination, but is confirmed by biopsy of the lymph nodes.

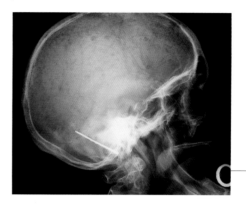

Left: Circular X-ray shadows typical of bone destruction by multiple myeloma.

Myeloma tends to be of less dramatic onset and can be quite advanced before causing symptoms of bone pain, from destruction of bone, and anaemia. There are many subtle biochemical changes due to high levels of calcium in the blood stream and kidney function may be impaired, but the resulting symptoms are rather non-specifically those of vague malaise. The diagnosis is made by demonstrating large quantities of abnormal protein in the blood or the urine.

TREATMENT

There are many subtypes of lymphoma and so treatment is tailored as appropriate, but in all cases involves radiotherapy, chemotherapy or both (see pages 338 and 339). A bone marrow transplant may sometimes be appropriate (see page 331). The outlook depends on the particular subtype; survival can be expected to be measured in years and a significant number of people are cured.

In the case of myeloma, treatment is complex, requiring chemotherapy to damp down the disease, radiotherapy to deal with bone invasion, and kidney support. Bone marrow transplantation is now being used more often, and is pushing up survival times to a number of years.

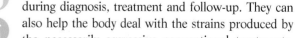

Complementary Treatment

Complementary therapies cannot cure either lymphoma or myeloma. However, many can offer support during diagnosis, treatment and follow-up. They can also help the body deal with the strains produced by the necessarily aggressive conventional treatments. **Chakra balancing** can help promote relaxation, symptom control and pain relief. **Massage**, **aromatherapy** and **reflexology** can be particularly beneficial. *Other therapies to try: see STRESS.*

SICKLE CELL DISEASE

An abnormality of the haemoglobin molecule that alters the shape and stability of red blood cells.

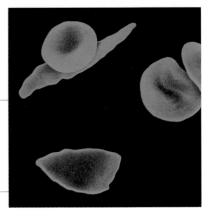

Right: Long, flat sickled red blood cells mingle with normal round red cells.

CAUSES

One of the basic processes of living creatures is to absorb oxygen from the air or from fluids and to transport it to cells where it fuels metabolism. In humans this is achieved by the haemoglobin molecule, carried in millions by each red blood cell. The haemoglobin molecule is like a nest cocooning iron in a special structure, which avidly takes up oxygen but gives it up into the cells. The proteins twist and turn so as to give a particular shape to the molecule, enhancing this function.

In sickle cell disease, there is an abnormality of haemoglobin caused by a single genetic error that substitutes one amino acid for another. This tiny slip makes the haemoglobin molecule less soluble and the red blood cell more rigid. It loses its bi-concave shape and instead looks curved, hence the term sickle cell. For much of the time the red blood cell gets by, but in certain conditions the abnormal haemoglobin becomes even less soluble and the cells more likely to sickle. These conditions include experience of cold temperatures, infection and lack of oxygen at high altitude.

Unlike normal red blood cells, which slip and glide through the narrowest capillaries, rigid sickled cells block small blood vessels and starve surrounding tissues of oxygen. As well as causing pain, this also reduces the life span of red blood cells – normally four months – and causes persistent **anaemia**.

For reasons not understood sickle cell is extremely common throughout Africa and in populations of African origin, for example Afro-Americans. It is not uncommon in Asians and in the Middle East but is rare in Caucasian populations.

SYMPTOMS

The symptoms of sickle cell disease are mainly the result of blockage of blood vessels – pain that can be anywhere in the body, even abdominal pain. Interference with blood flow in the fingers or long bones can lead to stunted growth and irregularly shaped fingers or toes. The persistent anaemia causes tiredness and increased susceptibility to infection. Eventually there may be kidney and brain damage, too.

The severity of symptoms is highly variable, depending on how much normal haemoglobin the individual also has. Those least affected by the disease have few symptoms except in severe infections or lack of oxygen, whereas those most affected suffer constant pain and anaemia.

TREATMENT

Many people with sickle cell disease require no treatment and simply need to be aware of the risks that they face. During any surgical procedures it is important for the anaesthetist to give high levels of oxygen via a face mask. Sickle cell disease may be an explanation of otherwise obscure pains.

People suffering sickle cell crises – acute and severe pain due to blockage of blood vessels, usually in the bones or the spleen – need urgent management in a specialized centre to control pain, infection and dehydration from tissue damage.

The anaemia of sickle cell disease cannot be treated in the normal way with iron. Blood transfusion might be necessary in cases of extreme anaemia. Research may, in the future, find a way of getting the body to switch to production of other more benign forms of haemoglobin.

QUESTIONS

Why is sickle cell so common?
Such a common genetic variant invites questions as to why the disease persists. The best guess is that people with sickle cell trait enjoy some protection against malaria.

Who is at risk?
Anyone of African origin should have a sickle cell blood test, especially if a family member is affected. The test will show how severely affected you are. This is important information to tell doctors during any serious illness and before surgical procedures.

 Complementary Treatment
No complementary treatment can cure sickle cell disease so do not abandon conventional approaches. However, many therapies do have a role in helping you cope. If you are sensitive to touch, you could benefit from the non-touch techniques of **chakra balancing**. **Yoga** and **tai chi/chi kung** are gentle forms of exercise that can help.

SYSTEMIC LUPUS ERYTHEMATOSUS

◆

An auto-immune condition, commonly abbreviated to SLE.

CAUSES

◆

The cause of SLE is an attack by the body against its own tissues. The fundamental attack is against the DNA and RNA molecules, which are at the very heart of the cell's structure. (DNA carries genetic information and RNA is involved in protein synthesis.) This explains why SLE affects organs all over the body. It is not known what triggers this auto-immune attack. Research is looking at whether a viral infection could trigger the body to react first against the virus and by extension against its own proteins, but this has not been established.

There is a strong hereditary element; if you have an affected sibling your chances of SLE are about five per cent as opposed to one in a thousand of the general population. There are certain racial groups in which it is much more common, for example Afro-Americans. In a few cases SLE follows drug treatment with hydralazine, used for high blood pressure. Women are affected far more than men – about nine to one. The disease is very rare in children and adolescents.

SYMPTOMS

◆

Any body system could be affected but the most common early symptoms are pains in the joints or a butterfly-like facial rash – so-called because of its symmetrical spread across the cheeks. Pain in the joints is of sudden onset and without blood tests could be thought due to **rheumatoid arthritis**. There may be a sensitivity to sunlight, **fever**, odd tender patches on the fingers and Raynaud's phenomenon (see RAYNAUD'S DISEASE). Many other organs are affected, for example the lungs, kidneys and heart, but these rarely cause symptoms at the time of presentation.

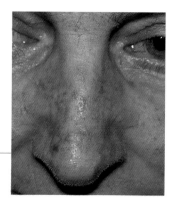

Right: A red butterfly-shaped rash on the face is suggestive of SLE.

The diagnosis is established by showing a certain number of symptoms plus blood tests that reveal antibodies to DNA.

If the disease progresses there is a risk of **stroke**, personality change and kidney damage. However, these represent the most severe end of the spectrum, at the other end of which there are many people with a relatively benign form of SLE.

TREATMENT

◆

People with SLE who become tired and have frequent rashes but are otherwise well need only anti-inflammatory drugs for flare-ups of pain in the joints; for much of the time they need no medication at all. In more serious disease, with increasing kidney damage, steroids are necessary by mouth in a dosage enough to bring things under control. If this is not sufficient chemotherapy is used (see page 339) with drugs such as cyclophosphamide or azathioprine – drugs used to treat cancer that work by reducing the activity of the immune system.

Typically, with SLE there are fluctuations in its severity. Doctors need to recognize a deterioration early enough to begin appropriate treatment while balancing the side effects of the treatment against the damage done by the illness.

QUESTIONS

What is the outlook for SLE?
The liberal use of steroids has improved the five-year survival to at least ninety-five per cent. There is evidence that if serious problems are going to occur it will be in the first few years of the illness, which thereafter takes a more benign course.

Can I still get pregnant?
Pregnancy can go ahead but with an increased risk of high blood pressure and miscarriage. Taking aspirin reduces the risks of miscarriage. The outcome is good in four out of five pregnancies.

       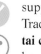

Complementary Treatment
It is important to maintain conventional treatment alongside complementary approaches. **Nutritional therapy** – try switching to a diet rich in fish oil, and supplementing with vitamin E and selenium. Traditional Chinese approaches (**herbs**, **acupuncture**, **tai chi/chi kung**) and **Western herbalism** can help by boosting your immune system. **Ayurveda** might advise detoxification, oil **massage** and specific **yoga** practices.

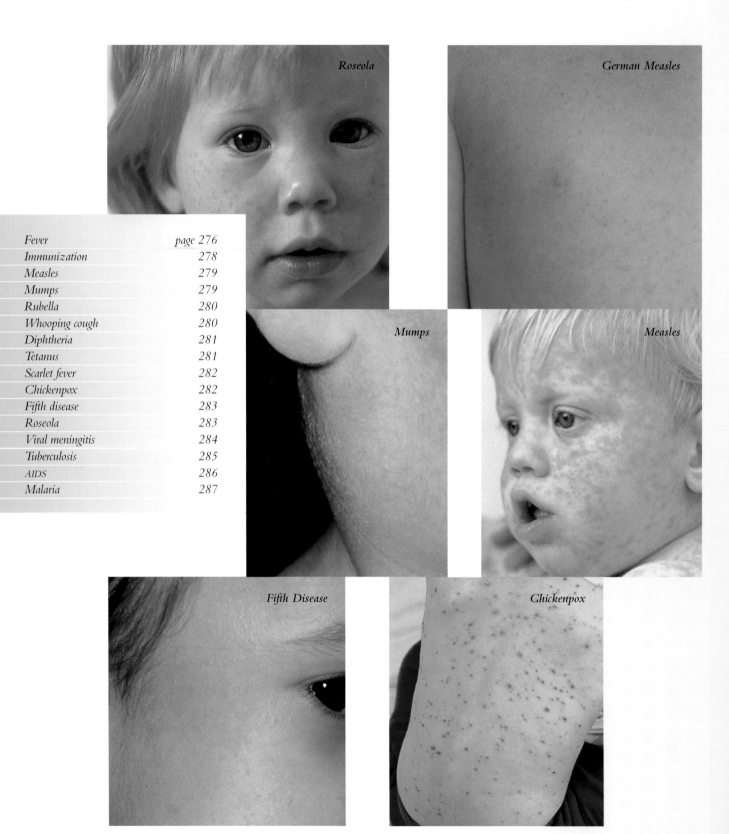

Roseola

German Measles

Mumps

Measles

Fifth Disease

Chickenpox

Infection is the single largest threat to health during much of the human lifetime and the range of infections is quite vast. Old infections change their character and new infections emerge regularly, making infection control a constant problem.

INFECTIOUS DISEASE

THERE IS A MULTITUDE of different types of micro-organisms that can cause infection, and while the body's sophisticated and ubiquitous defence systems can deal with many of them, some are so virulent that medication will be needed to destroy them.

Infecting micro-organisms

Viruses are particles so small that they are only visible through electron microscopes. They contain little other than enough genetic material to make more viruses. They rely on invading another organism to survive, taking over its internal metabolism and diverting it into producing more viruses. Because viruses are so intimately involved in the vital processes of cells, it is difficult to eradicate them with medication, although there are now a few antiviral drugs. The mainstay of defence against viruses is **immunization**. Important viral illnesses are, or were, **measles**, **mumps**, **viral meningitis**, smallpox, herpes and **AIDS**.

Bacteria are much larger organisms, visible under conventional microscopes. They are capable of independent existence and reproduction and cause many major and minor infectious illnesses, such as chest infections, blood poisoning and **bacterial meningitis**. Antibiotics have proved successful in controlling bacteria by poisoning a vital aspect of their metabolism, most often destroying the wall of the bacterium. Bacteria can mutate into forms resistant to antibiotics.

Protozoa are single-celled creatures, often parasitic – meaning that they grow within a host but without necessarily causing disease. They are, however, responsible for several serious illnesses such as **malaria** and sleeping sickness.

Fungi are organisms that grow slowly by throwing out filaments. Many are benign and even useful (penicillin was discovered in fungus). The illnesses they cause are usually more of a nuisance than life-threatening, for example **thrush**.

Other micro-organisms include *rickettsia* and *mycoplasma*, which are responsible for severe illnesses and often respond to an antibiotic.

Defence

The body maintains very complex systems to guard against infection. The mainstays are lymphocytes, a type of white blood cell, and antibodies, which are proteins shaped in a particular way that recognize the outer wall of invading micro-organisms. These components can recruit additional defensive cells and biochemicals to destroy viruses and bacteria, such as interferon, complement, leukotrienes, polymorphs and more.

How infection causes illness

Our bodies are continually being challenged by micro-organisms, most of which are recognized and destroyed rapidly. More established infection causes the release of toxic chemicals by both the invader and the defensive forces, accounting for **fever**, sweating, shivers, muscle pains, falls in blood pressure and fluid loss. Recovery occurs as these micro-organisms are destroyed.

Micro-organisms may cause disease through direct destruction of healthy tissues, such as lungs by **tuberculosis** or blood cells by malaria. Others release poisons called toxins, for example **diphtheria**, diarrhoeal illnesses and **tetanus**. Others destroy the immune system – AIDS is now the major example.

Left: Rashes and skin changes that reflect the ongoing struggle of the body against infecting micro-organisms.

FEVER

◆

A raised temperature is universally recognized as a sign of illness.

CAUSES

◆

The body functions within a narrow band of temperatures, shedding or increasing heat if the temperature strays outside the normal range (see below). Fever is mainly the result of an infection triggering defensive white blood cells to release a substance called endogenous pyrogen. Pyrogen affects the hypothalamus in the brain and turns up the body temperature. Pyrogen may also be released through tissue damage, accounting for some of the more unusual causes of fever.

Infectious causes

Fever is the usual response to invasion by infection for the reasons given above. However fever is only a marker of illness and not a diagnosis. Sometimes it is clear from the outset what is causing fever – a cold, a cough or symptoms of a urinary infection. Therefore, presented with fever alone, doctors go through systematic questions and examinations to determine what the cause may be, moving from the commonplace possibilities to the rare.

Incubation periods

In general, fevers of rapid onset are likely to be due to infection, but it often takes a few days for the infection to identify itself. Fever during those few days reflects the struggle within the body in which defences – white blood cells, antibodies and tissue destruction factors – battle with the infecting agent. If the body wins, the fever abates and you get better. If the infection wins then you eventually exhibit the features of an illness, be it a common cold at one extreme or **malaria** at the other.

The length of this battle varies greatly; the incubation period of common **colds** is two to four days, of **chickenpox** eighteen to twenty-one days. Fever is unlikely for all this time.

Prolonged fever

Unexplained fever lasting more than a week is called pyrexia of unknown origin. It can be a major diagnostic challenge, because the possibilities range through more exotic infections into other generalized illnesses (see below). Possible illnesses are those with a long incubation period – hepatitis A or unusual types of **pneumonia**. After recent foreign travel, malaria, typhoid or leishmaniasis need to be considered.

If fever lasts for weeks, thoughts turn to **tuberculosis**, heart infections, chronic abscesses within the abdomen or non-infectious causes.

Fevers not caused by infection

These bear consideration in someone with prolonged unexplained fever. They include auto-immune conditions such as **rheumatoid arthritis** or **systemic lupus erythematosus**, cancers – especially **Hodgkin's disease**, **cancer of the kidney** or **leukaemia** – and also reactions to drugs. It must be emphasized that these illnesses are unlikely in the case of acute fever and become a likelihood only after weeks if not months of unexplained fever.

SYMPTOMS

◆

Fever makes you feel hot and shivery despite the temperature. You will sweat and you may experience drenching night sweats. Associated symptoms include muscle aches, pains in the eyes, a headache – everything we all understand by saying 'I feel unwell'. Some infections cause rigors – intense shivering plus a high temperature. The symptoms may give the clue to the cause: a cough, a bad throat or a characteristic rash.

Measuring temperature

The glass or electronic thermometer is a good guide in adults; normal mouth temperature is 36.5–37.5°C/97.7–99.5°F. Mouth temperature is affected by hot or cold food for about a quarter of an hour after eating.

Temperature can be measured under the armpit, which gives readings half a degree centigrade lower, or rectally, which is half a degree centigrade higher than mouth temperature. It is often safer to measure temperatures of children in these ways. Increasingly common are special thermometers placed in the ear, which give a reliable result in seconds.

Investigations

These are neither useful nor needed in common feverish illnesses where the likely cause is a viral illness, which will be finished by the time the results are back. In some cases a doctor might want to take a throat swab and test a sample of urine, especially in children in whom a urinary infection may cause fever alone (see URINARY PROBLEMS).

The longer a fever lasts the more investigations become advisable. After a week the next step might be a chest X-ray to detect unusual forms of pneumonia, and a blood count. The number of white cells in a blood count indicates whether infection is of viral or bacterial origin; measures called ESR or C reactive protein help indicate the severity of infection.

Further information may come from faecal tests, blood tests for blood infections (septicaemia) or unusual infections such

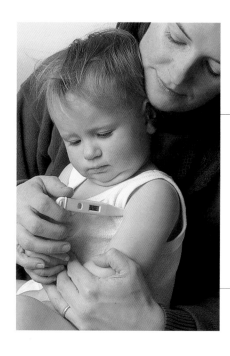

Left: It is safer and easier to measure the temperature of children under the arm rather than in the mouth.

as brucellosis and sophisticated immunological tests, which indicate the likely infection, whether viral or bacterial. You will be questioned about medication, as sometimes drugs cause fever. You may require scanning of the heart to detect infection (subacute bacterial endocarditis), the abdomen (for kidney disease or a liver abscess), or CT and MRI scans to search for unexpected cancers or deep-seated infections.

The pace of investigation is influenced by the condition of the individual: a feverish person who is seriously ill with confusion and low blood pressure needs everything urgently. An adult who is able to work, is eating and maintaining weight but sweating at night can have more leisurely investigation.

Many prolonged fevers resolve without anything abnormal being found.

TREATMENT

Even though fever is believed to be beneficial, treatment makes the person feel more comfortable, decreases the aches and aids rest. Fever greatly increases the body's metabolic rate and demand for energy, another reason to get it under control.

Discard excess clothing and do not swaddle children. It is better for them to be naked or at most wear a light vest and be covered with light bedding. Fanning is comforting, especially in summer. Tepid sponging reduces temperature rapidly, which is important in children, even if a little uncomfortable.

Febrile fits

If anyone's temperature rises high or fast enough, there is a risk of provoking a febrile fit. This is a common and potentially serious hazard in children, which is why there is such emphasis on reducing their temperature (see FEBRILE FITS). The risk in adults is extremely low.

Drugs to reduce temperature

The most widely used drug is paracetamol, which is safe for all ages. It is important not to exceed the recommended dosage as damage can be caused to the liver.

Aspirin is an alternative. Although ideal for adults, aspirin must not be used in children under the age of 12 as it can, in rare cases, cause a type of liver and brain damage called Reye's syndrome. Ibuprofen is as effective as paracetamol and safe for children.

Additionally, of course, the underlying cause of the fever should be treated as appropriate.

QUESTIONS

Is it harmful to go out with a fever?
Going into a cooler environment will help reduce fever. Parents often feel that children with fevers must stay at home, but no harm will come to them if they go outside.

Can people simulate a fever?
It is not unusual for puzzling fevers to prove to be due to deliberate deception, for example by putting a thermometer into a hot drink – this is something to consider if blood tests that should support serious infection remain normal.

Complementary Treatment

Western herbalism – catmint will cool you down. Make an infusion with 1 teaspoon per cup and drink freely. Many herbs promote sweating during fever, for example elderflower, ginger, hyssop and yarrow. Echinacea will boost your defences. Many herbs are warming, for example garlic, cayenne and cinnamon. **Homeopathy** – a whole range of remedies are available, for example belladonna and aconite. Their use depends on the specific details of your case and you should seek the advice of a registered homeopath. **Aromatherapy** – a few drops of oil in tepid water can be used to soothe fever. Lavender and Roman chamomile are especially soothing. Antiseptic oils include tea tree, myrrh, thyme. **Ayurveda** encourages regular detoxification to prevent infections attacking the body. If fever strikes, it offers herbal medications. **Nutritional therapy** – during convalescence eat plenty of fruit, vegetables and wholefoods. *Other therapies to try: Chinese herbalism; reflexology; Bach flower remedies.*

IMMUNIZATION

A medical technique that stimulates the body into producing resistance against infectious diseases.

BACKGROUND

There can be few advances in society that have provided so much good to so many people at so little cost as immunization. Less than a century ago infectious disease was a major killer at all ages, especially in childhood. Such diseases are now almost eradicated in the developed world. Other factors have contributed, but immunization is still of great importance.

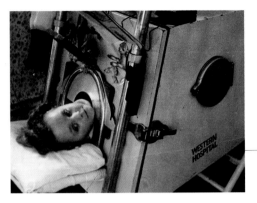

Left: One of the thousands of victims once paralysed by polio, inside an artificial lung.

Infection and the immune response

The 'trick' of immunization is to deceive the body into thinking it is meeting a disease before it actually encounters the real thing. In this way the body is stimulated to produce immune protection ready for when the real germs invade, so that it recognizes and destroys them on first contact.

When an organism invades the body, it is soon recognized as being 'non-self' by proteins that latch on to its unusual protein surface. These proteins, called antibodies, have the ability to call up additional resources to deal with infection. These are white blood cells that have been primed to attack organisms, either through direct recognition or by flowing to where antibodies have pinned down infection. The white blood cells and the antibodies inactivate germs by destroying their surface coating or by engulfing them and digesting them.

It takes a few days for the defences to be rallied, during which time bacteria or viruses may cause great damage and may tip the balance against the body being able to eradicate them. Previous immunization shortens this process by making possible swift recognition and destruction of the infection.

VACCINES

Immunization is achieved by giving the body a vaccine – a substance swallowed or, more usually, injected that is related to a serious infecting organism but has been rendered harmless. In the case of bacterial vaccines, it is extracts of killed bacteria that are enough to generate an immune response. In the case of viral vaccinations, it is usually a strain of the virus made harmless through modification and extended breeding.

Vaccination is given from infancy in order to stimulate antibodies well before the child is at risk of actual infection.

Many countries have vaccination programmes against illnesses such as **measles**, **mumps**, **rubella**, **tetanus**, polio, **diphtheria**, **whooping cough**, haemophilus and **tuberculosis**.

There are many additional vaccines kept for people at special risk, for example hepatitis A, typhoid and yellow fever for travellers, and hepatitis B for healthcare professionals. It is usual to have a first injection that stimulates a basic immune response and booster injections to trigger the full response. Booster injections may be advisable every few years, the precise details depending on the vaccine involved.

QUESTIONS

What are the overall risks of vaccination?

Before a vaccine enters use it must be shown that its serious risks are enormously less than those of the illness itself. Public concern justifiably pushes for ever safer vaccines, often forgetting that worldwide preventable infectious diseases still kill millions of unvaccinated children each year.

Who should not be vaccinated?

There is a separate list for each vaccine, generally including those with a current febrile illness, or who are on steroids, have reduced immune capability (for example leukaemia patients) or are allergic to components of the vaccine such as egg.

Complementary Treatment

The orthodox position is that there are no alternatives to immunization against the common infectious illnesses, especially those of childhood. However, **homeopaths** claim to offer effective substitutes. If you are considering immunizing your children and are interested in this option, discuss it with your doctor and a registered homeopath before reaching a final decision. **It is the author's opinion that children should be given conventional vaccinations.**

MEASLES

Once a feared childhood illness, now rare in the developed world.

CAUSES

The virus causing measles is in the same family as **flu** and **mumps**. Although measles is not a trivial illness, its effects are greatly reduced if the person is in otherwise good health.

SYMPTOMS

Measles spreads through the air and incubates for up to two weeks. It starts with high **fever** plus symptoms similar to **colds** – a streaming nose, cough and red eyes. After about four days a rash appears on the face, which rapidly spreads to the whole body. The blotchy rash fades to brown over a week, during which time the fever and malaise continue.

TREATMENT

Often a child with measles is put on an antibiotic; although this cannot influence the course of the viral illness it reduces the chances of a serious chest infection. Complications are uncommon in the developed world but are common and dangerous in malnourished people – for example **pneumonia** and heart disease are the main causes of death through measles.

There are rare but tragic instances of permanent brain damage through measles **encephalitis,** but thanks to routine vaccination, measles is now an avoidable disease.

QUESTION

How safe is a measles vaccination?
Even in the developed world, measles kills one in five thousand sufferers – one hundred and thirty children died in a recent epidemic in the United States – and leaves another one in five thousand with permanent brain damage. In Third World children the death rate is up to fifteen per cent. The latest estimates of the risks of vaccination are of less than a one in one hundred thousand chance of brain damage and no substantiated deaths.

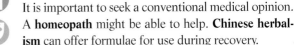

Complementary Treatment
It is important to seek a conventional medical opinion. A **homeopath** might be able to help. **Chinese herbalism** can offer formulae for use during recovery.

MUMPS

A viral infection that causes swelling of the salivary glands.

CAUSES

The mumps virus is spread through sneezing or saliva. Mumps has effects throughout the body beyond the typical enlargement of the salivary glands in the cheeks, affecting the pancreas, testicles, ovaries and brain. Mumps is infectious two to three days before the facial swelling appears and for three to five days afterwards.

SYMPTOMS

Mumps incubates for 18 days before producing typical viral symptoms of **fever**, **headaches** and muscle pains. Then there is enlargement of the parotid salivary glands – the ones lying over the angle of the jaws below the ears. The face becomes distorted – hamster-like is as graphic a description as any. The swelling lasts for about five days.

There may be pain in the testicles due to inflammation; girls can experience abdominal discomfort through inflammation of their ovaries. Temporary **deafness** is not uncommon but there is a less than a one in three hundred risk of permanent deafness. There is a small risk of **viral meningitis**.

TREATMENT

Only fluids, rest and painkillers are needed. Even mumps meningitis can be expected to settle within two weeks. The risk of mumps causing sterility is very small. Rarely, **encephalitis** can occur, with a coma lasting months or even permanently. Mumps is preventable by vaccination in infancy.

Complementary Treatment
Nutritional therapy – supplements of vitamins and minerals can boost your immune system. **Western herbalism** – see FEVER. **Chinese herbalism** can offer formulae to help. A **homeopath** might be able to help.

RUBELLA

Also called German measles, rubella is an infection that is minor for the patient but catastrophic for foetal development.

CAUSES

The rubella virus spreads through coughing or saliva. In a pregnant woman it passes to her foetus. The risk of damage is greatest during the first four months of pregnancy while the organs are forming. The child may be born with **deafness**, heart valve disease, **cataracts** and brain damage.

SYMPTOMS

After two to three weeks' incubation rubella begins with **fever** and enlarged lymph glands, especially at the back of the neck. A brownish rash appears after a few days, soon fading. Short-term joint pain is common; other complications are rare.

TREATMENT

There is no special treatment for rubella, other than taking aspirin or paracetamol to reduce fever or discomfort. For women who are in the first four months of pregnancy, it is essential to have a diagnosis of the illness confirmed by blood tests and then to consider the risks to the baby. These can be as high as a 30% chance of damage, with 20% of babies dying in early infancy. Many countries will offer abortion in these tragic circumstances.

QUESTION

How is rubella controlled?
In the United Kingdom vaccination against rubella is given with measles and mumps vaccinations. All pregnant women are checked for immunity to rubella. Thanks to these measures there were only 12 children born in the United Kingdom with congenital rubella in 1990, while only 10 abortions were needed for at-risk mothers, compared to the hundreds that were done as recently as the 1970s.

Complementary Treatment

Make sure you and your children are immunized. **Western herbalism** and **aromatherapy** – see FEVER. **Homeopathic** remedies include phytolacca and pulsatilla, but their use depends on a number of variables.

WHOOPING COUGH

Bacterial infection noted for causing a persistent cough in children.

CAUSES

Bordetella pertussis is the organism responsible for this highly infectious illness, once so common in childhood. The incubation period is seven to ten days. Vaccination has rendered the illness rare, with newer non-bacterial vaccines believed to be far safer than getting whooping cough.

SYMPTOMS

In its early stages whooping cough is like an ordinary **cold**, with a runny nose, red eyes and **fever**. The cough begins after a week; it consists of paroxysms of coughing that the child cannot stop until he or she desperately sucks in air, giving the characteristic whoop. In older children or adults, whose airways are wider, whooping is not likely, but they still suffer from the paroxysmal cough.

Complications of whooping cough include the collapse of part of the lung with permanent damage and starvation of oxygen leading to convulsions. The diagnosis is confirmed through swabs taken from the nose and the throat.

TREATMENT

If the illness is suspected within the first week, the infectivity is reduced by taking the antibiotic erythromycin. Once the full extent is known, treatment is with moisturized air, nursing care to keep up fluid intake and vigorous treatment of complications. The cough can last for months afterwards.

Complementary Treatment

Seek a conventional opinion. **Western herbalism** expectorants include horehound and thyme. Relaxants include lavender and hyssop. **Homeopathy** offers a variety of remedies; seek advice. **Chinese herbs** can be helpful.

DIPHTHERIA

A serious and sometimes fatal bacterial throat infection.

CAUSES

The infection is caused by a micro-organism called *Corynebacterium diphtheriae*; it is spread through coughing, sneezing and saliva. The infection grows in the throat or larynx into a tough membrane that restricts breathing. The bacteria produce a blood-borne toxin affecting the heart and nerves.

SYMPTOMS

A membrane can be seen in the throat and in the nostrils. The child, at first mildly unwell with **fever** and sore throat, soon deteriorates and has difficulty in breathing, becoming increasing blue from oxygen starvation. The effect on the heart is to cause heart failure with increasing breathlessness and collapse of the circulation, carrying a high risk of death.

TREATMENT

This is of the utmost urgency for a child with diphtheria – injections of antitoxins together with high doses of penicillin must be given once the illness is diagnosed. However, even with these measures the risks of the illness are high and may even appear several weeks after apparent recovery.

In the developed world vaccination has rendered the disease extremely rare, but it remains a significant risk in many less fortunate parts of the world. In the United Kingdom a few cases are diagnosed in immigrants who have come from developing countries.

QUESTION

What is the role of vaccination?
There is no substitute for vaccination if you want prevention for your children. In the United Kingdom vaccination is given at two months with monthly boosters over the next two months. Contacts of known cases should have injections of antitoxins. Travellers to countries where diphtheria has re-emerged, such as Russia, should consider having booster vaccinations.

Complementary Treatment
Complementary approaches are not appropriate as treatment. During recovery, **aromatherapy massage** could be very soothing for adults and children alike.

TETANUS

A very serious infection leading to spasms of the muscles, commonly called lockjaw.

CAUSES

Tetanus occurs if spores of the *Clostridium tetani* organism, which lives in the soil, get through a cut in the skin. Tetanus was common until vaccination became routine, and is still an important health hazard in undeveloped countries.

SYMPTOMS

Symptoms begin days or weeks after infection. The first muscles affected are those that close the jaws, which go into a rigid spasm – hence the name lockjaw. Spasm of the back muscles causes arching of the back. There may be **fever** and sweating. Mild cases can recover, but there is a poor outlook if the muscles of breathing or of the heart are affected.

TREATMENT

Any dirty wound is a risk for tetanus and you should have an injection of antitetanus toxin if there is any doubt about your vaccination status.

The illness is treated by intensive nursing care in a quiet environment, since stimuli set off spasms. Muscle relaxants are given to reduce the spasms and also artificial ventilation if needed. Even so the risk of death in serious cases is 20–60%.

In the United Kingdom the antitetanus vaccination programme, which begins in infancy, has made tetanus virtually extinct. Boosters are recommended every ten years for adults, especially those who work with soil (gardeners and farmers).

Complementary Treatment
Complementary approaches are not appropriate for treatment. Any of the therapies discussed under STRESS could help during the recovery period.

SCARLET FEVER

A once notorious bacterial throat infection.

CAUSES

Many throat infections are caused by the streptococcus bacteria, one strain of which is responsible for scarlet fever – now often called scarlatina. However the bacteria, while still causing the same symptoms, has lost its capacity to cause permanent damage, possibly through improvements in general health.

SYMPTOMS

The throat feels painful and there are enlarged neck glands and **fever**. After a day or two a fine red rash spreads all over the skin, from which the illness gets its name. The rash tends to spare the area immediately around the mouth, which looks pale by contrast. The tongue goes from having a white coating with red dots to looking raw. Later, skin may peel from the fingers and the toes. The appearance is typical and the diagnosis can be confirmed by throat swabs and blood tests.

TREATMENT

Penicillin is given for ten days, during which time individuals should use their own utensils; other isolation is unnecessary. Rest, fluids and paracetamol are also recommended.

QUESTION

What was the significance of scarlet fever in the past?
It was associated with rheumatic fever, which led to heart disease, kidney damage and severe infection. These complications made scarlet fever a leading cause of childhood death in the 19th century, whereas now it virtually never has any long-term consequences.

 Complementary Treatment
Chinese herbalism – treatments are offered to ease symptoms and help the body fight off infection. *Other therapies to try: see FEVER.*

CHICKENPOX

A viral infection characterized by a blistery rash.

CAUSES

In childhood, chickenpox is a relatively mild illness. The virus responsible is varicella zoster, which in later life causes shingles. Chickenpox is highly contagious from just before the blisters appear until they are all crusted over.

SYMPTOMS

After two to three weeks' incubation the illness begins with **fever** and aching. Tiny clear-headed blisters appear after two to three days, spreading within hours all over the body, including the scalp and mouth but not the palms and soles.

TREATMENT

The main problem is itching, eased by antihistamines such as chlorpheniramine, and soothing lotions like calamine lotion. It is important not to scratch blisters off or they will leave a scar. After about ten days all the blisters become scabbed and disappear over another two to three weeks. Chickenpox affects the lungs so a worsening cough should be treated with an antibiotic. Adults feel more ill and many doctors give them an antiviral drug such as acyclovir to reduce the severity. Vaccination against chickenpox may soon become available.

QUESTION

Is chickenpox serious?
Complications in children are very rare. About one in a thousand adults develops a form of encephalitis and requires more intensive treatment. In the uncommon event of catching chickenpox in early pregnancy, the mother is likely to have complications and the virus may affect the foetus; urgent medical advice should be sought.

 Complementary Treatment
Bach flower remedies – impatiens for irritability and crab apple for cleansing the skin may both be applied to the skin diluted. All itchy childhood rashes may be relieved with chicory, hornbeam or cherry plum.

FIFTH DISEASE

A benign viral illness, mainly affecting children, and notable for the red facial appearance it causes; hence 'slapped face' disease.

CAUSES

Medically known as erythema infectiosum, fifth disease is caused by a tiny virus, the parvovirus. Parvoviruses are responsible for many non-specific viral illnesses. It is thought to be spread by coughs; the incubation period is up to 18 days.

SYMPTOMS

The illness begins in the usual viral way with **fever** and muscle pains. After a day or two the child's cheeks become bright red with a fine rash, which then spreads elsewhere on the body, but with a more lace-like appearance.

TREATMENT

The only treatment necessary is something to relieve muscle aches and to reduce any fever. Paracetamol syrup is usually sufficient to do this.

In many cases the child remains well or only a little unwell and may require rest and fluids. The rash may reappear over the course of the next few weeks.

QUESTION

Why it it called 'fifth' disease?
Doctors tend to keep mental checklists for many conditions, including childhood illnesses with rashes. When presented with a patient with a rash, the doctor mentally reviews all of the possibilities. However, what constitutes the first four diseases with a rash varies from doctor to doctor. This author considers the following: measles, German measles, scarlet fever and roseola. This leaves erythema infectiosum as number five.

Complementary Treatment
Bach flower remedies – Rescue Remedy. **Aromatherapy** – bathing and **massage** are soothing, particularly with lavender or Roman chamomile. *Other therapies to try: see* FEVER *and* CHICKENPOX.

ROSEOLA

Common childhood illness with a rash, often confused with measles.

CAUSES

The virus responsible for this condition was only recently identified as another of the ubiquitous herpes viruses. It is almost always confined to children; most adults are immune.

SYMPTOMS

There is a high temperature, listlessness and runny nose, continuing for several days. In these respects it resembles **measles** before the rash appears. After four to five days the rash spreads, then the **fever** abruptly falls and recovery occurs.

TREATMENT

Treatment is simply a matter of taking fluids plus paracetamol to reduce the fever. Once the rash has appeared the child will be back to normal within two to three days. It is highly

unusual for the illness to follow other than an uncomplicated course. It is quite probable that the many 'allergic reactions' to antibiotics given for feverish illnesses are actually rashes that are due to roseola or similar viruses.

QUESTION

How does roseola differ from measles?
Measles tends to cause higher temperatures and more illness in the child; also red eyes are common. Otherwise the clinical picture is very similar. The difference is that in roseola the appearance of the rash signals recovery, whereas in measles it signals another few days of high temperatures and misery.

Complementary Treatment
Nutritional therapy – during convalescence children should eat plenty of fruit, vegetables and wholefoods. *Other therapies to try: see* FEVER *and* CHICKENPOX.

VIRAL MENINGITIS

A form of brain infection caused by a virus. It is relatively benign and rarely causes serious illness.

CAUSES

There is no one virus that causes viral meningitis; the most common ones are those that also cause the routine infections of childhood such as gastroenteritis (see DIARRHOEA AND VOMITING) or upper respiratory infections. Meningitis can accompany other well-known viral illnesses such as **mumps** and **glandular fever**.

The viruses gain access to the brain through the blood stream, having escaped the normally vigorous defences that keep infection away from the brain. Unlike the bacterial causes of meningitis, viral infection does not transmit easily from person to person.

Viral infection of the brain causes inflammation of the fine tissues covering the brain called the meninges, hence the term 'meningitis'. In contrast with bacterial infection, viral infections do not generally spread from the meninges into the brain and so do not often cause swelling nor lead to deposits of pus. These consequences make **bacterial meningitis** very serious and, conversely, make viral meningitis normally follow a much more benign course.

SYMPTOMS

All types of meningitis affect children more often than adults. Early in what appears to be a routine viral illness, the child will start to complain about severe and persistent **headaches**; he may vomit, and grumble about bright light irritating his eyes, and also a stiff neck. The child is feverish and unhappy, irritated at being handled in any way. This is the fully developed illness, but it is probable that many viral illnesses are accompanied by a mild meningitis causing similar, although less pronounced, symptoms.

TREATMENT

Although doctors may feel fairly certain that they are dealing with a case of viral as opposed to bacterial meningitis, it is essential to confirm the diagnosis by hospital admission for investigation. Doctors will be guided by blood tests that show changes more suggestive of a viral cause.

If there is the slightest doubt about any ill child, then a lumbar puncture will be performed to sample the cerebrospinal fluid that surrounds the brain and spinal cord. The fluid is then scrutinized to see if it contains any infection and for changes in the cells in it that reflect the type of meningitis. The identity of the virus responsible is established by further analysis of the blood and cerebrospinal fluid.

If the diagnosis is viral meningitis every one can breathe a sigh of relief, in the virtually certain knowledge that recovery can be expected over the next few days. Should recovery be delayed or the illness worsen, then the diagnosis may have to be reviewed or the child may have developed one of the relatively rare complications. Fortunately, fewer than one in a hundred meningitis sufferers develop **encephalitis**, with drowsiness, worsening headaches and possibly epileptic fits.

It normally takes seven to ten days for full recovery, and hospital care is not necessary once the diagnosis is certain. It is common for headaches to recur for several weeks after the illness and this in itself should not cause concern.

See also BACTERIAL MENINGITIS.

QUESTIONS

How can I recognize meningitis?
The generally agreed symptoms for viral meningitis are as given earlier – abnormal headaches, stiffness of the neck, discomfort from bright lights, unusual drowsiness and vomiting. The more serious bacterial meningitis has the additional symptom of causing a blotchy purple rash. However, the diagnosis of meningitis is not always straightforward and medical opinion should be sought even if it seems to be a remote possibility.

What is the role of antibiotics?
Viral illnesses do not respond to antibiotics. Many doctors would nevertheless prescribe antibiotics even though the diagnosis is viral meningitis – just to be on the safe side.

Complementary Treatment
Complementary approaches are not appropriate for treatment. However, many therapies could help during recovery. If the patient is a child, check that your chosen practitioner is experienced in treating children. Traditional Chinese medicine (**acupuncture**, **herbs**, **tai chi/chi kung**) can be helpful. **Reflexology** supports recovery by giving special attention to areas according to the specific characteristics of the personality and the symptoms. *Other therapies to try: see STRESS.*

TUBERCULOSIS

◆

Slow-growing infection that can spread from the lungs throughout the body. Its seriousness depends on the victim's general health.

CAUSES

◆

Tuberculosis (TB) follows infection with the organism mycobacterium tuberculosis, which gains access to the lungs by close contact with others coughing up the bacteria. In otherwise healthy individuals, infection is unlikely to progress further and will be eradicated by the body's own defence mechanism. Otherwise the bacteria lie relatively dormant causing few if any symptoms.

The disease then becomes reactivated months or years later, when the individual's resistance falls through other reasons such as malnutrition or **AIDS**. This secondary disease can spread throughout the body, affecting the lungs, brain, bones, joints and more.

Much of the increase in TB in the developed world has been through the spread of AIDS. This illness diminishes the immune response and leaves the individual susceptible to many other infections as well as TB.

SYMPTOMS

◆

If the initial infection causes any symptoms they are temporary vague ill health and a cough that settles in a few weeks. Symptoms from reactivation depend on which parts of the body are affected. The most common are recurrence of cough, which becomes chronic, persistent malaise, weight loss and night sweating. The phlegm often contains blood. At this stage enlarged lymph nodes may appear, typically in the neck.

Aggressive TB

This is called miliary TB and is the result of the spread of the bacterium throughout the blood stream, like a septicaemia. The individual is at first unwell in a vague way but rapidly becomes very ill indeed and may well develop meningitis. Miliary TB is a risk even several years after initial infection, but it is uncommon except in debilitated individuals.

Other effects

These are all fortunately now uncommon in the developed world. Bones are a favourite lodging site for TB and it is still considered in anyone with persistent bone pain. The infection slowly destroys the bone, which eventually collapses. This was previously a common cause for collapse of spinal vertebrae and distortion of the back. Chronic infection of the

intestines can lead to abdominal pain. Other organs that can be affected are the womb, causing pain, heavy bleeding and subfertility, the kidneys, causing chronic kidney infection, and the testicles. Tuberculous meningitis is particularly difficult to diagnose and is a dangerous form of the illness.

The diagnosis of TB depends on seeing typical changes on a chest X-ray, analysing enlarged lymph nodes, identifying the bacterium in sputum and examining tissue biopsies.

TREATMENT

◆

For six months, people with TB need to take daily tablets of the antibiotics rifampicin and isoniazid, and additional antibiotics depending on the individual case. Longer courses are given for bone, brain or gynaecological infection – up to a year. These drugs have proved to be effective and have few side effects. Cure can be virtually guaranteed in those who take the treatment reliably. There is, however, a problem of resistance to these drugs which is a worrying new phenomenon.

Aggressive therapy is required in the treatment of both miliary TB and tuberculous meningitis.

QUESTIONS

Who is at risk of TB?
TB is predominately a disease of poverty, malnutrition, overcrowded housing and self-neglect. Alleviation of these factors was responsible for the virtual eradication of TB in many countries. Immigrants from underdeveloped countries are still at significant risk.

What is BCG vaccination?
This is an inactivated strain of TB given by injection and providing about 70% immunity to TB. It stands for Bacille Calmette-Guérin, the French researchers responsible for this important vaccine.

Complementary Treatment
Remain with your conventional treatment regime and tell your doctor about any complementary approaches you choose to explore. Traditional Chinese medicine (**acupuncture**, **herbs**, **tai chi/chi kung**) can help the body fight off infection, but with TB the effects will be only partial. **Chakra balancing** and **hypnotherapy** can offer support during the long treatment schedule, and help relieve many of the symptoms. *Other therapies to try: see STRESS.*

AIDS

◆

AIDS kills by reducing a person's immune capability.

CAUSES

◆

AIDS (acquired immune deficiency syndrome) is caused by one of two viruses: HIV I, found in most of the world, and HIV II, found mainly in Africa. HIV stands for human immuno-deficiency virus. These viruses probably arose through spontaneous mutation in Africa in the 1950s; some believe they have been around much longer but only recently became aggressive.

AIDS as a specific medical condition was recognized in 1981 and the virus identified in 1983. The virus spreads through semen and blood products and especially through homosexual practices, for example anal intercourse, and intravenous drug abuse. It can be passed from mother to unborn child. Heterosexual spread is far less common in populations with good nutrition, although statistics suggest that heterosexual sex will eventually become the most important means of transmission over the next few decades. The disease has begun to spread rapidly through India and South-East Asia.

SYMPTOMS

◆

On initial infection the virus causes a non-specific viral illness with **fever** and enlarged glands. It continues to live in the body, but causes no symptoms. This is what is meant by being HIV positive. A person who is HIV positive will almost certainly eventually develop AIDS and show symptoms. This may take as little as six months or more than ten years.

The virus damages the immune system so that the later symptoms are from infections – recurrent **thrush**, **diarrhoea**, sweating, shingles, profound weight loss and malaise. Other features highly suggestive of AIDS are chest infections with unusual organisms; characteristic skin tumours such as Kaposi's sarcoma (see SKIN CANCER); **tuberculosis** in a young person and premature dementia. Many other infections and tumours result and, until recently, a progressive decline was inevitable. The illness is diagnosed by the clinical picture and by blood tests demonstrating the presence of the HIV virus.

TREATMENT

◆

The average survival time of AIDS patients has improved from six months to two years, reflecting the progress in treatment. Currently this is with a number of drugs, including zidovudine (AZT) and saquinivir, which together inhibit viral growth. They are very expensive, have many side effects and would normally be regarded as experimental, were it not for the special nature of AIDS. Other infections are treated as appropriate with antibiotics, chemotherapy, antifungal drugs and so on.

Recently it has been found that giving combinations of antiviral drugs to HIV positive people reduces their chance of developing AIDS. This may become the standard treatment for HIV in the future. There are also reports of a promising new anti-HIV vaccine.

QUESTION

How can HIV/AIDS be avoided?
Unprotected casual sex is dangerous; always use a condom, especially if you are having sex with multiple partners. Anal intercourse and intravenous drug use are high-risk behaviour for HIV. Oral sex may carry a risk if you have any sores or cuts in your mouth. If you are travelling abroad, bear in mind that Western standards of blood transfusion may not apply in all countries.

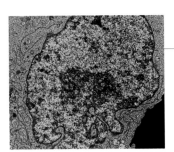

Left: A round HIV virus attacks a white blood cell.

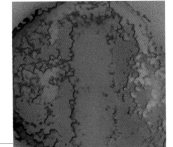

Right: The infected cell produces many more HIV viruses.

Complementary Treatment

Complementary therapies offer support, not cures. **Chakra balancing** – non-touch techniques are ideal and can help with relaxation, symptom control and insomnia, and also stimulate appetite. **Hypnotherapy** can relieve many of the symptoms such as depression and anxiety. Traditional Chinese medicine (**acupuncture**, **herbs**, **tai chi/chi kung**) offers a variety of immune-boosting preparations. **Nutritional therapy** – your practitioner will try to improve your assimilation of food. *Other therapies to try: Ayurveda; Western herbalism: see also STRESS.*

MALARIA

A parasitic infection, spread by mosquitoes. Malaria is probably the most significant and deadly infectious disease in the world.

CAUSES

Malaria is caused by four different types of a parasitic micro-organism, called plasmodium. Each type leads to a slightly different pattern of disease and requires different treatment.

Plasmodium enters humans by the bite of the anopheles mosquito, ubiquitous in hot, humid regions of the world. The parasite's eggs live in the mosquito's salivary glands. When the infected mosquito bites a human, eggs enter the human host and rapidly travel through the blood stream to the liver (see diagram, right). After some time the parasites escape into the blood stream again, this time invading red blood cells and multiplying until the cells rupture. The free parasites then circulate within the blood plasma, awaiting a bite by a mosquito, which sucks up the infected blood ready for the parasite to complete its life cycle, and to infect the next host. A number of parasites remain in the liver; their escape every few days or months accounts for the chronic and repeated nature of malaria.

SYMPTOMS

Depending on the type of infection it takes from ten days to six weeks before symptoms begin. An attack progresses within hours through three distinct phases, corresponding to stages of invasion of the blood stream. First there is sudden intense shivering and feeling cold, despite a **fever**; this merges into several hours of high fever with possible confusion and ends with drenching sweats and feeling better. The pattern repeats itself with variations, depending on which type of malaria parasite is responsible, for example every two days to a more irregular pattern. The illness can become chronic with persistent **anaemia** and ill health. At another extreme it may progress rapidly to **kidney failure**, coma and death.

TREATMENT

The parasite can be seen on blood samples. This is how the diagnosis is confirmed, the type identified and cure monitored.

Once the type of parasite is known, the appropriate drug is given usually by mouth or by intravenous drip in severe cases. The drugs – chloroquine, mefloquine and primaquine – act very quickly even in severe infection, where improvement can begin after just a single dose. Other measures are intravenous quinine, fluids and paracetamol or aspirin to reduce fever.

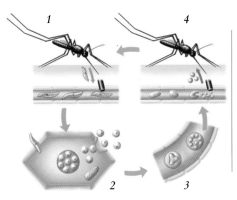

Left: 1) Mosquito injects parasite into blood stream. 2) Parasites multiply in liver; 3) invade blood stream and 4) are sucked up by mosquito which later infects new host.

Preventing infection

Before travelling to a potential malaria zone – especially countries too poor or unstable to maintain the necessary public health measures – get up-to-date advice about the health hazards, including the risk of malaria. There are many help lines and medical publications providing information about the drugs you should take. It is essential to begin the drugs a week before travel, to take them regularly during your stay and to continue for six weeks after you return. Even if your exposure to malaria may only be overnight on a stopover, you should consider taking preventive medication. Additional precautions are to wear clothing that covers exposed skin, use insect repellents, sleep under mosquito netting and avoid going out at times favoured by mosquitoes, for example at dusk.

QUESTION

How dangerous is malaria?
Between two and three hundred million people contract malaria each year, of whom two to three million die, many of them children. Certain forms are extremely dangerous, with collapse of blood pressure, kidney and brain damage and delirium.

Complementary Treatment

It is folly to travel into malaria-infested regions without following conventional medical advice. If you do catch the disease, follow your orthodox doctor's treatment programme, but remember that people living in countries where malaria is endemic traditionally use **Ayurvedic** medications and Chinese approaches, especially **Chinese herbalism**, to treat this disease. Consult the relevant practitioners if you are interested in exploring these options.

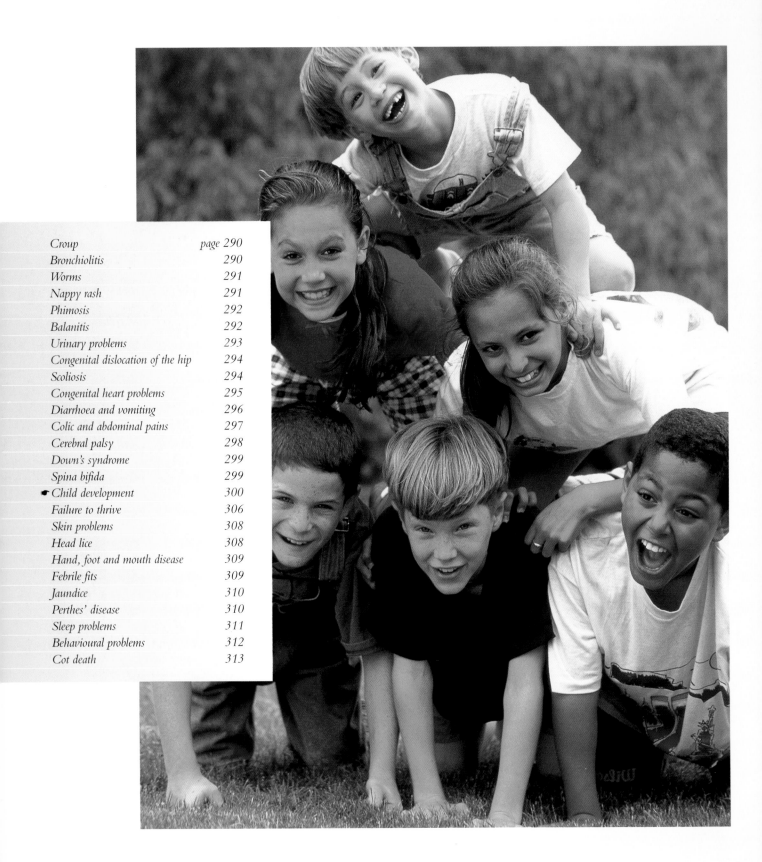

The realization that children are not simply little adults is a relatively late concept in medicine. The illnesses they get, their symptoms and their response to treatment are often quite unlike adult ill health. The speciality of paediatrics has only emerged in the second half of the 20th century.

CHILDREN

THE HUMAN BABY is helpless to a unique degree in the animal kingdom, requiring total support for feeding, warmth and grooming. This helplessness led to the belief that the baby was a blank sheet on which parents and society could write personality and abilities. This we now know is incorrect and babies are in fact already preprogrammed mentally and physically. Research increasingly shows the importance of prenatal influences on growth and high blood pressure.

Many systems are 'switched on' significantly for the first time at birth, especially parts of the heart and circulatory system, the liver, the bowel and the senses. Most of these systems function as intended immediately but medical checks in the first few weeks after birth ensure that all is working normally.

Learning and doing

The learning process includes the obvious things, such as recognising familiar people's faces, and the less obvious ones such as gauging distance. This is not a random process; babies have instinctive preferences for learning, for example they prefer to look at face-shaped objects and they appreciate the sound patterns of language from just a few weeks of age.

The helpless baby is soon reaching, rolling over, crawling, standing, cruising, walking and talking. This implies more than the acquisition of muscular control. It reflects desires and needs, which in turn imply that consciousness is maturing somewhere beneath that cute baby bonnet smeared with carrot purée. We do not really understand exactly how this process happens.

Growing

Babies are born with many of their organs in an immature state. These mature and grow during childhood, especially the brain, the skeletal system, the liver and the eyes. Growth is therefore one of the fundamental ways of judging the health of a child and much child healthcare involves measuring and monitoring the rate of growth.

Nurturing

Paediatric medicine and the many allied specialities aim to let all children attain their full potential. This means ensuring a healthy life within the womb, free from infection and trauma. Birth is managed to reduce brain damage and other injury. The newborn baby is scrutinized for the abnormalities that affect about one in fifty children so that treatment can be planned if required. There are guidelines for infant feeding, weaning, immunization, education and general development. Emotional and psychological influences on growth and development are crucially important.

General health

There is no one definition of 'normality' in childhood, be it the age of first speaking or the frequency of bowel actions. Your child's general health and development is of more significance than minor variations in attaining particular milestones.

Remember that children born in the developed world enjoy an expectation of health and development unimaginable to children in much of the rest of the world. When reading in the following pages of the things that may go wrong, do bear in mind that really serious ill health in childhood is uncommon.

Left: Children carry our hopes; their physical and psychological health is naturally a high priority for parents.

CROUP

Infection that narrows the airways, causing characteristic noises.

CAUSES

Many viruses can invade the upper respiratory tract and make the lining of the larynx and trachea swell, hence the medical term for croup – laryngo-tracheo-bronchitis. This swelling obstructs the smooth flow of air and leads to the croup sound when breathing out and stridor, which is noise on breathing in. Infection often spreads further down into the lungs. Croup mainly affects children between one and three years of age.

SYMPTOMS

Starting as a **fever**, cold and cough, croup worsens into hoarseness and a cough like a sea lion's. Serious deterioration is relatively uncommon but is suggested by an increasing rate of breathing, increasing stridor, lethargy and pallor.

TREATMENT

Treatment involves ensuring that the child stays quiet and rests, because any increased effort will increase the airways' obstruction. Make the child comfortable in a warm moist atmosphere such as a steamy bathroom or kitchen. This will rapidly give relief from the croup. For severe cases, steroids may be given in a nebulized mist. The worst of croup usually goes within 24–48 hours.

QUESTION

Why might children suffering with croup occasionally be admitted to hospital?

This may be necessary in a case of severe airway obstruction when the child is very breathless, increasingly lethargic and exhausted. Sometimes the diagnosis of croup might be in doubt and some other reason is suspected for obstructing the airway. For example, a foreign body might in fact be the cause of abrupt stridor in an otherwise well child.

Complementary Treatment

Aromatherapy – try dispensing lavender oil via a room humidifier. **Homeopathy** – a variety of remedies is available, including aconite, spongia and hepar sulph; their use depends on the details of your child's condition. See also BRONCHIOLITIS.

BRONCHIOLITIS

A viral infection in babies that causes coughs and wheezing.

CAUSES

Of several viruses causing bronchiolitis, the most common is respiratory syncytial virus (RSV), which provokes inflammation throughout the lungs and is highly contagious.

SYMPTOMS

Bronchiolitis mainly affects babies aged two to six months and begins as **colds** do, with a runny nose and wheezy cough. Many children remain only modestly unwell, but in some the illness becomes rapidly worse over a few hours. The child becomes lethargic. Breathing exceeds 30 breaths a minute; the ribs appear to suck in with each breath and the child is too breathless to feed. Blueness around the lips suggests severe lack of oxygen and needs immediate medical assessment.

TREATMENT

Mild cases need fluids and rest, and protection from smoke and fumes. It helps to put the child in a warm moist atmosphere such as a steamy bathroom or kitchen. Since the illness can deteriorate rapidly, doctors send any but the most mildly affected children into hospital for oxygen and close nursing.

About ten per cent of children develop **pneumonia**, so antibiotics are usually prescribed, even though the basic viral infection will not be affected by an antibiotic. The illness lasts three to five days. There is some evidence that children who keep getting bronchiolitis may later develop **asthma**.

Complementary Treatment

WARNING: Tai chi/chi kung is not suitable for children under ten. Children respond well to **acupuncture** (some acupuncturists specialize in treating children), **shiatsu-do** and **Chinese herbs**. See also CROUP.

WORMS

*Threadworms (*Enterobius vermicularis*) are the likeliest worm infection in temperate zones, where other worm infections are rare.*

CAUSE

Children playing may pick up soil containing the eggs then suck their fingers, as children do. The swallowed eggs hatch inside the large intestine and appear on the motions.

SYMPTOMS

At night worms congregate around the anus to lay eggs, provoking intense itching. Itching leads to scratching, scratching leads to eggs under the fingernails, fingers are sucked and the cycle is repeated. The worms may crawl into the vagina, causing itching there, too. The worms and tiny white eggs can be seen around the anus or on the motions, the former looking like strands of white thread, 0.5 cm/¼ in long and very thin.

TREATMENT

Suitable drugs include piperazine or mebendazole (the latter also kills several other types of worm apart from threadworms). Usually a single dose is enough but a repeat treatment after two weeks is advisable. Ideally the whole family should take treatment at the same time. However, do not treat children under two without taking medical advice on safety. The risk of re-infection is reduced by keeping fingernails short and by encouraging frequent handwashing. Since eggs are laid at night, a morning bath or shower will wash these away.

QUESTION

Are threadworms serious?
They hardly ever cause problems other than itch. In very rare cases, large numbers live within the appendix, discovered if the appendix is removed. The unpleasantness of the itch should not be underestimated as it can drive children (and adults) to distraction. Therefore they are well worth treating, especially in families and close communities where threadworms spread rapidly.

 Complementary Treatment
Nutritional therapy – raw garlic is toxic to worms, but it can be difficult getting children to eat it; carrots and pumpkin seeds also help clear infection. *Other therapies to try: Western herbalism; Ayurveda; homeopathy.*

NAPPY RASH

Raw red rashes in the nappy region affect all infants at some time.

CAUSES

The warm and wet conditions under a nappy favour colonization by **thrush**. Urine irritates the skin, creating **eczema** and letting in infection. A rubbing nappy may cause rawness. Children with **diarrhoea** are likely to get a rash.

SYMPTOMS

The skin is red and inflamed across the nappy region and raw in places. The edge of the rash is quite sharp. Thrush is likely if the rash extends deep into all the skin creases. A rash sparing the skin creases is typical of inflammation from urine, which has not penetrated the creases. The baby may be mildly irritated; parents are usually more upset by nappy rash than the infant. Considering the unhygienic conditions prevailing under nappies, the risk of serious skin infection is extremely low. In theory, a nappy rash might cause serious ulceration of the skin, scrotum and vagina but this rarely happens in practice unless the rash has been grossly neglected.

TREATMENT

Nappy rash is less common in this era of disposable nappies, which should be frequently changed and should contain no detergent to sensitize the skin. The many creams available contain an antifungal, an antiseptic and substances that protect the skin from urine. Ideally, the nappy should be left off.

 Complementary Treatment
Homeopathy – use calendula cream. **Aromatherapy** – add one drop of one of the following to 15 ml of carrier oil and apply to the affected area: Roman chamomile, lavender or yarrow.

PHIMOSIS

An unusually narrow opening of the tip of the foreskin.

CAUSE

Boys may be born with this slight abnormality, or the foreskin might be scarred by repeated **balanitis**. Ill-advised attempts to roll back the foreskin can traumatize it and lead to narrowing.

SYMPTOMS

There may be no symptoms; the boy's parents simply notice the small tip. The foreskin cannot be rolled back, but this is quite usual in boys until three to five years of age anyway. In significant phimosis the foreskin balloons out when urinating and urine dribbles out rather than exits in a stream; this needs a medical opinion. Balanitis under the phimotic foreskin is common and it can be hard to decide which is cause or effect.

TREATMENT

Treatment may not be necessary, in the expectation that the foreskin will stretch as the boy gets older. Where there is clear obstruction or repeated balanitis, surgery is appropriate. It may be enough to dilate the foreskin under anaesthetic. Afterwards the parents should show the child how to roll back the foreskin regularly to prevent renarrowing. Circumcision, if requested by the parents or advised by the surgeon, will of course cure the problem for good.

QUESTION

Is circumcision a good thing?
Opinion on this vexed question predates modern medicine, with views going back to biblical times. There is good evidence to suggest that circumcised men are much less likely to get cancer of the penis. Since non-ritual circumcision requires an anaesthetic, most surgeons try to avoid it in children unless recurrent infection or phimosis make it unavoidable.

 Complementary Treatment
Homeopathy – to reduce itching, bathe the foreskin and head of the penis with a solution made from five drops each of mother tincture of hypericum and calendula in 300 ml/½ pint of cooled boiled water.

BALANITIS

Infection under the foreskin, a problem closely related to phimosis.

CAUSES

Almost inevitably, sweat and secretions get under the foreskin and can become infected. Whereas adults can roll back the foreskin and clean beneath it, in children it is natural that the foreskin will not roll back until the boy is about five years old and attempts to do so may lead to scarring and **phimosis**. The latter adds to the problem in a chicken-and-egg way.

SYMPTOMS

The tip of the foreskin becomes reddened and inflamed; it can swell alarmingly, but harmlessly, because the skin is so lax. Infection often spreads to around the penis, the tip of which becomes inflamed. There is a discharge of pus from under the foreskin. After repeated attacks the foreskin becomes thickened, cracked and phimotic.

TREATMENT

Early mild infection is helped by bathing the penis in warm salty water and gently irrigating under the foreskin. More severe infection requires medication: creams that usually combine an antifungal and an anti-inflammatory agent as well as an antibiotic. This is because **thrush** often invades balanitis and adds to the inflammation. The very soreness and narrowness of the foreskin makes it difficult to get the cream inside, which is why oral antibiotics are often necessary, too.

Repeated balanitis is very uncomfortable for the boy and will cause the narrowing of phimosis. In such cases surgical dilation may be advisable, if not circumcision.

   Complementary Treatment
Children do generally respond extremely well to both **acupuncture** and **Chinese herbs**. Some acupuncturists specialize in the treatment of children. **Homeopathy** – see PHIMOSIS.

URINARY PROBLEMS

Malformations and infections of the urinary system occur quite frequently and predispose to kidney trouble in adult life.

CAUSES

The urinary system comprises the kidneys, where urine is made, the ureters (the tubes through which urine flows to the muscular bladder), the bladder itself and the urethra, through which urine exits in front of the vagina, or via the penis.

Malformations

There are many anatomical abnormalities, the most serious of which occur in boys, some of whom have posterior urethral valves. These are flaps of skin within the urethra which impede the outflow of urine from the bladder. They lead to great back pressure of urine into the kidneys and permanent damage. Many urinary system malformations are detected only on investigation of urinary infection.

Infection

In girls the urethra is short enough to allow bacteria to ascend fairly easily from the perineum into the bladder. As a result of this about five per cent of girls get urinary infections during their first two years. Bacteria find it much more difficult to gain access via the penis and the infection rate in boys is correspondingly lower at one to two per cent.

Infected urine may ascend (reflux) from the bladder into the kidneys, causing permanent damage, which in later life increases the risks of **high blood pressure** by 20%. Furthermore, about one-third of cases of **kidney failure** are believed to originate in kidney damage due to childhood infection. The risks are not huge – kidney failure is rare – but it may be partially avoidable (only partially, because a tendency to reflux is probably genetically determined).

SYMPTOMS

Childhood urinary infection is rarely accompanied by the classic symptoms experienced by adults – burning when passing urine and needing to go frequently. More likely, the child is simply feverish or 'off colour'. A child previously dry at night might become incontinent again and might also complain of stomach ache. Boys with posterior urethral valves tend to dribble urine rather than pass a proper stream.

It can be difficult to confirm urinary infection because it is so awkward to obtain a good sample from children, who do not obligingly 'pee to order' into a specimen bottle.

TREATMENT

Any infection is treated with an antibiotic. Many specialists recommend further investigation after even a single proven infection. Investigation has been greatly simplified by high-definition ultrasound and scans of the kidney, which display many malformations and existing kidney scars.

It may be necessary to have specialized X-rays in order to see whether urine is refluxing into the kidney and scarring it. If this is the case, the child needs to have both long-term antibiotics to reduce the chances of further infection and regular checks of kidney function. It is possible to reduce reflux by re-implanting the ureters into the bladder in a position that is less likely to reflux. The value of such surgery is debatable and is done only where infection is not controlled by antibiotics and where there is clear evidence of progressive scarring of the kidney.

QUESTIONS

Should all ill children be tested for urinary infection?
This is an unrealistic ideal. However urinary infection should be considered in any child who remains unwell or feverish for more than a few days.

How serious is a first infection?
It is not actually known how often infections go undetected; they may be more common, and therefore of less significance, than believed. On present evidence they should be taken seriously.

Can problems be detected before birth?
Many can be detected from just 18 weeks, including posterior urethral valves. A drainage tube can be inserted into the bladder before birth and the abnormality fully corrected surgically after birth. It is not known whether all abnormalities are a problem in later life.

Complementary Treatment

Treatment depends on the specific details of your child's problem. Always check the practitioner is experienced in treating children. **Western herbalism** works on the urinary system and reduces tension. Children respond well to **Chinese herbalism** and **acupuncture**. A **homeopath** will build up a picture of your child and should be able to help. **Chakra balancing** improves the immune response.

CONGENITAL DISLOCATION OF THE HIP

An abnormality at birth, which if undetected in infancy may cause the child to have a permanent limp.

CAUSE

The femur (thigh bone) should fit securely into a socket of the hip bone; in congenital dislocation of the hip (CDH) the femur is dislocated or slips out easily. Girls are affected six times more than boys and there is a higher incidence in breech-born babies. CDH is probably due to failure of the hip socket to grow normally; it affects about one in five hundred children.

SYMPTOMS

A baby should have symmetrical skin creases around the buttocks; in CDH these are asymmetrical. With time the affected leg looks shorter and turns outward. Doctors check for CDH at birth and again at six to eight weeks of age. They twist and press the hips to see if they will dislocate. Also they look at the skin crease around the buttocks with the baby lying on its front. If there is doubt, the child should have an ultrasound scan of the hips. Any hip that feels 'clicky' or fails the test should be assessed by an orthopaedic surgeon.

TREATMENT

The child has to stay in splints for some months to keep the top of the femur pressed into the cup of the hip, so encouraging the socket to grow properly. The few children who do not respond to this may need surgery to fix the femur in place.

QUESTIONS

Why is CDH missed despite examination?
The standard tests miss at least 30% of CDH. Evidence is also increasingly suggesting that the condition can develop in hips previously passed as normal. There is an argument for screening for CDH using ultrasound scans of the hip. Otherwise it may be detected only when the child limps when she starts to walk.

Complementary Treatment
Rolfing can improve the muscular balance around the hip joint. **Chakra balancing** can help relax an irritable child and reduce pain. *Other therapies to try: cymatics; shiatsu-do; Alexander Technique.*

SCOLIOSIS

A permanent side-to-side curvature of the spine.

CAUSES

For unknown reasons, scoliosis in the developed world is mostly congenital, i.e. an abnormality present at the time of birth. Occasionally disease of the muscles around the spine causes the twist. Poliomyelitis used to be a common cause.

SYMPTOMS

Scoliosis often only becomes apparent with the growth spurt of puberty, especially in girls. From behind, the spine should look almost straight. In scoliosis a sideways twist throws the ribcage on one side into prominence. If muscle imbalance is the cause, there may be weakness down one side of the body. Poor posture may resemble a fixed scoliosis but the abnormal curve goes when the child straightens or bends forward. In true scoliosis the curve remains however the child moves.

TREATMENT

It takes great judgement by an experienced surgeon to decide whether and when to treat scoliosis. Repeated review and measurement of the degree of scoliosis aid this judgement. The decision is more straightforward if the scoliosis is severe enough to compress the lungs or heart.

The surgery, called spinal fusion, involves fixing a number of vertebrae together so no further twist is possible. Other measures include wearing firm frames (braces) or inserting a rod into the vertebrae to prevent progression; the value of these techniques is more controversial.

Complementary Treatment
Chiropractors can advise on good exercises to do. If there is back pain, the child can be treated using specific manipulative and mobilizing techniques. **Rolfing** allows the spine to lengthen by relaxing both it and the soft tissues around it.

CONGENITAL HEART PROBLEMS

Abnormalities of the heart, many of which are minor, affect one per cent of children at birth.

CAUSES

The heart develops by a rather beautiful series of twists that transform an initially straight tube into the complex heart, but with a high risk of malformations. Before birth the heart does not have to pump blood around the lungs, oxygen instead being supplied via the placenta. At birth all this changes as the lungs expand for that first cry. This is a time when many serious abnormalities first show themselves.

Heart problems are generally divided into those that cause a blue baby (cyanotic heart disease) and those that do not. In cyanotic heart disease the abnormality allows blood that is low in oxygen, and therefore blue, to mix with blood from the lungs. In non-cyanotic conditions blood circulates through the lungs in the normal way, but problems arise through leaks and abnormal pressure of flow. Both types may end in **heart failure** or in disease of the lungs.

Common congenital heart defects

There are a number of common congenital heart defects (congenital meaning an abnormality present at birth). While most serious ones are apparent at birth, a few cause minimal symptoms and may not be apparent until later in childhood.

Ventricular septal defect (VSD): There is a hole between the right and left ventricles – the larger beating chambers – of the heart. When the powerful left ventricle pumps, it squeezes blood through the hole into the right ventricle.

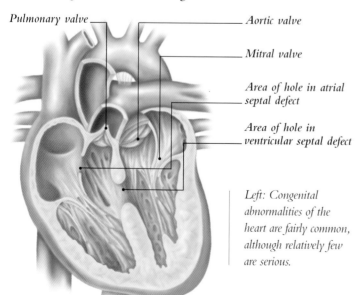

Pulmonary valve
Aortic valve
Mitral valve
Area of hole in atrial septal defect
Area of hole in ventricular septal defect

Left: Congenital abnormalities of the heart are fairly common, although relatively few are serious.

Atrial septal defect (ASD): There is a hole in the wall between the atria, smaller chambers that hold blood before it passes into the powerful ventricles. The effect is similar to a VSD.

Fallot's tetralogy: This is a cyanotic heart condition where there is gross malformation of the heart with a large VSD and a narrowing of one of the heart valves.

Hypoplastic left heart: In this serious condition the whole of the left heart has failed to form properly. The baby cannot survive more than a few days without major surgery.

Coarctation of the aorta, patent ductus arteriosus, pulmonary stenosis: These are abnormalities of major blood vessels around the heart, the significance of which varies.

SYMPTOMS

Some conditions cause symptoms at or around birth, for example cyanosis (blueness), breathlessness and a variety of murmurs over the heart – unusual sounds heard through a stethoscope and caused by turbulent blood flow. Badly affected babies rapidly go into heart failure, unable to feed properly and requiring resuscitation. Less badly affected children have heart murmurs but are otherwise reasonably well, although they may get breathless easily. Congenital heart disease is a major reason for **failure to thrive**.

The majority of minor heart conditions are detected as a murmur, the exact diagnosis defined by echocardiography and possibly angiography (see Modern investigations, page 48).

TREATMENT

Many congenital heart conditions will correct themselves during the first few years of life, for example 50% of cases of VSD, or require no surgical treatment at all. Some extreme forms require immediate surgical treatment and even a heart transplant (see page 331). Several other serious conditions can be corrected in a number of operations spread over a few years.

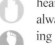

Complementary Treatment

Complementary therapies cannot correct congenital heart problems. They can have a supportive role, but always check the practitioner is experienced in treating children. A sick child may benefit from the sense of wellbeing generated by **aromatherapy** with **massage**. **Reflexology** can also be supportive.

DIARRHOEA AND VOMITING

Usually minor illness caused by stimulation of the gastrointestinal tract by viruses and bacteria, acquired by chance or by food poisoning. Also called gastroenteritis.

CAUSES

Among children in the developed world, most diarrhoea and vomiting episodes are caused by viruses, usually rotaviruses, which irritate the gastrointestinal tract. Here it is rarely more than an inconvenience and few children become severely ill. Globally, however, gastroenteritis is a major killer of debilitated young children who lack access to simple but effective treatment. Breast-fed babies are less likely to contract gastroenteritis, thanks to the inherently sterile milk supply and the protection from antibodies within the mother's milk.

Vomiting

Initiated by a vomiting centre within the brain, vomiting is a non-specific reflex reaction to many infections or pains. It has presumably evolved to get a possibly poisonous substance out of the stomach as soon as possible. Children and babies vomit readily since it is under less conscious control than in adults.

Diarrhoea

The intestinal tract normally absorbs fluid very efficiently; diarrhoea occurs because infection irritates the lining of the intestines so they fail to absorb carbohydrate. This has the effect of retaining excessive quantities of fluid within the bowel, hence diarrhoea. Another influence may be toxins from infections that paralyse the normal activity of the bowel.

SYMPTOMS

The child often has a cough and cold, suggesting a viral origin for the gastroenteritis. Food poisoning is suggested by abrupt vomiting in a previously well child, diarrhoea soon following. Vomiting frequently precedes diarrhoea and ends before it. Diarrhoea can begin without forewarning. Abdominal cramps are common but diarrhoea and vomiting with severe pain suggest an abdominal problem that needs urgent medical assessment. Most gastroenteritis settles within three to seven days.

TREATMENT

Gastrointestinal upsets are a normal feature of childhood and need cause no immediate alarm. The treatment principle is to replace fluid in small but frequent amounts, using electrolyte mixtures containing salt and sugar in concentrations similar to the natural fluids within the body. These widely available drinks are better absorbed than plain water and are pleasant to drink. Do not give the child sugary drinks, which tend to make diarrhoea worse. There are no recommended anti-diarrhoea drugs for children.

Once the vomiting phase has passed the child can eat if he wishes. Do not be alarmed if eating provokes a bout of diarrhoea. This is not 'food going straight through' but simply a reflex bowel action, which is normal after eating. Give the child bland food like rice or eggs, not milk or dairy products, which may worsen the diarrhoea.

It is important to monitor the child for dehydration (see box below). Most children can be managed at home unless dehydration becomes apparent, when they may need hospital treatment with intravenous fluids. This is more likely with babies, who become dehydrated much more quickly than older children.

WARNING SIGNS WITH GASTROENTERITIS IN CHILDREN

- *Blood or mucus in the diarrhoea*
- *Persistent or severe abdominal pain*
- *Vomit stained yellow with bile*
- *Reduced urine output – dry nappies for several hours*
- *Increasing lethargy*
- *Sunken eyes, sunken fontanelles (soft spots in the baby's skull)*
- *Pallor and cold skin*
- *In children below the age of one, symptoms continuing for more than 24 hours*

These suggest significant dehydration or another serious cause for the symptoms.

 ### Complementary Treatment

Complementary therapies have much to offer, but do check the practitioner is experienced in treating children. **Western herbalism** – peppermint or blackberry tea may help shorten recovery time. Several **homeopathic** remedies are available; the one to use depends on many variables. Diet – rest the digestive system by offering only liquid for a while; a **naturopath** could give specific advice. *Other therapies to try: acupuncture; Chinese herbalism; shiatsu-do; Ayurveda.*

COLIC AND ABDOMINAL PAINS

Abdominal pain in children has physical and emotional origins.

CAUSES

Children do get pains for serious reasons but frequently their pains are recurrent, non-specific, less easily categorized and settle without treatment. In an otherwise well child, maintaining weight and eating, a serious cause is unlikely and emotional problems at school and at home should be explored.

Colic

Colic means pain due to distension of a hollow internal organ, typically the intestine, to which children are especially prone. Colic rises to a crescendo then diminishes, the process repeating every few minutes. For some reason, babies aged between one and three months commonly go through a phase of recurrent colic at night, despite being well for the rest of the day.

A **hernia** in the groin will cause colic if it becomes trapped. Other causes in older children may be **constipation** or worry.

Inflammation of an internal organ

This is always the number one worry for both parents and doctors. The most common serious inflammation is appendicitis. Children occasionally get general inflammation of the bowel called colitis, **indigestion** or even a peptic ulcer. Boys may have a **twisted testicle**. Inflammation caused by **urinary problems** is notorious for causing abdominal pain in children. Diarrhoea is frequently accompanied by abdominal pains (see DIARRHOEA AND VOMITING).

Mesenteric adenitis/abdominal migraine

These are efforts at explaining the many abdominal pains where other causes are excluded. A sore throat is thought to cause painful glands within the abdomen as well as the neck, which accounts for many pains. Headaches in children are often accompanied by abdominal pains, as they are in adults.

SYMPTOMS

Older children complain of pain. Babies cry, appear distressed, curl up their legs and may vomit. More serious is pain accompanied by vomiting yellow bile or bleeding from the back passage. Other serious accompanying symptoms are **fever**, a raised pulse and coated tongue. Doctors look for another infection – **tonsillitis**, **ear infection** or chest infection.

Appendicitis usually starts over the belly button, shifting within hours into the lower right abdomen, plus fever,

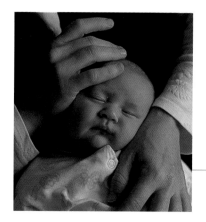

Left: Babies with colic often respond well to gentle cranial osteopathy, which is very calming.

vomiting and great abdominal tenderness. It can, however, present without these symptoms and even in the lower left abdomen. It may be diagnosed only by exploratory surgery.

The examination of the child's tummy is an art, assessing tension of the abdominal muscles, pain on releasing the abdomen, the sounds from the intestines. Doctors also check for a hernia or twisted testicle and test urine for infection.

TREATMENT

For babies suffering from colic, ensure they are well winded. If you are bottle feeding, experiment with changing the milk and timing of evening feeds. Paracetamol syrup can be given.

Suspected appendicitis, twisted testicle or intestine, trapped hernia and other serious internal problems require surgery. Exploratory operations are not undertaken lightly as surgeons prefer to operate with a definite diagnosis in mind.

Pains apparently due to infection elsewhere, such as tonsillitis, should settle as the infection goes. This leaves many instances where there appears not to be a serious cause for pain. Then it is reasonable to give a painkiller such as paracetamol and plenty of fluids and await spontaneous recovery, always being prepared to reassess the child if pains persist.

Complementary Treatment

Complementary therapies have much to offer, but do check the practitioner is experienced in treating children. **Homeopathy** – see DIARRHOEA AND VOMITING. **Aromatherapy** compresses and inhalations can help; oils are chosen according to the case. **Osteopathy** can be extremely helpful, especially some of the cranial techniques. *Other therapies to try: Western herbalism; acupuncture; shiatsu-do; Chinese herbalism; chakra balancing; naturopathy; cymatics; Ayurveda.*

CEREBRAL PALSY

Brain damage at the time of birth or occurring soon thereafter.

CAUSES

The natural hazards of birth can, in a few cases, damage brain cells enough to cause cerebral palsy. Prematurity is a major risk: about ten per cent of premature babies are affected. Infection after birth may damage the delicate brain.

At least half of the cases are due to developmental problems within the womb or infection during pregnancy such as **rubella**, although the latter is now very rare. For many children with cerebral palsy there is no obvious explanation and the assumption is that the child's brain simply failed to develop properly within the womb. Cerebral palsy affects one to two children per thousand in the developed world but is a much larger hazard in the underdeveloped world where pregnancy and childbirth are more dangerous.

SYMPTOMS

Children affected with cerebral palsy have some degree of weakness and abnormal stiffness of the muscles down one side of the body, called a hemi-paresis, or of all limbs – a quadriplegia. Symptoms can range from stiffness and clumsiness to complete paralysis of one side. There is an increased risk of **epilepsy**. Because of the muscle imbalance these children often develop distorted backs (**scoliosis**) or limbs.

At the worst extreme the baby may clearly be abnormal at birth, unusually floppy, breathing badly, not moving its limbs properly – all symptoms that are suggestive of major brain damage. The worst-affected children may never become continent or indeed capable of independent existence. At the other extreme there may be just a barely detectable difference in strength between the two sides of the child's body or slight developmental delays.

Many cases are recognized because the child fails to reach the 'milestones' of development, for example there is delay in sitting, walking, talking and social development. The diagnosis in mildly affected children often is not considered until rather later as a result of queries over school progress, unusual clumsiness or difficulty in reading.

It is important to review the pregnancy: perhaps the mother contracted rubella or **chickenpox** or had **high blood pressure**. Was the birth difficult? Was the child premature? Did the child have **jaundice** or a severe infection soon after birth? Further investigation would most likely include genetic analysis and tests for a biochemical abnormality.

TREATMENT

Although the diagnosis of cerebral palsy is a parent's dread, it is important to remember two things. First, a baby's brain can overcome brain damage that would be permanent and devastating in an adult. Although the baby may not ever fully recover, her final abilities may be much better than thought at the time of diagnosis. Second, cerebral palsy does not necessarily mean that the child's intelligence is affected.

Great changes have been made in treatment in recent years, aiming to help all children suffering from cerebral palsy make the most of their abilities, with physiotherapy to keep all muscle groups working, speech therapy to aid articulation, aids for speech or walking and constant stimulation. Operations may be advisable to correct twisted limbs.

Most children with cerebral palsy can attend a normal school and only a minority need special schooling or are too badly affected to benefit at all.

SEE ALSO CHILD DEVELOPMENT, PAGE 300.

QUESTIONS

Do children develop at the same rate in all areas of learning?
No, it is quite normal for a child to be advanced in one area and to lag in another, but a generalized delay in development should be further assessed medically.

What is the real outlook?
It may not be until the child is ten years old or more that the full extent of their abilities is clear. Unfortunately this is often a period of enormous strain on the parents, not knowing if their child will ever lead an independent existence.

Complementary Treatment

Programmes providing intensive stimulation have received much publicity in recent years, and it is now accepted that increased stimulation improves development. **Arts therapies** could have a role here. Any therapy that works the tissues – **osteopathy**, **chiropractic**, **rolfing**, **Hellerwork** or **massage** – could be beneficial. **Chakra balancing** could be supportive. The entire family could benefit from stress-reducing therapies such as **yoga** or **aromatherapy**.

DOWN'S SYNDROME

A genetic fault that causes heart and brain abnormalities.

CAUSES

Chromosomes that carry the genetic information normally exist in pairs. In Down's syndrome chromosome 21 exists as a triplet, hence the condition's alternative name trisomy 21. The defect arises when the fertilized egg begins to divide but the fundamental reason is unknown. There are other rarer genetic reasons for the defect.

Down's syndrome affects one in seven hundred children who are born live, the risk rising according to the mother's age: for example about one in three hundred and fifty at the age of thirty-five and one in twenty-five to thirty by the age of forty-six. Many affected foetuses die pre-term.

SYMPTOMS

Among numerous Down's syndrome features there is a prominent fold in the eyes as is found normally in Asian races, which accounts for the old term 'mongolism'. The tongue is large and the skin coarse. Heart abnormalities are common and ten per cent have **epilepsy**. Intelligence is invariably reduced but the range is wide. Since the baby will show the typical Down's syndrome features at birth it is unusual for there to be a delay in making the diagnosis.

TREATMENT

The condition cannot be reversed. The child is prone to chest infections that need vigorous treatment, as may heart disease. Some are intelligent enough to lead a semi-independent existence eventually and hold down a simple job, while others require constant monitoring. Few Down's syndrome adults live beyond 50 but their life can be a relatively happy one.

QUESTION

What screening is available?

The usual current method is amniocentesis (see page 324), which means drawing fluid from the womb, for genetic analysis of cells shed by the baby and measurement of certain biochemicals associated with the condition. As amniocentesis may itself provoke a miscarriage expert guidance is needed as to when this risk is outweighed by the risk of an affected baby. The parents must then decide if they wish a termination of pregnancy.

Complementary Treatment

Down's syndrome children could benefit from any **massage**, including one with **aromatherapy**. Check the practitioner is experienced in treating children.

SPINA BIFIDA

Failure of the foetus's spinal bones to fuse, associated with damage of the spinal cord and brain.

CAUSE

In embryonic life the bones of the vertebral column fuse together, enclosing the delicate spinal cord. This fails to happen in spina bifida, leaving part of it exposed. It is associated with hydrocephalus, increased pressure in the fluid surrounding the brain. It now affects about one in six thousand births.

SYMPTOMS

The child may be born with an obvious opening at the base of the back. The skull swells because of hydrocephalus. There are many degrees of spina bifida, all of which are serious.

TREATMENT

The spine must be immediately protected or surgically covered against infection. If there is hydrocephalus a tube is fitted within the skull to drain fluid from the brain to the heart, keeping pressure down. People with spina bifida are often paralysed below the waist and subject to urinary infection, **incontinence**, pressure sores and reduced life expectancy. Yet the top half of the body is normal, as is intelligence.

The risk of spina bifida is greatly reduced if the mother takes 0.4 mg folic acid daily, before and in early pregnancy.

Complementary Treatment

If you are planning a baby, a **naturopath** or **nutritional therapist** could advise on preconceptual diet, focusing on your intake of vital nutrients, including folic acid.

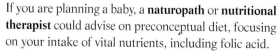

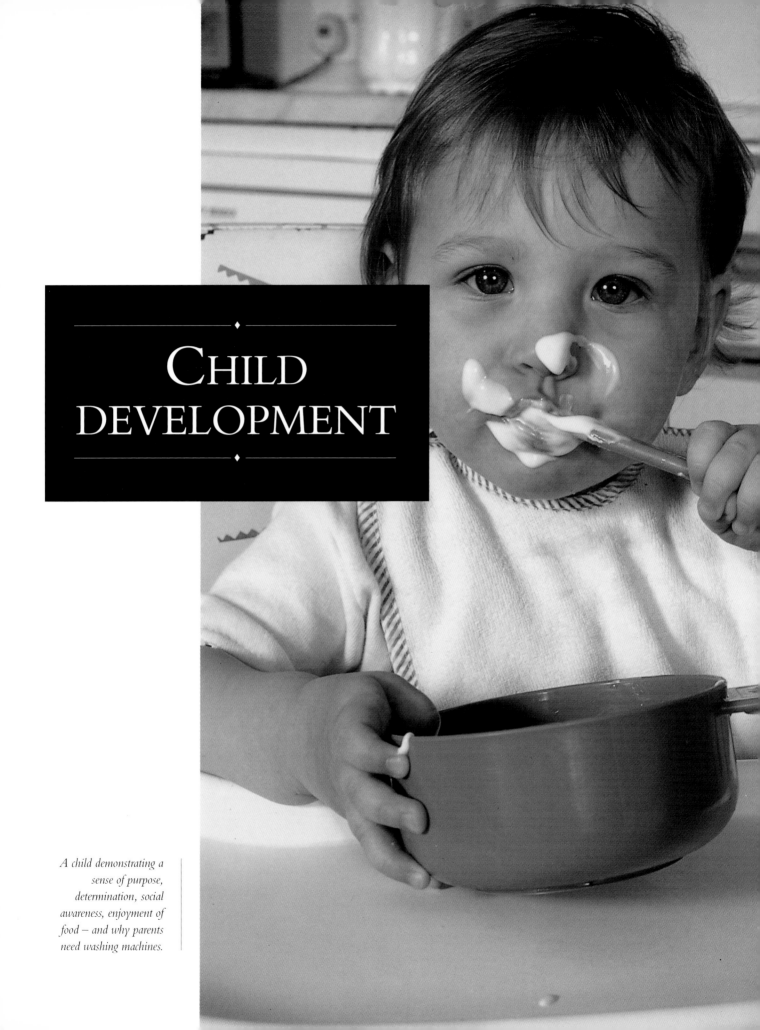

CHILD DEVELOPMENT

A child demonstrating a sense of purpose, determination, social awareness, enjoyment of food — and why parents need washing machines.

THE PLEASURE AND WORRY OF bringing up children is in watching them change from helpless babies to self-reliant teenagers. At each step parents naturally want to reassure themselves that there is normal development and full expression of their child's capabilities, and this process is monitored by child development assessments.

The details will vary from country to country, but certain general principles are described below.

Abilities

Abilities fall into physical and mental capabilities. Physical capabilities include usage of limbs, manipulation, walking and running and the senses of hearing and vision; mental capabilities include responsiveness, speech, social behaviour and play. Each category can be further analysed.

Milestones

These are the means of monitoring behaviour such as speech or motor skills – for example, it is a milestone to be babbling at eight months and to be speaking in formed sentences by three years. Milestones can cause anxiety or pride in parents but they are only theoretical averages and children may leap them or dawdle between them without being abnormal.

The following page shows examples of important developmental milestones at six weeks, eight months, one year and three years. They follow the usual United Kingdom development assessment and are greatly simplified.

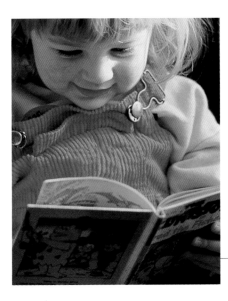

Left: Computers still cannot match the intelligence that lets a child learn to read.

'NORMAL' AND 'ABNORMAL'

It is unusual to categorize a child as 'normal' or 'abnormal' on the basis of a single assessment or test. It is the child's overall performance compared to that of the average child that is important in making such a judgement.

What is average?

This is judged by reference to other children brought up in the same culture and sharing the same opportunities for physical and mental development. What is the usual age at which children in that society talk, walk and play games of increasing sophistication?

What lies within the range of 'normal'?

While most children are walking at 15 months, it can be normal to walk at 9 months or to continue to shuffle on the bottom until 2 years. That same child who is a late walker may be advanced in speech or manipulation. Physical defects are abnormal, for example a heart murmur or a large birthmark. Even so, it is often not possible to give a firm opinion on their significance until the child has grown; this is especially the case with cerebral palsy (see page 298), where the child's ultimate capabilities are difficult to judge.

Measuring normality: centiles

This is a statistical way of showing how a child compares to all others. For example the third centile for height means that three in a hundred children fall below that measure, while ninety-seven in a hundred lie above it. This can be shown as a graph. What is important in such graphs is not so much where the child lies but that he or she is following an appropriate centile curve, whether for height or weight. Growing either too fast or too slowly suggests a possible problem.

Six weeks post-natal

Behaviour:	*Alert; responding to parents; starting to smile*
Language:	*Beginning to make sounds*
Vision:	*Fixing on objects*
Hearing:	*Startle reaction to noises and turning eyes to sound*
Motor:	*Some head control, not totally floppy*

CAUSE FOR CONCERN: *Unresponsive to sounds or sights; floppy; constantly irritable.*

Eight months

Behaviour:	*Sitting and manipulating toys; playing simple games; searching for hidden toys. Taking weight on legs for a few moments*
Language:	*Babbling happily, although meaninglessly*
Vision:	*Looking around and responding to visual cues*
Hearing:	*Responding to sounds presented to either ear*
Motor:	*Picking up small objects*

CAUSE FOR CONCERN: *A squint; failure to use one limb; no babbling; still floppy and not sitting.*

One year

Behaviour:	*Responding to questions; showing understanding*
Language:	*Speaking three to four words*
Vision/hearing:	*As above*
Motor:	*Standing if hand is held; cruising supporting self on furniture*

CAUSE FOR CONCERN: *Failure to sit unsupported; complete lack of speech; unresponsive to simple commands.*

Three years

Behaviour:	*Dry by day; dresses self. Drinks from cup; eats with spoon and fork*
Language:	*Speaks in sentences*
Vision/hearing:	*As earlier*
Motor:	*Copes with stairs; can build towers with bricks*

CAUSE FOR CONCERN: *Not running; unable to climb; unintelligible speech.*

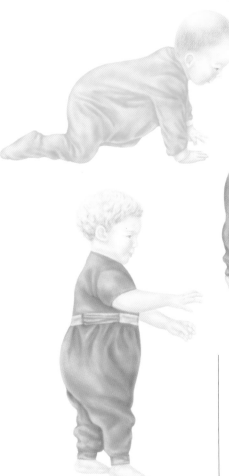

Left and above: On average a baby rolls at two and a half months, sits at six months, crawls at ten months, cruises at one year and walks by eighteen months.

After three

While physical and mental development do not end at the age of three, social development is more noticeable. From three years children increasingly learn to play in groups and to cooperate within a group setting. Working in groups is a fundamental skill in most societies because it means that individuals learn to control their immediate desires in order to achieve some common goal. Of course this should not be at the expense of individualism. This is nurtured by giving children special responsibilities and encouraging them to demonstrate any special skills.

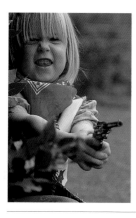

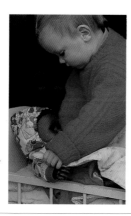

Left: Toddlers spend much time role playing and learning physical skills.

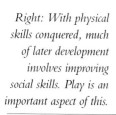

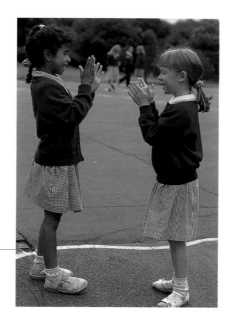

Right: With physical skills conquered, much of later development involves improving social skills. Play is an important aspect of this.

Much child development is through imitation, initially of parents but also of older children and other significant figures such as teachers or TV and film characters. If we could arrange such things we would probably want our children to identify with some social reformer or upstanding figure, but something within their brains steers them instead to identify with racing drivers, 'blobs' from beyond Mars and 'Hulks' of a variety of forms. Identifying with such figures suggests that children are keen to share in whatever their role model appears to be enjoying. Parents should not be at all surprised that children are seeking admiration and power, desires that come more naturally – and are usually rewarded better – than service, self-denial and altruism.

Achievements of childhood By the age of nine or ten children should have resources to last throughout their life. They should have a strong sense of their own identity, their uniqueness and their self-worth, as well as an awareness of their obligations within their family unit and within society at large.

The child will have experienced, it is to be hoped, love and protection but also responsibility, discipline and education. It is easy to see how failure to achieve these fundamentals may influence the child as an adult, although more difficult to explain or predict exactly how.

Things that go wrong These include irresponsibility, lack of control, cruelty, non-cooperation, lying, stealing and destructiveness. Children can develop neurotic traits such as obsessions or frequent nightmares. Such behaviour is not necessarily abnormal in itself, becoming so only through the degree and persistence of these traits. Occasionally children may become depressed or severely mentally ill, or show features of autism – this is where a child is completely unresponsive to people, including parents, emotionally 'flat' and uninterested in socializing with other children.

The treatment of such childhood behavioural problems takes time, patience and subtlety and, even so, is often unsatisfactory. It is assumed that a disturbed child reflects some wider family disturbance and therefore therapy begins by exploring family tensions, relationships and attitudes. It is difficult for other members of the family to open up about such matters, while many parents find it hard to alter what have become automatic methods of behaviour, possibly influenced by their own childhood experiences.

For the most disturbed children there are special schools where teachers attempt to encourage better behaviour, often using behavioural techniques such as ignoring undesirable behaviour and rewarding or praising desirable behaviour.

Personality

Children have differing personalities – something that is evident from a few months, if not just weeks, after birth. It is not known the extent to which personality is genetically determined, as opposed to being learnt, and therefore open to influence. Personality is also influenced by things such as birth order and sex.

In later childhood, parents and educators hope to see a happy combination of individuality and social cooperation, but it is not always an easy ride and there is a sneaking suspicion that the slightly awkward child may grow into a more self-reliant adult than the compliant child.

Puberty and adolescence

Puberty is the time when physical and mental changes turn children into men and women. In girls, this comprises the development of breasts and the external genitalia, contouring of the body and menstruation. In boys it consists of growth of the penis and testicles, production of sperm, deepening of the voice and muscular development. In both sexes there is the appearance of pubic hair. Accompanying these hormone-driven changes are a swirl of emotions and maturation of sexual feelings.

Puberty coincides with a growth spurt but, contrary to popular supposition, puberty eventually halts growth. It is for this reason that children who go into puberty early tend to be shorter than those who enter puberty later.

Cause for concern Girls, on average, begin a growth spurt at ten and menstruate at twelve to thirteen years. The average age for boys to enter puberty is twelve to fourteen years. Puberty before those ages or after about sixteen may be abnormal through hormonal disorders.

The true facts of adolescence What happens in adolescence? Physically, the child becomes an adult in appearance, with new bits appearing – the functions of which may be puzzling, pleasurable or intriguing, but somehow 'off limits'. Mentally, adolescents are hit by powerful emotions such as lust, aggression and love, the power of which comes as a surprise. They have no yardstick to judge how appropriate the emotion is. They test these emotions by flirting and having crushes and attachments that seem more eternal than the sun yet are as transient as dew.

Similarly they question the old order, rebel and espouse unusual or private causes, be they pop groups or fashions. This gives a sense of identity clearly different from the adult

Right: She is queen of the class, he is top of the heap; then puberty arrives. Adult emotions hit personalities still lacking confidence and direction. After the uncertainties, angst, turmoil and false starts, the adult emerges.

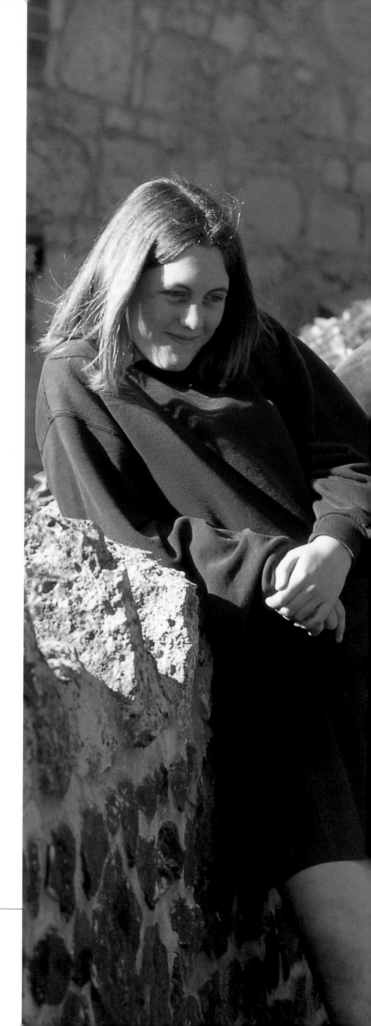

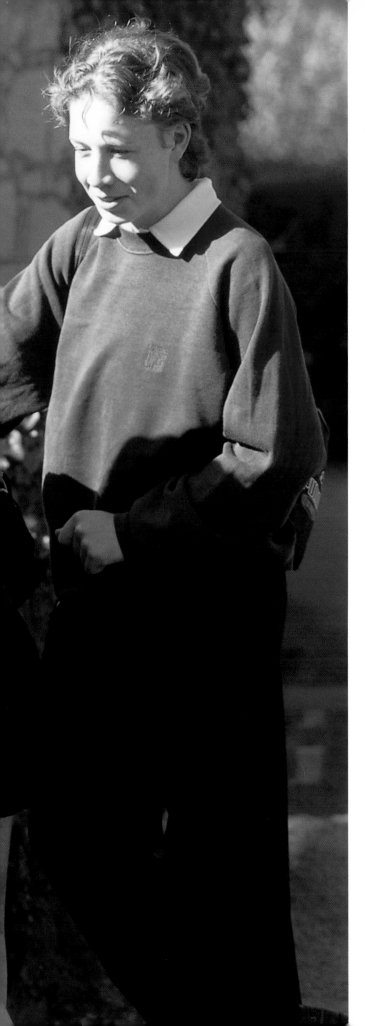

world and an idealism untainted by realism, which adults may envy – although they would not tell this to their teenagers!

Socially adolescents inhabit a nether world where they appear to enjoy adult privileges but where they are still dependent through school, family discipline and the facts of economic life. These considerations are fundamentally incompatible so the surprise is not that adolescence is usually stormy, but rather that families survive it at all.

Adolescence – the good Adolescence is when offspring are finding their own voice, while not totally disregarding everyone else's, and exploring their capabilities without trampling on everyone else's rights. It is a period for testing the limits while learning to acknowledge the restrictions demanded by society. It is a time of rebellion physically and mentally, usually petty, although interspersed with the occasional 'cold war'.

Adolescence – the bad There is generally an exaggeration of normal traits, for example extra aggression or extra negligence for others' rights leading to confrontation. Some adolescents do go right off the rails, however, and are subject to depression, eating disorders and even suicide. Deep unhappiness should be taken seriously.

Adolescence – the ugly The adolescent has many well-known problems such as **acne** and awkwardness through rapid growth or a voice that does odd things. This does not help the self-image and, although apparently trivial, such problems may haunt an adolescent well into the early adult years.

Must it be so?

In some societies the transition from childhood through adolescence is less stormy. It is marked by initiation ceremonies and brings the adolescent boy or girl immediately into a significant role in the society. This is not a realistic option in most developed societies, where childhood is greatly extended through tertiary education and training so that it may only be in the mid-20s that the young adult achieves real socio-economic independence. The developed world appears to make heavy weather of adolescence.

FAILURE TO THRIVE

A concept unique to paediatric practice, this means failure to gain weight and is a sensitive indicator of serious illness or of emotional deprivation in children up to about two years of age.

CAUSES

Children differ fundamentally from adults in that they are growing constantly. Growth continues throughout childhood, although there will be times when it is imperceptible. During the first two years of life growth should be especially rapid and sustained. Any serious illness interrupts growth by diverting the energy that would go towards growth into fighting the disease. Failure to thrive is therefore a challenge rather than a diagnosis and all aspects of the child's physical and emotional health need to be examined to discover the causes.

What counts as failure to thrive? Even a trivial illness interrupts growth briefly; babies' weight in particular may swing alarmingly. These brief perturbations are normal and should only raise concern if growth is interrupted for several weeks.

Inadequate nutrition

The rapid metabolic rate of children demands adequate energy input, lack of which is one of the most common reasons for problems. It is often a matter of mismanagement rather than deliberate misfeeding, for example a teat that is too narrow to let milk out or continuing to feed a baby solely on milk beyond the time when it is ready for solid food. Many babies do go through periods of faddy eating, if not food refusal, and their weight may fluctuate wildly at such times.

Emotional mishandling

It may come as a surprise to learn that children fail to grow if they are unhappy but this is certainly the case. The emotional neglect has to be severe – not being allowed to watch a certain programme on TV does not count. Emotionally deprived children are likely to be delayed in overall social and emotional development as well as in growth.

Intestinal disease

Constant vomiting will lead to weight loss for obvious reasons. This happens in pyloric stenosis, where an abnormal band narrows the duodenum, preventing food from leaving the stomach. That said, many babies vomit both small and large amounts of food without having any underlying physical abnormality. Other gastrointestinal possibilities are malabsorption through **coeliac disease** and chronic parasite infection, for example with hookworm.

Heart and lung disease

Serious **congenital heart problems** such as cyanotic heart disease cause failure to thrive through chronic oxygen starvation. Similarly, chronic lung diseases – severe **asthma**, cystic fibrosis or chronic lung infection – make the child constantly breathless, starve the body of oxygen and take energy. Ordinary coughs and **colds** are negligible but severe **pneumonia** or **bronchiolitis** might reduce growth for a few weeks.

Metabolic conditions

This covers a range of disorders in how the body handles energy. They range from the relatively uncommon such as **kidney failure** or an underactive thyroid gland (see THYROID PROBLEMS) to the downright rare, for example glycogen storage disease or liver disease.

Miscellaneous

Children born with **cerebral palsy** tend not to grow as well as normal children. The same applies to children born with genetic disorders of any type, **Down's syndrome** being the most common. Failure to thrive is unlikely to be the first indication of a problem, as these children will either be diagnosed at birth or will exhibit generalized delay in development of which failure to thrive is just one aspect, for example delay in language, manipulation or walking.

Certain premature babies remain small and fail to thrive throughout childhood, presumably because of permanent disruption of their potential for growth.

SYMPTOMS

While no one individual child grows at an average rate, by following large numbers of children average growth rates have been established to produce growth charts. These are not single figures but show a range – for example by six months it is normal for a child to weigh double its birth weight, but this could be anywhere from 6 to 9.5 kg/13 to 21 lb. These growth charts are specific for particular populations – the expected growth of affluent European children is quite different from that of children in the developing world. Moreover, the average changes over time, as children have tended to grow bigger and heavier, and also rates are different for boys and girls. Height and weight are the fundamental measures of growth. Babies also have head circumference measured.

It is important to realize that a single abnormal reading means very little – unless it is grossly extreme. This is because the weighing process may be affected by such things as wear-

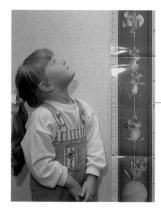
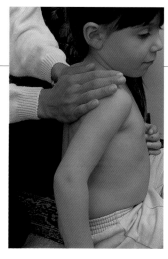

Above: Height gain is a basic measure of health in children.
Right: Massage helps children to feel loved.

ing different clothes, or even whether the child has a full bladder or not. What is important is to take several measurements over several weeks or months in order to plot growth curves.

Patterns of abnormal growth

Two types emerge: there is the child who was growing normally but whose growth then declines. This suggests a new and serious problem. Then there is the child whose height or weight start abnormally low and remain low, the implication being a congenital problem interfering with growth from the start. Most children have rather zigzag curves, with minor variations reflecting minor childhood illnesses.

Tests

A careful full examination is essential, when the doctor will look especially for signs of heart or lung disease, malnutrition (for example loose skin folds and thin buttocks), bruising or parental attitudes suggestive of emotional and physical abuse.

Blood tests establish the state of health of the kidneys and liver and detect whether there is **anaemia**, vitamin deficiency or the abnormal results that accompany malabsorption and **diabetes**. Additional basic tests might include a chest X-ray and testing a urine sample for infection. Many additional tests are available, depending on the suspected problems, for example a biopsy of the bowel might be used to establish **coeliac disease** or stool samples examined for malabsorption, chronic parasitic infection and metabolic diseases.

Measuring emotion

The paediatrician needs an insight into the usual emotional climate surrounding the child and so takes note of how you handle her. Does the child appear at ease with you or does she appear wary or apprehensive? Some parents truly interact with their child and respond to them; others pick them up and put them down like playthings. Is the child appropriately

dressed and reasonably groomed? This said, however, dirtiness or old clothes no more indicate neglect than a pristine child in designer gear signifies parental concern.

TREATMENT

Reasons for serious failure to thrive are generally rapidly established and treated. This also applies to the child growing normally but who then loses weight rapidly. More difficulties surround the child who is not severely unwell but whose growth is unsatisfactory without being disastrously bad. Many paediatricians, having established the child has a reasonable diet, will keep a watching brief, weighing and measuring the child monthly while waiting for a pattern to establish itself.

QUESTIONS

Can growth recover?
Most children will catch up after illness at up to three times the normal rate. The exceptions are chronic illness, for example kidney disease, or children suffering prolonged severe malnutrition, who may always remain smaller and lighter.

What about height?
Many of the influences on weight affect height, too. Investigation and treatment are largely the same except that the influence of heredity is greater and problems may not become apparent until the child is much older.

Complementary Treatment
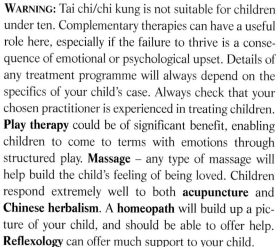
WARNING: Tai chi/chi kung is not suitable for children under ten. Complementary therapies can have a useful role here, especially if the failure to thrive is a consequence of emotional or psychological upset. Details of any treatment programme will always depend on the specifics of your child's case. Always check that your chosen practitioner is experienced in treating children. **Play therapy** could be of significant benefit, enabling children to come to terms with emotions through structured play. **Massage** – any type of massage will help build the child's feeling of being loved. Children respond extremely well to both **acupuncture** and **Chinese herbalism**. A **homeopath** will build up a picture of your child, and should be able to offer help. **Reflexology** can offer much support to your child.

SKIN PROBLEMS

◆

Problems in young skin – mostly eczema or minor infections.

CAUSES

The newborn baby's skin is virgin territory for germs and irritants, which invade from the instant of birth. This is not through lack of cleanliness but is a natural and inevitable process. **Eczema** often causes rashes from an early age. Birth marks are extremely common (see box right). Other causes, for example **psoriasis** and **acne**, are unusual in children.

SYMPTOMS

Most babies get a few spots after birth, usually around the face, from germs picked up from family members. Some babies have milia, tiny shiny dots around the nose due to blocked sweat glands, that go spontaneously. Few babies escape **nappy rash**, just as few older children escape **warts**. Older children have **boils**, **impetigo** and eczema, too.

TREATMENT

The principle of treating skin problems is to use the mildest skin preparation that controls the problem. Many, especially eczema, respond to simple moisturizing creams and emollient bath oils, keeping steroid creams for more resistant cases. Antibiotic creams are sufficient for minor infections and only occasionally are antibiotics by mouth required for such problems. (See WARTS for treatment details.)

QUESTION

What are birth marks?
Birth marks are coloured patches and lumps that are persistent, unlike the temporary bruises caused by the trauma of birth. Strawberry naevi are deep red raised lesions, which enlarge for a year or two before nearly always disappearing by the time the child is about five years old. Although many birth marks require no treatment, a few do. See your doctor for an opinion.

Complementary Treatment
Ayurveda is a therapy that is very successful with skin problems; treatment is through *panchakarma* detoxification. **Chakra balancing** promotes healing of the skin and pain control. *Other therapies to try: homeopathy; shiatsu-do; acupuncture; aromatherapy.*

HEAD LICE

◆

Small insects that thrive in hair, whether it be clean or dirty.

CAUSES

Head lice are 3–4 mm/⅛–³⁄₁₆ in long and feed on the rich blood supply of the scalp. A typical infection involves only five to ten lice, each laying up to three hundred eggs during its four-to six-week lifetime. The eggs are cemented to the hair shaft; the lice may similarly cement themselves or go roaming. Infection spreads through close contact and the sharing of combs or brushes. There is evidence that lice prefer longer hair and warmer weather.

SYMPTOMS

Itching is the main symptom, caused when the lice feed. You may notice the white eggs, called nits, adhering to hair shafts or spot a louse on an excursion. It is uncommon for any additional infection to enter the scalp unless the skin is greatly damaged by scratching. Itchy scalps are common so do not automatically assume head lice without definite evidence.

TREATMENT

Many regions have policies on which antilouse application to use in order to avoid spread of resistance. Standard medication includes malathion, carbaryl and permethrin in a wide range of brands and applications. A single treatment is highly effective; it is essential to treat all members of the family and to follow the instructions for use precisely. Some treatments affect asthmatics so do check the label.

Complementary Treatment

Aromatherapy – add one drop of one of the following oils to your child's shampoo: lemon, rosemary or tea tree. Use the shampoo in conjunction with a nit comb.

HAND, FOOT AND MOUTH DISEASE

A viral infection, typified by a rash covering the above areas.

CAUSE

This is not to be confused with foot and mouth disease, which is a different illness and caught from pigs, sheep or cattle. The virus responsible for hand, foot and mouth disease is called Coxsackie, although occasionally other common viruses may cause a similar picture. The illness is mainly confined to children and occurs in outbreaks in all parts of the world.

SYMPTOMS

The illness begins with mild **fever** and a sore throat. The typical rash appears after a couple of days as tiny red painful spots on the tongue, gums and lining of the mouth. A day or two later a rash consisting of tiny fluid-filled spots called vesicles appears on the palms of the hands and the soles of the feet.

The rash is uncomfortable and the child may go off her food because of discomfort and even be reluctant to walk because of the pain from the rash on the feet. The illness lasts seven to ten days and has no long-term health consequences.

TREATMENT

All that is needed is to give painkillers as appropriate, for example paracetamol syrup, and drinks. Avoid acidic fruit juices as these will make the mouth sting.

Complementary Treatment

Ayurveda treatments are available, according to the details of the case. Ayurveda believes this disease could be linked to faulty digestion, and offers appropriate dietary advice.

FEBRILE FITS

Convulsions triggered by high temperatures, affecting about one child in twenty-five.

CAUSES

Anyone whose brain is heated rapidly and high enough will eventually have a fit. The brains of babies and children are more sensitive to modest rises in temperature, whatever the reason for the **fever**, hence the febrile fits. The chances of **epilepsy** in later life are higher than in unaffected children, but only very slightly.

SYMPTOMS

The hot child suddenly becomes unresponsive and begins to twitch. The child's eyes roll up and the limbs jerk rhythmically, which may last for several minutes. After the fit the child is drowsy but otherwise normal.

TREATMENT

Try to prevent a fit in a very hot child by reducing his temperature by removing clothing and with paracetamol, fans and tepid bathing. During a fit place the child on his front but otherwise leave the child until the fit ends. Call for help if it is a first fit or if the fit is prolonged and the child remains unresponsive. Hospital admission is advisable for a first fit and also in babies to exclude conditions such as meningitis. Thirty to forty per cent of children have recurrent fits; their parents can give diazepam rectally to stop them.

WARNING SIGNS

Children with these features need urgent medical attention:

- ♦ *A first fit (to confirm the diagnosis)*
- ♦ *A fit occurring in a child less than six months and more than five years (febrile fits are unlikely)*
- ♦ *A non-feverish child (other causes are likely)*
- ♦ *A fit lasting more than ten minutes (needs sedation)*
- ♦ *A fit following a head injury (possible brain damage)*
- ♦ *Associated with headaches and aversion to light (meningitis)*

Complementary Treatment

If your child has a persistently high temperature, or a fit, he should quickly receive conventional medical attention. Many complementary therapies give advice on lowering transiently high temperature. See FEVER.

JAUNDICE

A yellow tinge to the skin caused by liver problems.

CAUSES

'Normal' jaundice is when, for one to two weeks after birth, the immature liver fails to handle fully the yellow pigment bilirubin from the normal breakdown of red blood cells, which therefore leaks into the skin. High levels of bilirubin may cause permanent brain damage.

Also, before the mother's milk flows plentifully, a newborn baby may get slightly dehydrated, which is believed to account for jaundice. The child remains lively and well.

'Abnormal' jaundice is jaundice occurring within 24 hours of birth, probably from destruction of blood cells through rhesus incompatibility, although this is now rare. This is when a rhesus negative mother carrying a rhesus positive baby produces antibodies that destroy the baby's red blood cells. The mother's liver handles the resulting bilirubin during pregnancy. After birth, however, the baby's liver cannot cope, resulting in jaundice.

Jaundice persisting beyond two weeks may reflect abnormal drainage in the liver, called biliary atresia, or an underactive thyroid gland (see THYROID PROBLEMS). Other causes include severe general infection or hepatitis (see LIVER PROBLEMS).

SYMPTOMS

The jaundiced baby looks tanned and the whites of the eyes turn yellow. The blood level of bilirubin indicates whether treatment is necessary or not. In 'normal' jaundice, the baby remains well; in 'abnormal' jaundice the baby is often feverish, breathing rapidly, and has other signs of illness as well.

TREATMENT

The treatment in the case of 'normal' jaundice that does not improve spontaneously after a few days is to put the baby under ultraviolet light; this breaks down bilirubin in the skin. Give extra drinks to a slightly dehydrated breast-fed baby who is otherwise well, unless blood levels of bilirubin rise high, which is relatively uncommon.

In severe or 'abnormal' cases the baby needs blood transfusion plus treatment of the basic cause.

 Complementary Treatment
Let your child sleep by an uncurtained window, to receive maximum light. A **Chinese herbalist** will be able to offer help. During the recovery period children may respond to **shiatsu-do**.

PERTHES' DISEASE

Abnormal growth of the hip joint leading to pain and a limp.

CAUSES

This is a problem caused when growing bone outstrips its blood supply, so that some of the bone dies. Perthes' disease involves the head of the thigh bone (the femur) and affects mainly boys between the ages of five and ten. Several similar disorders affect bones elsewhere in the body and are generally the scientific explanation for 'growing pains'.

SYMPTOMS

With Perthes' disease pain in the affected hip begins mildly but becomes constant. The child starts to limp. X-rays will show the typically abnormal appearance of the hip joint in Perthes' disease. (Although hip pain is common in childhood do not ignore it, especially if accompanied by a limp.)

TREATMENT

Usually the blood supply will re-establish itself enough for bone to regrow, although it may take two years before the final result is clear. Should this fail to happen, the affected child is likely to have a permanent limp and a higher risk of developing **osteoarthritis** of the hip later as an adult.

During the painful period, the child has to rest in bed but generally no other treatment is necessary. If the deformity is permanent, then surgery is performed in order to set the head of the femur in a better position in the hip joint.

 Complementary Treatment
Do not abandon conventional approaches here. **Rolfing** can improve the muscular balance around the hip joint. **Chakra balancing** can be beneficial by helping relax an irritable child and reducing pain. *Other therapies to try: Alexander Technique.*

SLEEP PROBLEMS

Children refusing to sleep or waking at night cause great stress for parents and solutions are rarely easy or perfect.

CAUSES

The newborn baby sleeps most of the time, reducing to two or three sleeps by the age of one year. By three years old many children have two sleeps, having dropped an afternoon nap. Children tend to wake naturally between 5.00 and 6.00 am. It is also normal for children above 18 months to lie awake at night talking or amusing themselves.

Refusal to go to bed or frequent waking interferes with parents' peace after a day of mayhem and with their full night's sleep before another demanding day. Common contributing factors are: too much daytime sleep, which reduces the need for sleep at night; a poor routine for getting the child off to bed; fears on the child's part about being alone or separated from her parent, feelings which are at a maximum between 18 months and 2½ years; and disturbances, which might include traffic noise, loud television and parental arguments.

SYMPTOMS

The child cries at night or sleeps only briefly before waking and crying or attempting to get up. This behaviour might be constant or might have appeared very recently. Older children may wake early and talk or cry. The child may be sleepy in the day but still doggedly refuses to go to bed at night.

TREATMENT

First review the child's physical comfort. Check whether the child is hungry or thirsty, too hot, too cold, damp, dirty or irritated by noise. These are more relevant in the young baby, less so in children above about one year old.

Sleep patterns and bedtime routines
Try to keep the child awake during the day or keep any nap brief. Help the child to know bedtime is coming and, by implication, what is expected of him. Instill a routine such as a bath, a cuddle, reading a story and settling into bed with favourite toys.

Controlled crying
Babies normally cry for a few minutes on settling. You must resist the temptation to go back to give another cuddle. Older children, being cunning, will extend their crying until a parent

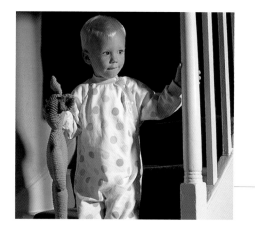

Left: Dealing with children's sleep problems calls for firm though caring handling.

reappears. Resist this also for five to ten minutes, then briefly enter to reassure the child and leave. Let the child cry for ten minutes, re-enter, reassure and leave, repeating as long as you can and letting the child cry for longer each time.

There is no reason to believe that crying can do psychological harm. Most experts agree that it is better to attempt to discipline children within a loving and consistent environment, rather than give inconsistent messages in an atmosphere of resentment from parental sleep deprivation.

Crying during the night should be handled in a similar way, checking first on physical discomfort, then leaving the child to cry. How long can this go on? As long as your nerves hold. Most experts agree that the worst will usually be over after four days, although individual children may stay difficult and go on much longer and louder. Be reassured that sleep problems rarely extend past about five years of age.

Medication
There comes a point when medication is reasonable to give the parents a break, for example when on holiday. Medication available includes chloral and trimeprazine. It should be seen as a last resort used for only a day or two at a time.

Complementary Treatment
Bach flower remedies depend on the cause of the problem, for example agrimony for children who keep their worries to themselves. If the problem follows change such as a new school, try walnut. Olive can help overcome tiredness. **Aromatherapy** – try one drop of Roman chamomile or lavender in the pre-bedtime bath or on the pillow. **Play therapy** could be of benefit if the problem has an emotional cause. *Other therapies to try: most have something to offer.*

BEHAVIOURAL PROBLEMS

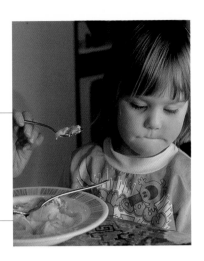

Right: Children will eat if they are hungry. Remember this before turning meals into battlegrounds.

The child is capable of better behaviour but seems driven to act otherwise. The diagnosis and management is complex.

FEEDING PROBLEMS

Causes: Many children aged between about nine and fifteen months are faddy eaters and refuse foods. Some children simply dislike the taste and texture of solid food.

Symptoms: These include outright refusal, sticking to one food, throwing food and spitting it out.

Treatment: With a thriving child there is little harm. Offer varying textures and flavours, praising 'good eating'. Remove food left after 20 minutes but do not allow sweets or snacks.

TEMPER TANTRUMS

Causes: The 'terrible twos' may last until four years of age! Tantrums are normal, but likelier in children from disturbed families, neglected children and those with chronic illness, especially **cerebral palsy** and speech disorders.

Symptoms: These are shouting, biting, scratching and breaking things in response to frustration or failure to get their way. Tantrums much beyond four years are abnormal.

Treatment: Ignore the tantrum – if possible by leaving the room. If this is impossible and, for example, you are in the middle of a supermarket, attempt to distract the child or hold the child tightly. Do not give in with a reward.

HYPERACTIVITY

Causes: This is a controversial subject in both diagnosis and cause; dietary factors are unproven. Theories include children at the extremes of normality, inappropriate learnt behaviour or minimal brain damage.

Symptoms: The child is impulsive and inattentive, rapidly switching activity and easily distracted, fidgeting and running around. Specialists vary greatly in how readily they make the diagnosis. Hyperactivity rarely lasts beyond adolescence.

Treatment: A medical assessment should detect any neurological damage, **epilepsy** or hearing disorders. Inconsistent parental handling may be affecting the child's behaviour. Behavioural techniques are used which basically attempt to ignore unacceptable behaviour and reward 'good' behaviour.

Try avoiding strong colouring in food, especially tartrazine, but there is no good evidence for extreme diets. Medication is used infrequently in the United Kingdom, although widely used elsewhere, for example Ritalin (methylphenidate).

BED-WETTING (ENURESIS)

Causes: There are emotional and strong hereditary influences.

Symptoms: The child wets the bed when deeply asleep. Children previously dry who start to wet may have a urinary infection (see URINARY PROBLEMS). Children who never achieve continence should have a urological assessment.

Treatment: Any parental or family tension needs resolving. Restricting drinks before bed and lifting the child in the night are practical measures. A pad in the bed that triggers a buzzer when wet works for children above the age of about six. The drug desmopressin reduces urinary output during the night.

INCONTINENCE OF FAECES

Causes: Apparent incontinence of faeces is often actually **constipation** with leakage of faeces. Sufferers from cerebral palsy are liable to incontinence. Deliberate incontinence suggests severe psychological disturbance.

Symptoms: Leakage of faeces together with embarrassment typify constipation with overflow or other physical problems. Secreting faeces around the house or deliberate soiling are different and typify psychological causes.

Treatment: Constipation with leakage requires taking laxatives until regular motions are achieved. Other causes need specialist assessment and often psychological help.

See also CHILD DEVELOPMENT, PAGE 300.

Complementary Treatment

Bach flower remedies depend on the cause of the problem, for example cherry plum for loss of control. **Homeopathy** can succeed in overcoming school phobia. **Hypnotherapy** is very helpful since in the state of hypnosis the child will be able to express the underlying issue – the child must be over three. **Play therapy** is useful if the problem has an emotional cause. *Other therapies to try: most have something to offer.*

COT DEATH

Sudden death of apparently healthy baby for no obvious reason.

CAUSES

The term cot death covers all unexpected infant deaths. Of those, a number will eventually be explained on post-mortem, when a few babies are shown to have a previously unsuspected abnormality of their heart or lungs and some may have a rare metabolic disorder. Those that remain unexplained are technically called sudden infant death syndrome (SIDS).

It is likely that SIDS is caused by a number of factors, rather than by one single cause. Some current theories are that babies are being kept too hot, that viral infection suddenly halts breathing or that allergic reactions are produced by environmental stimuli.

Following an unexpected infant death the police must be involved and invariably the possibility of deliberate harm must be considered, although this accounts for less than one in twenty-five cases in the United Kingdom.

Children at greatest risk of SIDS are between one and six months old; it is a little more frequent during winter, in boys, in babies of low birth weight, in babies living in poor socio-economic circumstances and in babies whose parents smoke.

SIDS is the most common reason for infant deaths after one month of age. In the United Kingdom about ten children a week die from it. This apparently high incidence is because other causes of death in infancy are now so rare, for example infections, accidents and **leukaemia**. Cot death is extremely uncommon after the age of one year.

SYMPTOMS

In most cases the child appeared well, fed normally and slept normally. Sometimes they had a minor infection. Children have been known to die just after being settled down, just after feeding or even in their parents' arms on a routine day.

TREATMENT

Every effort should be made to revive the baby, looking especially for food stuck in the throat. If efforts fail, the police and coroner must be informed and a post-mortem carried out.

Twins and other siblings

It is a sad but important fact that the surviving twin is at great risk of sudden death and a period of observation is recommended after one twin has died through cot death.

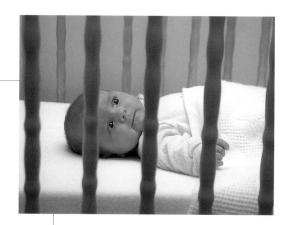

Above: Babies should be placed to sleep on their backs on a firm mattress, with their feet to the foot of the cot. Do not use pillows, duvets and cot bumpers.

Other siblings have a very slightly increased risk, too small to require any action, although it is understandable to be extra vigilant about minor illnesses until they reach one year of age.

Counselling

After such a tragedy parents have to cope with guilt, anger, fears about the health of remaining children and apprehension about another pregnancy. Such unresolved emotions can and do lead to the disintegration of the family. Parents experiencing a cot death should seek specialized counselling and consider joining one of the excellent support organizations.

Prevention

The 'Back to Sleep' campaign has been very effective in reducing the incidence of cot death worldwide. The simple message is to let babies sleep only on their backs. Other steps are not to smoke near a baby and not let the baby get over-hot (keep bedrooms within a degree or two of 18°C/65°F). Also, ensure the baby's head cannot be covered by bedding by making up their bed with their feet at the foot of the cot, which prevents them from wriggling down under the covers. Campaigns based on these messages have contributed to reducing by two-thirds the number of cot deaths since 1988 – decreasing in the United Kingdom from 1500 a year to 500 and still falling.

Complementary Treatment

No complementary therapy can prevent a cot death. Ensure you follow the preventive advice above. During mourning deep relaxation techniques can help parents and other children. See BEREAVEMENT; also STRESS and ANXIETY. If you decide to try for another baby, **hypnotherapy** could help reduce anxiety about the progress of the pregnancy, and the health of your next baby.

DIAGNOSTIC TECHNIQUES

D IAGNOSIS IS AT THE CORE of medicine, for without it it would be impossible to plan treatment. Diagnostic tools include everything from simply looking at your tongue to more complex studies using high-tech equipment to monitor the blood flow around your heart. This section covers many diagnostic procedures you may come across or undergo yourself, what they are used for, how they are performed, any risks they may have and likely future developments.

Low-technology medicine

Glancing through a textbook of medicine, you may be struck by the many entries named after doctors from the 18th and 19th centuries. These include Paget's disease, Heberden's nodes, Broca's area and Parkinson's disease (see page 83) to name just a few. Although these great doctors lacked modern diagnostic tools, they used their acute powers of observation to name the parts of the body and to recognize patterns of symptoms signifying specific diseases. They had nothing to go by but touch, smell and listening to the patient.

High-technology medicine

Modern medicine tries not to overlook the importance of observation in arriving at a diagnosis. There is still a great emphasis in medical training on teaching the skills of both history taking and physical examination (see pages 326 and 327), but this is increasingly being overshadowed by sophisticated investigations.

Investigations

At the simplest, an investigation might mean testing a sample of urine for sugar (glucose), and at the most complex having an MRI scan (see page 319). With easy access to investigations, doctors find it tempting to test for many things almost routinely, rather than thinking of probable diagnoses and doing the relevant tests. Since many tests are automated, it is relatively easy to do this.

However, there is a balance between the risks or discomfort of an investigation and the benefits that are to be accrued. The area most often involving risk is X-rays (see page 316). Although the risk is small, an X-ray is still a dose of radiation, which is why doctors may try to avoid them in circumstances where the X-ray is unlikely to make any difference to treatment, for example in uncomplicated lower back pain (see page 246).

Other tests carry disturbing implications. Antenatal tests for foetal abnormality fall into this category, posing a possible decision about terminating the pregnancy. This is why counselling is used before certain tests to be sure that you understand the decisions you will be faced with if a test proves abnormal. Genetic testing (see page 325) will certainly become one of the most controversial areas of medicine in the next few years.

Interpreting results

The more tests are done, the more likely an abnormality will appear, requiring a decision about further investigations. In arriving at this decision the doctor takes account of your general health, other symptoms and the pattern of abnormality as shown in the test. Unfortunately, this uncertainty is bound to generate anxiety on the patient's part, but without investigations there would be even more anxiety about illness.

Normal and abnormal Few investigations are absolutely 'normal' or abnormal; more often there is a large grey area of results ranging from possibly abnormal to probably 'normal'. Once again the interpretation has to take account of the history, the examination and the results of other tests. For this reason doctors will often repeat tests, especially the simple blood and urine tests, until the results become more definite. Interpreting the results from all of the diagnostic tests takes up a great deal of a doctor's thinking in order to come to an accurate diagnosis.

Right: Observation, touch and analysis are the fundmentals of diagnosis, helped by increasingly powerful investigative tools. The Physician's Visit by Jan Havicksz Steen (1625/26–79).

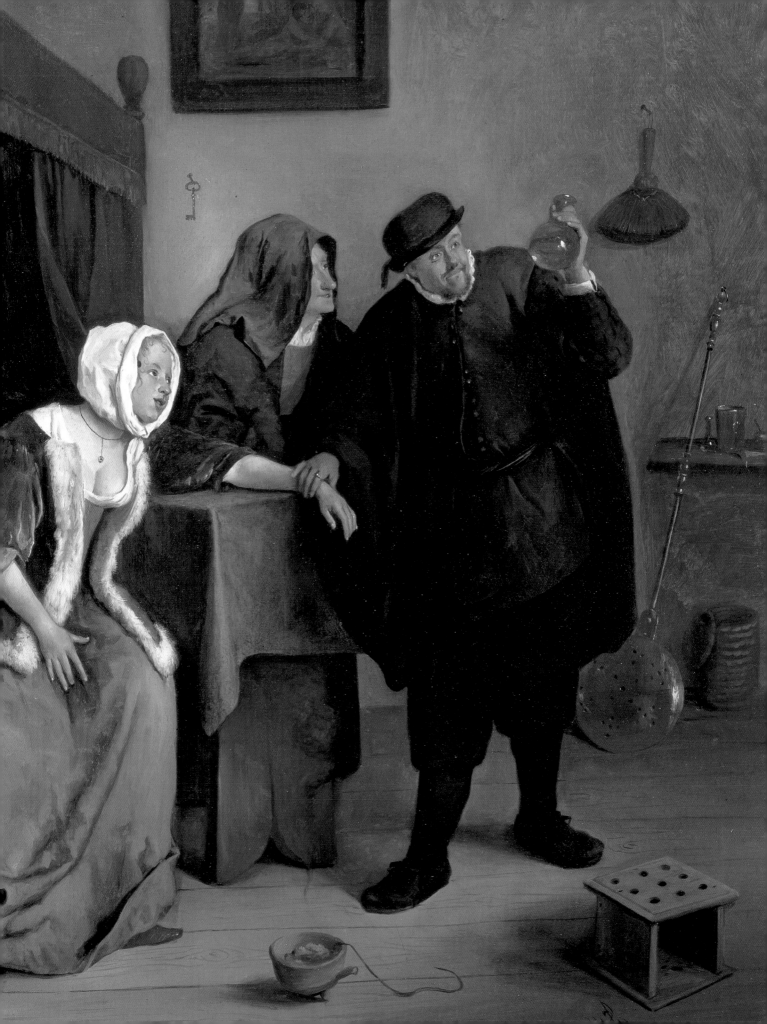

X-RAYS

Discovered by chance by Roentgen in 1895, X-rays are waves of electromagnetic radiation that are in the same family as light and radio waves. Their very short wavelength (much shorter than visible light) lets them penetrate solid material. Variations of density within the material show up as X-ray shadows similar to light shadows. X-rays are captured on photographic plates as negative films. They are taken by radiographers, skilled in positioning patients to get the most informative views and calculating the exposure needed. The interpretation of X-rays is done by radiologists, doctors who also perform a wide range of investigations using X-rays.

What X-rays can detect

X-rays are good for detecting abnormalities in bones, especially fractures (see page 249), and problems in the lungs. They are not good at detecting abnormalities in soft tissues, for example in the brain or the intestines. This is because X-rays penetrate these parts too well to show much detail and because everything they pass through casts shadows on the photographic plate, thereby blurring the image. X-rays can detect gross changes, such as whether the heart is enlarged or there is paralysis of the bowels. They may not give the precise diagnosis but they are enough to show that something is seriously wrong.

How an X-ray is performed

The X-ray equipment is brought close to the part of you being studied while you stay very still for the fraction of a second required. Some studies call for a series of photos, such as X-rays of the kidney, or a continuous film as in coronary artery angiography (see below). It takes a minute or so to develop the film.

X-ray films are nearly always photographic negatives where dense material, such as bone, shows white, and less dense material such as muscle shows grey.

Other forms of X-ray

By using materials that appear white on an X-ray, radiologists can improve how well soft tissues show up. For example, dyes can be injected into the blood stream to show blood flow within internal organs. When used in the kidneys, this is called an intravenous pyelogram; in the heart it is called coronary angiography (see below).

Barium studies Barium liquid is another material that is widely used, since barium does not dissolve in water and passes harmlessly out of the body. A barium swallow or barium meal outlines the gullet, stomach and intestine, and is used to detect ulcers, cancers and narrowing of these organs. A barium enema involves pumping barium into the rectum, then manoeuvring the patient around to coat barium on the walls of the bowels. A barium enema is used to investigate abdominal pains and bleeding from the back passage and for detecting cancers, diverticular disease and inflammatory bowel disease (see page 182).

Coronary artery angiography A very thin tube called a catheter is fed to the heart via a large artery or vein, usually in the groin. Under X-ray control the tip is brought close to the heart's own arteries, the coronary arteries. A harmless dye is pumped into the blood stream, while taking a rapid series of X-rays showing how blood flows around the heart. This will detect blockages and determine whether a person should have coronary artery bypass surgery (see page 43). A similar

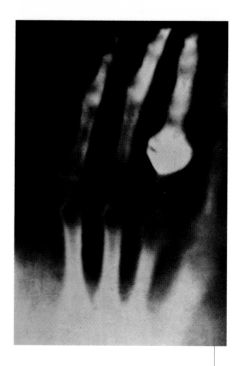

Above: An X-ray by Roentgen of his wife's hand. X-rays are among the most important diagnostic aids ever invented.

technique can demonstrate blood flow through the arteries of the abdomen and legs, if arterial disease is suspected.

Safety

X-rays can burn in overdose, which is why the early specialists, not knowing this, frequently developed cancers of their hands. Modern X-rays are very low dosage, thanks to finely focused equipment and sensitive photographic plates. For example, a chest X-ray involves a dose of radiation similar to that received naturally during a transatlantic plane journey. Legal guidelines limit the annual exposure to medical X-rays to an amount equivalent to six months' natural exposure to radiation. They should be avoided altogether during pregnancy unless essential to protect life.

ULTRASOUND

This is a technique in which high-frequency sound waves penetrate the body, casting sound shadows, which are then analysed. It is called ultrasound because the sound frequency is much too high to hear (the frequencies are well above 30,000 cycles per second). Each time the sound beam passes through a different material (blood, water, flesh and bone) the signal changes slightly. These tiny variations in the transmission and reflection of sound are detected by sensitive microphones. The pattern is further analysed by computer to generate a picture of the internal organs as grey shadows on a TV screen. The display is a continuous one, unlike most X-rays (see opposite), and reveals a world of internal movement and structure.

How ultrasound is performed

A watery gel is rubbed on to the skin in order to improve the transmission of the ultrasound beam. The source of ultrasound, shaped like a flat probe, is held against the skin. The operator focuses the ultrasound beam and moves it around. The resulting echoes are electronically analysed as pure sound, such as the baby's heartbeat, or into pictures showing structures, which is technically called echosonography.

What ultrasound can detect

Ultrasound is good at showing hollow internal organs. This has made it the method of choice for monitoring the growth of the unborn baby by taking measurements of the diameter of the skull or the baby's length (see page 132). Other uses for ultrasound are in looking at the kidneys or bladder and abdominal organs

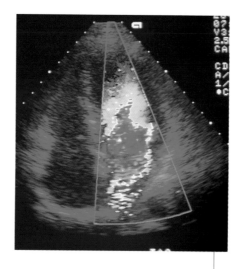

Above: An ultrasound view across the heart. The colours reflect the speed of the blood flow through one of the valves – red for slowest, blue for fastest.

such as the liver and gall bladder. Ultrasound is also helpful for detecting disease in the prostate gland (see page 120) or the breasts.

Gynaecological uses of ultrasound include detecting disease of the ovaries, such as cysts, and diseases of the womb, such as fibroids (see page 160). Ultrasound has made the diagnosis of an ectopic pregnancy (see page 136), where the fertilized egg settles in the Fallopian tube rather than the womb, much more reliable. It is also used in investigating bleeding in early pregnancy to see whether the foetus is still alive or has miscarried (see page 146).

Ultrasound images look rather like a television picture with a lot of interference. It takes a trained eye to see the detail, but with modern equipment the degree of it is remarkable.

Echocardiography

Ultrasound examination of the heart has become one of the most important applications of the technique and is revolutionizing the understanding of heart function and heart disease. The ultrasound beam is shone between the ribs (a constant nuisance in imaging the heart) to focus on

each chamber of the heart (the atria and the ventricles) and the heart valves (the aortic, mitral, tricuspid and pulmonary valves). Measurements can be electronically analysed to give the work capacity of the heart, to show how efficiently the valves are performing, whether any of them are leaking and whether the heart muscle is healthy. Ultrasound is now the best way of confirming whether someone has heart failure, valve disease and aneurysms (abnormally swollen blood vessels with fragile walls). What ultrasound cannot yet do is to show actual blood flow around the heart. For this you will still require X-ray coronary artery angiography (see opposite).

Other forms of ultrasound

Some other applications of much higher energy ultrasound make use of its heating effect, as applied in sports physiotherapy. Similarly, lithotripsy (see page 337) is a means of shattering kidney stones by employing sound waves at a much higher and more focused level of energy.

Safety

Ultrasound has been exhaustively tested for safety. There is no evidence that the doses used in ultrasound imaging do any harm at all, even to the unborn baby, which is why it is used so extensively.

CT SCANNING

Computed tomography (CT) is a means of using X-rays (see page 316) plus powerful computing to generate images of the interior of the body. When X-rays pass through the body, the shadows from everything they pass through lie superimposed on top of each other. The result is a flat image of the actual three-dimensional structure of the body, just like a television picture is a flat image of reality. However, if an X-ray is taken from a slightly different position (called an X-ray cut) all these shadows shift slightly and they shift once again when another 'cut' is taken. The breakthrough of CT scanning was in harnessing computers to analyse the tiny variations in each of the X-ray cuts in order to reconstruct an image of the interior of the body.

The technique was not entirely new. It was called tomography, but the results were a blurred image of one part of the body and not much else. In CT scanning the computers allow a reconstruction of any part of the body caught in the X-ray beam. Thus for the first time it was possible to see details of soft structures of the body, especially the brain and the abdomen, without painful or hazardous injections or operations. Indeed, the technique revolutionized the investigation of brain disorders, which until the 1970s had often been extremely unpleasant and not very revealing. CT scanning was an amazing advance in X-ray technology, for which the inventor Godfrey Hounsfield was awarded a Nobel Prize.

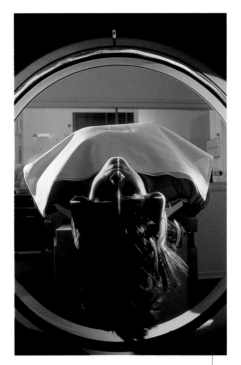

Above: A patient lying still within a CT scanner. Newer CT machines are not so bulky and intimidating and take less time to perform the scan.

How a CT scan is performed

All the work is carried out by the X-ray apparatus; the person being scanned just lies there as still as possible. Every few seconds the equipment takes a fresh X-ray cut through the body, moving on a few millimetres before taking the next cut. The process takes between ten and twenty minutes depending on how much is being scanned. The images can be improved by giving an injection of a contrast material which shows up better on X-ray; this is particularly useful for images of the brain. The very latest scanners take their photos much faster and are able to cope with moving organs such as the heart.

Safety

The total X-ray dose is larger than an ordinary X-ray but is still very small and no important side effects have emerged. Some people get claustrophobic in the apparatus or they cannot lie still enough for good images so it is not useful for people who cannot cooperate or for children, unless they are sedated beforehand.

What CT scanning can detect

Modern CT scans can detect abnormalities of less than 1 cm/⅜ in diameter. When scanning the brain, CT can investigate headaches, confirm strokes and detect brain tumours and features of multiple sclerosis. Another major application is in scanning the abdomen to investigate abdominal pain and possible cancers, in particular cancer of the pancreas, which is otherwise difficult to diagnose.

A further application has been in imaging the spinal bones and the spinal cord to investigate back pain or slipped discs. CT scans – and MRI scans even more so (see opposite) – are shedding new light on disease of bone (see page 257) and joints elsewhere, replacing exploratory surgery.

High-speed CT scanners can be used to investigate the heart, providing high-quality images and giving useful information about the muscles and valves. However, the scans do not give such good information about blood flow or atherosclerosis (see page 42), although research may improve this application. Other invaluable applications of CT scans are in investigating lung, liver and kidney disease.

MRI SCANNING

The letters MRI stand for magnetic resonance imaging, the latest and so far the most spectacular way of showing images of the interior of the body. The concept behind MRI is basically simple, although the physics and computers needed are very complex.

The technique relies on the fact that atoms in certain circumstances behave like tiny magnets. Hydrogen atoms are the best ones to show this property and are found throughout the body in fluids, fat and soft tissues such as the brain. Placing someone in an extremely powerful magnetic field makes many of their hydrogen atoms line up in relation to the magnetic field. The next step is to push those atoms out of alignment using a beam of radio waves. When that beam is switched off, the hydrogen atoms realign in the magnetic field, emitting a radio signal as they do so. By analysing that radio wave it is possible to build up an image of the hydrogen-rich parts of the body and turn this into photographs.

How MRI is performed

To achieve the very high magnetic field, you have to lie inside a bulky apparatus during the 20–30 minutes it takes to perform the scan. Some people find this claustrophobic, much more so than with CT scans (see opposite). Because of the magnetism, you must remove all metal objects such as jewellery from your body. People who have implanted metallic objects such as heart pacemakers or metallic clips from surgical operations cannot therefore be scanned.

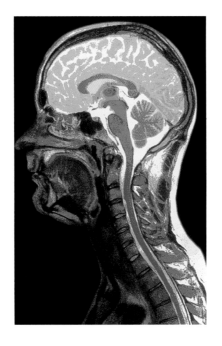

Above: An MRI scan showing the brain and spinal cord in anatomical detail.
Above right: A section through the brain and eyeballs.

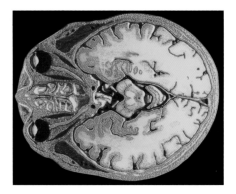

Safety

Intense magnetic fields and radio waves produce temporary changes in the body but so far none that appear to cause any serious effects. Until this is certain, there are restrictions on how long people are exposed to the magnetic fields. Scanning appears to be safe during pregnancy, but under current guidelines it is not routinely used until more research has been done.

What MRI can detect

The scans provide brilliant images of the brain for diagnosing tumours (see page 94), strokes (see page 82) and multiple sclerosis (see page 84). They show up slipped discs and narrowings in the spinal canal that may be the cause of back pain (see pages 246 and 254). So successful and reliable is MRI scanning for these conditions that it is gradually replacing CT scanning, even though it is still much more expensive.

Joint problems are another success story for MRI scanning, whether in the neck, shoulder or, especially, the knee, where MRI can reveal whether the internal ligaments are damaged and various other causes of knee pain. In all of these joints it shows muscle damage and bruising far better than any technique hitherto available. Probably MRI scanning will replace arthroscopy (looking inside the joint under anaesthetic) in the near future as a means of diagnosis, although arthroscopy will continue as a means of treatment.

Scans are also performed on the abdomen and the heart. Using rapid scanning, it is becoming possible to image the abdominal organs in detail to investigate abdominal pain or possible cancers, for example in the liver, pancreas, womb, ovaries and gall bladder. Scans of the heart can visualize the valves, the muscle of the heart walls and blood clots from previous damage, such as a heart attack. It is not yet possible to see blood vessels well enough to tell if they are narrowed with atherosclerosis (see page 42), but this may well occur in the next few years, transforming the ease of investigating coronary artery disease.

The future

This is a rapidly evolving technology, still just ten years old. Exciting future prospects are to improve the images of blood vessels in the heart and brain and to focus on the activity of the brain by giving injections of materials taken up by its active parts.

NUCLEAR MEDICINE AND PET SCANS

Although viewed by many with suspicion, radioactive techniques have a long-established role in medical investigation and treatment.

What is radioactivity?

Atoms are usually stable particles that do not break down. Radioactive atoms are unstable; they break down into their component parts, such as neutrons, protons and electrons. Many substances contain a small percentage of naturally radioactive forms called isotopes, which are therefore unavoidable in the environment, whether in food, water or the rocks and atmosphere around us. These contribute to what is called background radiation. For the purposes of nuclear medicine, isotopes are selected which are rapidly excreted from the body and which pose minimal risk of radiation damage. Radiation techniques are not used in pregnancy and are avoided in people of reproductive age unless it is essential.

Safety

Safety has to be uppermost in using radioactive substances. The dosages used are carefully regulated and there are maximum annual amounts that can legally be given. While it is true that there is no absolutely safe minimum dose of radiation, the risks are much lower than the risks of other investigations that they can replace, for example bone biopsy under anaesthetic or coronary artery angiography, and are actually comparable to the natural background radiation to which we are all exposed.

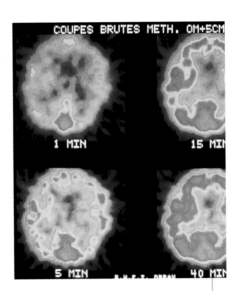

Above: Consecutive PET scans; the red marker spreads to areas of high brain activity.

How radio scans are performed

The idea behind radio scans is to label with a radioactive isotope something that is concentrated in the part of the body to be investigated. To do this, a few days or immediately before scanning, a radioactive substance is either taken by mouth or injected into the body. In the case of the thyroid gland this is radio-labelled iodine; for the heart it is the elements thallium or technetium, which are absorbed by the heart muscles. The radioactivity given off is measured by detectors and the results can be shown as a scan.

Heart Radioactivity scans are much less detailed than CT or MRI scans (see pages 318 and 319), but they do give important information on whether particular organs are working and how efficiently. For example, radio scans of the heart show whether there is a problem with blood flow during exercise which is serious enough to justify going on to the more detailed but more hazardous coronary artery angiography (see page 316).

Lungs and bones Radioisotopes have an important role in detecting disease in lungs and bones more quickly and safely than taking biopsies.

The main use in lung disease is to detect a pulmonary embolus (see page 69). This is done by intravenous injection of a liquid isotope or by breathing in a radioactive gas. The resulting scan shows whether blood is reaching all parts of the lungs or is blocked by a blood clot.

Scanning is particularly used to see whether bone pain is from secondary deposits from cancer. This is an important investigation before starting intensive treatment, for example in breast cancer (see page 148), which may not be advisable if a bone scan shows that the disease is already widespread in the skeleton.

PET scanning

Positron emission scanning (PET) is a relatively new type of scan using isotopes that emit particles called positrons and gamma rays. The main use has been in brain scans. An injection is given of an isotope, usually absorbed into glucose (sugar), which is the brain's main fuel. By detecting where the glucose goes, the PET scan shows the levels of activity of different parts of the brain. This is useful in detecting brain damage.

As a research tool PET scans show what parts of the brain are involved when performing mental activities such as speech as opposed to mental arithmetic, when smelling something or performing a particular task, such as writing. Such scanning may eventually lead to more precise knowledge of how the brain is organized.

BIOPSY

A biopsy means taking a sample of living body material. This is often the only way to make a definite diagnosis for some conditions.

Types of biopsy

Even a simple blood test (see page 322) is a type of biopsy, since the blood contains living elements, but more usually two other types of biopsy are performed. The first involves cutting out a section of a tissue such as skin or muscle for analysis under a microscope. This is most commonly done with skin problems such as coloured lumps, the nature of which is not clear to the naked eye (see page 235).

Other forms of biopsy are taken with a specially designed needle. These are used to diagnose suspicious breast lumps (see page 148) and to take samples from the liver, kidneys or bone marrow. The needles are inserted under local anaesthetic and pick up a core of the material desired. After being withdrawn the core is pushed out into a preservative solution.

Biopsies can also be taken from the stomach, intestines and even the brain.

When is a biopsy performed?

Not every condition can be diagnosed by appearance alone, yet important decisions on treatment require a precise diagnosis. Rather than subject someone to an unnecessary major operation, it is more practicable to obtain a small sample of tissue first. This is common practice in dealing with coloured skin lumps and with lumps in or under the skin that have a suspicious feel to them. It is also carried out on the cervix after a suspicious smear test (see page 150).

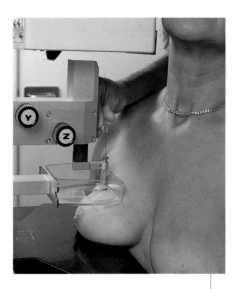

Above: A breast biopsy, using a frame to guide the needle precisely.

Persistently swollen lymph glands are one of the most common diagnostic dilemmas. Lymph glands in the neck or armpit are only doing their job if they swell up temporarily when there is an infection, but persistent swelling is abnormal and may be a feature of types of leukaemia (see page 270) or Hodgkin's disease (see page 264). In these cases, a diagnosis can only be arrived at by taking a biopsy of the gland.

At other times biopsies are taken as a kind of fishing expedition, for example, in investigating unusual bleeding from the womb or changes of bowel habit. In the case of bleeding from the back passage, although the lining of the bowel may look normal, a biopsy may indicate features of inflammatory bowel disease (see page 182). Certain obscure illnesses affecting nerve or muscle may prove a complete mystery until a sample of muscle can be analysed.

Lastly, after surgery for cancer, it is common to take a sample from the margins of the tumour that has been removed to make quite sure that none has been missed at the very edges of the growth.

How the material is analysed

Normally the tissues or cells are analysed under the microscope. To be seen well a biopsy usually has to be stained to show the cells, the nuclei of the cells and other tissue components. Staining takes time, after which the material has to be carefully cut into thin fragments small enough to be spread on a microscope slide. Interpreting the slides is done by a pathologist, skilled in recognizing different types of tissues and deciding what is normal and what is abnormal.

Healing after biopsies

Often so little material is taken during a biopsy that you need nothing more than a protective plaster for a couple of days; sometimes you need a stitch or two. The linings of the stomach, bowels and womb heal extremely rapidly without the need for stitches.

Getting results

Having a biopsy generates unavoidable anxiety, and because doctors are aware of this they try to get results back rapidly. Ordinarily it takes a couple of days to perform the analysis, but occasionally biopsies are taken during surgery to guide the surgeon on whether he has completely removed a tumour. In these cases a pathologist will stand by to report on the tissue immediately.

BIOCHEMISTRY AND BLOOD TESTS

The blood is one of the most easily accessible parts of the internal workings of the body and at the same time one of the most informative. Just a few millilitres of blood is all that is needed for even the most sophisticated blood tests.

What blood contains

Blood comprises red and white blood cells and platelets, which all float in a pool of liquid called plasma. Plasma contains hormones, proteins, sugar and many other chemicals essential to the working of the body.

Taking blood

For routine tests, blood from a vein in the arm is acceptable. The large antecubital vein lies in the fold of the elbow and is prominent enough for easy access. A cuff is placed around the arm to make the vein swell, then a hollow needle is passed into the vein by the doctor, nurse or technician (phlebotomist). The operator draws back on a syringe to get the amount required, although some syringes are vacuum sealed and fill automatically. The cuff is released, the needle withdrawn and a swab kept over the site for a few minutes to stem any bleeding.

The blood is transferred into a sample bottle – there are various types depending on the tests required. Some have fluid at the bottom to stabilize components of the blood until it can be analysed.

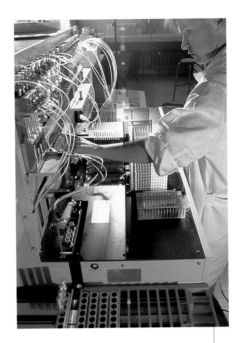

Above: Many blood tests are performed using sophisticated automated analysers.

Types of test

Blood chemicals The common ones measured are sodium, potassium, calcium and iron. These are fundamental to nerve and muscle function. Less often measured are magnesium, copper, zinc and many others that are important in rare medical conditions.

Biochemicals These more complex molecules are formed by the body, for example sugar (glucose), uric acid, ferritin, creatinine, albumin, alkaline phosphatase and many more. The commonly requested ones are grouped according to the organs most responsible for making them: liver function tests, kidney function tests, bone function tests and blood fats (cholesterol and lipids).

Hormones These are not measured as routinely. Examples are prolactin, thyroid-stimulating hormone, insulin, progesterone, testosterone and growth hormone. Frequently the test must be taken under more precise conditions – for example at a specific time of day, at rest, or mid-menstrual cycle.

Blood cells Tests analyse the quantities, types and appearance of the red and white blood cells and the platelets. Such information reveals anaemia or types of infection or explains unusual bleeding, among many other possibilities.

Miscellaneous Numerous proteins are tested if particular diagnoses are in mind, for example C reactive protein is a measure of inflammation within the body. The commonly requested ESR (erythrocyte sedimentation rate) is another measure of inflammation within the body whether from infection, arthritis or cancers and is measured by seeing how long it takes for a thin column of blood to settle into its component parts. Commonly measured vitamins include B_{12} and folic acid.

Arterial blood This might be analysed to measure oxygen concentrations for people with acute heart and breathing problems. The blood is taken by a more complex technique from the radial artery in the wrist or from the femoral artery in the groin.

Analysis

Most blood tests are now analysed through automatic blood sampling machines capable of working on very small quantities of blood. The analysis actually starts in the tube(s) the blood is put into, which are selected according to the tests required.

The analysis comes out of the analyser as a string of values, which can be compared to the normal range for that item, for example a normal level of blood protein can be 62–80 g per litre.

For haematology tests, as well as counting cell types it is also important to know the sizes and shapes of cells. Much of this can be also be done automatically, but sometimes a technician has to physically grade a sample of cells by examining them under the microscope.

ENDOSCOPY, COLONOSCOPY AND BRONCHOSCOPY

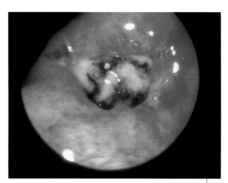

Above: Endoscopy of a stomach ulcer, showing black clotted blood and red fresh blood. Right: An endoscope being passed down the throat into the oesophagus and stomach.

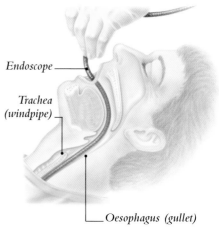

Endoscope —

Trachea (windpipe) —

— Oesophagus (gullet)

Endoscopy means looking inside the body through tubes in order to investigate abnormalities. The technique relies on narrow fibre tubes called endoscopes, which carry light efficiently and are highly flexible. A bright light source plus miniaturized operating devices allow both biopsies (see page 321) and manipulation of flesh. In electronic endoscopes fibre-optic bundles are replaced with tiny colour-sensitive electronic chips displaying a television image, which can be recorded and reviewed.

Endoscopes have flexible tips in order to get the best view and devices that squirt water and suck or blow air – also important for obtaining the best possible view.

The purpose of endoscopes

One of the major uses is in the examination of common intestinal symptoms, ranging from indigestion and stomach pains to bleeding from the back passage, constipation and chronic abdominal pains. Endoscopy has greatly simplified the exploration of these problems, for which the only earlier techniques were barium meals and barium enemas (see page 316), although these are still useful. One enormous advantage of endoscopy is that it allows the lining of the intestines to be seen and samples to be taken. Another important use of the technique is bronchoscopy, which looks inside the tubes of the lungs (bronchi) to investigate lung symptoms such as breathlessness and coughing blood.

Endoscopy

This is done under light sedation and after spraying a local anaesthetic on the back of the throat. The thin flexible tube is guided down the gullet and beyond. The operator twists the tip so as to inspect the walls of the gullet, then the stomach and as far as the duodenum, taking samples from suspicious-looking areas.

Instruments attached to the tip of the endoscope can be used to stop bleeding from veins in the gullet and to pass tubing up the ducts connecting the gall bladder to the duodenum. This latter technique is very important for visualizing the flow of bile from the gall bladder, to remove gall stones that are stuck (see page 186) and for investigating disease of the pancreas. The technique is called endoscopic retrograde cholangiopancreatography (ERCP). It is necessary to rest for an hour or two after undergoing an endoscopy.

Colonoscopy

Colonoscopy is done to inspect the lower bowel, from the anus through the rectum and along the large intestine. It may also be possible to reach as far as the caecum, where the small intestine joins the large intestine – an important region for cancerous growths and other diseases.

For a proper examination, bowel contents have to be cleared a day before examination by laxatives and possibly an enema. Patients are given a sedative plus a painkiller and drugs to relax the bowel. The flexible instrument is passed through the back passage and guided right around the large intestine. As with endoscopy, the operator sees the walls of the bowel and can sample suspicious-looking areas. Growths, called polyps, can also be removed. Because of the higher sedation, patients have to rest under observation for at least two hours after colonoscopy.

Bronchoscopy

This procedure is also done under sedation. The bronchoscope is passed via the nose down the trachea and bronchi, and biopsies are taken from the walls of the bronchi or the lung itself, which is more hazardous. The examination takes about 15 minutes.

Safety

The main risk is pushing the endoscope through the wall of the bowel; this is a very rare complication, estimated at one in every hundred thousand colonoscopies. In bronchoscopy, where a lung biopsy is taken, there is a risk of causing a pneumothorax (the collapse of one lung) so a postoperative chest X-ray is done routinely. The instruments are of course fully sterilized to eliminate the risk of cross-infection.

ANTENATAL TESTS

Increasingly sophisticated techniques are giving ever more information about the health of the unborn child. These possibilities are also raising ethical dilemmas about handling the results, which is why it is routine to offer counselling beforehand. This is so that parents understand the risks of the test, its reliability and what recommendations apply if an abnormality is detected. These tests are changing all the time; below are the currently used ones. Others are being developed using urine samples.

Blood tests

Rubella (German measles) This infection has devastating effects on the developing foetus if contracted during the first four months of pregnancy. A blood test in the first 16 weeks of pregnancy shows whether the mother is immune, in which case exposure to rubella (see page 280) carries no risk. If blood tests show no immunity, the mother must avoid exposure to rubella and ensure she is immunized after the baby is born well before any future pregnancy.

Alpha fetoprotein This is a substance released by a foetus with spina bifida (see page 299), which is detectable in the mother's blood stream. Finding high levels of alpha fetoprotein suggests either twins or a risk of an affected baby. The diagnosis must be further checked by detailed ultrasound scans (see page 317) and by amniocentesis (see below).

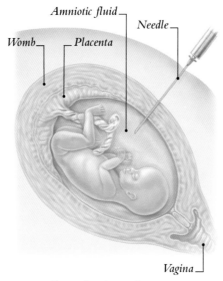

Womb — Placenta — Amniotic fluid — Needle — Vagina

Above: Amniocentesis – a sample of amniotic fluid being withdrawn at 16–18 weeks.

Tests for Down's syndrome These test several biochemical markers in the mother's blood stream; the usual ones are alpha fetoprotein, chorionic gonadotrophin and unconjugated oestradiol. They are a reliable indication of a number of foetal problems other than Down's syndrome (see page 299), including spina bifida, an undeveloped head (anencephaly) and, even rarer, an open abdominal wall (exomphalos). A firm diagnosis is not made on the blood tests alone; amniocentesis or chorionic villus sampling (see below) would also be offered.

Other tests

Amniocentesis It is possible to sample the amniotic fluid in which the baby floats, testing cells shed by the foetus into the fluid for abnormality. The test is done from about 14 weeks by passing a fine hollow needle through the mother's abdomen and drawing off fluid. The technique is used to confirm a diagnosis of spina bifida or Down's syndrome and for chromosome analysis. Amniocentesis carries a 0.5–1% chance of miscarriage, so it cannot be undertaken as a routine investigation. It takes about three weeks to get results.

Chorionic villus sampling This is another technique for deciding on the genetic make-up of the foetus. It can be performed from the tenth week of pregnancy. A needle is passed through the cervix or the mother's abdomen and guided, by ultrasound scanning, towards the placenta. The operator sucks up a small sample of the placenta, called chorionic villi, for analysis of the cells. The technique carries the similar 0.5–1% chance of causing a miscarriage. Results take just a few days but the technique does not detect spina bifida, anencephaly or exomphalos.

Ultrasound This can detect many cases of Down's syndrome by about 12 weeks but it is not yet accurate enough to replace other methods. In the second three months, ultrasound can detect spina bifida, abnormalities of the kidneys and heart and absence of a limb or fingers. Ultrasound is used to detect twins and to monitor the growth of the baby by measuring head size or length. It can establish the reason for bleeding in pregnancy, showing whether a foetus has survived a threatened miscarriage and whether there are abnormalities of the placenta, for example placenta praevia (see page 136). With newer techniques, such as scanning via the vagina, it is possible to detect foetal abnormalities by about 12 weeks. (See also page 317.)

Further investigations

Growth can be monitored by hormone blood tests and ultrasound of the baby's blood flow and heart rate. These tests help in deciding whether to let a high-risk pregnancy continue, for example if the mother has diabetes or high blood pressure (see page 137), or whether to induce labour or perform a Caesarean section (see page 141).

GENETIC ANALYSIS

The 'blueprint' of how to create life resides in the DNA (deoxyribonucleic acid) molecule (see page 134). DNA is organized into genes, sections of DNA which specify how to make each of the thousands of proteins on which life depends. Recent years have seen ever more detailed information about how genes are linked with disease.

Analysing DNA

From a blood sample, DNA is extracted using biochemical probes, which recognize particular sequences of DNA and break the molecule at those points. The fragments are separated by an electric current causing fragments to move at a rate dependent on their size.

Radioactive markers are then added which stick to known DNA sequences. By detecting the radioactivity on photographic plates, a picture of the DNA can be seen, showing whether particular fragments are present and thus whether the individual is susceptible to particular diseases or has abnormalities in his genetic make-up.

Polymerase chain reaction

This technique has opened up DNA analysis by 'amplifying' the minute amounts of DNA from just a single cell, for example as obtained from amniocentesis (see opposite). Biochemical probes targeted to the part of DNA of interest cause it to reproduce itself many times over, and after a few hours the technique produces millions of copies of an original DNA sequence, enough for more detailed analysis.

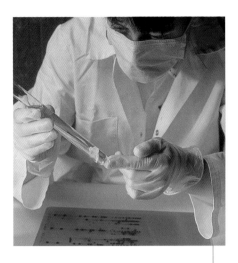

Above: A test tube of DNA over photographs of its genetic contents.

These are the techniques by which illnesses as diverse as breast cancer (see page 148) and schizophrenia (see page 86) are linked with particular DNA sequences.

Chromosomes

Humans have 23 pairs of chromosomes, including a pair of sex chromosomes that determine the individual's sex (see page 134). The chromosomes are revealed by staining cells and analysing chromosomes under the microscope.

The specialist looks for a full set of 23 pairs. Where there is a deficit or an excess of chromosomes, certain conditions can arise. For example, in Turner's syndrome, where there is a single female chromosome and no male chromosome, females are very short, have webbed neck skin and retarded sexual development. Extra chromosomes underlie conditions such as Down's syndrome (see page 299), where there is an extra chromosome 21, and Klinefelter's syndrome, where the presence of two female chromosomes plus a male one results in mental deficiency and abnormal male sexual development. Lack of a chromosome, apart from the sex chromosome, almost always causes gross physical abnormality and the death of the foetus.

Apart from being absent or duplicated, chromosomes may be misformed in numerous ways.

Genetic family trees

If genetic disease is suspected, it is important to plot who else in a family is affected. This establishes whether a genetic condition has arisen spontaneously, for example most forms of Down's syndrome, or whether it is inherited, such as haemophilia or cystic fibrosis. The family pattern also shows whether the gene responsible is dominant (always causes the condition), or recessive (causes the condition only if no normal genes are present, as with sickle cell disease, see page 272).

The specialist can then calculate the risk of other members of a family or future children inheriting the condition. This is vital when counselling on the advisability of amniocentesis or chorionic villus sampling (see opposite), procedures which themselves carry risks.

Most important is knowing the risk of conceiving a child with an invariably fatal or disabling condition such as Huntingdon's chorea (leading to paralysis and dementia) or Tay-Sachs disease (causing blindness, mental retardation and early death). Parents may then decide not to have children or to abort on the basis of antenatal tests.

These heart-rending choices will probably become more common when further discoveries are made about the genetic contribution to disease. Already the latest technology allows rapid genetic analysis for a wide range of conditions not traditionally thought of as being genetically determined, such as high blood pressure (see page 40), but where research suggests a genetic tendency. This is going to become one of the most controversial areas of medicine in the next few years.

COMPLEMENTARY DIAGNOSIS

Many complementary therapists arrive at a diagnosis in a similar way to conventional doctors, but with two major differences. First, such therapists concentrate on the whole person – the physical, emotional and psychological aspects, rather than only on the symptoms described and perhaps some personal factors. Secondly, each type of therapist will decide on a course of treatment based upon their individual speciality (see pages 341 and 368).

Consultations with therapists often last longer than with conventional doctors, sometimes up to an hour, especially if you are seeing the therapist for the first time. Usually consultations fall into two parts.

Assessing the whole person

The therapist, like a conventional doctor, will ask about your physical symptoms – when they began, if they are intermittent or continuous and when they appear. Again, as with conventional doctors, the therapist will ask relevant questions regarding your personal, family, sexual and medical history, but will then broaden this to build up a complete picture of you as a person. This may entail finding out about your personality, behaviour, relationships, work, diet, lifestyle and current mental state in order to assess your overall physical and emotional health.

Physical examination

The type of examination will depend upon the therapist's speciality. For example, an acupuncturist will look at your appearance and posture, the colour of your skin, the lustre of your eyes and the condition of your tongue to assess

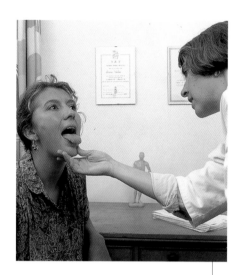

Above: A kinesiologist can determine a patient's health by testing her muscles.

whether there are energy blockages. A shiatsu-do practitioner will also look at these points but may feel parts of your body to see if there are underlying problems. Nutritional therapists may test hair, urine, sweat and muscles to see if there are deficiencies. A chiropractor will feel your spine and perhaps take some X-rays.

Diagnosis

The therapist will then discuss her findings with you, the treatment she proposes and the number of sessions needed.

HISTORY TAKING

During history taking, a doctor tries to obtain a precise description of your symptoms and form an overall picture of your state of health.

A doctor usually starts with open questions, such as 'What is troubling you?' or 'Tell me about this pain'. To complete a history he asks specific questions, such as 'Does coughing hurt?', 'Can you feel this?' or 'Do you feel depressed?'

Familiarity and fundamentals

In a long doctor–patient relationship a doctor already knows a great deal about you – problems you have had and your reactions to them. This helps decide on the significance of new symptoms and guides him through a physical examination (see opposite).

A doctor wants to know when the symptoms started, when they appear and what makes them better or worse. For pain, a doctor wants to ascertain its character, for example sharp or crushing, and whether it moves anywhere, for example from the chest into the neck. A doctor also wants to find out if there is anything else wrong, such as weight loss or fever.

Histories

Personal This concerns previous and current medical problems, your occupation, whether you smoke, drink or take drugs, and also whether you have done any recent foreign travelling.

Family Many illnesses run in the family, for example heart disease, so the health of parents, siblings and children is relevant.

Sexual It may be important to know whether you are at risk for AIDS or other sexually transmitted disease (see pages 124, 164 and 286).

Psychological This helps in assessing obscure symptoms or in deciding if depression or anxiety (see pages 72 and 74) may be causing physical symptoms, such as breathlessness or tiredness.

Diagnosis

At the end of history taking – which may take just a minute – a doctor should have a theory of what could be wrong and has probably decided upon the type of examination needed, the tests to be carried out and the likely diagnosis.

PHYSICAL EXAMINATION

Examining patients is one of the major skills doctors must master in order to arrive at a diagnosis.

A systematic approach

Doctors think in terms of body systems, for example the circulatory or cardiovascular system (see page 38) comprising the heart, arteries and veins, or the digestive system (see page 168) from the mouth to the anus. Examining each system follows procedures broadly the same worldwide.

Checking the circulatory system

These checks include:

- ◆ *Skin colour (blueness of fingers or tongue from lack of oxygen)*
- ◆ *Breathlessness*
- ◆ *Pulse rate (rapid, slow, irregular)*
- ◆ *Heart size (by feeling the chest wall)*
- ◆ *Heart sounds (regularity and any murmurs from abnormal blood flow)*
- ◆ *Blood pressure (see page 40)*
- ◆ *Veins in the neck (which distend in heart failure)*
- ◆ *Blood flow in arteries of the legs*
- ◆ *Ankle swelling (a feature of heart failure, among many other things)*

Detailed refinements are used if an abnormality is detected.

Physical examination in practice

Often patients complain of symptoms which span several systems. For example, breathlessness may result from heart, lung, hormone, kidney or psychological

causes. It is inefficient and tedious to go through each of these systems in turn. Instead doctors make a general examination, probably starting at the head and working down, which they mentally analyse into the individual systems while they are thinking about possible causes.

With practice, a physical examination can be performed very rapidly – it takes just a few minutes to check the heart, lungs, abdomen and nervous system, although a very thorough total examination takes at least half an hour.

Looking and listening

Experienced doctors watch and listen to patients carefully and examine in a focused way, homing in on the likely problem area. While listening to your account of your symptoms and asking the questions posed during history taking (see opposite), the doctor is observing among many things:

- ◆ *Colour (the blueness from low oxygen, the pallor of anaemia or the yellow of jaundice)*
- ◆ *Gait, tremors and ability to use limbs*
- ◆ *Sweating or features of weight loss*
- ◆ *Features of pain (sweating, paleness or grimacing)*
- ◆ *Skin changes of eczema, psoriasis or acne*
- ◆ *Clubbed (highly curved) nails (typical of serious lung and heart disease)*
- ◆ *Mood, ability to speak, coherence and memory*

Basic tools

As well as the basic tools below, others are a sphygmomanometer to measure blood pressure and biochemically coated strips for testing blood for sugar (glucose) or urine for sugar, protein and blood. All of these help doctors reach reasonable conclusions about most symptoms.

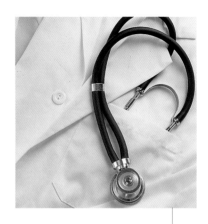

Above: Doctors rely heavily on their stethoscopes for diagnosis.

Stethoscope This is a device that amplifies sounds from the heart, lungs and intestines. Abnormal heart sounds or murmurs are found in heart disease and heart failure (see page 50). Taking blood pressure requires listening to sounds from the artery in the elbow as a pressure cuff is inflated and released. Lung sounds include the wheezing of asthma or bronchitis (see pages 59 and 60), the crackles of infection or fluid, or the absence of sound from a collapsed or fluid-filled lung. Listening to the abdomen may pick up a murmur from a diseased artery, the tinkling bowel sounds of obstruction, or the ominous absence of bowel sounds of peritonitis (infection within the abdomen).

Auroscope This bright light with ear pieces is used to inspect the ear, nose and throat.

Ophthalmoscope This is a bright light source with lenses to focus on the different parts of the eye. An opthalmoscope is used to check eye movements, reactions of the pupils and the health of the retina at the back of the eye.

Tendon hammer This is a stick with a weighted tip, which is used to test reflexes in the arms and legs. Variations in reflexes are an important sign of neurological disease, especially strokes (see page 82).

TYPES OF TREATMENT

HUMANS, IT HAS BEEN SAID, are a pill-taking animal. One hundred years ago, with modern surgery in its infancy, pills were almost the only choice of treatment. Today, people can be given treatments involving not just pills but electron beams, X-rays, sound waves, microscopic drills and transplantation of real and artificial organs. Even drug therapy has changed: now there are new ways of getting medication into the body, including implants, skin patches and hormone gels. And on the horizon there are smart drugs that will travel to targeted cells on specially designed molecules that latch on to tissues.

Behind these advances is an ever-more detailed knowledge of how the body works and increasingly sophisticated means of localizing the site of illness. This should allow doctors eventually to tailor treatments more exactly to the illness and deliver them more precisely to where things are going wrong.

This section reviews the major treatments possible. Many are exciting medical developments because they can reduce symptoms or cure serious illness as no other treatments in the past were able to do. This section also contains information about some complementary therapies.

'First, do no harm . . .'

Whatever the promise of a new treatment, doctors must bear in mind these words from Hippocrates 2500 years ago. The benefits should always outweigh the side effects. Treatments of all types are closely regulated by statutory authorities and need to prove their safety before they become accepted. The search for breakthroughs continues, but patient safety must always remain the number-one priority.

Advances and breakthroughs

The development of techniques such as surgery and treatments for cancer is slower because it takes both courage for specialists to use untested procedures and time to use these new procedures on enough people to produce evidence of the benefits and drawbacks. Whereas drugs can be thoroughly tested in animals or in healthy volunteers, surgery and cancer therapies cannot be tested in the same way. The techniques can be trialled, but ultimately the only test is on ill people.

That said, certain medical advances are so clearly worthwhile that they become accepted rapidly. This has happened with laser and key-hole surgery and with surgical implants, all of which are revolutionary – the first two as less invasive treatments and the third as a means of prolonging or enhancing the quality of a person's life.

True breakthroughs are unusual, despite the headlines. Behind such reports there is likely to be one of two things.

The first is an advance in technology which can be applied to medicine, for example improved scanners. The second is a treatment which shows promise, but which is still years off full evaluation, such as a vaccine against cancer.

And yet true breakthroughs do occur and no more so than in the last 30 years. The most outstanding ones are transplantation of organs, ultrasound treatment for kidney problems and key-hole surgery as already mentioned. These will be described in detail in this section.

Other forms of treatment evolve through steady, careful research, achieving minor changes which, over time, together add up to big improvements. These include intensive care and drug therapy in general, both which are also covered here.

Treatment menus

For serious illnesses, medical care is now likely to involve a combination of treatments. For example, heart disease may begin with medication to reduce cholesterol, move to angioplasty to open up blocked coronary arteries, then end with a heart transplant and chemotherapy to keep rejection at bay. Cancers are often removed surgically, then treatment may continue with a combination of radiotherapy and chemotherapy. Treatment menus such as these appear to be the path of the future.

Right: We approach the 21st century with treatments that were unimaginable at the beginning of the 20th century. The Surgeon by Jan Sanders van Hemessen (c.1504–66).

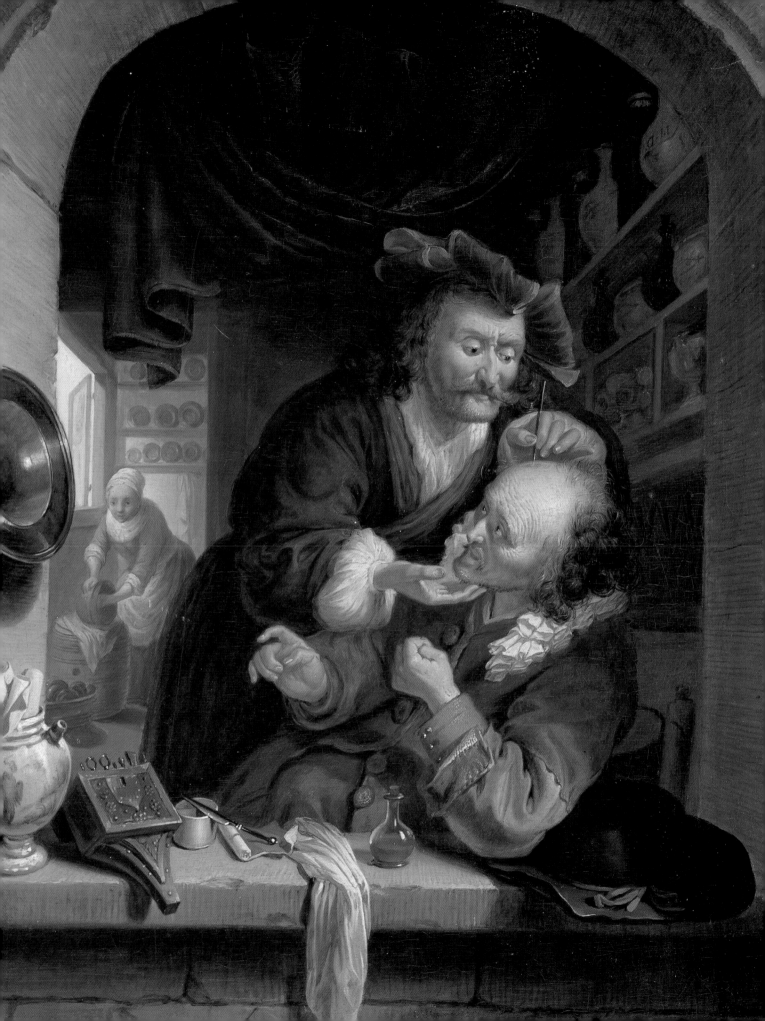

SURGICAL IMPLANTS

Living tissue is in some ways remarkably strong and resilient, but in other ways it is very delicate and easily damaged permanently. Over the centuries surgeons have used crude artificial replacements for damaged tissue, such as metal limbs, but the 20th century has seen particular advances in such techniques.

The great advantage of an artificial implant is that the body is unlikely to reject it, since rejection is what bedevils transplant surgery (see opposite). The following are the most common implants.

Artificial joints

Hips Hip replacement surgery started in the 1960s. Since then techniques have been refined to provide a wide choice of artificial hips.

There are two parts to the artificial hip: a plastic cup is set into the pelvic bone and the upper femur (thigh bone) is replaced by a metal tip, cemented into the rest of the femur.

Artificial hips last for ten to fifteen years. The main complications are infection, loosening and dislocation. Artificial hips can be replaced in an operation that is technically demanding.

Knees Implanting artificial knees is increasingly the treatment for severe pain. Part or all of the knee can be replaced with metal and plastic components, hinged to give a good range of back and front and side-to-side movement.

Other joints There are good results from the replacement of the whole shoulder joint and the small joints of the hand. These are likely to become more widely available operations in the future.

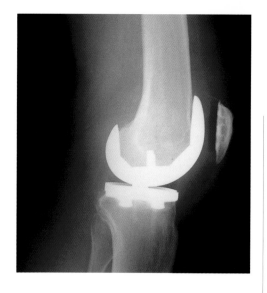

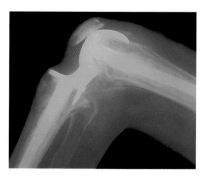

Above and left: Two of the many types of artificial knee joint available; different surgeons have their favourites.

Heart implants

Heart valves Valves damaged by atherosclerosis (see page 42), rheumatic fever or simply age cause breathlessness or heart failure. The Starr-Edwards valve, a ball within a cylinder, is still, after 30 years, the most widely used artificial valve. The flat Bjork-Shiley valve is another type. After implantation the patient must stay on an anticoagulant drug to prevent blood clots forming around the new valve.

Using valves from a pig's heart makes anticoagulation less of a necessity. The pig valves are treated so as not to provoke an immune reaction in the human recipient.

Artificial hearts Various pumping devices can assist the heart, using compressed carbon dioxide as a power source. Other devices support the heart while a patient is awaiting a heart transplant. The completely artificial, electrically driven heart has yet to be perfected. One major problem is getting power to the artificial heart without running wires through the chest wall by which infection can enter. This will probably be achieved using motors that generate electricity through magnetic induction across the chest wall.

Pacemakers These electronic devices are implanted under the skin of the upper chest (see page 51). Electrodes run from the pacemaker up veins into the heart, positioned under X-ray control. Pacemakers are sophisticated devices that deliver an electric shock to make the heart beat at a desired rate. They sense the natural beat of the heart and will therefore not 'fire' in competition with the heart. They can also vary the rate in reaction to exercise or stress. Pacemakers take about an hour to position, usually under a local anaesthetic, and their batteries last for five to ten years. There are very few hazards to wearing a pacemaker.

Other implants

A patient with cataracts (see page 201) can have the opaque part of the lens replaced with an artificial lens. Cochlear implants are artificial electronic sound detectors. Placed in the skull, they restore hearing reasonably well (see page 208).

The arteries to the legs and the great aortic artery within the abdomen commonly become blocked with atherosclerosis or are diseased in some other way. The affected part can be replaced with artificial fibre grafts.

The future

A challenging prospect is treating leg paralysis after spinal cord injuries. Experimental work is showing how electrodes in the spine could amplify natural nerve impulses to make the legs work again.

TRANSPLANTATION

Transplanting organs from a donor to another person (the host) is a relatively young science – the first successful heart transplant took place only in 1967. Transplantation raises important ethical as well as scientific issues. Transplants include the kidney, heart, liver, skin, bone and bone marrow. More ambitious transplants involve the lungs and heart combined or even a complete intestinal system. Timing is critical because donated organs survive just a few hours once detached from their blood supply.

The immune response and rejection

The body distinguishes its own cells from someone else's. By using special molecules called immunoglobulins and cells called lymphocytes, the host attacks transplanted tissues and can destroy the donor organ rapidly. The transplanted organ may itself react against its host. The great problem for transplant surgery has been to develop a means of reducing these immune rejection responses. Several drugs dampen the immune reaction, the best known of which is prednisolone. This is used with other drugs, the most effective being cyclosporin, which has relatively few side effects.

The ideal transplant tissue

This would be a duplicate of the damaged part of the body. Skin grafting, for example, transplants the patient's own skin on to the damaged area. It is beyond present capabilities to do this with more complex organs. It is easier to breed animals that provoke only a weak immune response in humans, for example pigs are bred for their hearts to be used as transplants.

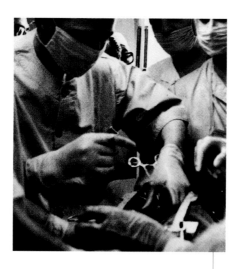

Above: Christian Barnard performing the first heart transplant. Risky and revolutionary in 1967, it is now an established treatment for serious heart disease.

The donor

A suitable transplant donor has a genetic make-up closely resembling that of the host so that less medication is needed to control rejection. Identical twins or close family are therefore often suitable donors.

Examples of transplantation

Kidney A kidney transplant has as good an outlook afterward as surviving on dialysis (see page 335) and is far more convenient for the patient.

Heart This is an option for people with diseased heart muscle, perhaps after infection or with congenital heart defects (see page 295). Four out of five people survive for a year after a heart transplant and many of these survive for more than five years. Most return to some kind of work and full activity.

Heart–lung Candidates for this surgery often have high blood pressure in the lung circulation. The results are almost as good as heart transplantation alone. It is impossible to transplant successfully lungs on their own without the heart.

Bone marrow This is used in forms of leukaemia (see page 270) and rare childhood diseases of the bone marrow. Without treatment these patients become severely anaemic, bleed profusely and succumb to trivial infections. This transplantation calls for the most careful matching of donor and host.

Liver, pancreas and intestine Liver transplants are used in treating liver cancer, chronic liver infection after hepatitis B and C or cirrhosis of the liver (see page 184) or, in children, congenital abnormalities of the liver. Liver transplants are quite successful, transplants of the pancreas and intestines less so.

Other Bone grafting has long been successfully performed. Close matching is not important because the transplant serves as a framework along which the host grows new replacement bone.

In the eye, corneal grafts are well known as a replacement for a cataract. Rejection is not a problem because there is no blood supply to that part of the eye and so no way for immunoglobulins and lymphocytes to destroy the graft.

Ethical issues

The donor of an organ loses it forever (except in the case of bone and bone marrow transplantation). The only organ a donor can survive giving is a kidney; otherwise for someone to have a new organ, someone else has to die. Tragically these potential donors are often young victims of accidents. Their families have only one or two hours in which to decide about donation while trying to cope with their tragedy. The increasing use of donor cards and 'advance directives' in wills may help reduce the trauma of what at present appears unseemly haste.

MICROSURGERY

Microsurgery is the general term for techniques that allow for surgery on very small or fragile parts of the body. The structures being operated can be a millimetre in diameter or less, and include nerves, arteries and veins. Microsurgery is particularly well established in operating on the eye.

The scope of the speciality has broadened with the development of operating microscopes and miniaturized equipment for cutting, probing and sewing. These are refinements of techniques first used in eye surgery. Microsurgery other than on the eyes took off from the 1960s, when it was first shown that it was possible to reimplant a thumb, and then other amputated limbs.

Equipment

The surgeon uses an operating microscope, which gives a magnified and full three-dimensional view of the operating field. The operating instruments include jewellers' forceps, electrodes to stop bleeding, fine probes and scissors. Of greatest importance was the development of ultrafine needles with nylon thread already attached to allow sewing of fragile structures without damaging them.

How microsurgery is performed

The surgeon works his way through each structure, cleaning, removing dead flesh where required, then repairing the site being operated on. After injury, such as an amputation, the first structures to be repaired are the blood vessels, because these are the most critical to the survival of the injured limb.

Each major vein and artery is identified, the ends brought together and painstak-

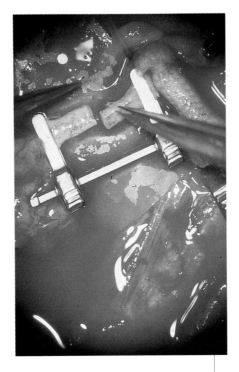

Above: Clamps holding the two ends of a cut blood vessel close enough for the surgeon to repair it.

ingly sewn. Then the surgeon finds the cut ends of nerves and carefully stitches them together. The tendons, muscles and bone are repaired similarly. The surgeon can see almost immediately whether the repair of blood vessels is successful, whereas it can take several months to know if repair of nerves has succeeded.

Uses of microsurgery

Nerve repair This is needed following accidental cuts, crushing or even amputation of a limb. After amputation of a hand or forearm, thumb and fingers, time is of the essence. The amputated part must be kept cooled, and it will then remain repairable for between six and twenty-four hours, depending on how much of the limb is injured.

Plastic surgery A common problem is the need to replace skin lost after trauma or surgery. This can now be done by transferring a whole segment of flesh with its skin from elsewhere in the body where

its loss is not so critical, for example transferring skin from the back to the face, or using a big toe to replace an amputated thumb. The procedure needs two teams of surgeons: one team removes the donor flesh, the other prepares the site where it is to go. The surgeon joins the various components – nerves, blood vessels and muscles – as detailed above. Often it is the scalp that requires reconstruction, but many structures around the face, including the cheeks, neck, floor of the mouth and jawline, also lend themselves to this type of surgery.

Gullet replacement This can be repaired using a section of intestine, joining the blood vessels by microsurgical techniques.

Brain tumours Certain rare tumours within the brain (see page 94) can be approached using miniature instruments. The tumour is cut out under microscopic control, reducing the chances of damage to surrounding brain material. Other uses are to repair aneurysms (arteries within the brain that bleed), abnormal blood vessels (haemangiomas) and spinal tumours.

Gynaecological surgery Microsurgery can unblock Fallopian tubes, the blockage of which is a cause of subfertility (see page 162). This blockage is often due to infection or tubes that have been tied previously or clipped for sterilization. Ovarian cysts are a common problem; their removal must be done delicately to preserve future fertility.

Safety

Bleeding is a problem in microsurgery, because just a small amount of blood may completely obscure the view. Although surgeons can use tiny scalpels, they also use lasers (see opposite) with very finely controlled beams that cut and stop bleeding at the same time.

LASER SURGERY

Since the 1970s, lasers have found a role in many parts of medicine. The thin, high-intensity beams of light offer a precise and bloodless operating tool.

Laser, which stands for light amplification by stimulated emission of radiation, is a beam of light with a high energy level. All the particles of the beam, called photons, move in precise step with each other and in a narrow beam that does not spread as an ordinary beam of light does. Different types of laser react on flesh in different ways, for example lasers of a certain type will pass through normal tissue yet burn tissue of a different colour because it absorbs the beam.

Laser beams can be fed through fibre-optic cables, and therefore can be manipulated into difficult positions in the throat, gullet, stomach and rectum.

Uses of laser surgery

Eye surgery Lasers are well established for operating for glaucoma and cataracts (see pages 200 and 201). They can deal with diseased blood vessels of the retina at the back of the eye which threaten vision, a common problem in diabetics. Ophthalmic surgeons use lasers to burn away blood vessels that look as if they may bleed, in a way that was impossible before lasers.

Gynaecological surgery Uses include unblocking Fallopian tubes (see page 162), cutting out cysts from the ovaries, removing the lining of the womb as a treatment for heavy periods (see page 154) and removing suspicious areas of the cervix (see page 150).

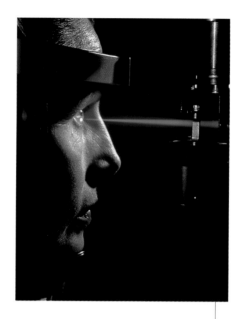

Above: A patient undergoing ophthalmic laser treatment. The laser is aimed using a retinal camera and its beam is delivered in a series of pulses.

Skin problems Lasers can remove small growths and coloured patches of skin. So-called tunable lasers are used for large patches of discoloured skin where scarring must be avoided, such as port-wine stains on the face. They emit light at wavelengths that are most absorbed by, and therefore destroy, coloured skin and cause little damage to less highly coloured normal skin nearby.

Tattoos, applied in haste and regretted at leisure, are another use for lasers. The laser emits very high energy for extremely short periods of time, enough to vaporize carbon, the black pigment in tattoos. However, the results are rarely as successful as would be desired.

Control of bleeding Bleeding from peptic ulcers is controlled by laser; small growths in the bowel or gullet can be removed by laser. These are not curative operations, but more to relieve symptoms, such as difficulty in swallowing, in otherwise inoperable illness. The laser can tunnel through the obstructing tumour in a way that could not be done by conventional cutting, because of all the bleeding that would be caused. Lasers can also cut out small cancers of the larynx and vocal cords.

Removal of prostate gland The laser burns away the prostate tissue, immediately relieving obstruction. This technique will probably become more widely used in future and may even make some prostate surgery (see page 120) an outpatient procedure.

Arterial and heart surgery Lasers initially appeared ideal for unblocking leg arteries obstructed by atherosclerosis (see page 42), but early enthusiasm has unfortunately not yet been matched by success. Using lasers to unblock coronary arteries is a more promising technique and will no doubt be improved over the next few years.

Safety

The main risk is from scarring nearby tissue. This is avoided by selecting the right lasers for the job, as mentioned above.

There is a risk of cutting through tissue, for example cutting through the stomach wall when operating on the stomach lining, but again this risk is reduced by selecting lasers which destroy only a millimetre or so of depth at a time.

The future

Photodynamic therapy is an exciting prospect, using the fact that lasers are absorbed differently by tissues of different colours. The patient swallows a photosensitizer that is taken up especially in cancerous tissues. When an appropriately coloured laser beam is shone on the affected area, it destroys only the cancerous cells, leaving the normal cells untouched. This remarkable advance is under intensive research.

DRUGS

Drugs are substances that affect the working of the body. (See also page 366.)

The modern drug industry began with aspirin, which is just a hundred years old. The first synthetic drug and one of the most successful ever, aspirin is a good example of how drugs are researched. A substance is found that appears to affect the body beneficially. For aspirin this was extracts from willow bark, which even the ancient Egyptians knew reduced pain and fever. The active ingredient is then identified, purified and tested to prove it works, and to check its dosage and side effects. Researchers can alter the ingredient biochemically to reduce side effects, and make the drug cheaper or more effective.

Dosage takes account of the patient's age and size, seriousness of the illness and function of the kidney and liver, the organs that usually get rid of drugs. Drugs rapidly eliminated by the body must be given frequently, hence penicillin is given every six hours whereas the antibiotic cefixime need be given only once a day.

How some common drugs work

Antibiotics These affect some unique part of the biochemistry of bacteria. For example, penicillin-type drugs destroy the cell wall of bacteria, making them burst.

Sedatives These alter brain chemistry, probably by interfering with neurotransmitters – biochemicals that pass from one nerve cell to another.

Painkillers Morphine-type painkillers attach to chemical receptors that normally respond to natural painkillers within the body (enkephalins and endorphins). Aspirin and other non-steroidal

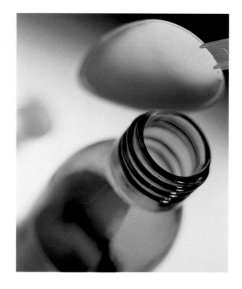

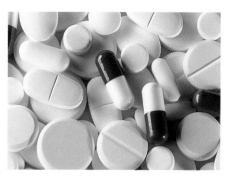

Above and right: It is difficult to imagine life now without drugs for pain relief and control of illness.

anti-inflammatory drugs (NSAIDs) such as ibuprofen affect biochemicals called prostaglandins, which regulate many body functions apart from pain.

Drugs for high blood pressure

Calcium-channel blockers (nifedipine and amlodipine) block calcium from entering muscle cells, letting blood vessels relax and reducing blood pressure (see page 40). ACE inhibitors (captopril and lisinopril) affect the uptake of potassium and sodium in the kidneys, thereby reducing blood volume and blood pressure. Beta-blockers (atenolol and metoprolol) have many not entirely understood actions on the blood vessels, kidneys and heart.

Taking drugs

By mouth (orally) These must taste acceptable and survive an attack by stomach acid. Drugs unable to resist this have to be given by other means. One of the best known is insulin, which has to be given by injection.

By injection Injected drugs work more rapidly than oral drugs, for example for rapid pain relief. Quickest of all is to inject drugs directly into the blood stream (intravenous therapy), which is used for intensive treatment of serious infections.

By patches, creams and ointments Drugs can be absorbed through the skin. This is a convenient method of administering them and allows the drug to bypass the liver at first, which would otherwise destroy much of the drug at the beginning of its journey in the blood stream. This route allows quantities lower than those taken by mouth to be used for hormone replacement therapy (HRT) or pain relief.

By suppository This method is very effective, working almost as fast as an injection. It is used to give painkillers and antiepileptic drugs rapidly, for example to someone having a prolonged epileptic fit.

Risks and benefits

Doctors are always weighing up possible side effects against possible benefits. This is why they advise against drug therapy for self-limiting problems or they select drugs with a low risk of side effects. However, for serious illness it is justifiable to use potent drugs such as gentamicin, despite there being a higher risk of side effects. Side effects vary from minor rashes and diarrhoea to the very serious – internal bleeding or liver damage. Always report possible side effects to your doctor.

Resistance

Over time germs become resistant to commonly used drugs. This is a serious problem with antibiotics and another reason why doctors try to limit drug use to essential circumstances only.

DIALYSIS

An estimated 500,000 people worldwide rely on dialysis to keep kidney failure (see page 114) under control. For some it is a temporary measure until a kidney transplant (see page 331) can be done, but for others it is a permanent way of life.

What dialysis is for
The kidneys perform many functions, one of the most important being the clearing of poisonous substances from the blood stream. These are accumulated waste products from metabolism which would otherwise cause kidney failure, with high blood pressure, anaemia, itching, general malaise and ultimately convulsions, heart disease and death.

Dialysis is a way of artificially filtering the blood stream to remove these substances. Additional medical treatment and careful diet can preserve many of the other functions of the kidneys.

The decision to begin dialysis is not straightforward and has to take into account social, personal and economic factors over and above purely medical considerations. It also depends on the local availability of kidney transplants, which varies greatly around the world. In the United Kingdom about half of the people with chronic kidney failure are maintained on dialysis.

How dialysis works
The kidney patient's blood is fed through a device that contains thousands of extremely thin-walled tubes of cellulose or plastic. The tubes rest in a liquid called the dialysate, which contains water with precisely calculated quantities of sodium, potassium, salt, sugar and other chemi-

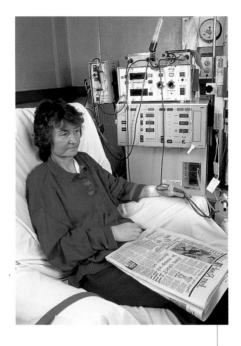

Above: While never routine, kidney dialysis can be fitted around everyday activities.

cals. With the blood flowing in one direction and the dialysing fluid flowing in the other, chemical forces called diffusion make waste products move from the blood stream across the membrane of the tubes and into the fluid, which is then pumped to waste.

How dialysis is performed
Once someone is judged as needing regular kidney dialysis, a surgeon fashions a permanent shunt called a fistula, usually in the patient's arm. This links a large artery to a large vein; the vein grows so it can be easily accessed by a needle. This allows a large blood flow to be taken rapidly every two to three days, the filtered blood being returned via another needle further down the shunt.

Blood at about 300–500 ml/approx 10–17 fl oz per minute flows through the dialysing machine, the whole sequence taking about five hours for an adult. The technology is largely automated, allowing many patients to have a dialysing machine at home and to deal with their dialysis themselves. However it is a complex technology and often patients prefer to be treated in a hospital setting.

This dialysing method is suitable for people with long-established kidney failure (chronic renal failure). Other dialysing techniques are suitable for people who go into sudden kidney failure (acute renal failure) as a result of serious blood loss or extensive burns.

Peritoneal dialysis
Conventional dialysis takes up a major part of a kidney patient's time and ability to work. Peritoneal dialysis is an attempt to reduce this burden. Instead of using an artificial membrane and machine, peritoneal dialysis uses the natural filtering properties of the lining of the abdomen, called the peritoneum.

Access is secured by fitting a permanent catheter tube, through which 2–3 litres/3½–5 pints of dialysing fluid is poured into the patient's abdomen, and let out again after an hour or two. In between changes the patient can be mobile. Again, there are refinements and some automated delivery systems.

Problems
The main potential problem in peritoneal dialysis is infection via the access sites; this can be extremely serious and difficult to manage. Despite this, death from peritonitis is rare as long as it is treated aggressively. In machine dialysis there is a risk of removing too much fluid, leading to low blood pressure with light-headedness and weakness. Some people understandably cannot cope with the technology or with the associated anxiety. Otherwise the outlook with dialysis is good, with patients managing on it for 20 years or more.

INTENSIVE CARE

Intensive care units are wards that are equipped to deliver intensive medical and nursing care to the seriously ill.

Those patients who require intensive care treatment include victims of serious accidents or illness, such as burns, head injury, heart attack, lung infections or major trauma with multiple injuries; those who are recovering from heart or abdominal surgery; and people who have taken drug overdoses. These patients all share the risks of collapse of blood pressure, infection, poor lung function and biochemical disturbances leading to heart irregularities and epileptic fits. They will be in pain and often unconscious, and will be disorientated when they regain consciousness. It is a carefully considered decision to put someone on intensive care; sometimes medically there is no point because of brain death or irreversible physical damage.

Intensive care is delivered by specialized doctors and nurses, skilled in relieving pain and dealing with infection and who know when to call in experts in kidney or heart diseases. They are also experienced at keeping relatives informed of progress and breaking bad news.

The first priority in intensive care is to keep the patient's circulation going with blood plentiful in oxygen.

Equipment used in intensive care
Central venous pressure (cvp) line A tube is inserted into a large chest or neck vein and is connected to a display unit. This measures the pressure of blood returning to the heart, indicating how well the heart is working and whether there is enough blood and fluid to keep the patient's circulation going.

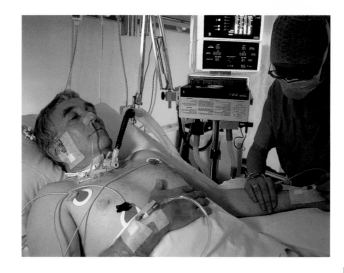

Pulmonary artery pressure line This is a catheter in the pulmonary artery, which supplies blood to the lungs. It is inserted from a vein in the groin and guided up to the chest.

Drips These feed fluids and drugs directly into the blood stream, enabling rapid therapy for sudden bleeding or collapse of blood pressure. A hollow needle in an arm vein is connected by tubing to a fluid-filled bag and the fluid is delivered at the desired rate. There may be two drips, one for blood and one for other fluids and medication.

Ventilators (artificial respiration) These machines push air and oxygen into the lungs. A tube is guided down the throat into the trachea (main airway), then connected to the ventilator. The type of ventilator varies greatly: some do all the work for a patient who cannot breathe at all, while others work in between the patient's own breaths. Once someone can breathe by themselves, they can have oxygen via a face mask.

Tests
Blood oxygen The simplest technique is called pulse oximetry. This is a device placed on the finger or ear lobe that shines bright light through the skin; the redness of the transmitted light is related to the amount of oxygen in the blood.

In addition, blood samples are taken from arteries in the wrist or groin.

Left: A patient with a nasogastric feeding tube, a drip attached to one hand, a tracheostomy for breathing, a CVP line and ECG electrodes.

Blood tests These monitor such critical things as potassium, sodium, sugar (glucose), kidney function, levels of medication and signs of infection.

Kidney function This is absolutely critical after a collapse of blood pressure. It requires frequent blood samples and accurate measurement of urinary output from a urinary catheter, a tube passed into the bladder that drains urine continuously into a bag.

Brain function It is a constant worry whether a serious illness has critically damaged the brain. There are scoring systems that rate responsiveness to stimuli, such as touch or commands, pupil dilation in response to pain, choking reflexes and the ability to breathe.

Leaving intensive care
Guided by tests and examination, specialists gradually wean people off the various devices, starting with the respirator then abandoning drips and catheters. Some people remain deeply unconscious, unable to exist without artificial input. The management of such cases involves difficult ethical issues; a decision to switch off support will be made jointly by doctors, the nursing staff and relatives.

LITHOTRIPSY

Developed in Germany in the 1970s, this technique has revolutionized the treatment of stones in the urinary system.

Kidney stones, which are very common, cause excruciating pain and possible damage to the kidney (see page 113). The preferred treatment is to allow the stone to pass spontaneously down the ureter, which happens in 50% of cases. However, many stones are too large or irregular to pass through the ureter to the bladder and out. Such cases formerly required surgery to expose the kidney and to remove the stone, or else to pass a tube up from the bladder to encircle the stone and pull it out. Both methods were unpleasant and traumatic.

How lithotripsy works
The term means wearing away of stones. The idea is to create a shock wave of energy which is focused on to the stone. The energy is created by a spark plug device, a piezo electric effect (compressing a ceramic plate) or something like a very powerful loudspeaker. The energy source rests within a specially shaped container which focuses the energy where it is needed. For technical reasons, the earlier lithotripsy devices required the energy source to be in water, so the patient had to sit in a water-bath. Newer devices still require water around the energy source, but are portable and the patient no longer has to sit in water.

Each shock wave causes tiny bubbles to form on the surface of the stone. When those bubbles collapse they release an enormous amount of energy and heat that crumbles the stone. A course of treatment may involve as many as two thousand rapid shocks.

How lithotripsy is performed
The apparatus is positioned very close to the affected kidney and precisely focused under X-ray guidance. The shocks are given automatically, in rapid succession. As originally designed, the shocks were powerful enough to be painful, and therefore lithotripsy was performed under general anaesthetic. Second-generation machines are deliberately less powerful, avoiding the need for a general anaesthetic. On the other hand, this means that it can take several treatments to shatter the stone.

Success and safety
Lithotripsy works very well for stones within the kidney, upper ureter and bladder, and less well if the stone is in the lower ureter. It may cause bleeding around the kidney, although this is rarely of any significance. People feel as if they have been bruised around the kidney, but again, rarely to any great degree. Occasionally the fragments of stone fail to pass so that further surgery is needed.

Other applications
Ultrasound lithotripsy This is a refinement using an ultrasound generator. Under anaesthetic the surgeon guides this tube device to the bladder and up the ureter to the stone, or he can insert it directly into the kidney through a cut in the loin. The probe vibrates vigorously and shatters the stone, as if it were being hammered. The instrument includes a suction device to suck up the fragments of stone. Ultrasound lithotripsy is used to shatter very hard stones resistant to the usual form of lithotripsy.

Laser lithotripsy The laser is guided in a tube up the ureter then focused against the stone. The high energy from the laser shatters the stone and the fragments pass out in the urine.

Gallstones It was natural to try to apply the same lithotripsy technology to destroying gallstones (see page 186), which are even more common than kidney stones. Surgeons have used ultrasound lithotripters guided to the gall bladder from the small intestine, with the patient under light sedation. However, the shattered fragments do not pass out as reliably as do the fragments from kidney stones. With the advent of key-hole gall bladder surgery (see page 340), gallstone lithotripsy is rarely used.

RADIOTHERAPY

In the 1920s scientists showed that radiation could affect cancerous cells more than normal cells. With that realization a search began for ever-more selective forms of radiation. The goal is still to find treatments that affect cancerous cells as much as possible but have the minimum effect on normal cells.

The selection includes X-rays (see page 316), which are the most common, and gamma rays, electron beams and neutron beams, which are the least used. Radiotherapy may be given by implanting radioactive material within the tumour, a technique especially used in treating cancer of the cervix and womb (see pages 150 and 151).

How radiotherapy works

Radiotherapy uses high-energy atomic radiation. X-rays and gamma rays interfere with the electrons orbiting around atoms, whereas proton and neutron beams destroy the nucleus of atoms and tend to have more devastating effects. Radiotherapy interferes with the normal working of the cell, stopping the cell reproducing, destroying vital proteins and altering DNA structure (see page 134).

Each type of cancer responds differently to radiotherapy. This depends upon many factors, including how quickly the tumour grows, how good its blood supply is and how quickly the tumour cells can repair damage from radiotherapy.

Uses of radiotherapy

Destroying cancers Radiotherapy is most effective for cancer of the cervix, the bladder (see page 115), the head and neck (the larynx and tongue), the prostate (see page 120), Hodgkin's disease (see

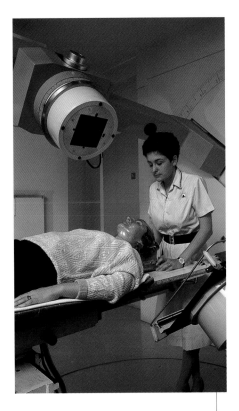

Above: Rotating radiotherapy equipment maximizes radiation on the target, minimizing damage elsewhere.

page 264) and cancer of the testicles (see page 122). It may be curative for these cancers. Radiotherapy alone does not cure leukaemia (see page 270), but it is often used before giving chemotherapy (see opposite) to destroy deposits of leukaemia at sites chemotherapy may not reach, such as the brain and spinal cord. Radiotherapy is also used with surgery for breast cancer (see page 148).

Radiotherapy is unlikely to cure cancers of the brain, lung (see page 68) and gastrointestinal system, including the bowel and stomach (see pages 180 and 181), but it may still help to relieve symptoms.

Relieving symptoms Even though a cancer is incurable, relief of symptoms may be valuable, especially if a tumour is causing pain or pressing on nerves in the spine. Radiotherapy shrinks the tumour enough to give relief, making it an extremely important application of the treatment.

Other uses An overactive thyroid gland (see page 107) is treatable using radioactive iodine. The thyroid gland takes up iodine and the concentrated radioactivity slowly destroys just those cells.

Planning treatment and the amount necessary

The tumour must be precisely localized. This is straightforward if it is visible on the surface, but often the tumour is deep within the body. Modern scanners have greatly improved localization, for example, CT and MRI scans (see pages 318 and 319). The radiotherapist needs to know the type of the tumour, the position and its volume in order to aim the radiotherapy and calculate a total dose.

Often radiotherapists use a plastic shell, which the patient wears and which allows rapid realignment for each treatment. The point to be aimed at may be marked by a tattoo or a light beam.

It is normal to have several sessions of radiotherapy, each lasting for just a few minutes. Treatment may be every day for a couple of weeks or weekly sessions for a couple of months. The schedule is calculated so as to reduce the risk of damage to normal tissue, while hitting the cancerous tissue at its most vulnerable time as it recovers from the previous session. This varies greatly from tumour to tumour.

Side effects

Common side effects include nausea, tiredness and burns where radiation beams pass through the skin. These occur immediately or within a week or two of treatment. Long-term effects include damage to the organ where the cancer lies, such as inflammation of the lung. It is always difficult to weigh side effects against the benefit of therapy. This is best done by complete honesty and discussion with patients.

CHEMOTHERAPY

This type of cancer treatment uses medication taken by mouth or by injection. Researchers believe that chemotherapy ultimately offers more hope for curing some forms of cancer than either surgery or radiotherapy (see opposite).

How chemotherapy works

The drugs used in chemotherapy are, for all practical purposes, poisons because they interfere with normal cell function. Among the first chemotherapy agents and still very important are those drugs that work by destroying the structure of DNA. Examples of these are cyclophosphamide and melphalan. Such drugs were originally developed for chemical warfare. Other drugs work by blocking normal metabolic pathways in cancerous cells. Examples are methotrexate, 5-fluorouracil and doxorubicin. Platinum is a metal which, in certain forms, can disrupt DNA, so it is put in some drugs. Finally, there are several drugs derived from plants which disrupt DNA or the internal structure of cells. Examples are vincristine, from the periwinkle, and taxol, from the bark of the Western yew.

Suitable cancers

The most responsive cancers are those that are fast-growing. This is because fast-growing cells take up the poisonous agents much more than normal cells, which means that side effects can be limited. Such cancers include leukaemia (see page 270), Hodgkin's disease (see page 264) and childhood cancers.

Then there is a group of less rapidly growing tumours where chemotherapy is still effective. Examples are breast cancer (see page 148) and cancers of the ovary (see page 152), bladder (see page 115), head and neck.

Certain cancers do not respond particularly well to current chemotherapy, such as cancer of the pancreas, lung, bowel and stomach (see pages 68, 180 and 181).

Deciding on the suitability of chemotherapy very much depends on the appearance of the tumour's cells under the microscope, the age and general health of the patient and whether the kidneys and liver are healthy enough to excrete the chemotherapy.

How chemotherapy is given

Usually the medication is given intravenously into the blood stream to avoid the patient immediately vomiting up the dose. Typically, treatment is given every three to four weeks to cause the maximum damage to the tumour while at the same time as little upset to the patient as possible. It has been found that chemotherapy is most effective if several types of drug are given at the same time, even at the risk of more side effects. This is called a 'cocktail' of drugs, and many cocktails are standardized for particular forms of cancer.

Side effects

While it is true that side effects are to be expected, modern chemotherapy is much less likely to cause these than was the case even as recently as the 1980s. Nausea can be controlled by the latest drugs such as ondansetron, with the result that therapy that entailed an overnight stay in hospital can now be given on an outpatient basis.

Hair loss is a feared side effect of chemotherapy. It is sometimes avoidable by the selection of drugs but often it is not. Cancer centres will advise on a temporary wig, but the hair always regrows after therapy.

The major side effects from a medical viewpoint are destruction of the bone marrow, leading to risk of infection, anaemia (see page 265) and bleeding, and damage to the liver and kidneys from the medication. Regular blood tests should detect these problems to allow for an adjustment of dosage or more intensive care in hospital.

Combinations of treatment

Often chemotherapy is one of several types of treatment given for cancer. This is the case in both breast cancer and cancer of the bowel. Surgery removes the obvious tumour and radiotherapy destroys cancers not visible at operation; then chemotherapy destroys deposits of cancer spread elsewhere in the body (metastases).

The future

Many experts believe that future developments in chemotherapy will make it much more specifically targeted to the cancer cells and less toxic elsewhere. This will be achieved by drugs using antibodies to cancerous cells that carry chemotherapeutic drugs with them, or with new forms of chemotherapy that directly target the growth of cancer cells.

KEY-HOLE SURGERY

Surgeons have long been able to look inside the body with a variety of tubes, such as cystoscopes for the bladder and bronchoscopes for the lungs (see page 323). A technique called laparoscopy, which uses a single rigid tube as opposed to flexible tubes, is well established for operations on the prostate gland (see page 120) and in gynaecological surgery for sterilization and inspection of the womb.

The breakthrough leading to key-hole surgery came with the availability of small television cameras that pick up the images from fibreoptic probes guided inside the body. This means that the electronic image could be magnified on to a television screen in full colour and detail, displayed for the surgeon and his assistants. Coupled with miniature instruments and bright illumination, key-hole surgery has rapidly become the method of choice for several common operations and is especially suitable for abdominal ones. The technical term is endoscopic surgery or minimally invasive surgery.

How key-hole surgery is performed

Most key-hole operations require three tubes inserted into the body. One tube carries the lighting and the optical equipment. At present these use fibreoptics, but soon they will have miniature cameras at the tip. The other two are access tubes. These are pushed through the surface and positioned close to the operation site. Once these are in place the surgeon passes the actual operating instruments through the access tubes to probe, cut, sample and staple. These operating instruments have long handles for manipulation; often they are disposable.

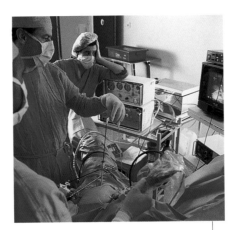

Above: In key-hole surgery the surgeon manipulates the instruments, watching the results on a television monitor.

In abdominal operations, in order to create room to operate, gas (usually carbon dioxide) is pumped inside the abdomen during the operation. Afterwards the gas dissolves harmlessly within the tissues. Some parts of the body are natural cavities, such as the sinuses of the face, so inflation is unnecessary.

Key-hole *versus* conventional surgery

Key-hole surgery is totally different from conventional open surgery, posing a considerable challenge to surgeons. Some traditional procedures do not work well – for example a conventional cut produces so much blood that it obscures vision. Therefore new instruments and methods have been devised to allow cutting with electrical currents (diathermy) or lasers that seal blood vessels as they cut. Conventional stitching with needle and thread is virtually impossible; instead surgeons use stapling instruments, clips or specially designed needles.

Patients benefit from smaller surgical cuts and scars, quicker healing and less time spent in hospital or recovery. This also has economic benefits for hospitals. On the other hand, there are the high costs of training surgeons and of expensive instruments.

Training for key-hole surgery is difficult: surgeons have to learn to look in one direction (the television monitor) while moving the instruments elsewhere. There are sophisticated training workshops to teach the skills. Some people think that the next generation of surgeons will learn the techniques more easily, having grown up with computer games.

Uses of key-hole surgery

The first and still most accepted operation is cholecystectomy, the removal of the gall bladder (see page 186). It is remarkable that this now universal use was first achieved in just 1987. Other abdominal operations are removal of the appendix, removal of part of the bowel and surgery around the stomach. Key-hole techniques are used to repair hernias in the groin (see page 176), operate on the sinuses and even pass small endoscopes into the skull. The benefits of all of these procedures are accurate surgery, minimal cutting and a rapid recovery for the patient.

The future

The fast-developing field of key-hole surgery is being carried along on a wave of enthusiasm. However, it may be that some operations are simply not worth doing through a key hole. For example, a key-hole hernia repair turns a simple, highly effective procedure into a difficult and more hazardous one. As with any new technique, it will take time to reach agreement about situations where key-hole surgery is suitable.

COMPLEMENTARY TREATMENTS

The type and length of treatment depends on the therapy used; the severity of symptoms and whether the condition is acute or chronic; whether the practitioner is performing the therapy or teaching you how to do it yourself; and whether follow-ups are required. Note that some therapies can be used to treat a variety of different conditions. Below are some typical complementary treatments. See page 368 for more detailed information.

Circulatory and respiratory disorders

High blood pressure (see page 40) can in part be controlled by stress reduction methods (see below). Naturopaths can also devise a low-fat, low-sodium, high-fibre diet. Autogenic training is particularly good for dealing with negative emotions that raise blood pressure.

For respiratory disorders homeopaths recommend herbal dilutions like phosphorus to relieve the coughing and breathlessness of bronchitis (see page 59). Acupressure can help the wheezing of asthma (see page 60) if you press on a specific pressure point. Autogenic training can show you how to prevent attacks. Reflexology can relieve symptoms and yoga reduces stress that starts an attack.

Mind, brain and nerve problems

Therapies to reduce stress (see page 76) include using acupuncture to release energy; putting aromatherapy oils in a bath or inhaling them from a bowl of hot water; taking Bach flower remedies such as rock rose to reduce anxiety; using biodynamics to release tension; chakra

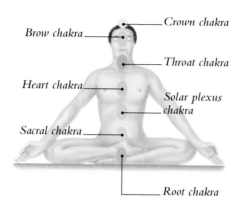

Brow chakra —
Crown chakra
Throat chakra
Heart chakra —
Solar plexus chakra
Sacral chakra —
Root chakra

Above: Chakras are energy centres in the body and are linked to the nervous and endocrine systems.

balancing for relieving energy blocks; and trying Hellerwork to realign the body. Other stress-relievers include massage with oils and creams to help relax the muscles, hypnotherapy, shiatsu-do for tension relief and yoga. Relaxation techniques such as meditation, deep abdominal breathing and progressive muscle relaxation have also proved beneficial.

Other mental and emotional problems can be helped by arts therapies, biodynamics, Chinese herbalism, healing, play therapy, tai chi and yoga.

Urinary and digestive problems

For cystitis (see page 111), nutritional therapists will recommend dietary changes. Herbalists will prescribe infusions to soothe the bladder.

Some stomach problems result from stress, others may be symptomatic of other conditions. For heartburn and indigestion (see pages 178 and 179), Ayurvedics prescribe alterations to lifestyle and diet; naturopaths recommend changes to the diet; both Chinese and Western herbalists offer stomach-calming infusions made with herbs; and nutritional therapists will investigate your diet

and recommend changes to your eating habits. Autogenic training may help with irritable bowel syndrome. For food allergies and intolerances (see page 187), naturopaths can recommend food-elimination diets to ascertain the cause.

Musculo-skeletal problems

Back, joint and muscle pain can be stress related or symptomatic of other conditions. Therapies for pain relief include the Alexander technique, which teaches you to move smoothly so that your body is put under less stress, chiropractic to manipulate joints and vertebrae and massage to relax muscles. Osteopathy, which releases strain in tissues, muscles and joints, is especially good for RSD (see page 256). Rolfing is beneficial for body realignment, shiatsu-do for easing joint pain and yoga for improving muscle tone. Acupuncture, acupressure and auricular therapy can also help to control pain.

Skin disorders

Dry or chapped skin, on its own or as a result of eczema or allergic reactions, can be soothed by creams, ointments and infusions recommended by a Western herbalist. Naturopaths will suggest dietary changes.

Infections

Aromatherapists suggest soothing a sore throat by inhaling steam from a bowl of hot water which contains eucalyptus and sweet thyme oil. For colds and flu, acupressure may alleviate symptoms generally. Chinese herbalists suggest specific infusions to reduce fever and encourage sweating, relieve mucus and ease sore throats, while homeopaths offer remedies that deal with these symptoms or boost the immune system, reducing the chances of future infection. For sinusitis, both Chinese herbalists and homeopaths prescribe remedies to relieve pain and eliminate the underlying infection.

ALTHOUGH ILLNESS IS NEVER ROUTINE, there are circumstances when it is particularly worrying – in the cases of children and the elderly and when someone requires hospital care. The following section contains information about dealing with illness in these circumstances.

The old wisdom

The fundamentals of caring for the sick have not really changed much over the centuries, although the technology and range of medication available have expanded enormously. Sick people still need reassurance during their illness and rest while recovering. Comfort, fluids, light food and amusement are still the cornerstones of care. These are best delivered by carers familiar with the individual who combine compassion with competence, who recognize when the sick person wants company and when not, and when to intervene and when to let nature heal.

Children

We worry about our children at the best of times, but especially when they are unwell. Children are more likely than adults to fall ill repeatedly, so some familiarity with how to nurse them back to health is desirable. The basic principles are not difficult and may even seem common sense, but they are no less important for that. You can expect your children to experience many fevers, pains, episodes of diarrhoea and vomiting and minor injuries and accidents during their childhood. It might be tempting to have a medical opinion each time, but this is not a realistic option nor is it in your child's best interests. The more you can become experienced in dealing with 'routine' illness, the better you will recognize episodes of illness that may be out of the ordinary.

It goes almost without saying that all caring parents naturally fear for their children's health even when logically they realize that serious illness is uncommon. It is hoped that the information about childhood illness here and elsewhere in this book will help you to assess the severity of your child's illness with more confidence.

The elderly

On the whole, most elderly people are able to cope for themselves and remain reasonably active, both physically and mentally. But, like an old car, when one thing goes wrong everything else may go wrong at once. The reason is that the elderly do not have large reserves of stamina and strength to deal with illness. Even though the underlying illness may be relatively mild, such as a urinary infection or a chest

CARING FOR THE SICK

infection, they may very quickly neglect themselves, or they may fall, become confused or be unable to walk. The burden of seeing them through illness then falls on to their carers. Dealing with an elderly person who is ill can be especially draining, but by following basic guidelines you can make a potential crisis less likely and minimize the strain on yourself.

Hospital treatment

Although as a society we are healthier, large numbers of us go into hospital each year following accidents, for investigation or for planned surgery. Increasingly treatment is done on a day case basis, as evolving technology has reduced the need for in-patient care. But no matter how brave people say they are, few really are immune to the anxieties generated by the unfamiliar hospital setting and the sense of vulnerability that comes with being in someone else's hands.

Hospitals run on routines; it is easy for staff to forget that what is familiar for them is an exceptional experience for a patient. This section explains what being a patient entails on a practical and psychological level and describes the basics of care in order to better prepare you for hospital treatment.

Right: A comforting and caring attitude is as important as ever, whatever the wonders of modern medicine. Sweet Dreams by Thomas Brooks (1818–91).

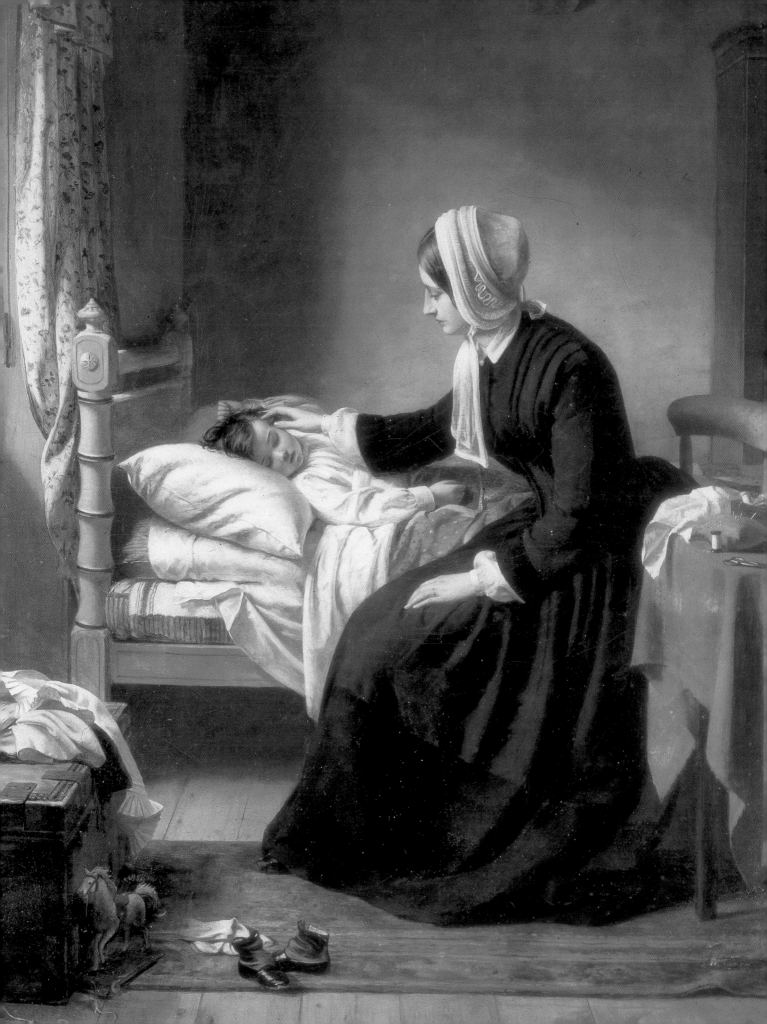

HOSPITALIZATION

Going into hospital is an important life event, regardless of whether it is for the removal of a benign lump or for further investigation of worrying, puzzling symptoms. Doctors and nurses are all now trained to be aware of the psychological effects on patients of hospitalization, but the following should be borne in mind.

Psychological factors

Entering hospital requires a considerable degree of trust. It is normal to have mixed feelings: apprehension, uncertainty and relief that things are going to happen. People can rapidly adopt what has been called the 'sick role' – acting the invalid, becoming passive and focusing on feelings of ill health. Enjoy this while you can. Modern speedy medical procedures mean you are likely to be back in your own home more rapidly than you expected.

Practicalities

The hospital staff will tell you what you need by way of clothing, washing equipment and so on. Bring a list of your medication and allergies. It may be comforting to have a relative escort you and remain there to listen to what the doctor or surgeon says. It is easy to forget things when you are in a state of anxiety.

Tell the hospital staff if you are on the contraceptive Pill or if you have had a problem with blood clots, for example, a deep vein thrombosis or a pulmonary embolism (see pages 53 and 69). The contraceptive Pill increases very slightly the risk of thrombosis, so you should stop taking it four weeks before major (abdominal, chest, heart or hip) surgery. Discuss this further with your doctor.

Being admitted

This is a formal procedure. The hospital staff have to know that you are who they think you are. They will check your age and address and make a note of your next of kin. A nurse will take a nursing history. This is a thorough document which includes social information, food preferences, nursing preferences, how you like to be addressed and an exploration of your feelings about your stay in hospital.

You will be medically admitted by a junior doctor. This involves reviewing the problems that have led to your admission, double-checking medication and asking about things that may affect treatment, such as previous thrombosis or allergies. You will be examined and this will possibly be very thorough, especially if you are being admitted for tests. You will probably be re-examined by other members of the medical team and at some point by the consultant.

Teaching hospitals

These are where both nursing and medical students learn their jobs, so students will be involved in some of your care. It is often a precondition of admission to such hospitals that you agree to this arrangement. If you have objections you should make this clear beforehand.

Tests

For procedures involving a general anaesthetic, some patients will require an ECG of their heart (see page 48), tests to check for anaemia, liver and kidney function to exclude diabetes and possibly a chest X-ray (see page 316). More detailed tests will be performed depending on the reason for the admission, for example scans or special blood tests (see page 322).

If you have been admitted because of a serious medical problem such as a suspected heart attack (see page 45) or a severe chest infection, it is normal to have an intravenous drip. This involves passing a hollow needle into a vein, normally in the arm, securing it in place, then running in fluid or blood. The reason for this is that you may require sudden urgent treatment with drugs directly into the blood stream via the drip, or there may be a risk of sudden bleeding or a drop in blood pressure requiring rapid administration of blood and other fluids.

Consent for procedures

All medical procedures require your informed consent. This means you agree that the procedures or surgery have been explained to you, including risks and side effects, and that you accept these. Simply entering hospital implies consent to many routine procedures. Before surgery a doctor, usually the junior doctor, will explain the procedure and ask for your written agreement. Ask questions about what is proposed until you feel satisfied.

Below: The inevitable anxieties of being in hospital can be reduced by discussion and explanation.

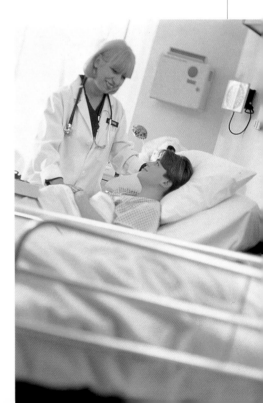

Preparation for surgery

You must not eat or drink for at least six hours before a planned operation under general anaesthetic. This is a very strict rule because eating increases the chance of vomiting during surgery and breathing stomach contents into the lungs, which is a very serious event.

The anaesthetist will visit you to satisfy himself that you are fit for surgery. The area to be operated on will be marked and possibly shaved. You will probably be given premedication – mild sedatives – by injection or tablet. These also reduce saliva flow during the operation.

Day surgery is increasingly the norm. You will be advised about whether you need to fast and any other preparations you should make, for example having a laxative to clear the bowel for bowel operations, and whether you need an escort to see you home.

Recovery from surgery

After surgery, you will come round in a recovery room where staff will monitor your blood pressure and breathing and check for any bleeding. Once you are stable they will transfer you to a ward unless you have had major surgery, in which case you will go into intensive care (see page 336) for a while.

Even after undergoing just a minor operation it is normal to keep a drip in place until you can swallow – usually just a few hours. After major surgery doctors will keep a drip going until you are out of the danger period.

Very often after major surgery you will have a urinary catheter, which drains urine directly from the bladder, and probably other tubes draining fluid from the operation site. Most tubes can be removed within a few days.

Preventing thrombosis

Blood clots in the legs and lungs are an important hazard after major surgery,

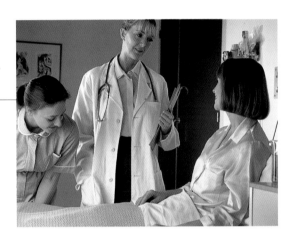

Right: Reassurance and explanation are aids to a patient's recovery; it is important that medical staff do not overlook this fact.

especially orthopaedic (for example for a hip replacement) and abdominal surgery. Therefore you may find that you are given compression stockings to wear to stop blood pooling in the leg veins, and injections of heparin to reduce the tendency of the blood to clot.

Pain relief

The many techniques include nerve blocks to provide long-lasting anaesthesia after the operation, epidural anaesthetics, painkillers in drips and syringes and of course painkillers by mouth. Be sure to let the staff know if you are in pain – pain relief is an important component of your care and enhances recovery.

The routine of the ward

You will be reviewed frequently by the nursing staff, so that they can check if you are comfortable and deal with medication, feeding, special diets, wound care and any problems you are having. Once or twice a day a junior doctor will review you, examining you and, in consultation with senior colleagues, adjusting medication, removing tubes and so on. You will probably see the consultant only once or twice; he will review the technicalities of your case, check the surgery and consider the results of tests.

Ward life tends to start early in the day

and finish early and it can be extremely wearing as a result of constant interruptions, emergencies and noises. For this reason many patients, once mobile and comfortable, actually look forward to leaving hospital.

Leaving hospital

You should have a clear idea of what has been done to you, what medication you need, when stitches need to be removed, what follow-up visits are required and any special instructions during recovery with respect to activity, diet and resuming sex. Many hospitals provide leaflets covering these topics.

Being a patient

Patients can expect to be treated with dignity and to be given clear and detailed explanations. Most authorities believe that keeping patients informed improves cooperation and reduces stress. Sharing the often inevitable uncertainties of medical treatment also improves patient satisfaction and incidentally reduces complaints if things go wrong or do not go as you would have wished. However everyone is an individual: some people want to be told everything, others nothing. Hospital staff are not mind-readers, so you should tell them if there is something causing you concern.

CARING FOR CHILDREN AT HOME

Illness is a normal part of childhood, and parents should get to know how to deal with the child who has a minor illness and when to call for help. The following guidelines apply to children with illness in the developed world where, thanks to immunization, good nutrition and good hygiene, serious illness is relatively uncommon.

Give comfort . . .

Ill children, even more than ill adults, want comfort, help and the knowledge that someone is at hand. Simply being there for your sick child is a major factor in relieving her discomfort.

You are the one best placed to know your child and how she responds to illness. Perhaps your child makes a fuss about being ill, groans, moans and demands attention. Or perhaps you have a child who curls up in a ball on the sofa and tries to make the best of things. As well as providing revealing insights into your child's character, it is important to know your child's normal reaction to illness as a means of judging when she is 'unusually' ill. When doctors talk about a parent's instincts, this is what they have in mind, and a wise doctor will take seriously a parent's instinct about illness.

. . . but do not make a drama out of illness

You would not be a responsible parent if you did not worry about your child being ill. However, children pick up parental panic and soon learn if illness gets them treats and extra attention. It is not in your child's long-term interest for her to learn that minor illness has compensations. Childhood illness in the developed world is usually no more than a nuisance and an inconvenience, to be handled with care and concern, but without going overboard on sympathy. Of course you will comfort, hug and reassure your sick child, but it is a mistake to let her see you worry over every trivial symptom.

Reduce fever

A high temperature is not an illness in itself, although parents often believe it is. Fever is no more than a symptom of illness, probably an infection, but on its own it does not allow a doctor to make a diagnosis (see page 276). Parents must develop confidence to cope with a feverish child and to allow time for other symptoms of illness to appear.

In the meantime, give paracetamol syrup or ibuprofen syrup (but not to asthmatics) in a dose appropriate to the child's age. These help regardless of the cause and can be given without masking other symptoms. Bear in mind that fever often persists despite medication and that fevers tend to rise at night.

Keep your child cool by removing layers of clothing. In summer leave her in a tee shirt in the shade; in winter put her in just enough clothes so she feels comfortable. The younger the child the more important it is not to let her get overheated, otherwise there is a risk of a fit (see page 309). If an infant remains very hot, cool her with a fan or sponge her brow with tepid water.

Give fluids

Give increased fluids, such as fruit cordials, low-sugar fizzy drinks allowed to go flat or water. A sick child should drink 1–2 litres/1¾–3½ pints a day depending on her size, and she should take small, frequent sips rather than large quantities all at once. Avoid milk and very sweet fizzy drinks, which distend the stomach and which the child is more likely to vomit. For babies there are specially formulated salt and sugar drinks, available from your pharmacist. Encourage your child to drink even if she is reluctant and especially if she has a fever or diarrhoea.

Do not worry about eating

Going off food is a basic symptom of illness. Save yourself frustration by recognizing this and not even bothering to serve up a tempting morsel. If your child is hungry, offer her a light snack such as bread, pasta, a biscuit or some soft fruit. If she can cope with that, you can give her something more substantial, but take it slowly and be prepared if a child who manages one bite of biscuit vomits up a rice pudding. Children will not starve through missing meals for a few days.

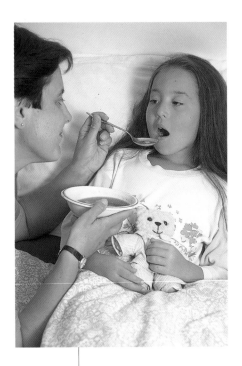

Above: Starting to eat again is a reliable sign that your sick child is recovering.

Let your child rest

Being ill takes energy: the child's body pours resources into fighting an infection and has less energy left over for the usual childhood mayhem. Brothers and sisters should leave their sick sibling alone, and if the child simply wants to sleep just let her. On the other hand, encourage a sick child to get up, to wash and to go to the toilet, perhaps with your help.

There will be times when an unwell child suddenly appears full of energy and begins to rush around; do not be fooled. Let her get it out of her system then encourage her to calm down again. It is especially common for a child to appear well again first thing in the morning only to wilt as the day goes on. So do not abandon your care on the basis of a single good hour.

Bed is not necessarily best

There is no reason for a sick child to stay in bed if she feels comfortable elsewhere.

Beds get hot, sheets get twisted; she may find it difficult to get out in a hurry to be sick or to go to the toilet. And it gets boring. Lying on a sofa is often more comfortable and convenient, and a carer can keep an eye on the child while going about other tasks.

Deal with boredom

For the first couple of days an unwell child will not need amusing, but she is likely to get bored as she starts to feel better. Some children will happily amuse themselves with books, magazines and games. Others prefer to watch television or a video. The healing powers of Disney are an under-researched area of medicine; half an hour giggling at cartoons can work wonders.

Giving medicine

If a doctor has decided that your child needs medication, you should give it to her. Drug manufacturers make their med-

icines palatable for children with sweeteners and flavourings – banana or strawberry are apparently guaranteed winners. Some children reject certain antibiotics but will accept others. Tell your doctor about this because often the exact choice of antibiotic does not matter and it makes sense to prescribe an alternative that the child prefers. You can disguise flavours by diluting medicines, mixing them in a cold drink or hiding a tablet in jam, but check the drug information leaflet first to be sure this is allowed.

What should you do with the child who refuses medication? You must try again and then again. Bribery? Offering a treat? Why not? But medication is not a game and illness is not a diversion, so you may have to insist she takes her medicine. If it all keeps ending in tears and tantrums, discuss it with your doctor. There may be another option or your doctor may judge that the child has had enough of a course and can stop.

Babies

Babies are different: they cannot tell you how they feel, they become ill more quickly and with fewer symptoms and they recover faster. It is entirely reasonable to seek advice about a sick baby, even if the only feature is vomiting, a rash, fever or constant crying. Your doctor can examine and reassure, prescribing medication only if it is really necessary. Your baby will have several minor illnesses during her first year of life, each of which is an opportunity to learn how your baby reacts during 'normal' illness so you become confident in recognizing when your baby is more than usually unwell (see page 12).

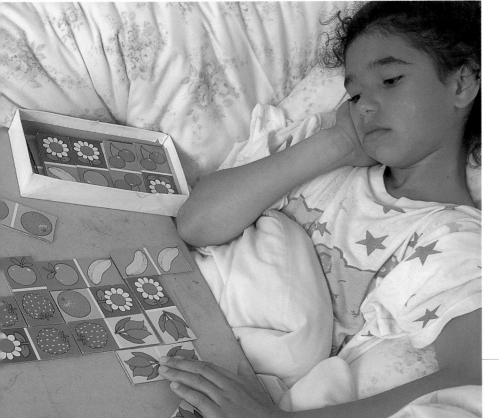

Below: Illness can be boring as well as unpleasant. Your child will welcome amusements while she recovers.

CARING FOR THE ELDERLY

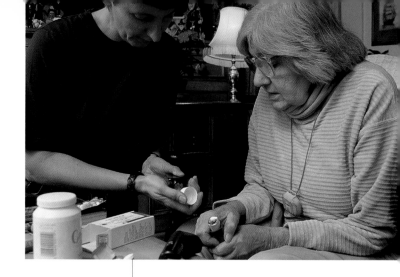

Above: In the elderly, 'a pill for every ill' can end up as a confusing array of drugs, calling for close supervision.

Unprecedented numbers of people in the developed world are now surviving into their 80s and beyond. Despite all you read about illness and dementia in the elderly, the majority do cope, with support from family, friends and care agencies.

This is the time of life when things can go seriously wrong and may do so very suddenly, the most common problems being chest pains, bleeding, strokes and immobility. While many illnesses show obvious symptoms, elderly people may have significant illness without any dramatic signs, although they may experience breathlessness, dizziness, falls or confusion or go off their food.

However, minor illness is still more likely than a serious one. Carers become familiar with an elderly person's normal health and mobility, allowing them to judge whether the person is significantly off colour. In this respect care of the elderly is similar to that of sick children.

Factors contributing to illness
The following may directly or indirectly cause illness in the elderly.

Accidents These are common. Elderly people become giddy, tripping and falling for no apparent reason. If, after a fall, an elderly person cannot walk or appears in pain, have him checked over for fractures. As a preventive measure, reduce the chances of accidents by making his home safer (see page 28).

Medication The elderly often take several medications, increasing the possibility of reactions to medication and accidental overdose. If an elderly person appears confused or falls, medication is one of the first things to consider.

Poor diet There is a temptation as one gets older to eat less and more simply, with a diet low in iron, protein, vitamins and fibre from fresh fruit and vegetables. Combined with lack of mobility, this can lead to malnutrition.

Lifestyle Although many elderly people keep active and interested, others allow themselves to become reclusive and take little exercise. This can degenerate into an isolated existence cut off from social activities, leading to and worsening the inevitable stiffness of old age. Such people may occupy only one room in a house which, through habit or lack of money, they keep inadequately heated.

Remaining at home: decisions and guidelines
A decision has to be made about whether a sick elderly person can stay at home. A few questions need answering before a decision is made. If he can cope, some guidelines must be followed to ensure that he is given the best care possible.

Is he safe? Critical factors are whether he can get to a toilet, prepare food, keep warm and not fall. Many communities and families can provide temporary home care for a week or two during recovery. Otherwise hospital admission is unavoidable (a so-called 'social admission'), even though the underlying medical problem may not be serious.

Will he take his medication? Another factor to consider is whether he can cope with medication at home – remembering, for example, to take tablets every eight hours. This can be made easier by drawing up a list or using a medication holder that holds the day's medication. The person should also be able to recognize if he is becoming more unwell and be capable of summoning help if this were the case.

Taking fluid Just as with children, it is important for the elderly to drink more fluids when unwell. They should have at least 3 litres/5 pints a day – more if they have a fever or diarrhoea. Dehydration in the elderly is difficult to be certain about, but you should suspect it if the person becomes more confused, passes little and concentrated urine, and has a dry tongue and sunken eyes.

Taking food Loss of appetite is inevitable during illness, so high-carbohydrate drinks that will provide a lot of energy in a small quantity are advisable. There are also many liquid feeds that can completely supply necessary nutrition during a prolonged illness.

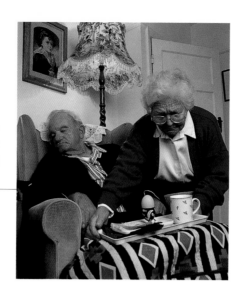

Right: The sick elderly person needs warmth and light, and nourishing food with plenty of fluids.

Rest A sick elderly person will naturally want to doze and will not feel inclined to do anything. Simply going to the toilet can be a major effort. It also takes longer for an elderly person to recover from even a minor illness. A cold or chest infection that a younger person recovers from within a week may leave an elderly person feeling debilitated for a month, without signifying any serious complication.

Warmth Body temperature control becomes poor in the elderly. Keep the house warm – 18–21°C/65–70°F is reasonable but be guided by the individual's preferences. It is vital to keep a good temperature in the evening by leaving heating on, because if an elderly person falls in a cold room during the night and is unable to move it could lead to hypothermia.

Amusement Illness is as boring at 90 as it is at 9. Television, radio and magazines can pass long and uncomfortable hours. Buy a daily newspaper as time disorientation can occur very quickly during illness.

Bed rest It takes only a few hours of resting heavily in bed for the skin to break down, so encourage the elderly person to sit in a chair. This is better both for the skin and for draining the lungs if there is a heart or chest problem. Resting in bed also leads to constipation (see page 171), a common problem anyway in the elderly.

Some elderly people find it more comfortable to sleep in a chair covered with blankets rather than in a bed, but they must keep warm during the night.

Aids Temporary aids can make all the difference in allowing someone to stay at home. Some of the aids available include a commode, soft bedding and air mattresses to reduce the chance of bedsores, raises placed under chair legs to make it easier to rise from a sitting position, meals on wheels, syringe drivers which supply medication continuously through the skin (especially useful for controlling severe pain) and incontinence devices such as pads and catheters.

Skilled help for the patient

It can be difficult to care for an elderly person who appears demanding and critical of the help they are given. While professional helpers are used to this, it can be extremely difficult for relatives. Try to accept that it is the illness causing this and discuss how you feel with other helpers you meet.

However devoted a helper you may be, you might need assistance from a district nurse to deal with dressings and bedsores. Call a doctor if you are in any way concerned about the condition of an elderly person in your care, because his symptoms may be minimal despite serious illness. It is also reasonable to ask for reassessment if the patient fails to improve within a few days, always remembering that full recovery can take a number of weeks.

Long-term care

Advances in medical care mean that large numbers of the elderly now survive with chronic disabling conditions. Examples are following strokes (see page 82), chronic bronchitis (see page 59) and severe arthritis (see page 244). This puts a great physical and psychological burden on their carers.

In coping with this you need to:

♦ *Have a routine – daily, weekly, monthly*
♦ *Get home aid assessment for showers seats, grab handles and stair lifts*
♦ *Investigate other services available, e.g. meals on wheels, district nurses and physiotherapists.*
♦ *See what government benefits apply, both for the individual and for you as a carer*
♦ *Let professionals know if the elderly person's condition changes*
♦ *Arrange respite care to give yourself a break*

In the United Kingdom these facilities are accessed via social services and the patient's doctor. Hospitals often provide a day centre to give both you and your elderly person a rest.

Guilt

This is normal for a thoughtful carer to experience. It may arise through your own feelings of inadequacy at the level of care you can provide, resentment at the demands made by the elderly person and how responsibilities encroach on your own life. Coping with a demented but otherwise well elderly person is draining. You should explore all means of having a break and consider long-term institutional care if the burdens are affecting your own physical and emotional health.

ALTHOUGH FIRST AID cannot be entirely learnt from books, you can learn certain basic techniques to deal with minor injuries and health problems. Anyone should be capable of dealing with minor cuts, wounds and burns, for example.

When it comes to skills such as artificial respiration, there is no substitute for proper training but there may be circumstances where it is better to have a go than not to do anything. Even a little knowledge of first aid will give you a confidence which will communicate itself to the casualty. That comfort alone is very worthwhile.

This section will give you some practical guidance for more common problems. It is not a complete first aid manual. For that, and especially to learn the physical techniques of resuscitation, enrol on a first aid course.

The principles of first aid

The important principles in administering first aid in any situation are as follows:

- *Do not endanger yourself*
- *Assess the situation*
- *Protect a casualty from further harm*
- *Attend to the most serious problem first*
- *Support life where possible*
- *Get help if necessary*

Do not endanger yourself Do not go into hazardous situations without thinking or without proper equipment. At fires, stay away; similarly, beware of exposure to chemical spillages and fumes. At a road traffic accident, put up hazard signs to keep other vehicles clear. If someone is drowning, be sure that you can stand the cold and swim strongly enough before attempting to help the victim.

Assess the situation Can you deal with the situation alone, or is your most useful action to call for help? Are there any people around who can assist? You could organize them to comfort the casualty, make dressings or go for help.

Protect a casualty from further harm Help those people who can move by themselves into a comfortable position, away from fire or fumes and so on. Otherwise do not move anyone unless it is essential for their further safety. If someone is unconscious, place them in the recovery position (see page 352), unless there is a possibility that they have a neck or spinal injury.

FIRST AID

Attend to the most serious problem first Check each casualty for breathing and pulse – if absent, the person will need resuscitation (see page 353) (unless obviously dead). Then deal with people who are unconscious, bleeding heavily, choking, breathless or who have fractures and so on. Finally, deal with the minor cuts and bruises and those who are emotionally shocked.

Support life where possible Give resuscitation (see page 353) until help arrives; it is for healthcare professionals to decide when efforts are hopeless. You may have to balance the risk of moving someone with a possible neck injury against the need to resuscitate.

Get help Many minor injuries can be dealt with perfectly well by first aid. You may need help for a fuller assessment, more intensive treatment or transfer to hospital. Call for help if in any doubt; do not attempt first aid beyond your capabilities or confidence unless the situation is absolutely desperate, in which case it is better to have a go rather than leave someone to their fate.

Right: It is reassuring, and potentially life saving, to learn a few basic first aid techniques. A painting by Issac Koedyck (Koedijck) depicting a barber surgeon tending a peasant's foot, c. 1650.

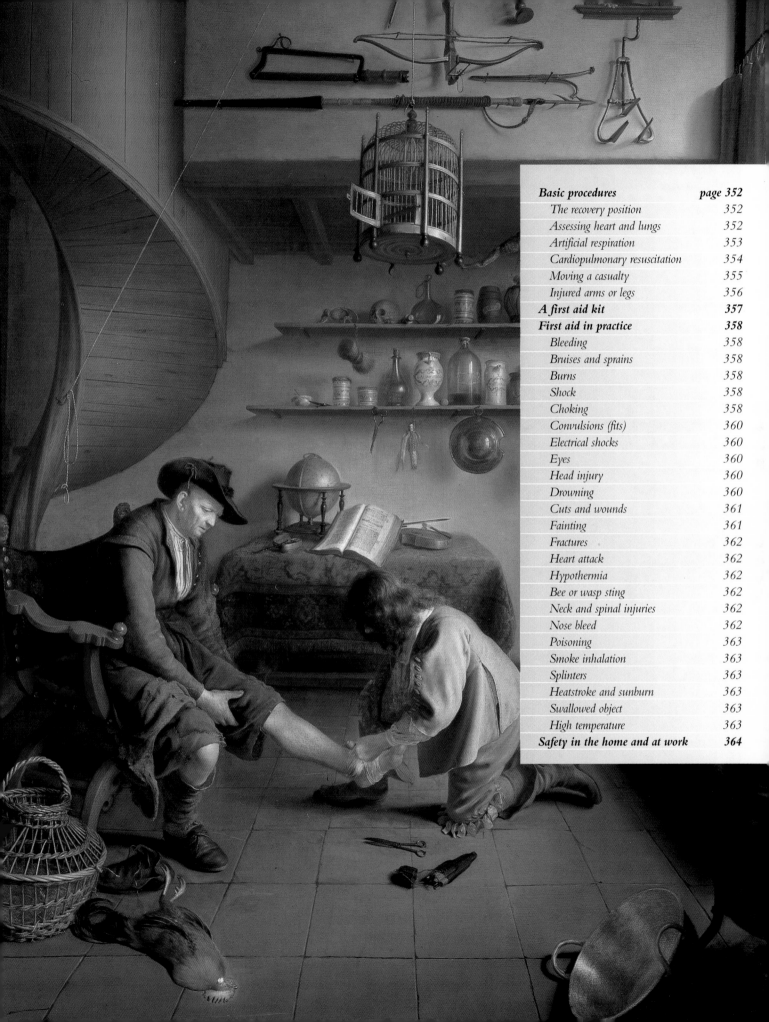

BASIC PROCEDURES

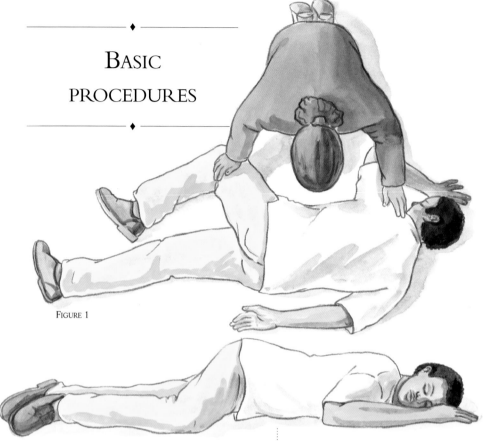

FIGURE 1

FIGURE 2

THE RECOVERY POSITION

Purpose: To prevent an unconscious or drowsy person from inhaling vomit; to allow drainage of material from the mouth. It is not necessary for someone who is conscious and who can move into a comfortable position.

WARNING: Do not use if there is the possibility of a neck or spinal injury.

To place someone in the recovery position, first roll the person on to his front (Figure 1). Turn his face to one side, resting against that hand. Place the other arm down his side (Figure 2).

> *To assess heart and lungs, check* **ABC:**
> **A**IRWAY
> **B**REATHING
> **C**IRCULATION

ASSESSING HEART AND LUNGS

Purpose: To make sure the casualty's heart and lungs are working. Check 'ABC': airway, breathing, circulation.

Airway (throat, windpipe)
Look for and clear away vomit, fluid, food, foreign body or a swallowed tongue. Tilt the chin upward.

Breathing
Check if the casualty's chest is moving and feel for breath. If he is not breathing start artificial respiration (see right).

Circulation
See if the heart is beating by feeling with two fingers for a pulse in the carotid artery in the neck (or in the inner arm above the elbow in a baby – the brachial pulse).

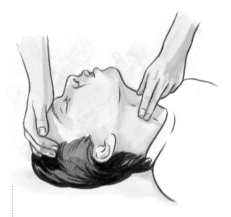

FIGURE 3

To check for a pulse in an adult or child, first feel for the Adam's apple. Move your fingers to one side and press gently over the artery (Figure 3). If no pulse is felt after ten seconds, assume the heart has stopped and start cardio-pulmonary resuscitation (see page 354).

ARTIFICIAL RESPIRATION (MOUTH-TO-MOUTH RESUSCITATION)

♦

Purpose: To breathe for the casualty.

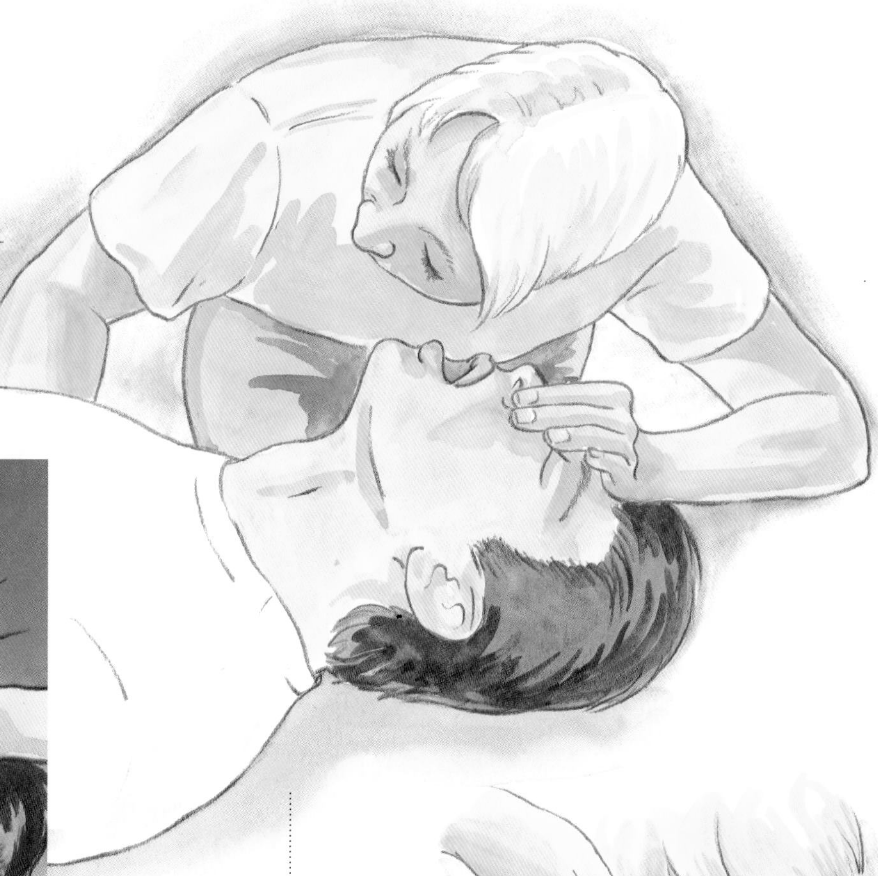

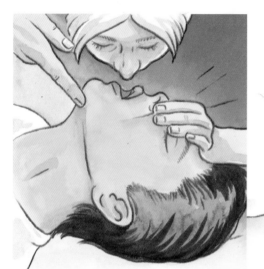

FIGURE 4

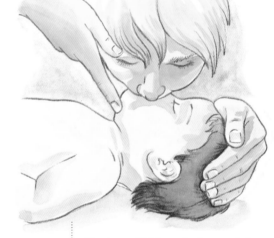

FIGURE 5

To give artificial respiration to an adult or child over the age of one year, keep the casualty on his back. Clear the airway, tilt back the chin and pinch his nostrils shut. Place your mouth over his and blow in for two seconds at a time (Figure 4). His chest should rise; if it does not, look again for an obstruction. Remove your mouth; the chest should fall (Figure 5). Repeat. Keep checking the pulse; if absent start cardiopulmonary resuscitation (see page 354).

FIGURE 6

To give artificial respiration to a baby less than one year old, keep the baby on her back. Clear the airway and tilt back the chin, as for an adult. Place your mouth over the baby's nose and mouth. Breathe into her nose and mouth (Figure 6) then let the baby's chest fall, allowing three seconds for this process of breathing into the baby and letting her chest fall. Keep checking for circulation, or else begin cardiopulmonary resuscitation (see page 355), giving one breath every five heart compressions.

CARDIOPULMONARY RESUSCITATION (CPR)

◆

Purpose: To keep the blood pumping if the heart has stopped. It always has to be combined with artificial respiration (see page 353), hence the name cardiopulmonary resuscitation (CPR).

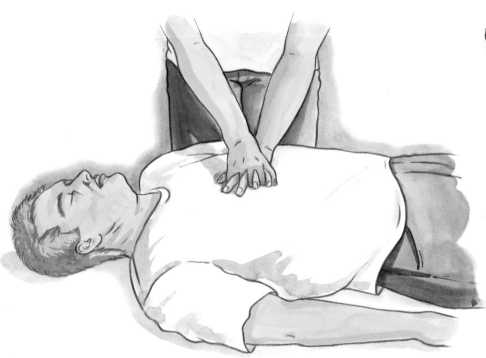

FIGURE 7

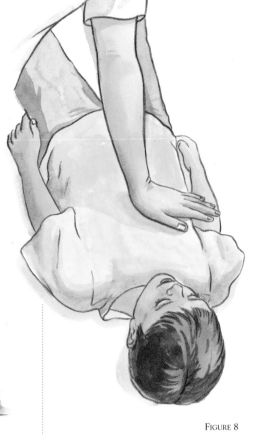

FIGURE 8

To administer CPR to an adult or an older child, keep the casualty on his back. Kneel over him, place the heel of one hand over the lower breastbone, place your other hand on top (Figure 7). With your arms straight, press down 4–5 cm/1½–2 in firmly at a rate of about 100 compressions per minute. Give 15 compressions, then 2 breaths and keep repeating. Check for a pulse after the first minute (see page 352) then every few minutes, until help arrives or the heart restarts.

For CPR in a child aged between one and seven years, position the child on his back and kneel over him. Place one hand over the lower breastbone (Figure 8). Using the heel of your hand, press the breastbone down to one-third of the depth of the chest at a rate of about 100 compressions per minute. Give one breath through the mouth every five compressions.

MOVING A CASUALTY

◆

Purpose: Move a casualty only if it is necessary to get the person out of danger and not at all if there is a possibility of fracture to the person's neck or spine. Take care not to strain your own back – if in doubt wait for help and equipment.

If the casualty has been electrocuted, do not touch her until the electricity has been turned off at the mains (see Electrical shocks, page 360).

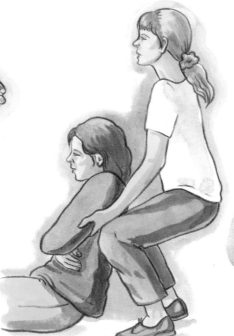

FIGURE 9

For CPR *in a baby less than one year old,* place two fingers over the lower breastbone (Figure 9). Press the breastbone down to one-third of the depth of the chest at a rate of about 100 compressions per minute. Give one breath (through the nose and mouth) every five compressions.

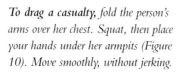

FIGURE 10

To drag a casualty, fold the person's arms over her chest. Squat, then place your hands under her armpits (Figure 10). Move smoothly, without jerking.

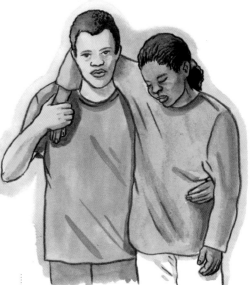

FIGURE 11

To support a casualty to walk, stand on her injured side – but if the arm is injured, stand on the opposite side. Place her arm across your shoulder and hold her hand. Place your other arm across her back at waist level, holding her clothing (Figure 11). Walk with small steps, starting off with your inner foot.

INJURED ARMS OR LEGS

◆

Keep the limb comfortable and supported until help arrives. Move it as little as possible, but check for bleeding from cuts. The injured limb will swell so do not hesitate to cut away anything that might constrict the swelling.

An injured arm

Purpose: To keep an injured arm or shoulder immobile and supported. Gently place the injured arm across the person's chest and improvise a support using bandages, clothing or a towel, tied behind the neck. In the case of an injured elbow do not use a sling if it is too sore to bend; instead keep it in the position of the least pain, tied against the body if possible.

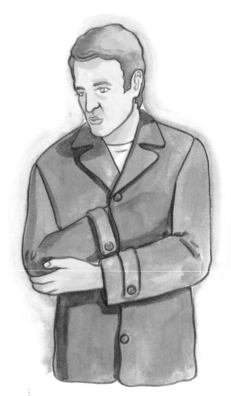

FIGURE 14

A sling can usually be improvised if a triangular bandage is not available. One method is to tuck the hand of the injured arm into a buttoned shirt or jacket at chest height (Figure 14).

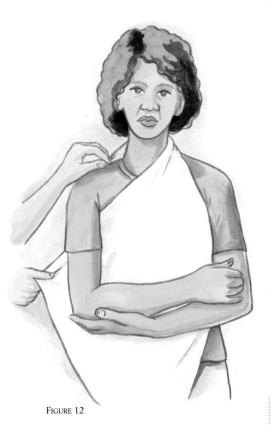

FIGURE 12

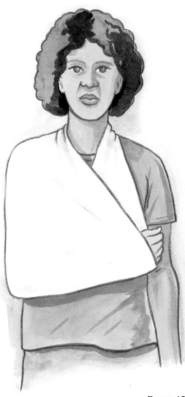

FIGURE 13

To make a sling using a triangular bandage, run one point of the triangle over the shoulder and around the neck (Figure 12).
Lift the lowest point of the bandage up over the forearm to meet the end at the shoulder. Knot these ends together just below the level of the shoulder. Tuck in the third point at the end of the elbow (Figure 13) and secure with a safety pin.

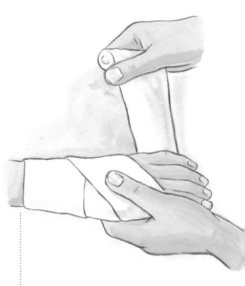

FIGURE 15

To bandage a hand, for holding pads to control bleeding or for support after a sprain, begin at the wrist (Figure 15).

An injured leg

Purpose: To keep the leg immobile in the position of the least pain and slightly elevated to reduce swelling.

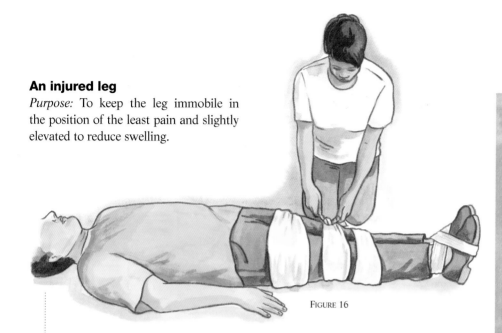

FIGURE 16

To immobilize a leg, *lay the casualty down. Move the limb only if it is essential for comfort. Place a support under the injured part, for example rolled-up clothing or a towel. Bandage the injured leg against the good one (Figure 16) if the ambulance is going to be delayed.*

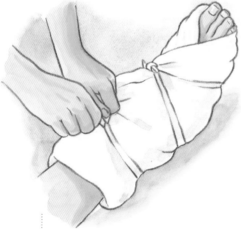

FIGURE 17

For an injured foot and ankle, *use a piece of cloth or a flat cushion secured with narrow bandages for support (Figure 17), until you can get professional help.*

A FIRST AID KIT

Keep a well-labelled kit where it is most likely to be used, for example the kitchen, the garage, the car or at work. Select items according to common sense. If you live in town, you probably need enough only for minor injuries; if you live, work or drive somewhere remote, keep a more comprehensive kit. Kits for public places such as offices and factories must meet approved standards – discuss with your health and safety representative or supplier. Replace things you use immediately, and discard anything that is out of date.

DRESSINGS
♦

Sticking plaster *of various sizes*
Sterile dressings *of various sizes (non-stick if possible) – to cover wounds*
Gauze pads *– for absorbency over cuts and burns*
Adhesive tape *– to fix pads and bandages*
Rolls of bandage *of various widths to hold dressings in place and support limbs*
Tubular bandages *plus applicator for injured fingers*
Triangular bandage *– to support an injured limb, bandage the head or pad large wounds*
Eye pad
Swabs *– for cleaning wounds*
Cotton wool *– for padding and washing, but not to be used directly on wounds*

MEDICATION
♦

Antiseptic cream *– for cuts*
Antiseptic liquid *– to clean wounds and skin*
Antihistamine cream *– for insect bites and stings*
Paracetamol tablets *(liquid for children), or* ***ibuprofen*** *– for fever or pain relief*

EQUIPMENT
♦

Tweezers *– for splinters*
Thermometer
Eye bath
Disposable gloves
Safety scissors
Safety pins

FIRST AID IN PRACTICE — WHAT TO DO WHEN

BLEEDING

Assuming this is from a minor injury, raise the bleeding limb or lay the patient down if the wound is on the body. Apply firm pressure over the bleeding point for two to four minutes. Once the bleeding has stopped, do not disturb the clot. Cover with a clean dressing.

Beware of the following: bleeding from a deep wound; arterial bleeding (spurts, bright red); heavy bleeding; the victim becoming pale and faint with rapid pulse. In such cases apply pressure or a pad to the bleeding point. Get the casualty to hospital immediately.

BRUISES AND SPRAINS

The swelling that accompanies these injuries is from bleeding under the skin and fluid in the tissues.

For bruises cool the area with an ice pack – a pack of frozen peas is ideal. Keep it there for ten to twenty minutes to reduce further bleeding under the skin. No other treatment is necessary.

A sprain is a pulled ligament – usually of the ankle or knee. The area is tender and you may not be able to walk properly. Carry out 'RICE': rest, ice, compression, elevation (see box, above right).

See a doctor for severe bruising, or if you cannot put weight on a sprain, since you may have torn the ligament.

---

*Carry out **RICE**:*

♦ **R**EST: *Stop walking or playing sport as soon as possible*
♦ **I**CE: *Put the injured part in ice-cold water for ten to twenty minutes, or apply an ice pack – a pack of frozen vegetables is perfect*
♦ **C**OMPRESSION: *After cooling, apply a compression bandage to reduce further swelling*
♦ **E**LEVATION: *Keep the injured part slightly raised for several hours after the injury*

BURNS

Remove the source of heat, i.e. fire or hot liquids. Remove hot clothing from the skin carefully – but do not attempt to remove anything that appears stuck to the skin. Cool the burn with cold water for 15 minutes to reduce tissue damage. Cover with a dry, non-stick dressing. Do not burst any blisters. If the burns are extensive, give the person drinks and keep him lying down and warm until help arrives.

Seek medical advice for any burn that is larger than 5 cm²/2 sq in, for severe blistering, charred skin and burns from chemicals or electricity.

SHOCK

Medical shock is a collapse of blood pressure caused by bleeding, heart attack, poisoning, burns or dehydration. Symptoms include cold clammy skin, weak pulse, feeling faint, going unconscious, blue lips and difficulty breathing. Lay the casualty down with her legs raised and keep warm. Do not give food or fluids. Be prepared to resuscitate until help arrives.

CHOKING

Food or foreign objects may stick in the throat, obstructing breathing. The victim may be coughing or clutching his throat, or has collapsed and looks blue.

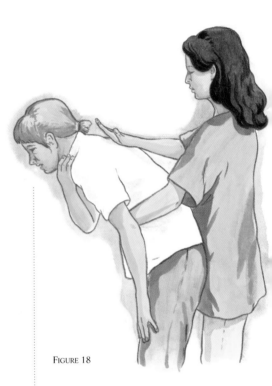

FIGURE 18

For choking adults and older children, first try to pull out the obstruction if it is obvious and can be done fairly easily. Get the person to bend forward and to try to cough. Slap firmly between the shoulder blades up to five times to try to dislodge the obstruction (Figure 18). If this does not work, perform the Heimlich manoeuvre (see far right).

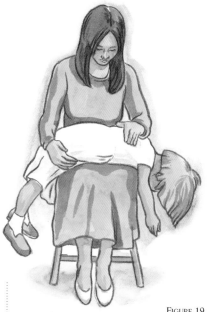

FIGURE 19

Lay a choking toddler face down over your lap (Figure 19) and give five quick slaps between the shoulders. If this fails, try the Heimlich manoeuvre (see right), then more back slaps if still choking. Keep checking if the obstruction has been dislodged and can be easily removed.

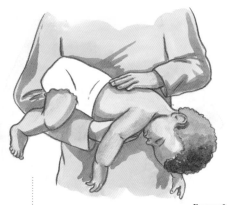

FIGURE 20

For a choking baby less than one year old, lay the baby face down across your knees or arm, head well down (Figure 20). Give up to five firm slaps to her back; see if the obstruction can then be removed easily. Otherwise, turn the baby on her back, head still down. With two fingers, push firmly several times over the lower breastbone. Repeat as necessary.

For victims of any age, give resuscitation if required until help arrives.

Performing the Heimlich manoeuvre

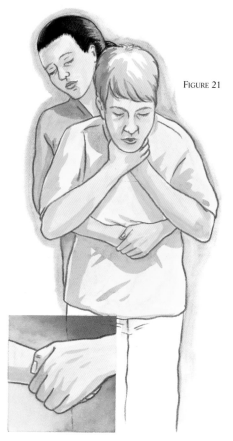

FIGURE 21

FIGURE 22

For the Heimlich manoeuvre in an adult, stand behind the person who is choking. Place your hands over her upper abdomen, just below the bottom of the breastbone (Figure 21). Link your hands and have one thumb pushing against her abdomen (Figure 22). Pull sharply in and upward five times, then slap her back. Repeat if necessary if the obstruction has not been dislodged.

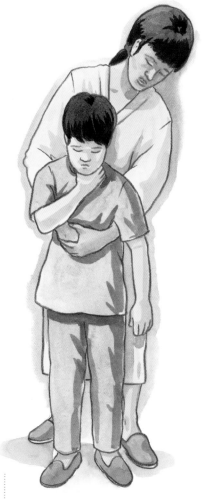

FIGURE 23

For the Heimlich manoeuvre in a child aged one to seven years, stand or kneel behind the child. Place your fist over the lower breastbone, your other hand over it. Thrust firmly in and upward five times, then slap her back. If there is no success, reposition your hands lower, over the upper abdomen (Figure 23). Give five thrusts upward, then slap her back. Repeat if necessary.

WARNING: Do not use the Heimlich manoeuvre on a child less than one year old.

CONVULSIONS (FITS)

Recognize a fit by the following symptoms:

♦ *Collapse*
♦ *A few seconds of clenched teeth and muscles, followed by jerking movements for several minutes*
♦ *Finally, drowsiness and a gradual return to consciousness*
♦ *Children may be very hot*

Lay the individual down; put him into the recovery position. Do not otherwise interfere. Do not put anything in his mouth, even though he might bite his tongue. Cool a hot child (see High temperature, page 363). Take the person to hospital if it is a first fit, if it lasts longer than ten minutes or if it keeps repeating.

ELECTRICAL SHOCKS

Turn the electricity off at the mains before attempting anything else. Do not endanger yourself by directly touching the appliance or the victim.

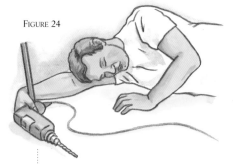

FIGURE 24

If you cannot turn off the electricity, you need to separate the casualty and the live electrical appliance: push away the appliance or the victim's limb with a broom or a wooden chair since dry wood does not conduct electricity well (Figure 24). Stand on a dry chair or paper while doing this – a telephone directory is a good insulator. Resuscitate the person if necessary, and treat any burns.

EYES

Foreign bodies or splashes in the eye cause irritation, watering and redness. Get medical help if the problem cannot be immediately sorted out or if vision remains blurred.

Foreign body in the eye

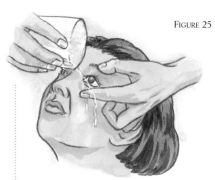

FIGURE 25

To remove the irritant, first locate it by pulling up the eyelid. Gently wipe away the object with a clean tissue or handkerchief. Otherwise pour cool water over the eye (Figure 25) or get the person to blink under water. Do not attempt to remove an object which appears embedded in the eye.

Chemical splashes in the eye

Wash out the eye immediately using running water or cups of water; continue for ten minutes. Apply an eye pad and have the patient checked at hospital.

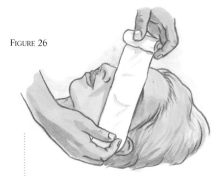

FIGURE 26

Protect the eye with a pad, held in place with a bandage (Figure 26), while transferring the casualty to hospital.

HEAD INJURY

Blows to the head can be serious, although minor knocks are unlikely to cause a problem.

If someone is knocked unconscious, put them in the recovery position (see page 352) and arrange for transfer to hospital. If someone is conscious, treat any cuts. Transfer them to hospital if any of the following occurs:

♦ *They cannot move all of their limbs normally*
♦ *They have a fit*
♦ *Their pupils are irregular in size*
♦ *They begin vomiting*
♦ *They become drowsy or unconscious*
♦ *They were knocked out*
♦ *They have amnesia (loss of memory)*

If the casualty seems all right otherwise, reassure her but she should seek professional help if any of the above features appear during the next few days.

DROWNING

The risks of drowning are from inhaled water and from chilling (hypothermia, see page 362) while in the water or once rescued. Rescuers also risk hypothermia and exhaustion, so attempt a rescue only if confident about your own safety – it may be better to manoeuvre a boat or raft, or wade out attached to a rope, for example.

Lay the victim in a sheltered area on his back, his head lower than his feet to allow water to drain out. Clear debris from his mouth, check 'ABC' (see page 352) and resuscitate if necessary. Once he is conscious, put him in the recovery position (see page 352) and keep him warm until help arrives – further assessment in hospital is always essential.

CUTS AND WOUNDS

Most minor cuts can be dealt with by first aid alone. Check the casualty's tetanus coverage – a booster may be required for a dirty or penetrating wound.

Wash dirt away from the injury with water or antiseptic solution. Put pressure on the injury until bleeding stops – two to four minutes. Then clean it more thoroughly, without dislodging the blood clot. Apply a plaster or a non-stick dressing.

Hand wounds

Wounds to the hand often bleed heavily, requiring padding.

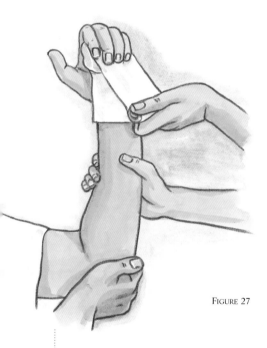

FIGURE 27

To treat a cut palm, put a clean gauze or handkerchief in the person's palm. Get the person to squeeze it and wrap the hand with a bandage (Figure 27). Get the person to hospital.

Embedded objects

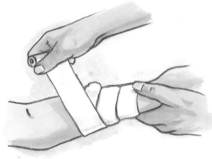

FIGURE 28

Bandaging around an object may be necessary in the case of deeply embedded objects such as glass (Figure 28). Do not pull out embedded objects since you may set off heavy bleeding. Get the patient to hospital.

Fish hooks

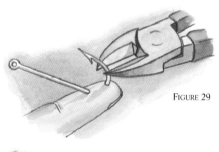

FIGURE 29

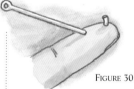

FIGURE 30

Removing a fish hook often requires hospital attention. Only attempt the following if it is unavoidable: if the barb has come completely through, cut it off (Figure 29) then withdraw the rest of the hook (Figure 30). If the barb is still buried, do not withdraw it. Attempt to push it quickly through and out of the flesh; cut off and withdraw as above.

FAINTING

Faints are common in people having to stand for long periods, especially in the heat, during pregnancy or after missing meals, and often even for no obvious cause. Blood pressure falls, the person feels light-headed and dizzy, then slowly collapses. She looks pale, sweaty and has a slow pulse.

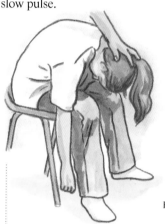

FIGURE 31

If someone feels faint, help them to lie down or to sit with their head between their knees (Figure 31).

FIGURE 32

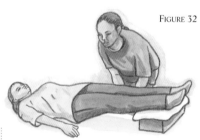

If someone has fainted, check that they have a pulse and are breathing – if neither, begin resuscitation (see page 352) and call for help. Lay the person down and raise her legs to a level above her head (Figure 32). She should recover within a few seconds but do not let her sit up or stand until she feels back to normal – ten to fifteen minutes. Give her a drink of water and a light snack if she has not eaten for some while. Get help if the victim is bleeding, has a fit or remains unconscious.

FRACTURES

Suspect a fracture if, after an accident, someone has pain over a bone, difficulty using that part of the body or deformity of a limb. Deal with any bleeding and cover any protruding bone or open wound. Do not let the victim put weight on a fracture. If an arm or shoulder is involved, support the limb with a sling (see page 356), then get the casualty to hospital.

HEART ATTACK

Suspect a heart attack if someone complains of chest pain and then has difficulty breathing, looks blue around the lips or collapses. Lay the person down; check for pulse and breathing – if absent begin resuscitation (see page 352). Arrange for immediate medical help.

HYPOTHERMIA

This is most likely to occur in the elderly, in outdoor enthusiasts, or in someone who has fallen into cold water.

The person feels cold, is confused or unconscious. Remove any wet clothing, and place the person in a warm or sheltered place. Warm him gradually with blankets or your own body heat. If conscious give him warm drinks – but do not give him alcohol. A mildly affected person can have a warm bath; someone severely affected must not – continue warming them gradually until help arrives.

BEE OR WASP STING

Brush the sting off; do not squeeze it. Use tweezers if available. Apply a cold dressing to reduce swelling. If stung in the mouth, suck ice cubes. Get help if there is severe swelling or difficulty in breathing.

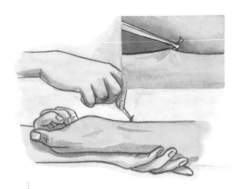

FIGURE 33

To remove the sting, place tweezers below the poison sac, as close to the skin as possible, then pull it out (Figure 33).

NECK AND SPINAL INJURIES

Such injuries happen after accidents and falls – often through sporting activities. Beware of paralysis, severe pain or tingling down the limbs. If these symptoms are present, do not allow any movement of the back; get urgent help. Keep the patient's neck well supported.

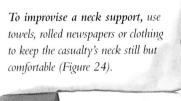

To improvise a neck support, use towels, rolled newspapers or clothing to keep the casualty's neck still but comfortable (Figure 24).

NOSE BLEED

Most nose bleeds are a result of inflammation of the lining of the nose through colds or the heat.

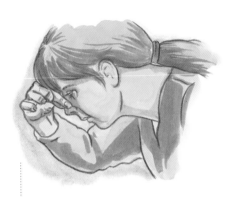

FIGURE 35

To deal with a nose bleed, lean forward. Firmly pinch the soft part of the nose just above the nostrils for ten minutes (Figure 35); breathe through the mouth. Do not wipe or blow your nose for several hours afterwards. If bleeding persists, seek hospital treatment.

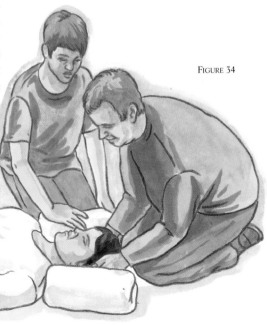

FIGURE 34

POISONING

Suspect poisoning if a child or adult becomes suddenly drowsy or unconscious; if there are chemical burns around the mouth or hands; or if someone has been drinking heavily or using drugs.

Give resuscitation if required. If someone has swallowed a caustic substance give artificial respiration (see page 353) only via a face mask. Do not make them vomit. Wash mouth burns with water. Wash chemical contaminants off the skin. Identify the poison or keep a sample of it and try to establish how long ago it was taken. Get medical help urgently. Keep the casualty safe until the antidote can be given. Remember alcohol is a poison, too; treat drunkenness as poisoning.

SMOKE INHALATION

Smoke causes damage by suffocation and by irritation of the lungs. Do not risk your own safety by entering smoke- or fume-filled areas without proper equipment.

Escape from smoke or fumes if possible. Otherwise find a room with a window; put towels or clothing at the base of doors to prevent smoke entering. Keep yourself low because smoke rises. Open the window to help you breathe.

Avoid opening doors or windows in a burning room since the incoming air will fan the flames.

SPLINTERS

Remove splinters as soon as possible, before the skin swells. Clean the area around the splinter. Use tweezers to grip the splinter where it meets the skin. Pull it out in the direction in which it entered. After removal, clean the wound more thoroughly with antiseptic solution.

HEATSTROKE AND SUNBURN

Heatstroke can appear within minutes in someone exposed to heat through exertion, illness or a hot atmosphere. Symptoms include nausea, a bad headache, confusion, a fast pulse and very hot skin. This is an emergency – call for help. Move the heatstroke victim into the shade, remove his clothing and fan him. Put wet clothing or towels on him to reduce temperature quickly. Resuscitate if necessary.

Sunburnt skin is red, hot and tender. Get the person out of the sun. Cool the skin with cool water or a cooling cream such as calamine. Give fluids. Seek help if the burns are extensive or blister.

Keep yourself low down in a smoke-filled area. Cover your nose and mouth with a wet cloth to keep out fumes (Figure 36).

FIGURE 36

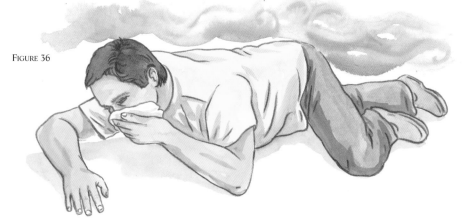

SWALLOWED OBJECT

It is unusual for swallowed coins or similar objects to cause problems unless they are sharp, for example fragments of glass or bones.

Give plenty of fluids. Seek hospital treatment if the object was sharp or large, i.e. more than 1 cm/½ in in diameter, or if the person was coughing and may have breathed it in. (An X-ray at hospital may be used to locate a swallowed object which fails to pass within 48 hours, is large or may have been inhaled.)

HIGH TEMPERATURE

A fever is almost always due to infection; it may be 48 hours or more before the cause is apparent. The younger the person, the more important it is to reduce temperature to avoid a fit.

Children

To take a child's temperature place a thermometer under the arm for one minute – never in the mouth. Normal underarm temperature is 36.5°C/97.5°F. An alternative is to use a fever strip which is placed across the forehead to measure skin temperature. Although a useful guide, this is not nearly as reliable as using a standard thermometer.

Give paracetamol syrup. Never give aspirin to children below 12 years of age. Remove clothing apart from a light vest. Use a fan if necessary or sponge the child's brow with tepid water. Give the child plenty of drinks.

Adults

Place a thermometer in the mouth, under the tongue, for one minute. Normal temperature is 37°C/98.4°F. Take paracetamol or aspirin. Wrap up or undress, whichever is more comfortable for you. Drink plenty of fluids.

SAFETY IN THE HOME AND AT WORK

Many accidents happen in the home through falls, cuts, burns, domestic chemicals and so on. Make your home a safer place by identifying and eliminating hazards before harm comes. Similarly, you can make your workplace safer, too, by reporting unsafe working practices and making suggestions for improvements.

In the bathroom

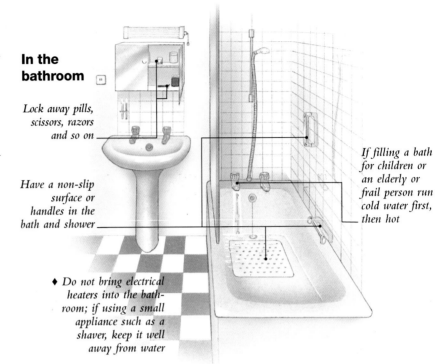

Lock away pills, scissors, razors and so on

Have a non-slip surface or handles in the bath and shower

If filling a bath for children or an elderly or frail person run cold water first, then hot

♦ *Do not bring electrical heaters into the bathroom; if using a small appliance such as a shaver, keep it well away from water*

In the kitchen

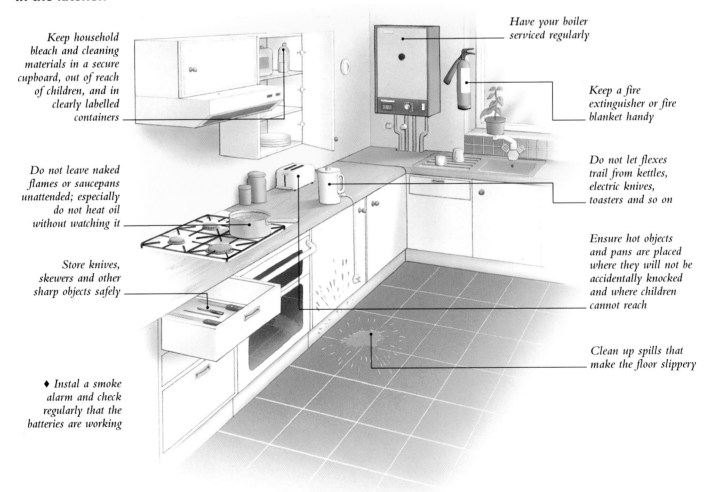

Keep household bleach and cleaning materials in a secure cupboard, out of reach of children, and in clearly labelled containers

Do not leave naked flames or saucepans unattended; especially do not heat oil without watching it

Store knives, skewers and other sharp objects safely

♦ *Instal a smoke alarm and check regularly that the batteries are working*

Have your boiler serviced regularly

Keep a fire extinguisher or fire blanket handy

Do not let flexes trail from kettles, electric knives, toasters and so on

Ensure hot objects and pans are placed where they will not be accidentally knocked and where children cannot reach

Clean up spills that make the floor slippery

In the garden

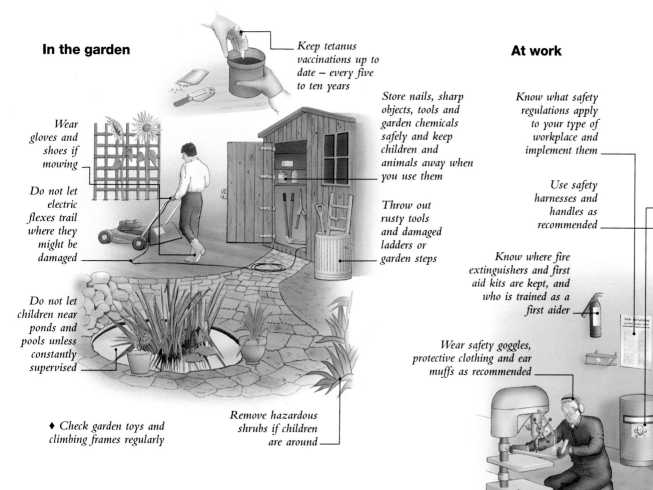

Keep tetanus vaccinations up to date – every five to ten years

Wear gloves and shoes if mowing

Do not let electric flexes trail where they might be damaged

Do not let children near ponds and pools unless constantly supervised

Store nails, sharp objects, tools and garden chemicals safely and keep children and animals away when you use them

Throw out rusty tools and damaged ladders or garden steps

♦ Check garden toys and climbing frames regularly

Remove hazardous shrubs if children are around

At work

Know what safety regulations apply to your type of workplace and implement them

Know what to do if contaminated by the materials you work with

Use safety harnesses and handles as recommended

Know where fire extinguishers and first aid kits are kept, and who is trained as a first aider

Wear safety goggles, protective clothing and ear muffs as recommended

Operate only the equipment you are trained to operate

Learn to lift safely (see page 246)

In the car

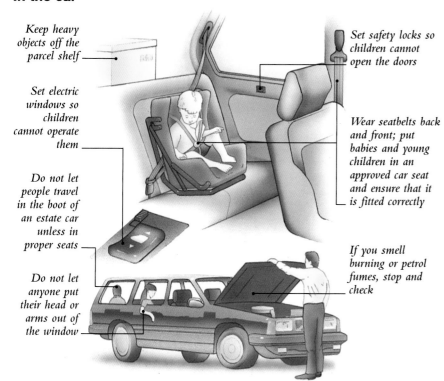

Keep heavy objects off the parcel shelf

Set electric windows so children cannot operate them

Do not let people travel in the boot of an estate car unless in proper seats

Do not let anyone put their head or arms out of the window

Set safety locks so children cannot open the doors

Wear seatbelts back and front; put babies and young children in an approved car seat and ensure that it is fitted correctly

If you smell burning or petrol fumes, stop and check

DRUG GLOSSARY

This glossary explains the more important or common types of drugs referred to in this book.

ACE inhibitors
Angiotensin-converting enzyme inhibitors. Angiotensin is a hormone involved in blood pressure. By blocking its action, ACE inhibitors reduce blood pressure and treat heart failure. Examples are captopril, lisinopril and enalapril.

Anaesthetics
Medication that reduces pain during surgery. Local anaesthetics, given by injection, deaden pain in a small area. General anaesthetics, in the form of injection or gas, make the patient unconscious.

Antacids
Substances that neutralize stomach acids. Many proprietary brands contain aluminium or magnesium hydroxide.

Antibiotics
Drugs that kill or damage microscopic organisms, especially bacteria, by affecting some vital part of their metabolism. Types include penicillin (amoxycillin and ampicillin), cephalosporins (cephalexin and cefaclor), tetracyclines (minocycline and oxytetracycline), 4-quinolones (ciprofloxacin), macrolides (erythromycin) and many others. Different infections respond to different antibiotics. Antifungal antibiotics include nystatin and clotrimazole. Viruses do not respond to conventional antibiotics (see antivirals).

Anticonvulsants
Drugs that reduce the chances of an epileptic fit. Examples are phenytoin, carbamazepine and vigabatrin.

Antidepressants
Mood-altering drugs that affect brain chemistry to relieve depression. The most widely used are tricyclics (amitryptiline, dothiepin and imipramine) and selective serotonin reuptake inhibitors, SSRIs, (fluoxetine and paroxetine).

Antihistamines
These block histamine, a biochemical involved in allergic reactions, itch and hay fever. Examples are chlorpheniramine, loratadine and cetirizine.

Antihypertensives
Medication to reduce blood pressure. Common types are diuretics, beta-blockers, calcium-channel blockers and ACE inhibitors (see entries).

Antiemetics
Drugs that reduce sickness and giddiness by sedating the organs of balance in the ear or the 'nausea centre' within the brain. Types include prochlorperazine and domperidone.

Antipsychotics
Sedatives (see entry) for the agitation, aggression or disordered thought of serious mental illness such as schizophrenia or manic depression. Examples are haloperidol and risperidone.

Antivirals
Fairly recently developed antibiotics effective against viruses. Not many are available and only for a few infections, for example acyclovir for herpes. Zidovudine (also called AZT) fights AIDS.

Aspirin
Aspirin reduces pain and fever; in a low dose it makes blood less likely to clot. It works via the prostaglandin system, biochemical substances involved in many basic body functions. Aspirin must not be taken by children under the age of 12, nor by people with severe indigestion or previous peptic ulcer.

Beta-blockers
Adrenaline is a substance produced by the body in response to stress. Beta receptors are nerves that respond to adrenaline in the heart, lungs, brain and blood vessels. By blocking these nerves, beta-blockers reduce heart rate and palpitations, ease anxiety, lower blood pressure and control migraine. They include atenolol, propranolol and labetolol.

Bronchodilators
Medication to make airways widen within the lungs, to treat asthma and chronic bronchitis. Available as aerosol sprays, tablets and injections. Examples are salbutamol and terbutaline.

Calcium-channel blockers
By affecting calcium metabolism in the muscles around arteries, these drugs make blood vessels dilate. A treatment for high blood pressure and angina. Common examples are nifedipine, amlodipine and diltiazem.

Clot busters

Drugs that dissolve blood clots within arteries or veins after pulmonary embolus, deep vein thrombosis or heart attack, allowing blood flow to recommence. Their use has greatly improved the outlook of these conditions. Examples are streptokinase and urokinase.

Contraceptives

Means of controlling fertility using hormones. Their actions include stopping the release of an egg each month and altering conditions at the cervix to prevent sperm from penetrating. The combined Pill is a mixture of oestrogen and progestogen (see entries); the minipill contains progestogen only.

Cough mixtures

Liquids that loosen mucus, often with a sedative to improve sleep as well.

Cytotoxics

Treatments for cancer that destroy cancer cells. They need specialist monitoring to minimize side effects. Examples are methotrexate, cyclophosphamide and fluorouracil.

Decongestants

Medication to reduce the flow of mucus by constricting blood vessels in the nose and sinuses during colds or sinusitis. They are advisable for a few days only. Examples are pseudoephedrine and xylometazoline.

Diuretics

Drugs that make the kidneys pass more urine. Useful in treating high blood pressure, heart failure and severely swollen legs. Types include bendrofluazide and frusemide.

H2 blockers

Substances that block histamine receptors in the stomach involved in acid production. They have revolutionized the treatment of chronic indigestion and peptic ulcers. Examples are cimetidine and ranitidine.

Hormones

Natural proteins, produced by glands, that circulate in the blood stream, having effects around the body. Examples are insulin, thyroid hormone and oestrogen.

Immunosuppressants

Drugs that reduce the immune response, important in transplant surgery. Examples are azathioprine and cyclosporin.

Laxatives

Substances that relieve constipation. Some (senna) stimulate the bowels to pass out material, while others (lactulose) hold fluid within the bowel.

Non-steroidal anti-inflammatory drugs (NSAIDs)

Drugs related to aspirin (see entry) that work similarly; especially useful for joint pain and minor injuries. They can cause indigestion and must not be taken by anyone with a peptic ulcer. Names include ibuprofen, diclofenac, naproxen.

Oestrogens

Hormones produced mainly in the ovaries, which cause female sexual characteristics and regulate the menstrual cycle. Oestrogens are used for contraception, menstrual disorders and hormone replacement therapy (HRT).

Opioids

Powerful painkilling drugs such as morphine, diamorphine (heroin), pethidine and codeine. They affect parts of the brain which normally respond to the body's natural painkillers. They are potentially addictive but, if properly used, are immensely helpful for relieving pain.

Paracetamol

A painkilling, fever-reducing substance, safe at all ages. In excess it causes liver damage so do not exceed the safe dose.

Progestogens

Hormones involved in pregnancy, which can regulate periods, act as contraceptives and are included in most HRT preparations.

Proton pump inhibitors

Recently available drugs that work on molecular pumps in cells involved in acid production, greatly reducing acid in the stomach. They are more powerful than H2 blockers (see entry). Examples are omeprazole and lansoprazole.

Sedatives

Drugs that reduce brain activity, relieving anxiety, agitation or major psychiatric disturbances such as mania. They include diazepam, chlorpromazine, chloral and certain antihistamines.

Sleeping tablets

Sedatives with a powerful, rapid action that induces sleep. Generally recommended only for short-term use. A common example is temazepam.

Steroids

Biochemicals that, by affecting cell activity, have many powerful actions on the body. They reduce inflammation in arthritis and skin disorders, dampen the immune response in asthma, are used in transplant surgery and to restore blood pressure after severe blood loss and collapse. Side effects after prolonged use at high doses include high blood pressure, weight gain and thinning of the skin. However, steroids, properly used, have transformed the management of many serious or chronic conditions such as asthma and eczema. Examples are prednisolone, dexamethasone, betamethasone and hydrocortisone.

COMPLEMENTARY TREATMENT GLOSSARY

Many of these therapies have a holistic approach, meaning that they treat the whole person and not just the symptoms, and rely on the body's self-healing process.
Some therapeutic techniques can be practised on one's own; others require the help of a skilled practitioner.

EASTERN THERAPIES

Acupuncture
One of the oldest forms of treatment. The Chinese believe that a vital force or energy, called chi, runs through our bodies along pathways called meridians. Acupuncture uses needles to stimulate points along the meridians to promote the flow of chi, thus restoring good health; acupressure uses the fingers. Acupuncture is especially good for pain control.

Auricular therapy
A form of acupuncture focusing specifically on the ear. It is an effective form of pain control and can help with changing unwanted patterns of behaviour.

Shiatsu-do
Practitioners uses their fingers, palms, elbows, arms, knees and feet to stimulate pressure points on the body. Shiatsu-do relieves tension and eases joint pain.

Chinese herbalism
Practitioners use herbs to maintain good health and prevent and treat ill health. This therapy can be used for a range of physical complaints, including eczema and digestive disorders, and it also helps to promote mental and emotional wellbeing. It is sometimes used in conjunction with acupuncture (see entry).

Ayurveda
The Indian science of life. Ayurveda provides a holistic approach to healing, which assesses individuals and all their circumstances, giving advice on nutrition, exercise and lifestyle, as well as offering medication.

Chakra balancing
This Indian therapy enables energy blocks to be relieved – the subsequent flow promotes healing. The effect of deep relaxation aids both mental and physical recovery.

MANIPULATIVE THERAPIES

Osteopathy and cranial osteopathy
Osteopathy uses gentle manipulation on the whole body to adjust the musculo-skeletal system and improve joint movement. It can help many conditions, for example repetitive strain disorder. Cranial osteopathy involves gentle palpation of the bones of the skull, and is often used effectively on children.

Chiropractic
Treatment for the musculo-skeletal system and supporting nerves, with particular emphasis on the spine. Practitioners offer a range of manipulative techniques, aiming to increase mobility in joints and overcome problems originating in the soft tissues.

Massage
The manipulation of the body's soft tissues by stroking, kneading, rubbing and other techniques, sometimes with oils or creams. Practitioners detect and treat problems in the muscles, ligaments and tendons. Massage can also alleviate stress.

Reflexology
Reflexologists believe that the body is divided into ten energy zones, running from the feet up through the body and down to the arms and hands. Pressure is applied to points on the feet and hands to stimulate the energy flow to a related muscle or organ, and thus promote healing.

NATURAL THERAPIES

Aromatherapy
This uses the essential oils of aromatic plants to promote vitality of the body and serenity of mind. The oils can be added to a bath, inhaled from a bowl of hot water, applied in lotions or in compresses, or vaporized in an oil burner. Aromatherapy alleviates stress, improves mood and is a treatment for many minor disorders.

Homeopathy
'Like may be cured by like' is the basic principle of homeopathy. A homeopathic remedy is one which produces the same symptoms as those the sick person experiences and stimulates the body's natural healing process. Remedies are based on animal, plant or mineral substances and are given as pills, solutions, creams and granules.

Nutritional therapy

This is based on the idea that a good diet can maintain good health, prevent illness and treat specific conditions, such as migraine. Issues addressed include food allergies, nutritional deficiencies and toxic overload.

Western herbalism

Practitioners prevent and treat illness by using plant remedies and extracts from a part of the whole plant (including roots and berries), which contains hundreds of active constituents. Remedies are made up into infusions, decoctions, tinctures, syrups, oils and creams.

Naturopathy

Naturopaths see disease as a natural phenomenon and believe that people should rely on their own body to cure itself of illness. Treatment might include a healthy diet and fasting in order to eliminate toxins, hydrotherapy, exercise and relaxation.

Bach flower remedies

These distilled floral essences can be used as a supportive therapy for any condition involving emotional issues, including despondency, anxiety and anger, and help counteract the effects of stress.

ACTIVE THERAPIES

◆

Alexander technique

This trains people to regain their natural posture and thus to use their bodies more efficiently. Great emphasis is placed on breathing. The technique is particularly helpful in dealing with problems of the musculo-skeletal, respiratory and nervous systems.

Hypnotherapy

Under trance, people bring to consciousness many subconscious fears, memories and emotions. This enables them to change unwanted patterns of behaviour. Hypnotherapy is effective for treating addictions, phobias and stress-related conditions.

Yoga

Originally an Indian therapy, yoga is an effective way of promoting flexibility and strength in the mind and body. It can improve posture, muscle tone and mobility and bring a sense of peace in a stressful world. It may also help strengthen the body's immune system.

Tai chi/chi kung

Gentle Chinese practices that use flowing exercises to help improve the flow of chi (energy) through the body, and thus maintain or improve physical, mental and spiritual health and wellbeing.

Autogenic training

A gentle, self-administered form of psychotherapy, this can relieve conditions such as asthma, high blood pressure and irritable bowel syndrome.

THERAPIES INVOLVING EXTERNAL POWERS

◆

Healing

Also known as spiritual healing or therapeutic touch. Energy is transmitted through the practitioner's hands to the patient to relieve mental and emotional problems as well as some physical illnesses.

Cymatics

A therapy based on the idea that each molecule of the body has its own individual sound pattern which, in an organ or tissue, builds into a complexity of harmonic frequencies. Any change to these frequencies causes pain and discomfort. Treatment is with natural frequencies of sound.

Biodynamics

Practitioners combine specialized massage techniques with psychotherapy to release physical or emotional tension and bring about healing.

Hellerwork

Practitioners believe that movement is stressful to a body that is structurally misaligned. Misalignment can occur as a response to bad postural habits or emotional stress. The aim is to realign the body and release the physical, emotional or mental patterns that led to misalignment.

Rolfing

The central premise of rolfing is that a structurally misaligned body experiences gravity as stressful, so movement and flexibility are limited. Practitioners help to realign the body and correct abnormal posture with hands, fingers, knuckles and elbows.

Arts therapies

Drama, art, music and dance are used to alleviate emotional and mental problems. Arts therapies are a valuable alternative to verbal psychotherapy for people who find it hard to talk about their emotions or who have speech difficulties.

Play therapy

This indirectly addresses a child's subconscious by using play as a medium of communication. It is suitable for children from three upwards for a range of problems linked to emotional development.

DIRECTORY

◆

CIRCULATORY SYSTEM

◆

British Heart Foundation
14 Fitzhardinghe Street
London W1H 4DH   Tel 0171 935 0185

Coronary Prevention Group
42 Store Street
London WC1E 7DB   Tel 0171 580 1070

The Raynaud's and Scleroderma Association
112 Crewe Road
Alsager
Cheshire ST7 2JA   Tel 01270 872776

RESPIRATORY SYSTEM

◆

Action Against Allergy
PO Box 278
Twickenham
Middlesex TW1 4QQ   Tel 0181 892 2711

Action on Smoking and Health (ASH)
16 Fitzhardinghe Street
London W1H 9PL   Tel 0171 224 0743

Cancer Information Service (BACUP)
3 Bath Place
London EC2   Tel 0171 613 2121
                   Counselling 0171 696 9000

Macmillan Cancer Relief
Anchor House
15-19 Britten Street
London SW3 3TZ   Tel 0171 351 7811
              Information line 0845 6016161

National Asthma Campaign
Providence House
Providence Place
London N1 0NT   Tel 0171 226 2260
                   Helpline 0345 010203
                   (Mon-Fri 9am-9pm)

MIND, BRAIN & NERVOUS SYSTEM

◆

Alcohol Concern
Waterbridge House
32-36 Loman Street
London SE1 0EE   Tel 0171 928 7377

Alzheimer's Disease Society
Gordon House
10 Greencoat Place
London SW1P 1PH   *Helpline* 0845 3000336

British Epilepsy Association
Anstey House
40 Hanover Square
Leeds LS3 1BE   Tel 01132 439393
                   Helpline 0800 309030

Cruse, Bereavement Care
Cruse House
126 Sheen Road
Richmond
Surrey TW9 1UR   Tel 0181 940 4818

Encephalitis Support Group
Pasture House
Normanby
Sinnington
York YO62 6RH   Tel 01751 433318

Migraine Action
(formerly British Migraine Association)
178a High Road
West Byfleet
Surrey KT14 7ED   Tel 01932 352468

MIND (National Association for Mental Health)
Granta House
15-19 Broadway
London E15 4BQ   Tel 0181 519 2122

Multiple Sclerosis Society of Great Britain and Northern Ireland
25 Effie Road
London SW6 1EE   Tel 0171 610 7171
                   Helpline 0171 371 8000
                   (Mon-Fri 10am-4pm)

Multiple Sclerosis Telephone Counselling Service
Tel 0171 222 3123 (London); 0121 476 4229
(Midlands)

National Meningitis Trust
Fern House
Bath Road
Stroud
Gloucester GL5 3TJ   Tel 01453 768000
              24-hour supportline 0345 538118

Parkinson's Disease Society
215 Vauxhall Bridge Road
London SW1V 1EJ   Tel 0171 931 8080
                   Helpline 0171 233 5373

Schizophrenia - A National Emergency (SANE)
1st Floor
Cityside House
40 Adler Street
London E1 1EE   Tel 0171 375 1002
                   Helpline 0345 678000
                   (2pm-midnight)

The Stroke Association
Stroke House
123-127 Whitecross Street
London EC1Y 8JJ   Tel 0171 490 7999

ENDOCRINE SYSTEM & METABOLISM

◆

British Diabetic Association
10 Queen Anne Street
London W1M 0BD   Tel 0171 323 1531
                   Careline 0171 636 6112

Hypothyroidism Support Group
Tel 01942 874740 (Mon-Fri 5pm-7pm)

URINARY SYSTEM

◆

Association for Continence Advice
Winchester House, Kennington Park
Cranmer Road
London SW9 6EJ   Tel 0171 820 8113

British Kidney Patient Association (BKPA)
Bordon
Hampshire GU35 9JZ   Tel 01420 472021

National Kidney Federation
6 Stanley Street
Worksop
Nottinghamshire S81 7HX   Tel 01909 487795

MALE REPRODUCTIVE SYSTEM

◆

Group B Hepatitis
Basement Flat, 7A Fielding Road
London W14 0LL

The Herpes Viruses Association
41 North Road
London N7 9DP   Tel 0171 609 9061

ISSUE: The National Fertility Association
114 Lichfield Street
Walsall WS1 1SZ   Tel 01922 722888

FEMALE REPRODUCTIVE SYSTEM

◆

The Amarant Trust
(information and advice on menopause and HRT)
Grant House
56-60 St John Street
London EC1M 4DT   Tel 0171 490 1644
                   Advice line 01293 413000
                   (Mon-Fri midday-7pm)

Association of Breastfeeding Mothers
PO Box 207
Bridgewater
Somerset TA6 7YT   Tel 0171 813 1481

Association for Postnatal Illness
25 Jerdan Place
London SW6 1BE   Tel 0171 386 0868

Breast Cancer Care
Kiln House
210 New Kings Road
London SW6 4NZ   *Helpline* 0171 384 2984
              Nationwide freeline 0500 245345

British Pregnancy Advisory Service
Austy Manor
Wootten Wawen
Solihull
West Midlands B95 6BX   Tel 01564 793225
                   Helpline 08457 304030

Family Planning Association
2-12 Pentonville Road
London N1 9FP   Tel 0171 837 5432
                   Helpline 0171 837 4044

Foresight (Pre-Concentual Care)
28 The Paddock
Godalming
Surrey GU7 1XD   Tel 01483 427839

Miscarriage Association
c/o Clayton Hospital
Northgate
Wakefield
West Yorkshire WF1 3JS   Tel 01924 200799

National Childbirth Trust
Alexandra House
Oldham Terrace
London W3 6NH   Tel 0181 992 8637
                             (Mon-Fri 9.30am-4.30pm)

National Endometriosis Society
50 Westminster Palace Gardens
Artillery Row
London SW1P 1RL   Tel 0171 222 2781
                           Helpline 0171 222 2776

Women's Nationwide Cancer Control Campaign
Suna House
128 Curtain Road
London EC2A 3AR   Tel 0171 729 4688
                           Helpline 0171 729 2229

DIGESTIVE SYSTEM
◆

Coeliac Society
PO Box 220
High Wycombe
Buckinghamshire HP11 2HY   Tel 01494 437278

Digestive Disorders Foundation
(formerly British Digestive Foundation)
PO Box 251, Edgeware
Middlesex HA8 6HG   Tel 0171 487 5332
                      (Please send sae for information)

National Association for Colitis and Crohn's Disease
4 Beaumont House
Sutton Road
St Albans
Hertfordshire AL1 5HH   Tel 01727 844296

EYES
◆

Royal National Institute for the Blind (RNIB)
224 Great Portland Street
London W1N 6AA   Tel 0171 388 1266

EAR, NOSE & THROAT
◆

British Dental Association
64 Wimpole Street
London W1M 8AL   Tel 0171 935 0875

Defeating Deafness (Hearing Research Trust)
330-332 Gray's Inn Road
London WC1X 8EE   Tel 0171 833 1733

Ménière's Society
98 Maybury Road
Woking
Surrey GU21 5HX   Tel 01483 740597

Royal National Institute for Deaf People (RNID)
19-23 Featherstone Street
London EC1Y 8SL   Tel 0171 296 8000

SKIN & HAIR
◆

Acne Support Group
PO Box 230
Hayes
Middlesex UB4 0UT   Tel 0181 561 6868
                  (Please send large sae for information)

Hairline International
The Alopecia Patients' Society
39 St Johns Close
Knowle, Solihull
West Midlands B93 0NN   Tel 01564 775281

National Eczema Society
163 Eversholt Street
London NW1 1BU   *Helpline 0171 388 4097*
             24-hour information line 0990 118877

Psoriasis Association
7 Milton Street
Northampton NN2 7JG   Tel 01604 711129

MUSCULO-SKELETAL SYSTEM
◆

Arthritis Research Campaign
Copeman House
St Mary's Court
St Mary's Gate
Chesterfield S41 7TD   Tel 01246 558033

Brittle Bone Society
30 Guthrie Street
Dundee DD1 5BS   Tel 01382 204446

Muscular Dystrophy Group of Great Britain and Northern Ireland
7-11 Prescott Place
London SW4 6BS   Tel 0171 720 8055

National Back Pain Association
16 Elmtree Road
Teddington
Middlesex TW11 8ST   Tel 0181 977 5474

National Osteoporosis Society
PO Box 10
Radstock
Bath BA3 3YB   Tel 01761 471771
                           Helpline 01761 474721

Repetitive Strain Injury Association
Chapel House
152 High Street
Yiewsley, West Drayton
Middlesex UB7 7BE   Tel 01895 431134

BLOOD, GLANDS & THE IMMUNE SYSTEM
◆

Leukaemia Care Society
14 Kingfisher Court
Venny Bridge, Pinhoe
Exeter EX4 8JN   Tel 01392 464848
                    24-hour supportline 0345 673203

Lupus UK
St James's House
Eastern Road
Romford
Essex RM1 3NH   Tel 01708 731251

Lymphoma Association
PO Box 275
Haddenham
Aylesbury
Buckinghamshire HP17 8JJ   Tel 01844 291479
                           Helpline 01844 291500

Myalgic Encephalomyelitis (ME) Association
4 Corringham Road
Stanford-le-Hope
Essex SS17 0AH   Tel 01375 642466
                   Information line 01375 361013

National Blood Service   Tel 0345 711711

Sickle Cell Society
54 Station Road
London NW10 4UA   Tel 0181 961 4006

INFECTIOUS DISEASE
◆

Children with AIDS
2nd Floor
111 High Holborn
London WC1V 6JS   Tel 0171 242 3883
              24-hour AIDS helpline 0800 567123

Malaria Information Line   Tel 0891 600350

Terrence Higgins Trust
52-54 Gray's Inn Road
London WC1X 8JU   Tel 0171 831 0330
                           Helpline 0171 242 1010

CHILDREN
◆

Association for Spina Bifida and Hydrocephalus (ASBAH)
42 Park Road
Peterborough PE1 2UQ   Tel 01733 555988

Cerebal Palsy Helpline   Tel 0800 626216

Community Hygiene Concern
(information on headlice and other parasitic diseases)
160 Inderwick Road
London N8 9JT   Tel 0181 341 7167

Down's Syndrome Association
155 Mitcham Road
London SW17 9PG   Tel 0181 682 4001

Foundation for the Study of Infant Death
14 Halkin Street
London SW1X 7DP   Tel 0171 235 0965
                 24-hour helpline 0171 235 1721

Hyperactive Children's Support Group
71 Whyke Lane
Chichester
West Sussex PO19 2LD   Tel 01903 725182

SCOPE (formerly Spastics Society)
6 Market Road
London N7 9PW   Tel 0171 619 7100
                                    Helpline 0800 626216

COMPLEMENTARY THERAPIES
◆

British Register of Complementary Practitioners
PO Box 194
London SE16 1QZ   Tel 0171 237 5175
          (Send large sae for a register of practitioners)

ACUPUNCTURE

British Acupuncture Association and Registrar
34 Alderney Street
London SW1V 4EU   Tel 0171 834 1012

ALEXANDER TECHNIQUE

The Society of Teachers of the Alexander Technique
20 London House
266 Fulham Road
London SW10 9EL   Tel 0171 351 0828

AROMATHERAPY

International Federation of Aromatherapists
Stamford House
2-4 Chiswick High Road
London W4 1TH   Tel 0181 742 2602

ARTS THERAPIES

Association for Dance Movement Therapy
c/o Arts Therapies Department
Springfield Hospital
61 Glenburnie Road
London SW17 7DJ   Tel 0181 672 9911

Association of Professional Music Therapists
38 Pierce Lane
Fulbourn
Cambridge CB1 5DL   Tel 01223 880377

British Association of Art Therapists
11A Richmond Road
Brighton
East Sussex BN2 3RL

British Association of Dramatherapists
5 Sunnydale Villas
Durlston Road
Swanage
Dorset BH19 2HY

AUTOGENIC TRAINING

British Association for Autogenic Training and Therapy (BAFATT)
Heath Cottage, Pitch Hill
Ewhurst, Nr Cranleigh
Surrey GU6 7NP

AYURVEDA

Ayurvedic Medical Association UK
17 Bromham Mill
Giffard Park
Milton Keynes MK14 5KP   Tel 01908 617089

BACH FLOWER REMEDIES

The Edward Bach Centre
Mount Vernon
Sotwell, Wallingford
Oxon OX10 0PZ   Tel 01491 834678

BIODYNAMICS

The Gerda Boyesen Centre
Acacia House
Centre Avenue
London W3 7JX   Tel 0181 743 2437

CHINESE HERBALISM

The Register of Chinese Herbal Medicine
PO Box 400
Wembley
Middlesex HA9 9NE   Tel 0181 904 1357
          (Send sae and £1.50 for the register)

CHIROPRACTIC

The British Chiropractic Association
Blagrave House
17 Blagrave Street
Reading RG1 1QB   Tel 0118 9505950

CYMATICS

The Bretforton Trust
c/o Dr Peter Manners, Bretforton Hall
Bretforton
Vale of Evesham
Worcestershire WR11 5JH   Tel 01386 830537

HELLERWORK

The European Hellerwork Association
c/o Roger Golten, The MacIntyre Gallery
29 Crawford Street
London W1H 1PL   Tel 0171 723 5676

HOMEOPATHY

The British Homeopathic Association
27a Devonshire Street
London WC1N 1RJ   Tel 0171 935 2163

The Society of Homeopaths
2 Artizan Road
Northampton NN1 4HU   Tel 01604 21400
          (Send large sae for a list of practitioners)

HYPNOTHERAPY

Central Register of Advanced Hypnotherapists
28 Finsbury Park Road
London N4 2JX   Tel 0171 359 6991
          (Send sae for a register of practitioners)

The National Register of Hypnotherapists and Psychotherapists
12 Cross Street
Nelson
Lancashire BB9 7EN   Tel 01282 699278
          (Send sae for a register of practitioners)

MASSAGE

Massage Therapy Institute of Great Britain
PO Box 27/26
London NW2 4NR   Tel 0181 208 1607
          (Send sae for a register of practitioners)

NATUROPATHY

The General Council and Register of Naturopaths
6 Netherall Gardens
London NW3 5RR   Tel 0171 435 8728
          *(Send sae plus £2.50 cheque or postal order
          for a copy of the register)*

NUTRITIONAL THERAPY

Society for the Promotion of Nutritional Therapy
PO Box 47
Heathfield
East Sussex TN21 8ZX   Tel 01435 867007
          (Send sae plus £1 for a copy of the register)

OSTEOPATHY

General Council and Register of Osteopaths
56 London Street
Reading
Berkshire RG1 4SQ   Tel 01734 576585

Osteopathic Information Service
PO Box 2074
Reading Rerkshire RG1 4YR   Tel 01491 875255

PLAY THERAPY

British Association of Play Therapists
PO Box 98
Amersham
Buckinghamshire HP6 5BL

REFLEXOLOGY

The Association of Reflexologists
Flat 6
Sillwood Mansions
Sillwood Place
Brighton
East Sussex BN1 2LH   Tel 01273 771061

ROLFING

Loan Tran
Neal's Yard Therapy Rooms
2 Neal's Yard
London WC2H 9DP   Tel 0171 379 7662

The Rolf Institute Headquarters
205 Canyon Boulevard
Boulder
Colorado 830302, USA

SHIATSU-DO

Shiatsu Society of Great Britain
5 Foxcote
Wokingham
Berkshire RG11 3PG   Tel 01734 730836

TAI CHI

The Tai Chi Union for Great Britain
102 Felsham Road
London SW15 1DQ   Tel 0171 352 7716

WESTERN HERBALISM

The National Institute of Medical Herbalists
56 Longbrooke Street
Exeter EX4 8HA   Tel 01392 426022

YOGA

The Iyengar Yoga Institute
233A Randolph Avenue
London W9 1NL   Tel 0171 624 3080

The Yoga Therapy Centre
Royal London Homeopathic Hospital
60 Great Ormond Street
London WC1N 3HR   Tel 0171 833 7267

AUSTRALIA
◆

Allergy Information Network
Suite 14, 370 Victoria Avenue
Chatswood
NSW 2067   Tel 02 419 7731

Australian National Association for Mental Health
PO Box 146
Kippax
ACT 2615   Tel 02 6278 3148

Cancer Information and Support Society
6/81 Alexander Street
Crows Nest
NSW 2065   Tel 02 9906 2189

Heart Support-Australia
PO Box 3940
Weston Creek
ACT 2611   Tel 02 6285 2357

COMPLEMENTARY THERAPIES

Association of Massage Therapists
18A Spit Road
Mosman
NSW 1088

Australian Institute of Homeopathy
Box 122
Roseville
NSW 2069   Tel 02 9415 3928

The Australian Medical Acupuncture Society
1/77 Albert Avenue
Chatswood
NSW 2067   Tel 02 415 3800

Australian Natural Therapists Association
7 Highview Grove
Burwood East
Victoria 3151

Australian Osteopathic Association
PO Box 699
Turramurra
NSW 2074   Tel 02 449 4799

Chiropractors' Association of Australia
319 Victoria Road
Brunswick
Victoria 3056   Tel 03 9387 9377

NEW ZEALAND
◆

Allergy Awareness Association
PO Box 12701
Penrose   Tel 09 303 22024

New Zealand Psychological Society
Level 2, Fogel Building
22 Garret Street
Wellington   Tel 04 801 5414

COMPLEMENTARY THERAPIES

New Zealand Homeopathic Association
PO Box 2929
Auckland   Tel 09 630 5458

South Pacific Association of Natural Therapy
28 Willow Avenue
Birkenhead, Auckland 10

CANADA
◆

Allergy Asthma Information Association
30 Eglinton Avenue West
Mississauga
Ontario L5R 3E7   Tel 905 712 2242

Heart & Stroke Foundation of Canada
Suite 200, 160 George Street
Ottawa
Ontario K1N 9M2   Tel 613 241 4361

National Cancer Institute of Canada
Suite 200, 10 Alcorn Avenue
Toronto
Ontario M4V 3B1   Tel 416 961 7223

COMPLEMENTARY THERAPIES

Acupuncture Foundation of Canada
3003 Danforth Avenue
PO Box 93688
Ontario M4C 5R5   Tel 416 752 3988

Canadian Chiropractic Association
1396 Eglinton Avenue West
Toronto
Ontario M6C 2E4   Tel 416 781 5656

Canadian Society of Homeopathy
87 Meadowlands Drive West
Nepean
Ontario K2G 2R9

College of Massage Therapists
1867 Yonge Street
Toronto
Ontario M4S 1Y5   Tel 416 489 2626

USA
◆

American Heart Association
7320 Greenville Avenue
Dallas
Texas 75231   Tel 214 373 6300

American Psychiatric Association
1400 K Street NW
Washington, D.C. 20005   Tel 202 682 6000

Asthma and Allergy Foundation of America
Suite 305
1717 Massachusetts Avenue
Washington, D.C. 20006   Tel 202 265 0265

National Cancer Institute
Cancer Information Service
NCU Building 31
Bethesda
Maryland 20205   Tel 800 422 6237

COMPLEMENTARY THERAPIES

American Association of Acupuncture and Oriental Medicine
4101 Lake Boone Trail Suite 201
Raleigh
North Carolina 27607   Tel 919 787 5181

American Chiropractic Association
1701 Clarendon Blvd
Arlington
Virginia 22209   Tel 703 276 8800

American Massage Therapy Association
Suite 100, 820 Davis Street
Evanston
Illinois 60201   Tel 312 761 2682

American Osteopathic Association
142E Ontario Street
Chicago
Illinois 60611   Tel 312 280 5800

National Center for Homeopathy
801 North Fairfax Street
Alexandria
Virginia 22314   Tel 703 548 7790

SOUTH AFRICA
◆

Cancer Association of South Africa
PO Box 2000
Johannesburg 2000   Tel 011 616 7662

Heart Foundation of South Africa
PO Box 7091
Roggebaai 8012   Tel 021 25 4572

South African Federation for Mental Health
PO Box 2587
Johannesburg 2000   Tel 011 725 5800

Stroke Aid Society
PO Box 51283
Raedene 2124   Tel 011 882 1612

COMPLEMENTARY THERAPIES

The Confederation of Complementary Health Associations of South Africa
PO Box 2471
Clareinch 7740   Tel 021 58 8709

Holistic Massage Practitioners Association South Africa
42 Emerald Road
Fish Hoek 7975   Tel 021 782 5909

South African Naturopaths and Herbalists Association
PO Box 18663
Wynberg 7824   Tel 021 797 8629

Western Cape Su Jok Acupuncture Institute
3 Periwinkle Close
Kommetjie 7975   Tel 021 783 3460

INDEX

◆

ACKNOWLEDGMENTS

◆

Authors acknowledgment:

My contribution to this book has been moulded by innumerable discussions with designers and editors in and outside the Octopus Publishing Group. In particular Jane McIntosh, who steered the whole project, Jo Lethaby, Arlene Sobel and Catharine Davey who handled much of the editing. My own 'Family Health' has been provided by my wife Marilyn and children Zoe and Daniel. However, the responsibility for errors and opinions rests with myself.

Complementary treatment consultants include:
Acupuncture: **Stuart Lightbody** MAc, MTAcS, MASTER OF ACUPUNCTURE
Alexander Technique: **Anthony Kingsley** BSc HONS, MA
Aromatherapy: **Denise Brown**
Auricular Therapy: **Oran Kivity** MBAcC
Ayurveda: **Shantha Godagama** DAMS, MBAc, A, MF (HOM), MAcF
Bach Flower Remedies: **Judy Howard** SRN, SCM, HV, BACH CENTRE
Chiropractic: **Susan Steward** DC
Cymatics: **Peter Manners** MD, MA
Healing: **Midi Fairgrieve**
Hellerwork: **Roger Golten** BA (HONS)
Homeopathy: **Dr Andrew Lockie** MB, CHB, MF HOM, DIP OBST, RCOG, MRCGP
Hypnotherapy: **Marisa Peer** DP PSYCH, C HYP, CMH, CAH, CA HYP, D HYP, MHEC
Kinesiology: **Brian Butler** BA
Massage: **Clare Maxwell-Hudson** DIRECTOR OF INSTITUTE OF HEALTH SCIENCES, PRINCIPAL OF CLARE MAXWELL-HUDSON SCHOOL OF MASSAGE
Naturopathy: **Roger Newman Turner** B AC, ND, DO, MRO, MRN, FBACA
Nutritional Therapy: **Linda Lazarides** DIRECTOR OF SOCIETY FOR THE PROMOTION OF NUTRITIONAL THERAPY
Play Therapy: **Nancy Secchi** MA, RDTH, PLAY THERAPIST
Relaxation: **Carol Horrigan** MSc, SRN, DIP N, RCNT, PGCEA, RNT, NURSE CONSULTANT IN COMPLEMENTARY THERAPIES EDUCATION
Reflexology: **Mo Usher** MAR, MGCP
Tai Chi: **Lam Kam Chuen** LAM CLINIC, LONDON
Western Herbalism: **Mark Evans** B. PHIL. and **Trudy Norris** BA, MNIMH, PGCE, INFORMATION OFFICER FOR NATIONAL INSTITUTE OF MEDICAL HERBALISTS
Yoga: **Janet Balaskas**

Thanks also to:
Dr Marion Newman, Dr Melita Brownrigg, Dan Smith, Ray Ridolfi, Colin Dove, Dr Lee Craig Brown, Rosemary Steel, Alison Barnes

The publishers wish to thank the following organizations for their kind permission to reproduce the photographs in this book:
Bridgeman Art Library, London and New York, detail from "Cataracts III", by Bridget Riley, 1967, emulsion PVA on linen canvas, 88" x 87 1/2", collection: British Council 195bBottom/"Cat in a Rainbow" by Louis Wain/Bonhams, London 86/Cheltenham Art Gallery & Museums, Gloucestershire 328/Johnny van Haeften Gallery, London 351/Noortman (London) Ltd 315/Phillips, The International Fine Art Auctioneers 343 **Bubbles** 26/Moose Azim 132 top/Paul Beard 90 top right/Andrew Compton 61 top/Jacoui Farrow 47 bottom/Angela Hampton 89

bottom/Perry Joseph 138, 211 top/James Lamb 91 bottom right/Claire Paxton 205/Frans Rombout 18/Peter Sylent 237/Loisjoy Thurston 9, 88, 143 left, 157 right, 229, 274 top left, 277, 297/Ian West 28, 143 right, 214, 312/Jennie Woodcock 207 right/Jenny Woodcock 233 **Collections**/Anthea Sieveking 74, 311. **Reed Consumer Books Ltd.**/Peter Myers front cover, back cover **Angela Hampton/Family Life** 13 left, 13 right, 14, 15, 16, 20, 27, 65 bottom, 90 left, 95, 239 bottom, 246, 300, 303 bottom, 303 top left, 303 top right, 304-305, 313, 347. **Robert Harding Picture Library**/M. Colonel 91 bottom left. **Trevor Hill Photos** 189, **Hulton Getty Picture Collection** 278, 331. **Image Bank** 23, 62/Daniel Arsenault 211 bottom/Barros & Barros 213 bottom/Derek Berwin 319 left/A Boccaccio 210/Chris Close 91 top left/Michael Downing 80/Steve Dunnel 267/Patrick Eden 236/P. Goetgheluck 93 bottom left/Steven Hunt 134-135 background/John P. Kelly 252 centre/Michael Melford 93 bottom right/Benn Mitchell 90 bottom right/Kaz Nori 250/Anne Rippy 216/William Sallaz 105 top left/Paul Simcock 132 bottom/Steven Wilkes 17 **King's Healthcare NHS Trust** 101. **Oxford Scientific Films**/Stephen Dalton 66. **Science Photo Library** 47 top, 182, 186 bottom, 234, 241, 316/Argentum 200, 203/Alex Bartel 175 Top/John Bavosi 208/Alex Bartel/Dr Beer-Gabriel 323/Tim Beddow 338/Biology Media 269 top/Biophoto associates 107/Biophoto 134/Martin Bond 212/Dr. Tony Brain 123/BSIP Laurent 325/BSIP LECA 340/BSIP VEM 81, 330 right/BSIP.LECA 322/Oscar Burriel 105 bottom/CEA-ORSAY/CNRI 320/Jean-Loup Charmet 11/Dr Ray Clark & Marvyn Goff 104 top/Mark Clarke 274 bottom right/CNRI 124 bottom/A.B. Dowsett 56 bottom, 179/CAMR/ A.B. Dowsett 175 bottom/Malcolm Fielding 336/Sue Ford 201/Simon Fraser 94, 335/Simon Fraser/Freeman Hospital, Newcastle Upon-Tyne 46/Simon Fraser/Royal Victoria Infirmary, Newcastle 264/GCa - CNRI 257/Lowell Georgia 274 centre right/Richard J. Green 106/Tim Hazael 256/Dr. Huntington Potter 92/Institute Pasteur/CNRI 184/James King-Holmes 29, 135/Dr P Marazzi 273, 274 centre left/Dr P. Marazzi 198, 230, 240 top, 240 bottom right, 240 bottom left, 274 top right, 274 bottom left/Jerry Mason 266/R. Maisonneuve 213 top/Tim Malyn & Paul Biddle 326/Eamonn McNulty 51 top/Will & Deni McIntyre 327/Dr Gopal Murti 272/NASA GSFC 65 top/NASA 194/National Institute of Health 333/Dr Yozgos Nikas 129/Omikron 269 bottom/Alfred Pasieka 56 top, 124 top, 319 right/Pascale Roche/Petit Format 141/Petit Format/Nestle 128/Philippe Plailly 318/Chris Pries 321/Princess Margeret Rose Orthopaedic Hospital 259/John Radcliffe Hospital 85/Dr H. C. Robinson 225/Dep. of Clinical Radiology, Salisbury District Holpital 249/Department of Clinical Radiology, Salisbury District Hospital 186 top/Science Source 286 right/Dr. Linda Stannard, UCT 111/James Stevensen 332/Sheila Terry 157 left/TEK Image 334 left/Alexander Tsiaras 49, 163, 195 top/Prof. P. Motta/Dep. of Anatomy/University 'La Sapienza', Rome 248 right/Prof. P.Motta/Dep. of Anatomy/University 'La Sapienza', Rome 248 left/Dr. E Walker 113/Hattie Young 252 bottom. **Tony Stone Images** 93 top/Bruno Astorg 239 top/Bruce Ayres 7, 21, 76 top, 100, 252 top/Chris Barry 253/Christopher Bissell 77/Anthony Blake 190/Warren Bolster 238/Tim Brown 345/Demetrio Carrasco 19/Julian Calder 251/David Chambers 334 right/Charles Thatcher 76 bottom/Joe Cornish 301/Patrick Cocklin 78/Donna Day 174/James Darrell 102/David Frazier 330 left/Ben Edwards 41/Carol Ford 153/John Garrett 172/Hans Gelderblom 286 left/Howard Grey 103/Sara Gray 89 top/David Hanover 344/Paul Kenward 91 top right/Mike King 24/Tony Latham 133/David Madison 47 centre, 105 centre/Gary John Norman 175/Dennis O'Clair 197 top left/Lori Adamski Peek 197 right/Steven Peters 104 bottom/Ed Pritchard 87/RNHRD NHS Trust 51 bottom, 245/Bill Robbins 197 bottom left/Rohan 25/Ian Shaw 349/Phillip & Karen Smith 144/Andrew Syred 265/Sheila Terry 22/Darryl Torckler 317/Roger Tully 288/Penny Tweedie 224, 348/Terry Vine 226/Spike Walker 167/Duncan Wherrett 63/John Willar 61 bottom/Keith Wood 64. **Wellcome Institute Library, London** 53, 165, 228, 271, 307 left